PERIOPERATIVE MEDICINE
Just the Facts

Notice

PERIOPERATIVE MEDICINE
Just the Facts

Editors

Steven L. Cohn, MD, FACP

Chief, Division of General Internal Medicine
Director, Medical Consultation Service
Clinical Professor of Medicine
State University of New York, Downstate
Brooklyn, New York
Steven.Cohn@downstate.edu

Gerald W. Smetana, MD, FACP

Associate Professor of Medicine
Harvard Medical School
Division of General Medicine and Primary Care
Beth Israel Deaconess Medical Center
Boston, Massachusetts
gsmetana@bidmc.harvard.edu

Harrison G. Weed, MD, MS, FACP

Professor of Clinical Internal Medicine
Division of General Internal Medicine
The Ohio State University College of Medicine
Columbus, Ohio
harrison.weed@osumc.edu

McGraw-Hill

Medical Publishing Division

New York Chicago San Francisco Lisbon London Madrid
Mexico City Milan New Delhi San Juan Seoul
Singapore Sydney Toronto

The McGraw-Hill Companies

Perioperative Medicine
Just the Facts

1 2 3 4 5 6 7 8 9 0 QPD/QPD 0 9 8 7 6

ISBN 0-07-144766-0

This book was set in Times New Roman by International Typesetting and Composition.
The editors were James Shanahan, Christie Naglieri, and Lester A. Sheinis.
The production supervisor was Catherine H. Saggese.
The text designer was Joan O'Connor.
The cover designer was Aimee Nordin.
The indexer was Alexandra Nickerson.
Quebecor Dubuque was printer and binder.

This book is printed on acid-free paper.

Library of Congress Cataloging-in-Publication Data

Perioperative medicine : just the facts / [edited by] Steven L. Cohn, Gerald W. Smetana, Harrison G. Weed.—1st ed.
p. ; cm.
Includes bibliographical references and index.
ISBN 0-07-144766-0 (softcover)
1. Therapeutics, Surgical—Handbooks, manuals, etc. 2. Surgery—Complications—Handbooks, manuals, etc. 3. Preoperative care—Handbooks, manuals, etc. 4. Postoperative care—Handbooks, manuals, etc. I. Cohn, Steven L. II. Smetana, Gerald W. III. Weed, Harrison G.
[DNLM: 1. Perioperative Care—Handbooks. WO 39 P4447 2005]
RD49.P462 2005
617'.919—dc22

2005051065

CONTENTS

CONTRIBUTORS

Majed Abu-Hajir, MD, Assistant Professor, Division of Hematology, Department of Medicine, Medical College of Wisconsin, Milwaukee, Wisconsin (Chapter 31)

Jeffrey R. Allen, MD, Associate Director, Medicine in Psychiatry Service, University of Rochester Medical Center, Rochester, New York (Chapters 18, 40, 62)

Ahsan M. Arozullah, MD, MPH, Assistant Professor of Medicine, Jesse Brown VA Medical Center and Sections of General Internal Medicine and Health Promotion Research, Department of Medicine, University of Illinois at Chicago, Chicago, Illinois (Chapters 25, 52, 54)

Martin J. Arron, MD, MBA, Assistant Professor of Medicine, Division of General Internal Medicine, Feinberg School of Medicine, Northwestern University, Chicago, Illinois (Chapters 38, 39)

Andrew D. Auerbach, MD, MPH, Assistant Professor of Medicine in Residence; Physician Director of Perioperative Performance Improvement Initiative, University of California, San Francisco, Department of Medicine, Hospitalist Group, San Francisco, California (Chapters 2, 4)

Margaret Beliveau-Ficalora, MD, Instructor in Medicine, Mayo Clinic College of Medicine, Rochester, Minnesota (Chapters 44, 62)

H. Jay Biem, MD, MSc, FRCPC, Associate Professor & Director of Day Medicine, University of Saskatchewan, Saskatoon, Saskatchewan, Canada, (Chapter 4)

Daniel J. Brotman, MD, FACP, Director, Hospitalist Program, Department of Medicine, Johns Hopkins Hospital, Baltimore, Maryland (Chapters 7B, 55)

Jeffrey L. Carson, MD, Richard C. Reynolds Professor of Medicine; Chief, Division of General Internal Medicine, Department of Medicine, University of Medicine and Dentistry of New Jersey–Robert Wood Johnson Medical School, New Brunswick, New Jersey (Chapters 30, 59)

Michael P. Carson, MD, Chief, Division of General Internal Medicine, Saint Peter's University Hospital; Assistant Clinical Professor of Medicine & Assistant Clinical Professor of Obstetrics, Gynecology, and Reproductive Sciences, University of Medicine and Dentistry of New Jersey–Robert Wood Johnson Medical School, New Brunswick, New Jersey (Chapter 45)

Vinky Chadha, MD, Assistant Professor of Medicine, Northwestern University Feinberg School of Medicine, Chicago, Illinois (Chapter 37)

Calvin L. Chou, MD, PhD, Director, SFVAMC Medical Consultation Service; Associate Professor of Clinical Medicine, University of California, San Francisco, San Francisco, California (Chapters 35, 60)

Steven L. Cohn, MD, FACP, Chief, Division of General Internal Medicine; Director, Medical Consultation Service; Clinical Professor of Medicine, State University of New York, Downstate, Brooklyn, New York (Chapters 1, 7A, 19, 20, 51)

Michelle V. Conde, MD, Audie Murphy Division/South Texas Veterans Health Care System and Division of General Medicine; Clinical Associate Professor of Medicine, University of Texas Health Science Center at San Antonio, San Antonio, Texas (Chapters 22, 24)

Gabriela S. Ferreira, MD, Assistant Professor of Medicine, Division of General Internal Medicine, Department of Medicine, University of Medicine and Dentistry of New Jersey–Robert Wood Johnson Medical School, New Brunswick, New Jersey (Chapter 30)

Shaun Frost, MD, FACP, HealthPartners Medical Group and Clinics, Regions Hospital; Assistant Professor, Clinical Scholar Track, Department of Medicine, The University of Minnesota Medical School, St. Paul, Minnesota (Chapters 2, 52)

William A. Ghali, MD, MPH, Professor and Canada Research Chair, Departments of Medicine and Community Health Sciences, and the Centre for Health and Policy Studies, University of Calgary, Calgary, Alberta, Canada (Chapters 21, 26)

Kenneth Gilbert, MD, MPH, Associate Professor, Division of General Internal Medicine, Department of Medicine, University of Western Ontario, London, Ontario, Canada (Chapters 3, 8, 20)

Adam J. Gordon, MD, MPH, Assistant Professor of Medicine, University of Pittsburgh School of Medicine, Center for Health Equity Research and Promotion, VA Pittsburgh Healthcare System; Mental Illness Research, Education, and Clinical Center, VISN 4; Center for Research on Health Care, University of Pittsburgh, Pittsburgh, Pennsylvania (Chapter 43)

David A. Halle, MD, Assistant Professor, Division of General Internal Medicine; Associate Program Director, Internal Medicine Residency, Boston University Medical Center, Boston, Massachusetts (Chapters 28, 45)

Amir K. Jaffer, MD, Medical Director, Internal Medicine Preoperative Assessment Consultation and Treatment (IMPACT) Center and the Anticoagulation Clinic, Cleveland Clinic Foundation, Cleveland, Ohio (Chapters 7B, 11, 46, 55)

Bruce E. Johnson, MD, FACP, Professor of Medicine, Brody School of Medicine at East Carolina University, Division of General Internal Medicine, Greenville, North Carolina (Chapters 13, 15, 42)

Scott Kaatz, DO, Co-Director, Anticoagulation Clinics, Henry Ford Health System, Detroit, Michigan (Chapters 7B, 46)

Peter Kaboli, MD, MS, Assistant Professor, Center for Research in the Implementation of Innovative Strategies in Practice (CRIISP) at the Iowa City VA Medical Center and Department of Internal Medicine, Division of General Internal Medicine, University of Iowa Carver College of Medicine, Iowa City, Iowa (Chapter 46)

Jennifer C. Kerns, MD, Assistant Clinical Professor of Medicine, Department of Medicine, Division of Hospital Medicine, University of California, San Diego Medical Center, San Diego, California (Chapters 26, 56, 57, 58)

Nadia A. Khan, MD, MSc, Assistant Professor of Medicine, Department of Medicine and Centre for Health Evaluation and Outcome Sciences, University of British Columbia, Vancouver, British Columbia, Canada (Chapters 21, 26)

Maninder Kohli, MD, Director, Medical Consultation Service, Department of Medicine, Stroger Hospital of Cook County; Assistant Professor, Rush Medical College, Chicago, Illinois (Chapters 34, 36, 57, 58)

Colleen G. Lance, MD, Assistant Professor of Medicine, The University of Texas M.D. Anderson Cancer Center, Houston, Texas (Chapter 32)

Valerie A. Lawrence, MD, MSc, Audie Murphy Division/South Texas Veterans Health Care System and Division of General Internal Medicine; Professor of Medicine, University of Texas Health Science Center at San Antonio, San Antonio, Texas (Chapters 22, 25)

Frank Lefevre, MD, Associate Professor of Medicine, Northwestern University Feinberg School of Medicine, Chicago, Illinois (Chapters 37, 61)

James B. Lewis, Jr., MD, Associate Professor of Medicine & Program Director, Internal Medicine, University of Tennessee Health Science Center, Memphis, Tennessee (Chapters 3, 12, 61)

Howard Libman, MD, Director, HIV Program, Healthcare Associates, Beth Israel Deaconess Medical Center; Associate Professor of Medicine, Harvard Medical School, Boston, Massachusetts (Chapter 33)

David S. Macpherson, MD, MPH, Vice President Primary Care, VA Pittsburgh Healthcare System; Professor of Medicine, University of Pittsburgh, Pittsburgh, Pennsylvania (Chapters 5, 7A)

Brian F. Mandell, MD, PhD, FACR, Professor and Vice Chairman of Medicine for Education, Center for Vasculitis Care and Research, Department of Rheumatic and Immunologic Disease, Cleveland Clinic Foundation, Cleveland, Ohio (Chapters 11, 42)

Ellen Manzullo, MD, FACP, Deputy Chair, General Internal Medicine, Ambulatory Treatment & Emergency Care; Professor of Medicine, The University of Texas M.D. Anderson Cancer Center, Houston, Texas (Chapter 32)

Seth McClennen, MD, Director of Arrhythmia Education & Instructor of Medicine, Harvard Medical School, Beth Israel Deaconess Medical Center, Boston, Massachusetts (Chapters 23, 53)

Sylvia C. W. McKean, MD, Medical Director, Brigham and Women's Faulkner Hospitalist Service; Assistant Professor of Medicine, Harvard Medical School, Boston, Massachusetts (Chapters 2, 10)

Donna L. Mercado, MD, FACP, Director, Medical Consultation Program, Baystate Medical Center; Assistant Professor of Medicine, Tufts University School of Medicine, Springfield, Massachusetts (Chapters 17, 40, 41)

Visala Muluk, MD, Assistant Professor of Medicine, University of Pittsburgh; Director, Medical Preoperative Evaluation Clinic, VA Pittsburgh Healthcare System, Pittsburgh, Pennsylvania (Chapters 10, 27)

Kevin J. O'Leary, MD, Assistant Professor of Medicine, Associate Division Chief for Inpatient Medicine, Division of General Internal Medicine, Feinberg School of Medicine, Northwestern University, Chicago, Illinois (Chapters 38, 39)

Mary H. Pak, MD, Clinical Associate Professor of Medicine & Director, General Medicine Consultation Service, University of Wisconsin, Madison, Wisconsin (Chapter 6)

Brent G. Petty, MD, Hospital Pharmacologist, The Johns Hopkins Hospital, and Associate Professor of Medicine, Johns Hopkins University School of Medicine, Baltimore, Maryland (Chapter 15)

Kurt Pfeifer, MD, FACP, Assistant Professor, Division of General Internal Medicine; Associate Program Director, Internal Medicine Residency, Department of Medicine, Medical College of Wisconsin, Milwaukee, Wisconsin (Chapters 14, 31, 59)

James C. Pile, MD, FACP, Assistant Professor of Medicine, Case Medical School; Director of Perioperative Services, CWRU/MetroHealth Medical Center, Cleveland, Ohio (Chapter 50)

Joann Porter, MD, FACP, Assistant Professor, Division of General Internal Medicine; Associate Residency Director, Creighton University, Omaha, Nebraska (Chapters 9, 13, 14)

Kaleem M. Rizvon, MBBS, FACP, Fellow, Division of Gastroenterology, Nassau University Medical Center; Assistant Professor of Medicine, State University of New York at Stony Brook, East Meadow, New York (Chapters 35, 60)

Gregory B. Seymann, MD, Associate Professor, Department of Medicine, Division of Hospital Medicine, University of California, San Diego Medical Center, San Diego, California (Chapters 28, 29)

Tariq Shafi, MD, FACP, Clinical Fellow, Division of Nephrology, The Johns Hopkins School of Medicine, Baltimore, Maryland (Chapters 19, 29, 51)

Vaishali M. Singh, MD, MPH, MBA, Director of Medical Affairs, Section of Hospital Medicine, Cleveland Clinic Foundation, Cleveland, Ohio (Chapters 8, 36)

Gerald W. Smetana, MD, FACP, Associate Professor of Medicine, Harvard Medical School; Division of General Medicine and Primary Care, Beth Israel Deaconess Medical Center, Boston, Massachusetts (Chapters 3, 5, 9, 24, 54)

Scott R. Springman, MD, Professor of Anesthesiology & Medical Director, Outpatient Surgery Center & Preoperative Anesthesia Clinic, University of Wisconsin, Madison, Wisconsin (Chapter 6)

Anjala V. Tess, MD, Hospitalist, Division of General Internal Medicine and Primary Care, Department of Medicine, Beth Israel Deaconess Medical Center, Harvard Medical School, Boston, Massachusetts (Chapters 18, 49)

Harrison G. Weed, MD, MS, FACP, Professor of Clinical Internal Medicine, Division of General Internal Medicine, The Ohio State University College of Medicine, Columbus, Ohio (Chapters 16, 32, 47, 48, 50)

William Wertheim, MD, FACP, Assistant Professor of Medicine, Stony Brook University School of Medicine, Stony Brook, New York (Chapters 27, 44, 63)

Tosha B. Wetterneck, MD, Assistant Professor of Medicine, Department of Medicine, University of Wisconsin Medical School, Madison, Wisconsin (Chapter 4)

Paul H. Willoughby, MD, Associate Professor of Clinical Anesthesiology; Director, Acute Pain Service, Department of Anesthesiology, Stony Brook University School of Medicine, Stony Brook, New York (Chapter 63)

Judi Woolger-Kraft, MD, FACP, Assistant Professor of Medicine, Director, Medical Consultation Service at Jackson Memorial Hospital and University of Miami School of Medicine, Miami, Florida (Chapters 12, 17, 41)

Peter J. Zimetbaum, MD, FACC, Section of Cardiac Electrophysiology, Division of Cardiology, Beth Israel Deaconess Medical Center, Harvard Medical School, Boston, Massachusetts (Chapters 23, 53)

PREFACE

People have performed surgery for thousands of years; however, it was only 150 years ago that inhalation anesthesia enabled relatively painless procedures. Even then, patients continued to die at alarming rates from surgery, anesthesia, and postoperative infection. With the subsequent development of the germ theory and antiseptic technique in the late 1800s, then blood transfusion, intravenous saline hydration, and antibiotics in the first half of the twentieth century, surgery became almost commonplace.

In the early 1960s, anesthesiologists standardized the assessment of perioperative risk based on general physical status, and research demonstrated that many perioperative deaths were attributable to cardiac complications. In the 1970s, Goldman and colleagues developed an index to more specifically predict a patient's risk of perioperative cardiac complications. Over the subsequent 25 years other investigators refined cardiac risk indices, developed new algorithms and guidelines, and introduced interventions to reduce the risk. At the same time, intensive physiologic monitoring and the development of safer anesthetics markedly reduced the risk of death attributable to anesthesia. With older and sicker patients now undergoing surgery, current perioperative morbidity and mortality is due primarily to medical complications rather than to surgery or anesthesia.

While some physicians, such as surgeons, anesthesiologists, and hospitalists, may spend a major portion of their clinical time caring for patients in the perioperative period, many other primary care physicians may feel less comfortable when asked to evaluate and manage perioperative medical conditions. The goal of this book is to provide a simple, direct guide to the medical (as opposed to the surgical and anesthetic) aspects of perioperative care. It is not intended to repeat information available in medical textbooks or to serve as a scholarly treatise. We have deliberately limited the number of references to keep the focus on the practical aspects of patient care. This book is intended for use by surgeons, anesthesiologists, hospitalists, general internists and specialists, and students and residents in-training who are caring for patients before and after surgery.

This book is divided into five sections. The first section addresses general aspects of perioperative care and considerations that apply to most surgical patients. The second section highlights aspects specific to different types of surgery, and the third concerns preoperative evaluation and management of concomitant medical conditions. The fourth section covers general prophylactic measures, and the fifth reviews evaluation and management of postoperative complications.

Medicine is constantly changing; new information often makes previous recommendations obsolete. Furthermore, errors, inaccuracies and omissions are an inevitable part of any human endeavor. Therefore, we advise readers to use this book in the context of clinical judgment and to confirm information contained in the book using other sources. This is especially important when prescribing or administering medications.

We would like to acknowledge the invaluable support of the publisher in bringing this book to life. We are indebted to the many physicians, most of whom are practicing internists and members of the Society of General Internal Medicine Medical Consultation/Perioperative Medicine Interest Group (*www.sgim.org*), who have authored chapters for this book. In addition, our patients, colleagues, and teachers have all contributed to what we are able to provide in this book.

Finally, without the love and encouragement of our families, this book would not have been possible. Dr. Cohn thanks his wife, Deborah, children, Alison and Jeffrey, and mother, Lynn, and dedicates this book in memory of his father, Leo, who passed away shortly before the book was published.

Steven L. Cohn, MD, FACP
Gerald W. Smetana, MD, FACP
Harrison G. Weed, MD, MS, FACP

PERIOPERATIVE MEDICINE
Just the Facts

Section I
INTRODUCTION TO PERIOPERATIVE MEDICINE

Harrison G. Weed, MD, Section Editor

1 THE ROLE OF THE MEDICAL CONSULTANT

Steven L. Cohn

INTRODUCTION

- Preoperative medical consultation is an important aspect of the clinical practice of internists, other primary care physicians, and various subspecialists. As more surgeries have shifted from the inpatient to the outpatient setting or to same-day admissions, preoperative consultations have also shifted to the outpatient setting. Hospitalists are increasingly frequently performing medical consultations for patients admitted to the hospital or undergoing nonelective surgery.
- Some consultants feel that they are inadequately trained to perform preoperative evaluations. Previously, most of the perioperative literature was published in a variety of specialty journals. Only in the past decade has more information appeared in the general medical literature.
- This chapter reviews the basic concepts and practical aspects of medical consultation pertaining to the perioperative setting.[1,2] The role of hospitalists in the medical comanagement of the surgical patient is discussed in Chap. 2.

GENERAL PRINCIPLES OF MEDICAL CONSULTATION

TEN COMMANDMENTS FOR EFFECTIVE CONSULTATIONS

◦ Goldman et al.[3] best described the basic principles of medical consultation:

1. Determine the question.
2. Establish urgency.
3. Look for yourself.
4. Be as brief as appropriate.
5. Be specific and concise.
6. Provide contingency plans.
7. Honor thy turf.
8. Teach with tact.
9. Talk is cheap and effective.
10. Follow up.

THE CONSULTANT'S PERIOPERATIVE ROLES

Preoperative

- Evaluate the patient's known medical problems, including the degree to which each problem is controlled and its surgery-associated risk.
- Recognize previously unrecognized or unacknowledged medical problems.
- Optimize treatment of the medical problems and the patient's general medical condition.
- Recommend risk-reduction strategies, including perioperative medication management.

Postoperative

- Follow up to reevaluate the medical problems.
- Anticipate, recognize, and treat postoperative complications.

Always

- Communicate and collaborate with the other members of the patient's health care team.

DETERMINING THE QUESTION

- Consultation requests are sometimes vague.
- The reason for consultation sometimes consists of no more than a request for "medical clearance." This might

be a request for advice, for perioperative management, or for the medicolegal assurance that another doctor is on the record as approving the patient for surgery.
- The consultant must determine what is being requested in order to respond appropriately.
- Direct verbal communication is the best way to accomplish this and to eliminate the potential for any misunderstanding.

ANSWERING THE QUESTION

- In addition to addressing any specific questions, determine whether the patient is in his or her "optimal medical condition for surgery." In order to do this, the consultant must answer a number of questions, including:
  - What are the patient's medical problems?
  - How severe are they?
  - Are they adequately controlled?
  - How do they affect surgical risk?
  - Are there any tests of these problems that would significantly improve estimates of surgical risk and alter management?
  - Are there any treatments for these problems that would significantly reduce surgical risk?
  - How urgent is the surgery?
  - Should the surgery be postponed?
- Based on these guidelines, recommend treatments known to reduce perioperative complications, such as prophylactic therapy to prevent venous thromboembolism, surgical-site infection, endocarditis, and cardiac ischemia.
- Also make specific recommendations for the perioperative management of the patient's medications.

WRITING THE REPORT

WHAT TO INCLUDE

- Include in your consultation report specific information regarding demographics, medical problems, medications, other history, pertinent physical findings, and test results. Once these data have been obtained, assess the patient's fitness for surgery and make specific recommendations for perioperative management.

HOW TO STRUCTURE THE REPORT

- A sample report, structured to highlight the key information for the surgeon and anesthesiologist, is shown in Fig. 1-1. On the first page are the reasons for consultation, pertinent medical problems, an impression as to whether the patient is in optimal condition for surgery, and recommendations for perioperative management. The remainder of the medical history, physical examination findings, test results, and additional discussion are presented on the second page.

DEMOGRAPHICS

- The patient's name, age or date of birth, medical record number, primary care physician, referring physician, and service should be noted.

MEDICAL PROBLEMS

PRESENT ILLNESS
- This is actually the surgical problem; the medical consultant does not have to explore this in detail but should focus on the pertinent past medical and surgical history.

PAST MEDICAL HISTORY
- Cover body systems commonly associated with perioperative medical complications, including cardiovascular, pulmonary, and hemostatic. Also include any disease, condition, or habit that affects perioperative risk or requires perioperative management. Common examples include hypertension, diabetes mellitus, dyslipidemia, cigarette smoking, obesity, thyroid disease, and renal insufficiency.

PAST SURGICAL/TRAUMA HISTORY
- List all prior surgeries including approximate date, type of anesthesia and any anesthetic, surgical or medical complications. In general, if a patient tolerated major surgery without complications within the past year or two and if there has been no change in his or her medical condition since that time, the patient will probably do reasonably well.

SOCIAL HISTORY
- To elicit accurate information, ask specific but nonjudgmental questions, such as "When did you most recently use tobacco (or alcohol or drugs)?" Many patients, when told they need surgery, may stop using these substances. If asked "Do you smoke?" they will answer no, since they had recently decided to stop.

MEDICATIONS
- Do not just copy the patient's medications from a list but ask the patient or caregiver what medications, vitamins, supplements, and herbs the patient actually takes.

- Ask about medication, food, or other allergies (including allergy to latex) as well as the route of administration and the type of reaction.

Family History

- In the preoperative evaluation of adults, this is usually of relatively minor importance. If the patient has not previously undergone major surgery, it is reasonable to inquire about a family history of malignant hyperthermia and bleeding disorders.

Review of Systems

- This should focus primarily on cardiac, vascular, and pulmonary symptoms. Note the presence of chest pain or dyspnea, but recognize that their absence in a sedentary patient is no reassurance that the stress of surgery will not precipitate these symptoms or other complications.
- Assess functional capacity with a standardized questionnaire or by asking the patient how many blocks he can walk or how many steps (or flights of stairs) he can climb without stopping. Try to determine usual activities and ability to perform activities of daily living.
- Other items of potential importance in the screening review of systems include any abnormal bleeding or easy bruisability, dizziness and loss of consciousness, and polyuria or polydipsia.

PHYSICAL EXAMINATION

- In general, the physical examination serves to assess and confirm positive findings in the history. New diseases may be diagnosed as well.
- Vital signs are vital. Check blood pressure yourself using a cuff of appropriate size. Note any abnormal or irregular pulse, tachycardia or bradycardia, tachypnea, hypertension, hypotension, and orthostatic changes.
- Head and neck exam: Evaluate the airway, thyroid gland, carotid pulses, and presence of bruits or jugular venous distention.
- Cardiopulmonary exam: Note any heart murmurs, gallops (especially S_3), rales, rhonchi, or wheezes.
- Abdominal exam: Note the presence of organomegaly, an aortic aneurysm, or bruits.
- Extremity exam: Note any edema, tenderness, or abnormal pulses.
- Neurologic exam: Assess the patient's mental status and note any gross motor or sensory deficits.

LABORATORY TESTS

- Recommendations for preoperative laboratory testing are discussed in Chap. 5.
- Note the results of all pertinent tests and address any abnormal findings.

IMPRESSION

- Based on the above information, make a statement about whether the patient is or is not "in his or her optimal medical condition for the planned procedure." Being in optimal condition for the procedure does not necessarily mean that there are no potential problems or that the patient is in perfect health; it means that the patient's medical problems have been adequately controlled, that additional testing or treatment would not substantially reduce the patient's risk of perioperative medical complications, or that the delay required for such treatment would worsen the patient's overall prognosis.
- Avoid using the expression "cleared for surgery," as this implies a guarantee that there will be no problems. It is best to be more explicit about your assessment of the patient's fitness for the specific procedure and the potential for complications.

RECOMMENDATIONS/DISCUSSION

- Advise the patient and surgeon how to manage the patient's medications in the perioperative period.
- Include specific recommendations for any indicated prophylactic medications, monitoring, or other measures. Examples include prophylaxis against deep venous thrombosis, surgical-site infection, endocarditis, or aspiration.
- It may also be helpful to include a statement to the effect that "additional testing is not indicated at this time."
- In the discussion, briefly describe pertinent findings and the reasons for your recommendations. Also mention whether the patient is at greater than usual risk for complications or poor outcome.
- Finally, specifically state whether you will follow the patient after surgery or be available to do so and provide contact information for questions and follow-up.

IMPROVING COMPLIANCE WITH RECOMMENDATIONS

- Although the physician who requested your consultation may choose not to follow your advice, there are several tactics[4] than can improve compliance with your recommendations (Table 1-1).
  - Answer the consultation in a timely fashion.
  - Address the primary reason for the consultation.
  - Be concise yet informative in your written report. Address all pertinent medical problems, assess overall

KINGS COUNTY HOSPITAL CENTER

PREOPERATIVE MEDICAL CONSULTATION

- 1 -

Doe, John

Name: Doe (inst), John (first) **MR #** 123456

Age: 70 **Race:** AA **Gender:** M

Referring Service: General Surgery **Surgical Procedure:** Hemicolectomy

Primary Reason for Consultation: HTN

MEDICAL PROBLEMS:

1. CAD - Class II; stable
2. HTN - 10 yrs.-Stage I
3. DM - 5 yrs.
4. Asthma
5.

Medications:

Clonidine 0.1 mg bid
Norvasc 5 mg qd
Vasotec 5 mg qd
Nitropatch 0.4 mg/hr
Ecotrin 81 mg qd
Glucotrol XL 5 mg qd
Albuterol inhaler PRN

Allergies: none known

IMPRESSION:

Pt. is in his optimal medical condition for the planned surgical procedure.

RECOMMENDATIONS:

- Withhold Glucotrol XL on AM of surgery; fingerstick periop and cover with Humulin regular insulin for glucose > 200.
- Stop Ecotrin one week prior to surgery.
- Continue other meds, incl. on AM of surgery, with a sip of water.
- Should pt develop bronchospasm periop, Rx with nebulized beta-agonists and steroids.
- DVT prophylaxis; surgical wound prophylaxis; incentive spirometry.
- No further cardiac workup is indicated at this time.

FIG. 1-1 Sample preoperative medical consultation report.

risk and whether or not the patient is in his or her optimal medical condition, and provide recommendations regarding perioperative medication management and risk-reduction strategies.

- Limit the number of recommendations (to five or fewer) and be specific.
- Prioritize recommendations and focus on central issues.
- Recommendations considered to be crucial or critical are more likely to be followed, as are those involving therapy as opposed to diagnosis.
- Provide follow-up.
- Communication (by phone or in person) with the requester and the surgical team is critical for ensuring awareness, understanding, and compliance with recommendations.

KINGS COUNTY HOSPITAL CENTER

PREOPERATIVE MEDICAL CONSULTATION

Doe, John

- 2 -

Other Pertinent Medical History:

Denies MI, CHF;

otherwise negative

Past Surgical History:

cholecystectomy-GA, 1990

RIH - spinal; 1992. R cataract-local

No anesth/surg complications

Social History:	Yes	No	Ex	
Tobacco:	☐	☐	■	Amount: 1 PPD x 20 yrs; D/C'd 10 yrs. ago
Alcohol:	☐	■	☐	Amount:
Drugs:	☐	■	☐	Specify:

Family History of problems with anesthesia/surgery? Yes (No) — circled
Specify

Review of Systems:	Yes	No		Yes	No
Chest pain: Exertional	■	☐	Orthopnea	☐	■
Resting	☐	■	PND	☐	■
			Edema	☐	■
Dyspnea: Exertional	☐	■	Cough	☐	■
Resting	☐	■			

Exercise Capacity: 5-6 blocks, 2-3 flights; minimal CP relieved by rest
Other: no polyuria, polydipsia; denies bleeding problem

PHYSICAL EXAM: BP 140/80 P 66 R 14 T 99

Head/Neck: no JVD, thyromegaly, bruits
Heart: S1S2 WNL; II/VI SEM@LSB; no gallop
Lungs: clear; no wheezing
Abd: soft, NT, no organomegaly, BS+
Ext: no edema or calf tenderness
Neuro: no focal deficits

LABS:

Hct 40.2 WBC 8.6 Plat 245,000
Na 142 K 4.8 BUN 18 Cr 1.3
Glucose 162
PT: 12.2 INR 1.1
LFT's: WNL PTT: 26.5

EKG: NSR, LVH; NS ST-T changes
CXR: NAPD

DISCUSSION: Pt with above probs: mild stable exertional angina, unchanged over past 2 yrs. Denies MI. Never hospitalized for asthma; last ER visit 1 yr ago; last attack 4 mos. ago; never intubated or on steroids. Glucose is mildly elevated, BP is adequately controlled for surgery. No evidence of bronchospasm. Based on this, pt is at somewhat increased risk for periop cardiopulm complications but is medically stable for surgery.

Name of Consulting Physician (Print)		Signature of Consulting Physician / Attending Physician Countersignature
Jones, Jeffrey		[signatures]
Title	**Beeper #**	**Date**	**Time**
PGY-III	917-123-4000	05/10/05	10 AM

FIG. 1-1 (*Continued*)

SUMMARY

- Perioperative medical consultation is a combination of art, science, and politics. The important theoretical concepts and the art of communicating have been reviewed here. The scientific basis for the consultant's evaluation and management of the surgical patient is discussed in the subsequent chapters.
- Being able, affable, and available can go a long way toward working well with colleagues and, ultimately, improving patient outcomes.

TABLE 1-1 Factors That Influence Compliance with Consultant Recommendations

Respond promptly (within 24 h).
Limit the number of recommendations (five or fewer).
Identify crucial or critical (as opposed to routine) recommendations.
Focus on the central issues.
Make specific, relevant recommendations.
Use definitive language.
Specify drug dose, route, frequency, and duration.
Follow up frequently, including writing progress notes.
Make direct verbal contact.
Make therapeutic (as opposed to diagnostic) recommendations.
If the patient is more severely ill, recommendations are more likely to be followed.

SOURCE: Adapted from Cohn and Macpherson,[1] with permission. For more information visit *www.uptodate.com.*

REFERENCES

1. Cohn SL, Macpherson DS. Overview of the principles of medical consultation, in Rose ED (ed): *UpToDate*. Wellesley, MA:2005.
2. Cohn SL. The role of the medical consultant. *Med Clin North Am* 87:1–6, 2003.
3. Goldman L, Lee T, Rudd P. Ten commandments for effective consultations. *Arch Intern Med* 143:1753–1755, 1983.
4. Sears CL, Charlson ME. The effectiveness of a consultation—compliance with initial recommendations. *Am J Med* 74: 870–876, 1983.

2 THE ROLE OF HOSPITALISTS

Sylvia C.W. McKean, Andrew D. Auerbach, and Shaun Frost

INTRODUCTION: WHY HOSPITALISTS?

- In the last 20 years, internists have become more involved in perioperative patient care due to a number of factors, including improved technology and anesthesia, which enables older and frailer patients with more comorbid disease to undergo surgery. These patients require more complex perioperative care.
- More recently, surgeons are spending more of their time in the operating room and are less available to respond to complex medical issues that arise with their patients. This situation is further aggravated by the work hours mandated by the Accreditation Council for Graduate Medical Education (ACGME) for surgeons in training at academic medical centers.
- The hospitalist movement initially developed as a method to reduce length of hospital stay, thereby reducing costs per patient admission and improving hospital fiscal performance.
- In addition, in some states, hospital closures forced the remaining hospitals to further reduce average length of stay and to discharge patients earlier in the day so as to enable them to accommodate more patients.
- The hospitalist movement then expanded into academic medical centers to fulfill many roles, including teaching, reducing length of stay, and caring for patients whose primary care physicians were unable to follow them to the tertiary hospital.
- As primary care physicians withdrew from the hospital in response to the increasing demands of their outpatient practices and the inefficiencies of travel, medical consultation became one of the roles assumed by hospitalists.

HOW DO HOSPITALISTS PARTICIPATE IN PERIOPERATIVE CARE?

- The roles of hospitalists are varied and have evolved from those of a traditional consultant in 1996 to the functions of a comanager in 2005.
- In general, hospitalists approach the care of surgical inpatients differently from traditional medical consultants.
  - Hospitalists are more likely to focus on hospital processes than are traditional medical consultants.
  - Hospitalists are more likely to be available to comanage patients, to see them in the recovery room, and to be available to respond promptly to the concerns of patients or family members.
  - Hospitalists typically focus on the entire hospital course from admission onward, anticipating problems during hospitalization and preparing for discharge.
  - Hospitalists can take the lead in coordinating care, including communicating with referring primary care physicians regarding test results, key discharge information, and preferred extended care facilities after discharge.
  - Hospitalists may improve care coordination and bridge performance gaps in the following areas:
    - Venous thromboembolism prophylaxis
    - Titration of perioperative beta blockers to heart rate and blood pressure targets
    - Tight glucose control

  - Pain assessment and treatment
  - Prevention and early identification of infection
  - Identification and prophylaxis of substance abuse
  - Early correction of abnormalities leading to renal insufficiency and states of fluid overload
- Prevention, appropriate use of resources including consultation, and addressing end-of-life issues are additional contributions often made by hospitalists.
  - Hospitalists are invested in making the hospital run more safely and efficiently.
  - They may play a role in developing comanagement models for selected surgical patients.
  - The hospitalist model markedly improves clinical efficiency without negatively impacting quality measures such as readmissions. In addition, there are now data supporting a possible mortality benefit from using hospitalists to care for inpatients. These same benefits may be extended to medical consultation.
    - Expertise, experience, and knowledge of the hospital coupled with enhanced availability represent a departure from the traditional consultant role, where the physician has competing outpatient obligations outside of the hospital.
    - Additional studies are needed to determine how hospitalists affect the quality of care in their role as medical consultants.

HOSPITALISTS IN PREOPERATIVE CARE

- Hospitalists perform preoperative medical consultations in a variety of locations, including outpatient clinics, emergency departments, and preanesthesia holding areas.
- Hospitalists perform preoperative medical consultations at varying times before surgery, even up to "the last minute."
- Preoperative clinics have arisen to centralize routine preoperative evaluations, but there is little evidence addressing the utility of preoperative evaluations.
  - It is likely that preoperative medical evaluations are not cost-effective in low-risk patients and that targeted evaluations yield the most benefit.
  - Anecdotal evidence reporting site-specific experiences with a "preoperative clinic" suggests benefits in terms of clinical outcomes, patient satisfaction, and surgeon satisfaction.
  - One randomized trial examined the effect of preoperative consultation by a medical specialist. Although this trial demonstrated that preoperative evaluations reduced canceled surgeries, patients in this group had more consultations in the postoperative period and no difference in length of stay.
- Evaluations for patients undergoing emergent procedures take place in the compressed time period immediately preceding surgery.
  - Hospitalists are often contacted because of their on-site availability.
  - Hospitalists seek to minimize risk and place emphasis on perioperative and postoperative care.
  - Hospitalists may take a leadership role in developing systems to facilitate effective preoperative evaluation.

INPATIENT CONSULTATION MODELS

- A 1998 national survey of hospitalists showed that, in addition to caring for general medical patients, more than 80 percent of hospitalists performed preoperative evaluations and more than 90 percent performed medical consultations on nonmedical services.
- The traditional medical consultant may not see the patient in the hospital postoperatively.
  - The primary responsibility for the management of medical conditions is left to the surgeon, who is not obliged to obtain additional postoperative consultation.
  - The goal of preoperative evaluation by traditional medical consultants is the prevention of adverse events through effective management of preexisting conditions and early detection of asymptomatic illnesses that might result in perioperative complications.
- A 1998 survey of hospitalists revealed that 44 percent of respondents were comanaging surgical patients regularly.
- The comanagement model represents a departure from the consultative model in that an internist is part of the patient care team, sometimes as the attending of record.
  - This role is a logical extension of the hospitalist model in that surgeons, like primary care physicians, are often physically unable to see patients repeatedly throughout the day.
  - In addition, trends in illness severity and increases in outpatient surgery have made surgical patients more "medical" than in the past.
  - A comanaging internist has the ability to order tests, medications, or therapies as an equal member of the team, with care being coordinated by daily collaborative contact with the surgical team.
  - From national survey data, we know that nearly half of hospital-based internists act as the attending of record for surgical patients.
- There are a variety of models, ranging from simple consultation to robust consultation (i.e., the consultant writes orders), to models where comanaging internists

round with the surgical team, write orders, and take responsibility for providing many elements of follow-up care.
  - Implementation depends on the complexity of the model chosen as well as site-specific requirements, such as the presence of a hospitalist system and local referral and consultative preferences.
  - Some models are service-based (e.g., all orthopedic patients), some are diagnosis-based (e.g., all patients undergoing spinal fusion and total knee replacement), and some are based on the severity of illness (e.g., all hip fracture patients with specific comorbidities).
    - MacPherson's comanagement model (order writing and daily rounding with the surgical team) reduced postoperative stay, total hospital stay, transfers to a medical service, the number of radiographic studies per patient as well as the number of medications at discharge, with no difference in hospital mortality.[1]
    - Huddleston's comanagement model for patients undergoing total knee replacement at the Mayo Clinic reduced minor postoperative medical complications, adjusted postoperative length of stay, and increased surgeon and nurse satisfaction without changing total costs.[2]
  - Accounting for the costs of the system must include physicians' fees for consultation, the costs of tests and procedures, and the costs of medical complications.

COMANAGEMENT: THE NEED FOR A CONTRACT

- The American College of Surgeons' "Statement on Principles Underlying Perioperative Responsibility" clarifies the role of the surgeon but is not sufficiently specific about hospitalist comanagement.
  - In most situations, hospitalists and surgeons will benefit from a contract to help them specify responsibilities, avoid pitfalls, ensure quality, and maximize efficiency.
  - A comanagement protocol should specify how the comanagers will coordinate care and establish mechanisms and expectations for communication.
  - Roles should be clearly defined, including who has primary responsibility for:
    - Requesting additional consultations
    - Ordering ancillary tests
    - Writing orders (admission, discharge, postoperative, routine)
    - Being available to nursing for first call
    - Providing case management liaison
    - Coordinating care and discharge planning
    - Completing records, paperwork/dictations of admission history and physical, and discharge
    - Managing the surgical site
    - Ordering physical therapy
  - Expectations should be clearly defined, including:
    - Level of medical comorbidity required to initiate referral (i.e., reason for referral)
    - Time to complete consultations
    - Location of consultation
    - Duration of hospitalist participation
    - Number and timing of postoperative surgical visits
    - Scheduled communication
    - Trainee and physician extender involvement
  - Mechanisms for communication should be defined, including:
    - How to initiate a referral
    - Protocol for transfer of primary service
    - Optimal time and mechanism to contact surgeon
    - Method to contact surgeon with urgent issues
    - Expected time for return of messages regarding nonurgent issues
  - The services offered should be specified, including:
    - Preoperative evaluation and postoperative care
    - Addressing nonsurgical but acute problems and the times of day when this service will be provided (e.g., regular hours, evenings, weekends)
    - Discharge planning
    - Pathway adherence
    - Paperwork
    - Family meeting coordination
    - Teaching
  - Patients and families should be informed about the comanagement model of care.
- Although there are few data describing its true effects, the comanagement model of perioperative care has theoretical parallels to practices that increase the availability of expert physicians' care for patients in intensive care units.
  - It has the potential to eliminate some known difficulties in consultative medicine, specifically delays in execution of recommendations and gaps in communication.
  - Even without specific guidelines, therapies, or educational interventions, a comanagement model in which the hospitalist makes daily rounds, writes orders, and initiates discharge planning is expected to reduce length of stay.
  - A comanagement model might also reduce transfers to medical services, which can be critically important at academic centers with limited house staff.
  - Reduction of laboratory and radiology use, mortality, and discharge medications would likely depend on the expertise and experience of the hospitalist.

- Role definition is critical to avoid conflict and ensure that patients do not "fall through the cracks."

- Despite a paucity of evidence demonstrating efficacy, comanagement of nonmedical patients by hospitalists is growing.
  - The presence of multiple specialists in a care system makes it mandatory that we research complex collaborative arrangements in perioperative care.

THE CARE OF SURGICAL PATIENTS POSTDISCHARGE

- Hospitalists are increasingly staffing extended care facilities, including rehabilitation facilities.
- As sicker patients are transitioned to other sites of care, the expertise, experience, and availability of hospitalists provides an opportunity to improve the care of these patients and to continue prevention protocols that were begun in the hospital.

HOSPITALISTS AS DRIVERS OF SYSTEM CHANGE

- The hospitalist movement is not only a response to economic and social changes in medicine but also an engine of changes in practice.
  - Hospitalists are now nationally organized through the Society of Hospital Medicine.[3]
  - As medical consultants participating in varied and evolving models of care, hospitalists lead initiatives to reduce the incidence of the perioperative medical complications that occur in up to 29 percent of patients by 30 days postsurgery.
  - Effective and timely communication with primary care physicians and medical specialists requires time and availability and is central to the hospitalist role.
  - Hospitalists can enhance continuity of care during transfers from one physician to another in a setting where everything happens faster.
  - Hospitalists can also take leadership roles in ensuring that their hospitals reach patient-centered and patient-safety goals in caring for patients in the perioperative period.
  - Hospitalists actively teach other team members, including surgical trainees and medical residents.
  - Hospitalists can develop triage or clinical prediction rules, which can be used in prospective studies to evaluate the effects of different models of consultation.
  - Hospitalists can lead, coordinate, or participate in the development of guidelines, critical pathways, and rapid cycle improvements to improve the care of postoperative patients.

REFERENCES

1. Macpherson, DS, Parenti C, Nee J, et al. An internist joins the surgery service: Does comanagement make a difference? *J Gen Intern Med* 9:440, 1994.
2. Huddleston JM, Long KH, Naessens JM, et al. Hospitalist-Orthopaedic Team Trial Investigators: Medical and surgical comanagement after elective hip and knee arthroplasty: A randomized, controlled trial. *Ann Intern Med* 141:28, 2004.
3. Website for the Society of Hospital Medicine. *www.HospitalMedicine.org*

3 ASSESSING PERIOPERATIVE RISK

Kenneth Gilbert, James B. Lewis, Jr., and Gerald W. Smetana

INTRODUCTION

- Estimating the risks of perioperative complications is an important part of evaluating patients who are anticipating surgery.
- Although perioperative risk assessment is based largely on experience and opinion, specific models address the risks of cardiovascular and pulmonary complications.
- This chapter covers the sources of perioperative risk, potential complications, and the preoperative evaluation.

SOURCES OF RISK

THE SURGERY

- Following is general information about perioperative risks of different types of surgeries. Refer to the surgery-specific chapters for more detailed information.
- Cardiac surgery carries the greatest risk of cardiovascular complications, including myocardial infarction, arrhythmia, congestive heart failure, stroke, and sudden death.
- Major vascular surgery also carries a relatively high risk of cardiovascular complications.
  - For example, the risk of procedure-associated stroke after carotid endarterectomy is approximately 3 percent for even the most proficient surgeons.

- Major abdominal surgery (e.g., bowel resection, lysis of adhesions, tumor debulking, and resection of all or part of a solid organ) is associated with cardiac, pulmonary, and infectious complications.
  - For example, the risk of surgical site infection is as high as 20 percent.
- Thoracic surgery (e.g., partial or total pneumonectomy) carries a high risk of pulmonary complication.
- Complications of intracranial operations (e.g., brain tumor resection, abscess drainage, aneurysm clipping) include cerebral edema, seizures, stroke, hemorrhage, and meningitis.
- Many different types of minor procedures are often performed in an outpatient or short-stay setting.
  - Such procedures include cataract removal, intraocular lens insertion, and excision of skin lesions as well as urologic, gynecologic, and even laparoscopic surgeries such as cholecystectomy.
  - Although these procedures are intrinsically low-risk, complications sometimes develop after patients have returned home.

THE PATIENT

- Advanced age is a risk factor for perioperative complications including cardiac, pulmonary, thromboembolic, infectious, and neurologic complications.
  - The contribution of age to risk is primarily due to the accumulation of comorbidities; healthy older patients have risks that are similar to equivalently healthy younger patients.
- Obesity increases the risk for some but not all postoperative complications.
  - Obese patients are at increased risk of surgical site infection and dehiscence and for thromboembolism.
  - Profound obesity can preclude adequate patient assessment due to technical limitations, thereby obscuring underlying risk factors.
    - For example, nuclear imaging and coronary angiography equipment usually has a patient weight limit.
- Cardiac disease, including coronary artery disease and congestive heart failure, confers a higher risk for postoperative cardiac complications.
- Chronic obstructive pulmonary disease (COPD) is the most important patient-related risk factor for postoperative pulmonary complications.
- Chronic renal insufficiency poses special challenges in fluid and electrolyte management (see Chap. 58).
  - Patients on dialysis must coordinate the timing of their surgery with their dialysis.
  - Patients with renal insufficiency are at greater risk for both volume depletion and overhydration.
    - Volume depletion can cause hypotension and poor perfusion of vital organs.
    - Overhydration can lead to pulmonary edema.
  - Perioperative stresses can exacerbate or precipitate electrolyte and acid-base disorders, including hyperkalemia, hypocalcemia, and acidosis (see Chaps. 56 and 57).
- The most common endocrine condition associated with increased surgical risk is diabetes mellitus (see Chap. 26).
  - Other endocrine disorders include hyper- and hypothyroidism, hyper- and hypoadrenalism, and pheochromocytoma (see Chaps. 27 and 29).
  - Selected patients who are chronically taking corticosteroid medication may require supplemental "stress" doses of corticosteroids in the perioperative period (see Chap. 28).
- Surgery increases the risk of venous thromboembolism through a variety of mechanisms, including venous stasis and the inflammatory response to surgical trauma (see Chap. 46).
- Bleeding disorders are usually apparent in the medical history of an adult or the family history of a child.
  - In rare cases, perioperative bleeding may be the first sign of a bleeding diathesis; however, there are no effective laboratory screening tests for bleeding disorders in the absence of suggestive history or physical findings (see Chaps. 5 and 31).
- Preexisting dementia and other forms of neurologic impairment (e.g., prior stroke) are risk factors for postoperative delirium (see Chap. 62).
- A careful medication history is a critical part of the preoperative evaluation (see Chap. 7).
  - For example, medications (e.g., aspirin, warfarin) can increase perioperative blood loss or other postoperative complications.
  - Specific advice prior to surgery about which medications to continue and which to discontinue can help to reduce perioperative risk.

ANTICIPATED COMPLICATIONS

MORBIDITY AND MORTALITY OF HEALTHY PATIENTS

- The physical status classification of the American Society of Anesthesiologists (ASA class), initially developed in 1941, is a robust estimate of perioperative risk based on the impact of underlying illness on a patient's capacities (Table 3-1).
  - Perioperative cardiac events are uncommon among ASA class 1 patients.
    - For example, only 3 of 14,609 ASA class 1 patients (0.006 percent) undergoing ambulatory surgery sustained a perioperative myocardial infarction.[1]

TABLE 3-1 Mortality Risk Associated with American Society of Anesthesiologists (ASA) Physical Status Classification

CLASS	DEFINITION	MORTALITY
1	A normally healthy patient	0.2%
2	A patient with mild systemic disease	0.5%
3	A patient with severe systemic disease that is not incapacitating	1.9%
4	A patient with an incapacitating systemic disease that is a constant threat to life	4.9%
5	A moribund patient who is not expected to survive for 24 h with or without operation	N.A.

SOURCE: From Prause G, Ratzenhofer-Comenda B, Pierer G, et al. Can ASA grade or Goldman's cardiac risk index predict peri-operative mortality? A study of 16,227 patients. *Anaesthesia* 52:203–206, 1997.

- In the cohorts of the revised cardiac risk index, no ASA class 1 patient developed a major postoperative cardiac complication.
- Morbidity among ASA class 1 and 2 patients is primarily due to factors related to the surgery or to the anesthesia, including adverse and idiosyncratic drug reactions, operator error, complications of endotracheal intubation, equipment failure, aspiration of gastric contents, and postanesthesia respiratory depression.
- Among ASA class 1 patients who are healthy and have no significant illness except for the surgical condition, the risk of perioperative mortality is below 0.2 percent.
  - In a study of 38,598 patients who underwent ambulatory surgery, 2 patients died of complications potentially related to the surgery; neither of these patients was in ASA class 1.[1]
- The three most frequent types of major perioperative complications are cardiac, pulmonary, and thromboembolic.

CARDIAC COMPLICATIONS

- Perioperative cardiac complications are a significant cause of perioperative morbidity and mortality.
  - Major perioperative cardiac complications include pulmonary edema, atrial fibrillation, ventricular fibrillation, heart block, myocardial infarction, and cardiac death (see Chaps. 19 to 23).
  - In the cohorts of the revised cardiac risk index, the rate of major cardiac complications ranged from 2.0 to 2.5 percent among patients 50 years or older undergoing major noncardiac surgery.[2]

PULMONARY COMPLICATIONS

- Postoperative pulmonary complications are more frequent than cardiac complications, and they substantially contribute to morbidity, mortality, and length of stay (see Chaps. 24 and 25).
- Major pulmonary complications include pneumonia, respiratory failure (prolonged mechanical ventilation), and bronchospasm.
- The rate of pulmonary complications after major noncardiac surgery is approximately 6 percent.[3]
- Procedure-related risk factors, particularly involving the surgical site, are more significant predictors of postoperative pulmonary complications than are patient-related risk factors.
  - Pulmonary complications occur even among apparently healthy patients who undergo high-risk surgeries, including upper abdominal, thoracic, and abdominal aortic aneurysm repair.

VENOUS THROMBOEMBOLISM (VTE)

- Postoperative deep venous thrombosis and pulmonary embolism are among the most common and serious complications of major surgery (see Chap. 46).
  - Although the risk of postoperative VTE increases with increasing patient-related risk factors, healthy patients are also at significant risk of postoperative VTE after some procedures.
    - For example, after major noncardiac surgery 10 to 20 percent of patients aged 40 to 60 years who have no other risk factors develop postoperative deep venous thrombosis and 1 to 2 percent develop pulmonary embolism.[4]
- Hip or knee arthroplasty and hip fracture repair are among the procedures that confer the highest risk of deep venous thromobosis.
- General surgery and major gynecologic and urologic surgeries confer moderate risk.
- Appropriate recommendations for VTE prophylaxis incorporate both patient- and procedure-related risk factors (see Chap. 46).

POSTOPERATIVE BLEEDING COMPLICATIONS

- Postoperative bleeding at the surgical site is a potential complication of any surgery (see Chap. 59).
  - The medical consultant should suggest strategies to minimize bleeding risk in patients with coagulation disorders (see Chap. 31).
  - In general, the management and treatment of postoperative bleeding is the domain of the surgeon rather than the medical consultant.

POSTOPERATIVE PAIN

- The management of postoperative pain is an important aspect of perioperative care (see Chap. 63).
  - Surgeons and anesthesiologists usually share this responsibility; in general this is not a role of the medical consultant.

DELIRIUM

- Postoperative delirium is common (see Chap. 62).
  - The major clinical elements of delirium include inattention, disorganized thinking, altered level of consciousness, acute onset, and fluctuating course.
  - Major risk factors include age over 70 years, vision impairment, comorbid major illness, preexisting neurologic disease, depression, renal dysfunction, anemia, infection, and abuse of alcohol or other drugs.

INFECTIONS

SURGICAL SITE

- Surgical site infections are an important source of morbidity for otherwise healthy patients.
  - Rates range from 2 to 5 percent for patients undergoing clean extraabdominal surgery to as high as 20 percent for intraabdominal surgery.
  - Strategies to reduce this risk include standardized protocols for surgical antimicrobial prophylaxis based on the proposed procedure (see Chap. 48).

CATHETER-ASSOCIATED

Vascular catheters Bacteremia is detected in approximately 0.6 percent of all hospital admissions.

- The incidence of bloodstream infection after placement of a central venous catheter is approximately 5 percent.
- In evaluating a patient with fever, examine all intravascular catheters and consider the diagnosis of a catheter-associated infection (see Chap. 50).
- Although signs of inflammation are usually present for patients with an infected peripheral intravenous line (including redness, warmth, tenderness, or a palpable cord proximal to the site), fever is often the only sign of an infected central venous line.

Urinary catheters Four percent of all patients undergoing major surgery develop a postoperative urinary tract infection, and 80 percent of postoperative urinary tract infections are due to indwelling urinary catheters.

ADVERSE MEDICATION REACTIONS

- A thorough history of medication allergies and adverse medication reactions should be obtained as part of every preoperative evaluation.

ALLERGIC

- Perioperative allergic reactions are common.
- Manifestations include rash and fever.
- Antimicrobials are most frequently implicated, but allergic reactions to heparin and to blood products also occur.
  - Because the immune system is complex, immunologic reactions have a variety of manifestations and occur at a variety of times after exposure.

MALIGNANT HYPERTHERMIA

- Malignant hyperthermia is a life-threatening metabolic derangement precipitated by inhalation anesthetics and depolarizing muscle relaxants (see Chap. 6).
  - It is manifest as fever, muscle rigidity, and metabolic acidosis.
  - The predisposition to malignant hyperthermia is inherited.

TOXIC

- Examples include hepatitis due to volatile anesthetics and antibiotic-induced interstitial nephritis.

PHARMACOLOGIC

- Expected pharmacologic adverse effects of perioperative medications can cause complications.
  - Examples include hypoventilation from sedatives, ileus and urinary retention from opioids, nausea and vomiting from volatile anesthetics, and gastrointestinal bleeding and acute renal failure from nonsteroidal anti-inflammatory drugs.

PREOPERATIVE EVALUATION

- There are no studies proving that preoperative medical consultation reduces perioperative morbidity and mortality; however, preoperative evaluations frequently result in significant changes in perioperative management.
- There are several standard aspects of the preoperative medical evaluation (Table 3-2).

HISTORY

HEART DISEASE

- The American Heart Association guideline on perioperative evaluation emphasizes the risks associated

TABLE 3-2 Sample Screening Preoperative Assessment Form

DATE:	TIME:	PATIENT NAME:
Age/Sex/Ethnicity:		
☐ History unobtainable due to:		
Reason for consultation:		
Requesting MD or Service:		
History of present illness (include anesthesia and bleeding history):		
Family history (include anesthesia, thrombosis/bleeding):		
Past medical/surgical history (include diabetes, hypertension, chronic heart, lung, liver, renal disease, prior hospitalizations, operations, cardiac procedures, transfusions):		
Medications (include herbals, eyedrops, recent steroids):		
Allergies (medications, latex, angioedema; indicate reaction):		

Review of systems (symptoms present in past 30 days):

	Y	N		Y	N
General			Respiratory		
Weight loss			Cough		
Fever			SOB		
Eyes			Wheezing		
Visual changes			GI		
Dermatologic			Abd. Pain		
Rash			Stool changes		
Pruritus			Nausea/vomiting		
ENT			Heartburn		
Hoarseness			GU		
Nose bleeds			Dysuria		
Snoring			Frequency		
Cardiovascular			Menstrual symptoms		
Chest pain			MSK		
Edema			Painful joints		
PND			Swollen joints		
Palpitations			Endocrine		
Neurologic			Polyuria		
Weakness			Polydipsia		

TABLE 3-2 Sample Screening Preoperative Assessment Form (*Continued*)

Review of systems (symptoms present in past 30 days):

	Y	N		Y	N
Seizures			Heat/cold intol.		
Paresthesias			Hematologic		
Hypersomnolence			Bleeding		
Psychiatric			Bruising		
Depression			Clotting		
Hallucinations			Anticoagulant use		

□ All other ROS reviewed and normal

Exercise tolerance:

Comments:

Social History (include sexual history, smoking, alcohol, substance abuse):

Physical Examination (circle normal findings, comment if abnormal):

Enter Vital Signs Below:

T°	HR	BP	R	Pulse Ox	Tilt

Comments/General Obs:

Eyes:	PERLA	EOMI	Conjunctivae pink	Anicteric
ENT:	N nasal mucosa	N oropharynx	N teeth/gums	
Neck:	Supple	No thyromegaly	No JVD/HJR	
Chest:	Resp. unlabored	Clear to P&A	N breath	
sounds				
	N breast symmetry	N breast palpation		
Heart:	N Apex	RRR	N S1S2	No MRG
	No edema	No cyanosis		N Carotids
Abdomen:	No bulging	N bowel sounds	No tenderness	
	No HSM	Liver span_____		
Lymph Nd:	No nuchal	No axillary	No inguinal	
MSK:	No clubbing	N power/tone	N ROM	
GU:	N ext. genitalia	No CVA tenderness		
Neuro:	Symm. DTRs	Sensory intact		
	CN II–IV intact	No muscle hypertrophy		
	No tremor	No weakness		
Skin:	N turgor	No telangiectasias	No rash	
Psych:	A&O X 3	N mood	N memory	cooperative

Laboratory & ECG:

Assessment and Recommendations:

with congestive heart failure, uncontrolled hypertension, coronary artery disease, valvular heart disease, and uncontrolled arrhythmias (see Chaps. 19 to 23).
   - Inquire about previous hospitalizations and operations, previous cardiac procedures, previous cardiac evaluations especially in the prior 2 years, irregular heartbeat, shortness of breath, chest discomfort, and exercise capacity.
   - Self-reported poor exercise capacity is associated with twice the risk of perioperative complications.[5]
     - Poor exercise tolerance can be defined as the inability to walk four blocks or climb two flights of stairs without stopping.

Lung Disease

- Factors that increase the risk of postoperative pulmonary complications include COPD, cigarette smoking, poor functional status, and, possibly obstructive sleep apnea (see Chaps. 24 and 25).
   - Inquire about cough, wheezing, snoring, daytime hypersomnolence, and any history of emphysema, asthma, or tuberculosis.
   - The smoking history should include total pack-years, current use, and date of cessation.

Hematologic Disease

- The medical history is the key to uncovering a bleeding dyscrasia (see Chap. 31).
   - Key questions include personal and family histories of a bleeding disorder; prolonged bleeding after an injury, dental extraction, or other surgical procedure; and frequent or severe nosebleeds or spontaneous bleeding at other sites.
     - Ask specifically about hemophilia, von Willebrand's disease, and "Christmas" disease.
   - Also obtain a careful medication history and seek a history of hepatic disease, renal disease, and hematologic malignancy.
   - Ask about previous thrombophlebitis and pulmonary embolism ("phlebitis" or "blood clots"), and previous use of heparin or warfarin (see Chap. 7A).
   - Obtain subspeciality consultation if the patient has hereditary angioedema. Prophylactic preoperative danazol may be indicated, because invasive procedures can precipitate a crisis.

Medications and Allergies

- Obtain a thorough history of the use of medications, including vitamins, nutritional supplements, and herbal preparations (see Chap. 7).
   - Ang-Lee and colleagues recommend that patients bring all of their medications, including herbal preparations, to the physician for identification, because patients may not know what they are taking.[6]
   - Seek a history of corticosteroid use within the past year to assess for the possibility of adrenal suppression (see Chap. 28).
   - In addition to medication allergies, inquire about other allergies, such as those to latex and radiocontrast media.
     - The most commonly reported allergic reactions are to antimicrobials, particularly penicillins and sulfa compounds; however, up to 85 percent of people reporting a prior allergic reaction to penicillin will have no reaction to skin tests and can usually safely receive a penicillin or cephalosporin.
     - Latex, extracted from the rubber plant, shares antigens with related plants including banana and kiwifruit. Therefore rash or other allergic reactions to these fruits can be a clue to a latex allergy.

Family History

- A family history of surgery or anesthesia-related problems may uncover risk for a bleeding disorder or malignant hyperthermia.

General Systems Review

- Review systems for evidence of liver disease, renal disease, endocrine disease (especially diabetes mellitus and adrenal insufficiency), gastrointestinal disease (reflux), rheumatologic disease, and neurologic disease (seizures, stroke).
- A history of alcohol or other substance abuse can affect perioperative care.
- Ask every woman of childbearing age about menstrual history and potential pregnancy.
- Inquire about HIV risk factors.
   - HIV patients with low CD4 cell counts are at risk for poor healing at the surgical site and opportunistic infections (see Chap. 33).
- Atlantoaxial subluxation can occur in patients with rheumatoid arthritis, ankylosing spondylitis, or Down's syndrome (see Chap. 42).
   - Symptoms may include neck, shoulder, or arm pain or weakness as well as abnormalities of gait, but instability of the cervical spine can also be asymptomatic.
- Dysphagia, hoarseness, or stridor may predict the presence of cricoarytenoid dysfunction in patients with rheumatoid arthritis.

PHYSICAL EXAMINATION

General Appearance

- Cachexia, obesity, cyanosis, dyspnea, anxiety, flat affect, Cushingoid features, dysmorphic facies, inappropriate behavior, and other findings on observation of a patient's general appearance can all have important implications for perioperative care.

VITAL SIGNS

- Persistent, unexplained tachycardia should be further investigated prior to surgery.
- Unexplained fever is a relative contraindication to elective surgery.
- Systolic blood pressures above 180 mmHg and diastolic pressures above 110 mmHg are associated with an increased risk of perioperative ischemia, arrhythmias, and blood pressure lability, but it is unclear if deferring surgery improves outcomes.
  - Avoid rapidly reducing mean arterial pressure more than 20 percent in the days immediately prior to surgery.[7]
  - Although this issue has not been studied systematically, it may be useful to test for hypovolemia and autonomic instability in selected patients by measuring blood pressure in both the supine and standing positions prior to surgery.

CARDIOVASCULAR

- An S_3 gallop, rales (fine, late-inspiratory crackles in dependent lung fields), jugular venous distention more than a couple of centimeters above the sternal angle, nonresolving hepatojugular reflux, and, less specifically, peripheral edema are signs of heart failure.
  - Heart failure is a risk factor for perioperative cardiac complications; it should be controlled prior to surgery to optimize tissue perfusion and oxygentation.
- Pathologic heart murmurs should be fully characterized prior to surgery.
  - The likelihood of aortic stenosis is greater if the patient reports exertional angina or syncope, if carotid upstrokes are slow or delayed, if S_2 is absent, if the murmur is louder, its peak is later in systole, or it has a musical component, and if there is evidence of left ventricular hypertrophy on electrocardiography or palpation of the apical impulse.
  - When in doubt, obtain transthoracic echocardiography, because aortic stenosis is a potent risk factor for fatal cardiac complications.
- A carotid bruit is neither a sensitive nor a specific indicator of significant cerebrovascular disease.
  - Nonetheless, many practitioners further investigate asymptomatic patients with carotid bruits using Doppler ultrasonography.
    - Most surgeries should not be postponed for investigation of an asymptomatic carotid bruit; however, it might be appropriate to further assess cerebral blood flow in patients undergoing surgery of the head or neck in which cerebral blood flow could be temporarily or permanently compromised.
- The presence of a peripheral arterial bruit is associated with a slightly increased risk of perioperative cardiac complications, but it is not an independent predictor.

PULMONARY

- Diminished breath sounds, prolonged exhalation, crackles, and wheezes are each associated with an increased risk of postoperative pulmonary complications.[8]
  - Wheezing in particular contraindicates elective surgery and, as time permits, should be further assessed and addressed prior to any surgery. For example, by optimizing asthma treatment, wheezing may be resolved.

ABDOMINAL

- Before surgery, examine patients for signs of chronic liver disease, including ascites, jaundice, testicular atrophy, gynecomastia, hepatomegaly, splenomegaly, and spider telangiectasias.
- Childs-Pugh classification stratifies the perioperative risk of patients with liver disease (see Chap. 35).

EXTREMITIES

- Clubbing of nailbeds can indicate significant cardiopulmonary or infectious disease.
- Fingernails stained by cigarette smoke are associated with lung disease and nicotine dependence.
- Joint deformities of rheumatoid arthritis are associated with cervical spine arthritis and with risk for atlanoaxial subluxation. (see General systems review above, and Chap. 42).

NEUROLOGIC

- Unexplained muscle hypertrophy or weakness is associated with an increased risk of malignant hyperthermia.
- In older patients, consider using a screening test for cognitive impairment, such as the Folstein Mini-Mental Status Examination, because cognitive impairment is associated with an increased risk for postoperative delirium (see Chap. 62).
- Be alert for undiagnosed Parkinson's disease (tremor, bradykinesia, expressionless facies) and muscular dystrophy (myotonia, weakness), because pulmonary complications are more frequent in patients with these conditions (see Chap. 54).
- Note physical findings that suggest prior stroke (focal weakness and hyperreflexia), because prior stroke is associated with increased risk for delirium, aspiration, and thrombophlebitis.

PREOPERATIVE CHECKLISTS

- A few studies have investigated the use of preoperative screening questionnaires to identify low-risk patients.
  - One study of a 13-question medical history in 200 patients found that, in self-assessed "healthy" patients, additional screening history, physical examination, and preoperative laboratory testing were not needed.[9]

- ◦ Anesthesiologists have proposed a similar screening questionnaire.[10]
- ◦ There are no studies validating these questionnaires in large numbers of patients.

SUMMARY

- Risk assessment of patients undergoing surgery depends upon the type of surgery and on the patient's medical illnesses.
- Carefully assess the risks of cardiac, pulmonary, and thromboembolic complications for all patients, since these are the principal sources of perioperative morbidity and mortality.
- Elicit a thorough medication history, including use of over-the-counter medications, nutritional supplements, and herbal preparations.
- Consider using a comprehensive preoperative assessment form or checklist to help ensure a complete assessment.

REFERENCES

1. Warner MA, Shields SE, Chute CG. Major morbidity and mortality with 1 month of ambulatory surgery and anesthesia. *JAMA* 270:1437, 1993.
2. Lee TH, Marcantonio ER, Mangione CM, et al. Derivation and prospective validation of a simple index for prediction of cardiac risk of major noncardiac surgery. *Circulation* 100:1043, 1999.
3. Smetana GW, Lawrence VA, Cornell JE. Preoperative pulmonary risk stratification for non-cardiothoracic surgery: A systematic review. *Ann Intern Med* 2005. In press.
4. Geerts WH, Pineo GF, Heit JA, et al. Prevention of venous thromboembolism. The seventh ACCP conference on antithrombotic and thrombolytic therapy. *Chest* 126:338S, 2004.
5. Reilly DF, McNeely MJ, Doerner D, et al. Self-reported exercise tolerance and the risk of serious perioperative complications. *Arch Intern Med* 159:2185, 1999.
6. Ang-Lee MK, Moss T, Yuan CS. Herbal medicine and perioperative care. *JAMA* 286:208, 2001.
7. Howell SJ, Sear JW, Foex P. Hypertension, hypertensive heart disease and perioperative cardiac risk. *Br J Anaesth* 92:570, 2004.
8. Lawrence VA, Dhanda R, Hilsenbeck SG, et al. Risk of pulmonary complications after elective abdominal surgery. *Chest* 110:744, 1996.
9. Hilditch WG, Asbury AJ, Jack E, et al. Validation of a pre-anaesthetic screening questionnaire. *Anaesthesia* 58:874, 2003.
10. Wilson ME, Williams MB, Baskett PJ, et al. Assessment of fitness for surgical procedures and the variability of anaesthetists' judgments. *Br Med J* 280:509, 1980.

4 QUALITY IMPROVEMENT AND PATIENT SAFETY IN PERIOPERATIVE CARE

Tosha B. Wetterneck, H. Jay Biem, and Andrew D. Auerbach

THE CHALLENGE OF HIGH-QUALITY PERIOPERATIVE CARE

Quality care is providing the right service (process) at the right time (access) in the right way (safety) for the right outcome (effective) at the right price (efficiency), so that patients are happy (satisfaction).

A medical error is an adverse event or near miss that is preventable with the current state of medical knowledge.[1]

Providing quality perioperative care is challenging, because it requires the coordination of several different types of providers in several different settings (Table 4-1). The risk of miscommunication is high.

The perioperative care team should focus on quality by creating systems to promote communication and other safe care practices.

Specific evidenced-based practices can reduce postoperative complications: for example, thromboembolism prophylaxis, surgical infection prophylaxis, and perioperative beta blocker to prevent cardiac ischemia.[2] Such interventions have become quality indicators for perioperative and hospital care and are promoted by national quality organizations and regulatory agencies; however, studies continue to show that these practices are underused.

QUALITY IMPROVEMENT

QUALITY CARE

The Institute of Medicine has defined quality care as care that is safe, timely, effective, efficient, equitable, and patient-centered.[3]

The quality of perioperative care can be assessed by these characteristics, which make up the mnemonic STEEEP.

- Safe: e.g., physician and patient are notified of abnormal test results, and patient allergy information is available to all providers.
- Timely: e.g., wait times for preoperative consultation appointments are appropriate.
- Effective: e.g., use of evidence-based deep venous thrombosis prophylaxis.

TABLE 4-1 Perioperative Transitions of Care

	PROCESS STEP	SETTING	PROVIDER
Preoperative	Plan procedure	Surgeon's office	Surgeon
	Optimize medical status, assess risk for surgery and plan for perioperative care	Internist's or surgeon's office	Primary physician, medicine consultant, and/or surgeon, surgical midlevel provider
	Assess risk for surgery and plan intraoperative care	Anesthesia clinic	Anesthesiologist, nurse anesthetist
Operative	Perform procedure	Operating or procedure room (outpatient surgery center or hospital)	Surgeon and anesthesiologist
Postoperative	Immediate care	Postoperative acute care unit	Surgical nurse, surgeon, anesthesiologist
	Convalescent care	Hospital, skilled nursing facility, patient home	Surgeon, anesthesiologist, medical consultant, primary physician, nurse, respiratory therapist, physical therapist, dietitian, specialist consultants, etc.

- Efficient: e.g., preoperative laboratory results are available to the surgeon and anesthesiologist on the day of surgery.
- Equitable: e.g., equivalent care is provided to patients regardless of socioeconomic, gender, racial, or other medically irrelevant characteristics.
- Patient-centered: e.g., patients are informed and included in decision making, and pain after surgery is well controlled.

A MODEL FOR QUALITY IMPROVEMENT

A useful model for quality improvement is based on four elements: aims, measures, ideas for change, and tests of change implemented in cycles of *plan, do, study, act*.[4]

The *aim* identifies the improvement to be accomplished, e.g., improve perioperative deep venous thrombosis prophylaxis.

- Aims commonly focus on processes, such as appropriate tests being obtained and appropriate medications being administered at appropriate times.

The *measures* determine whether the desired change has been accomplished: e.g., the proportion of patient meeting criteria who received prophylaxis for deep venous thrombosis (DVT).

- Measures may be of the *process* (as above) or of the *outcomes* (e.g., DVT events, cardiovascular events, mortality, length of stay, satisfaction).
- Measures should be important, easily determined, and reflective of change.

The *ideas for change* are the specific methods used to encourage the desired behavior: e.g., preprinted orders to facilitate use of DVT prophylaxis.

- A combination of different methods (e.g., reminders, auditing, feedback, and academic detailing) is usually most successful in producing change.[5] Passive provider education (e.g., mailing guidelines) is generally ineffective (Table 4-2).

Ideas for change are then *tested* through the "plan, do, study, act" process. Short-term pilot studies with frequent reassessment and refinement of the change process can promote rapid improvement.

- The *plan* identifies the changes that will be made to meet the improvement goal.
- *Do* is implementing the changes.
- *Study* determines whether the changes have been implemented and if there are indications that the improvement goal has been or will be met. Study may include auditing process and/or outcomes. If the changes have not been successfully implemented or it does not appear that the improvement goal is affected, then the reasons are sought and additional planning ensues to devise and implement different changes.
- *Acting* is the broad, often systemwide implementation of changes that have been demonstrated to produce the improvement goal.

SYSTEMS OF CARE

A *system* is a group of mutually dependent elements that interact to achieve a common function.

Systems can be categorized into macrosystems (e.g., a health care region) and microsystems (e.g., a nursing unit).

A work system is composed of (1) the people who work in it, (2) the technology and tools with which the work is done, (3) the tasks that need to be done, (4) the

TABLE 4-2 Interventions to Change Care Delivery

INTERVENTION	EXAMPLE
Clinical practice guidelines	Antibiotic selection for surgical infection prophylaxis
Policy and procedure	Policy on patients requiring preoperative consultation for patients with diabetes
Provider reminders	Chart flag or automatic order to remove urethral catheter
	Computerized reminder to order screening laboratories
Academic detailing	One-on-one education for provider
Checklists	Preoperative history and physical checklist
Standardized provider order sets	Preprinted order set for postoperative care
Automate the flow of patient information	Electronic medical records
Algorithms	Preoperative cardiac risk assessment algorithm
Nomograms	Heparin nomograms
Integrated care pathways	Postoperative hip arthroplasty pathway (outlines routine, standard, and time line for care)

environment in which the work is performed, and (5) organizational factors.[6]

Systems are often complex in that changes affecting one part of a system (e.g., introducing new technology) affect other parts of the system (e.g., new technology can require new people, eliminate tasks, or introduce new tasks). Therefore when a change is made, the entire system should be monitored to assess for unanticipated effects.

Some systems can promote a "silo" mentality, in which there is poor communication within the system. Strategies to manage the transitions of care, to improve information exchange, and to improve communication across the system can help to eliminate such silos. Strategies include electronic medical records, regular meetings of providers from different silos, and care coordinators whose contacts and responsibilities cross the separate silos.

PROVIDING QUALITY PERIOPERATIVE CARE

Specific evidence-based practices can reduce postoperative complications: appropriate antibiotic use can reduce surgical site infection, perioperative beta blocker can reduce cardiac-related morbidity and mortality, and DVT prophylaxis can reduce DVT and pulmonary embolism.[4] These interventions have become quality indicators for perioperative care and are promoted by national quality organizations and regulatory agencies; however, they remain underused.

Perioperative antibiotic use can be improved by a multifaceted approach that includes, (1) guidelines for procedure specific antibiotic prophylaxis, (2) physician leadership, (3) preprinted antibiotic order sets, and (4) computerized decision algorithms to aid in antibiotic selection.

Perioperative beta-blocker use can be improved by an order set with dose titration parameters that follows the patient through translocations of care, from the preanesthesia care area to the operating room to the postanesthesia care area and finally to the intensive care unit or ward. Preoperative beta-blocker use can be improved by (1) academic detailing of the providers in the preoperative clinic and (2) either beta-blocker samples or preprinted prescriptions for a beta blocker.

Glucose control after surgery can be improved by the routine use of a continuous insulin infusion protocol in the surgical intensive care unit.

Postoperative DVT prophylaxis can be improved by the routine use of risk-assessment protocols and preprinted or computerized postoperative order sets.

Perioperative risk assessment can be improved by the use of validated algorithms: for example, algorithms for preoperative cardiac risk assessment (Chap. 20).

Perioperative care can be improved by including a hospitalist physician on the perioperative management team.

QUALITY MONITORING

Routine monitoring of process and outcomes measures can help to ensure the quality of perioperative care and to identify areas needing improvement. Ideal measures should be important, easily collected, and reflective of change. Using automated systems such as administrative databases, electronic medical records, and computerized order entry systems can facilitate monitoring.

Sample process measures include:

- Time to next available or third available patient appointment for preoperative clinic consultation
- Rates of use of postoperative DVT prophylaxis in appropriate patients

- Proportion of patients receiving antibiotic within 1 h prior to the start of the procedure
- Proportion of patients receiving patient education materials
- Patient satisfaction

Sample outcome measures include:

- Operative and 30-day postoperative mortality rates
- Postoperative cardiovascular event rates
- Procedure specific length of stay, cost, and readmission rates

PATIENT SAFETY

Patient safety in the perioperative setting is jeopardized by the complexities of communication across multiple care settings and multiple providers, and by the underutilization of practices known to minimize nosocomial complications.

CONTINUITY OF PERIOPERATIVE CARE

Continuity of care is coherent care with seamless transitions between providers and settings. Continuity of care is essential for quality care and can be challenging in the perioperative period because of the number of different care providers in different disciplines and because of the transitions between settings (e.g., primary care clinic, preoperative clinic, operating room, recovery room, hospital nursing unit, extended care facility, home) (see Table 4-1).

- Continuity of care can be further challenged by a patient's comorbidities, including cognitive deficits affecting the patient's ability to collaborate and medical therapies that need to be stopped and restarted, such as anticoagulants.

There are three types of continuity of care:

- Relational (regular contact with the same providers)
- Informational (reliable, consistent communication)
- Managerial (coordination of multidisciplinary team)

Good continuity of care can be characterized by "the seven C's": *contact* (regular), *collaboration* with the patient (patient education), *communication* (clear, concise recommendations; patient information available to all caregivers), *coordination* of care (structured, reliable handoffs), *consistency* (fail-safe mechanisms, checklists, reminders), *contingency* (alternate contacts and care plans for problems or unusual care needs), and *convenience* for patients, families and providers.

Transitions of care jeopardize patient safety due to the increased probability of many types of errors, commonly including medication errors due to inadequate reconciliation and inadequate patient education.[7]

- Medication reconciliation can improve patient safety, especially when there is a transition of care, such as when the patient moves from one nursing unit to another or when the patient is discharged from the hospital. Medication reconciliation can ensure that there have not been mixups, that the patient is prescribed the right medications, and that there is a feasible plan for the patient to receive them. Common mixups include inadvertent discontinuation of usual medications and inappropriate continuation of perioperative medications, such as an antihypertensive that was substituted to conform to the hospital formulary or a diuretic that was intended for temporary postoperative use to mobilize excess fluid.
- Patient and family education at the time of transitions of care can be crucial, because the patient and family are usually involved in the care plan for disease and wound management. Education should include contact information for additional care or guidance.

Continuity across transitions of care can be improved by increasing communication and by designating responsibilities.

- Information flow can be improved by ensuring rapid completion and availability of consultation reports: for example, by using computerized patient records and faxes and by providing the patient with a copy of the report.
- A standardized preoperative history and physical data collection form can help ensure collection of crucial information.
- Personal contact, either face to face or via the phone, can help ensure good communication.
- Clinics and care teams should design the information flow system so that medications are always reconciled and diagnostic test results are always reviewed and addressed in a timely fashion.

OTHER PATIENT SAFETY IMPROVEMENTS

Safety efforts overlap with quality improvement efforts (e.g., deep venous thrombosis prophylaxis, falls avoidance, patient education). Prevention of nosocomial hospital infection occurs through prompt removal of urethral and venous catheters.

"Wrong person, wrong site, wrong procedure surgery," although rare, receives a lot of attention from regulatory agencies and the press. The consultant internist needs to be an active part of the process to help avoid such errors. The person, procedure, and site should be verified at the preoperative evaluation, whenever a transition of care

TABLE 4-3 Perioperative Errors

ERROR	COMPLICATION	PREVENTION
Commission		
Urethral catheter continued needlessly	Urinary tract infection	Protocol to remove urethral catheter after surgery
Intravenous fluids continued needlessly	Congestive heart failure	Protocol to stop fluids when patient is receiving adequate enteral intake or to monitor and address fluid balance
Intravenous access continued needlessly	Septic thrombophlebitis	Protocol to discontinue intravenous medications and remove catheters when not needed
Receiving heparin needlessly	Heparin-induced thrombocytopenia	Protocol to discontinue heparin when patient is ambulating adequately
Receiving a medication to which patient is known to have an adverse reaction	Adverse medication reaction	System to obtain and communicate an allergies and adverse medication reaction history and to modify it during hospitalization
Omission		
Perioperative beta blocker not given	Acute coronary syndrome	Routine orders for preoperative, intraoperative and postoperative beta blocker
Resuscitation against patient wishes	Inappropriate intubation and ventilation	Protocol for obtaining and charting advance directives and making them available during "codes"
No routine platelet count for patients receiving heparin	Heparin-induced thrombocytopenia	System for routine every-third-day platelet count for patients receiving heparin
Fall risk assessment not done	Postoperative fall	Preoperative assessment of fall risk and fall precaution implementation, scheduled toileting postoperatively
Alcohol withdrawal assessment	Delirium	Routine preoperative alcohol use assessment linked to preoperative care, including counseling, and postoperative withdrawal assessment and treatment
Patient not followed postoperatively	Complications that could have been avoided by follow-up	Computerized patient lists
Failure to address abnormal laboratory results	Anemia, Hyperkalemia, or Renal failure	Automatic physician notification of critical values by laboratory
Failure to initiate follow-up	Adverse drug event	Communication with primary care provider about new medications at discharge

occurs, and immediately before the procedure by using "time-out" verification.

Preventable, adverse events that occur commonly in the perioperative period are listed in Table 4-3.

ERRORS AS LEARNING OPPORTUNITIES

Errors should be seen as learning opportunities.

It is critical to avoid blame. People make mistakes. Blaming a person for a mistake will not improve the system and is likely to impair good flow of information. The system must be designed to minimize mistakes and to prevent people's mistakes from becoming errors.

Review of errors in quality grand rounds and morbidity and mortality seminars with a focus on system issues and avoidance of blame can raise awareness of patient safety issues and quality improvement efforts.

STRATEGIES TO ENSURE IMPROVEMENT

The success of improvement efforts, especially for large systems, can be maximized by the following:[8]

- Ensure that all disciplines involved in the process are represented on the quality improvement team.
- Provide the team with administrative support from the highest levels.
- Adjust clinical duties or arrange coverage to enable adequate participation on the team.
- Develop interdisciplinary consensus on improvement goals.
- Understand the organizational culture and choose ideas for change that are likely to work within the culture.
- Develop and encourage physician leadership for the change.
- Measure baseline data and provide timely feedback to stakeholders to maintain momentum for change.

THE SAFE, HIGH-QUALITY CONSULTANT

Communicate with the surgical team and other medical consultants, preferably verbally:
- After performing initial consultation
- After reviewing preoperative diagnostic testing
- On a daily basis in the hospital and at the time of any significant change in medical therapy

Communicate with the primary care provider and other physicians involved in postdischarge care:
- About complications and new developments
- About significant findings and new or discontinued medications at the time of discharge

Use clinical practice guidelines and institutional protocols to practice evidenced-based perioperative care.

Use or develop standardized preoperative evaluation protocols and algorithms for diagnostic testing and referral.

Utilize quality assurance monitors in the preoperative assessment clinic and inpatient consult service, and use the quality improvement process to meet and exceed quality assurance goals.

Develop or participate in multidisciplinary perioperative quality improvement projects.

Share systems errors and barriers to care with the hospital or health care organization for system improvement.

REFERENCES

1. Quality Interagency Coordination Task Force. *Report to the President on Medical Errors*. Available at: http://www. quic.gov/report/index.htm. Accessed January 15, 2005.
2. Shojania KG, Duncan BW, McDonald KM, et al. Making health care safer: A critical analysis of patient safety practices. *Evid Rep Technol Assess* (Summ) i–x:1, 2001.
3. Institute of Medicine Committee on Quality of Heath Care in America. *Crossing the Quality Chasm: A New Health System for the 21st Century*. Washington, DC:, National Academy Press, 2001.
4. Langley GJ, Nolan KM, Nolan TW, et al. *The improvement guide: A Practical Approach to Enhancing Organizational Performance*. San Francisco: Jossey-Bass, 1996.
5. Grimshaw JM, Shirran L, Thomas R, et al. Changing provider behavior: An overview of systematic reviews of interventions. *Med Care* 39:II-2, 2001.
6. Smith MJ, Carayon-Sainfort P. A balance theory of job design for stress reduction. *Int J Indust Ergonom* 4:67, 1989.
7. Coleman EA, Berenson RA. Lost in transition: Challenges and opportunities for improving the quality of transitional care. *Ann Intern Med* 140:533, 2004.
8. Lurie JD, Merren EJ, Lee J, et al. An approach to hospital quality improvement. *Med Clin North Am* 86:825, 2002.

5 PREOPERATIVE TESTING

David S. Macpherson and Gerald W. Smetana

INTRODUCTION

- Physicians often order "routine" tests before elective surgery.
- Testing is often driven by local policies and based on tradition rather than on evidence.
- The purpose of this chapter is to help physicians order preoperative tests more thoughtfully.

DEFINITION OF ABNORMAL TEST RESULTS

- Test results can be continuous (e.g., 0.00 to infinity), ordinal (e.g., 1, 2, etc.), or categorical (e.g., normal or abnormal).
- Most laboratory test results are continuous, and "normal" is defined as those values lying within two standard deviations of the mean. Therefore, 5 percent of test results will lie outside the normal range.
- When clinicians order several tests simultaneously, it is likely that at least one test will fall outside the normal range. For example, if 20 tests are ordered, that probability is more than 60 percent.
- When repeated, most of these "abnormal" results will be normal or will not indicate illness or disease.

DOES PREOPERATIVE TESTING ADD VALUE?

- The primary rationale for routine preoperative testing is to screen for clinically unsuspected abnormalities that would change prognosis or treatment.
- Therefore the first question to ask is whether the results of preoperative testing add incremental value to the risk assessment obtained by history and physical examination.
- The second question to ask concerns the probability of a clinically unsuspected abnormal result. If a test does not modify the likelihood of a potential complication compared with the prior probability estimated by clinical evaluation, the test should not be obtained.
- Several studies have evaluated the impact of panels of commonly ordered preoperative tests in unselected patients undergoing surgery. While a small proportion of individuals subjected to such screening have abnormal test results, these studies have uniformly found that the test results have little impact on perioperative management.

- In one of the most widely cited studies, investigators studied 2000 patients undergoing elective surgery and determined the proportion of preoperative tests that were not indicated and the proportion of these that were abnormal.[1] They analyzed the following commonly ordered tests: prothrombin time, platelet count, hemoglobin, total and differential white blood cell count, serum electrolytes, blood urea nitrogen, creatinine and glucose concentrations. Although 4.1 percent of the test results fell outside of normal range, only 0.4 percent of the results were both not indicated and abnormal and only 0.15 percent of the results were not indicated and yielded surgically significant abnormal results.
- In another study of patients ≥ 70 years of age, both the physical status index (ASA class) of the American Society of Anesthesiologists and procedure-related risk were stronger predictors of postoperative complications than were any preoperative tests or combinations of tests.[2] Serum sodium and creatinine were univariate predictors, but hemoglobin, potassium, platelet count, and glucose were not; in multivariate analysis, no laboratory test result was a significant predictor of postoperative complications.

PREOPERATIVE TESTS

HEMOGLOBIN

- Significant blood loss during surgery can lead to anemia, possibly impairing oxygen delivery to tissues and increasing perioperative cardiac stress.
- The prevalence of anemia in preoperative patients is about 1.8 percent, but it is higher in older patients and in menstruating women.
- Only a small number of studies have correlated preoperative anemia with perioperative morbidity; in these reports, the positive likelihood ratio was 3.3.
- Hemoglobin must be measured in patients undergoing surgeries in which significant blood loss is anticipated.
- Hemoglobin must be measured before surgery in patients who have a history of anemia or diseases known to cause anemia (e.g., cancer, kidney disease) or signs of anemia (e.g., resting tachycardia, conjunctival pallor).

WHITE BLOOD CELL COUNT

- The prevalence of abnormalities in the white blood cell count of preoperative patients is less than 1 percent.
- Although only a small number of studies have examined whether the finding of an abnormal white blood cell count influences management or increases perioperative morbidity, these investigations have found no alteration in management and no relationship to perioperative morbidity.
- Clinicians should not routinely obtain white blood cell counts before surgery.
- It is appropriate to measure the white blood cell count before surgery in patients who have symptoms of infection, signs of a myeloproliferative disorder (e.g., petechiae, purpura, splenomegaly, or lymphadenopathy), and in those who are taking medications or have conditions known to affect the white blood cell count.

PLATELET COUNT

- The incidence of an unanticipated abnormal platelet count is less than 1 percent among preoperative patients. Routine measurement of the platelet count changes perioperative management in only 0.02 percent of patients.
- We do not recommend routine measurement of platelet counts before surgery.
- Obtain platelet counts in patients with a history of platelet abnormalities, symptoms or signs of impaired hemostasis on history and physical examination, or myeloproliferative disorders and in those receiving medications known to commonly alter platelet counts (e.g., chemotherapy, heparin).

COAGULATION TESTS

Prothrombin Time/International Normalized Ratio

- A potential rationale for obtaining a prothrombin time/international normalized ratio (PT/INR) before surgery would be to identify patients at risk for postoperative bleeding.
- The PT/INR is one of the least helpful tests in the preoperative armamentarium. In a recent review, it was the perfect unhelpful test.[3] Abnormal results occurred in 0.3 percent of patients and, among a subset of studies that evaluated outcomes, abnormal test results did not affect management and were not associated with increased postoperative bleeding rates in any patients.
- Clinicians can generally predict which patients are likely to have an elevated PT/INR on the basis of clinical data. For example, patients with known chronic liver disease, malnutrition, or a history of bleeding tendencies are more likely to have an abnormal PT/INR than are unselected patients.
- A preoperative PT/INR should also be obtained for all patients who are taking warfarin, in order to help guide warfarin management.

Partial Thromboplastin Time

- Although an abnormal partial thromboplastin time (PTT) is more common than an abnormal PT/INR, this test is equally unhelpful.
- In one review, 6.5 percent of all PTT values were abnormal, but only 0.1 percent of all tests influenced management.[3]
- The PTT should not be used as a screening preoperative test.

Bleeding Time

- The bleeding time was commonly used in the past to assess perioperative bleeding risk, especially in patients taking aspirin or nonsteroidal anti-inflammatory drugs.
- However, a normal bleeding time does not predict a low risk for surgical hemorrhage, and an abnormal bleeding time does not increase the risk of hemorrhage.
- A bleeding time should not routinely be obtained before surgery.
- For a patient whose history and physical examination suggest impaired hemostasis and whose PT/INR, PTT, and platelet count are normal, a bleeding time may be an appropriate part of a more thorough hemostasis evaluation that includes consultation with a coagulation specialist.

ELECTROLYTES

- Most patients with abnormalities of serum sodium or potassium can be identified clinically. Abnormal findings are uncommon for patients without comorbidities or medications that could cause electrolyte abnormalities.
- Clinicians often order serum electrolytes to identify patients at higher risk for perioperative arrhythmia. In particular, hypokalemia can potentially increase this risk. How do these tests perform in actual clinical practice?
- Electrolyte abnormalities are more common than abnormalities in other commonly performed preoperative tests; the incidence was 12.7 percent in a recent review. However only 1.8 percent of all tests influenced management.[3]
- Contrary to generally held beliefs, an isolated finding of preoperative hypokalemia does not increase the risk of postoperative arrhythmia. For example, in a study of 447 patients undergoing major cardiac or vascular surgery, ventricular arrhythmias were no more common among patients with preoperative hypokalemia than among those with normal serum potassium concentrations.[4]
- Restrict preoperative serum electrolyte testing to patients who are likely to have abnormalities. For example, test patients with congestive heart failure or renal insufficiency and those taking diuretics, angiotensin converting enzyme (ACE) inhibitors, angiotensin receptor blockers (ARBs), digoxin, or other medications that increase the likelihood or risks of an abnormal concentration.

RENAL FUNCTION TESTS

- In contrast to the limited value of many commonly ordered preoperative tests, serum creatinine has value in identifying patients at risk for perioperative cardiac complications.
- In the revised cardiac risk index, serum creatinine >2.0 mg/dL was one of six independent risk factors for cardiac complications.[5] It predicted cardiac risk as well as established risk factors including coronary artery disease (CAD), congestive heart failure, and high-risk surgical procedures. Other studies have demonstrated the value of chronic renal insufficiency as a predictor for adverse outcomes after cardiac and vascular surgery.
- Renal insufficiency is often unsuspected by clinical evaluation. In a recent review, 2.6 percent of routine preoperative measurements of serum creatinine were abnormal and influenced perioperative management.[3]
- Serum creatinine should be measured in patients above 50 years of age; in those with diabetes, hypertension, renal insufficiency, cardiovascular disease; in patients undergoing major surgery; and in those who are taking medications that affect renal function.

GLUCOSE

- Although insulin-treated diabetes is a risk factor for postoperative cardiac and infectious complications, there is no evidence suggesting that previously undetected, asymptomatic hyperglycemia leads to increased rates of postoperative complications.
- Most abnormal preoperative serum glucose results are in those with known diabetes; the incidence of an unexpected abnormal blood glucose concentration that might influence perioperative management is 0.5 percent.[3]
- Serum glucose should not be obtained as a screening preoperative test in unselected patients. Serum glucose measurement is appropriate to screen patients with risk factors for diabetes, such as obesity, and to assess glucose control in patients known to have diabetes.

LIVER FUNCTION TESTS

- The most commonly obtained preoperative liver function tests are the serum transaminases. Alkaline phosphatase is not commonly obtained and should not be part of routine preoperative testing.

- Patients with hepatic cirrhosis have markedly increased perioperative morbidity and mortality. The risk is proportional to the severity of the cirrhosis as measured by the Childs-Pugh classification (see Chap. 35 for details).
- In contrast, no evidence suggests that liver function test abnormalities that are not associated with symptoms predict postoperative complications; the rate of unexpected abnormalities that influence management is 0.1 percent.[3]
- Clinicians should not obtain screening liver function tests on unselected patients as part of preoperative testing.

ALBUMIN

- Serum albumin concentration is a robust laboratory predictor of postoperative morbidity and mortality.
- In a study of 54,215 veterans, low serum albumin was the single strongest predictor of 30-day postoperative mortality among patients undergoing major noncardiac surgery.[6] A linear relationship existed: the risk of mortality began to increase with serum albumin concentrations <3.5 g/dL. For patients with serum albumin concentrations <2.1 g/dL, the perioperative mortality rate was 28 percent. In other studies, low serum albumin concentrations have also predicted postoperative pulmonary complications.
- Although conditions such as recent severe blood loss and nephropathy can cause hypoalbuminemia, it is most often an indication of undernutrition. A few studies have shown a benefit of delaying surgery to allow time for vigorous nutrition to increase serum albumin, but most studies have not suggested benefit. Therefore, while a preoperative serum albumin concentration may have prognostic value, it usually does not affect patient management.
- Serum albumin concentration should be measured if it is likely to be low (e.g., in patients with liver disease, nephropathy, enteropathy, recent severe illness, blood loss, or cachexia) and if the prognostic information is likely to affect the patient's care plan.

URINALYSIS

- One rationale for preoperative screening urinalysis is to identify patients with asymptomatic bacteruria, on the assumption that these patients are at increased risk for postoperative urinary tract infection or prosthetic implant infection. However, it is generally not beneficial to treat asymptomatic bacteruria; most patients receiving prosthetic implants should receive prophylactic antibiotic treatment at the time of surgery regardless of test results.
- Another rationale is to identify patients with clinically unsuspected diabetes mellitus. However, no evidence suggests that unsuspected diabetes increases the risk of postoperative complications.
- In practice, the urinalysis performs poorly as a preoperative test. In a review of 3666 patients undergoing preoperative urinalysis, 1.4 percent of tests were abnormal and influenced management.[3] The positive likelihood ratio for an abnormal urinalysis with regard to postoperative complications was 1.7; the negative likelihood ratio was 0.97.
- A urinalysis should not be obtained as a routine preoperative screening test.

ELECTROCARDIOGRAM

- Interpretation of the literature regarding the value of a preoperative, screening electrocardiogram (ECG) is complex, as many abnormalities may potentially influence management, including Q waves, atrial fibrillation, frequent atrial or ventricular ectopy, and conduction system disease.
- Evidence of CAD, such as Q waves, is often clinically unsuspected and confers an increased risk of postoperative cardiac complications. Such findings may lead to further preoperative testing or to changes in perioperative management.
- Although atrial fibrillation was a risk factor for postoperative cardiac complications in the original Goldman cardiac risk index, it was not an independent predictor in the more recent revised cardiac risk index.[5] Atrial fibrillation, however, can be asymptomatic and is likely to lead to additional preoperative testing.
- The common ECG findings of left ventricular hypertrophy, bundle branch block, and nonspecific ST-segment changes are also not independent predictors of postoperative cardiac complications.
- The rate of abnormal preoperative ECGs is high; it was 29.6 percent in a recent review, and 2.6 percent of all studies influenced perioperative management.[3] Whether the finding of an abnormal ECG influences the risk of postoperative cardiac complications remains unresolved. Several studies have shown no difference in event rates between patients with normal and abnormal preoperative ECGs.[7]
- It is reasonable to obtain a preoperative screening ECG for patients who are at increased risk for coronary artery disease and consequently for postoperative cardiac complications.
- A preoperative ECG should be obtained before major surgery for men above 40 years of age, women above 50 years of age, and younger patients with risk factors for coronary disease or who have established coronary disease. A preoperative ECG is not necessary before

minor surgery or procedures requiring only conscious sedation.

CHEST RADIOGRAPH

- One rationale for a screening preoperative chest radiograph is to identify patients at higher than average risk for postoperative pulmonary complications. Another is to provide a comparative baseline for postoperative radiographs. No evidence supports the latter rationale.
- Abnormal findings on screening preoperative chest radiographs are common; 21.2 percent had at least one abnormal finding in a review of 18 studies.[3] However, abnormal findings that are both unexpected and that change preoperative management are uncommon, occurring in from 0.1 to 3.0 percent of radiographs.
- Abnormalities are more common in patients who are older and who are known to have cardiopulmonary disease.
- A screening preoperative chest radiograph should be obtained for patients with a higher than average likelihood of abnormal findings that might affect perioperative management. This includes patients above 50 years of age, those with known cardiac or pulmonary disease, and those with a history or physical examination findings of cardiopulmonary disease.

SUMMARY RECOMMENDATIONS

- Table 5-1 summarizes recommendations for the use of preoperative laboratory tests and includes an estimate of the incidence of abnormalities that affect perioperative

TABLE 5-1 Recommendations for Laboratory Testing before Elective Surgery

TEST	INCIDENCE OF ABNORMALITIES THAT INFLUENCE MANAGEMENT (%)	LR+*	LR−	INDICATIONS
Hemoglobin	0.1%	3.3	0.90	Anticipated major blood loss or symptoms or signs of anemia
White blood cell count	0.0%	0.0	1.00	Symptoms of infection, myeloproliferative disorder, or myelotoxic medications
Platelet count	0.0%	0.0	1.00	History or signs of bleeding disorder, myeloproliferative disorder, or myelotoxic medications
Prothrombin time (PT)	0.0%	0.0	1.01	History or signs of bleeding disorder, chronic liver disease, malnutrition, recent or long-term antibiotic use
Partial thromboplastin time (PTT)	0.1%	1.7	0.86	History of bleeding disorder
Electrolytes	1.8%	4.3	0.80	Renal insufficiency, congestive heart failure, medications that affect electrolytes
Renal function	2.6%	3.3	0.81	Age > 50 years, hypertension, cardiac disease, major surgery, medications that may affect renal function
Glucose	0.5%	1.6	0.85	Diabetes (or strong family history), obesity, symptoms of diabetes
Liver function tests	0.1%			No indication for screening; consider albumin measurement for major surgery or chronic illness
Urinalysis	1.4%	1.7	0.97	No indication for screening
ECG	2.6%	1.6	0.96	Men > 40 years, women > 50 years, CAD or risk factors for CAD, such as diabetes and hypertension
Chest radiograph	3.0%	2.5	0.72	Age > 50 years, cardiac or pulmonary disease, symptoms or examination findings of cardiac or pulmonary disease

*LR+ = positive likelihood ratio. LR− = negative likelihood ratio.
SOURCE: Adapted from Smetana and Macpherson,[3] with permission.

management and the positive and negative likelihood ratios for postoperative complications.

OUTCOMES IN PATIENTS WHO HAVE UNDERGONE LIMITED TESTING

- In a study of over 1000 ASA class 1 or 2 patients undergoing minor surgery or diagnostic procedures, there was no morbidity or mortality.[8]
- A randomized trial of over 19,000 patients undergoing cataract surgery found that limiting routine testing did not worsen perioperative outcomes.[9]

HOSPITAL GUIDELINES ON PREOPERATIVE TESTING

- Most hospitals have written guidelines that establish local standards for preoperative testing.
- These guidelines should be based on evidence from the medical literature.
- Hospital or institutional guidelines on preoperative testing should recommend few routine preoperative tests.
- Guidelines should encourage physician discretion to limit testing and to selectively order tests based on the findings of the patient's history and physical examination.
- Guidelines, policies, and procedures should ensure that clinicians review preoperative test results and document this review in the medical record.
- A laboratory test result that is abnormal but ignored may pose more medicolegal liability than a test that is not ordered in the first place.

REFERENCES

1. Kaplan EB, Sheiner LB, Boeckmann AJ, et al. The usefulness of preoperative laboratory screening. *JAMA* 253:3576, 1985.
2. Dzankik S, Pastor D, Gonzalez C, et al. The prevalence and predictive value of abnormal preoperative laboratory tests in elderly surgical patients. *Anesth Analg* 93:301, 2001.
3. Smetana GW, Macpherson DS. The case against routine preoperative laboratory testing. *Med Clin North Am* 87:7, 2003.
4. Hirsh IA, Tomlinson DL, Slogoff S, et al. The overstated risk of preoperative hypokalemia. *Anesth Analg* 67:131, 1988.
5. Lee TH, Marcantonio ER, Mangione CM, et al. Derivation and prospective validation of a simple index for prediction of cardiac risk of major noncardiac surgery. *Circulation* 100:1043, 1999.
6. Gibbs J, Cull W, Henderson W, et al. Preoperative serum albumin level as a predictor of operative mortality and morbidity: Results from the National VA Surgical Risk Study. *Arch Surg* 134:36, 1999.
7. Tait AR, Parr HG, Tremper KK. Evaluation of the efficacy of routine preoperative electrocardiograms. *J Cardiothorac Vasc Anesth* 11:752, 1997.
8. Narr BJ, Warner ME, Schroeder DR, et al. Outcomes of patients with no laboratory assessment before anesthesia and a surgical procedure. *Mayo Clin Proc* 72:505, 1997.
9. Schein O, Katz J, Bass E, et al. The value of routine preoperative testing before cataract surgery. *N Engl J Med* 342:168, 2000.

6 ANESTHESIOLOGY FOR THE NONANESTHESIOLOGIST

Mary H. Pak and Scott R. Springman

ANESTHESIA

- The word *anesthesia* (from the Greek *an*, "without," and *esthesia*, "perception") was first suggested by Oliver Wendell Holmes.
- The function of modern anesthesiology is to provide analgesia ("without pain"), with or without unconsciousness and amnesia ("without memory"), in order to enable surgery and other procedures, to maintain and protect vital organ function through the stresses of surgery, and to treat acute and chronic pain.
  - Perioperative anesthesia care begins with preoperative assessment and includes both perioperative and emergency management of the airway, ventilation, fluids and blood, cardiohemodynamics, and cerebral perfusion and protection.
  - In addition to perioperative and emergency care, modern anesthesia care includes acute and chronic pain control.[1]
    - The analgesia repertoire includes traditional analgesics, newer pain-modulating drugs, special techniques such as neuraxial and peripheral nerve blockade, and implantation of nerve stimulators.
  - Anesthesiologists and their associate providers—including anesthesia assistants, nurse practitioners, and certified registered nurse anesthetists (CRNAs)—provide anesthesia care in many venues including preoperative assessment clinics, freestanding surgery centers, hospital operating rooms, labor and delivery suites, postanesthesia care units (PACUs), critical care units, and radiology and cardiology diagnosis and intervention suites.

PREOPERATIVE ISSUES

ASA CLASSIFICATION

- In the 1960s, the American Society of Anesthesiologists (ASA) developed a gestalt perioperative risk classification based on the physician's overall assessment of the medical history, physical examination, and laboratory findings.
  - This "ASA Physical Status Classification" has proven to be a robust predictor of perioperative complications and outcomes (Table 6-1).[2]
  - More specific indexes of perioperative risk have also been developed (see Chap. 3).

PREOPERATIVE FASTING

- Preoperative fasting reduces the incidence of pulmonary aspiration of gastric contents.
  - It is standard to ask adult patients undergoing elective procedures to fast from food for 8 h prior to surgery.
    - Patients are asked to fast longer after a meal of fatty food or if they have delayed gastric emptying, although there are no studies demonstrating improved outcomes.
  - Patients should fast from clear liquids for at least 2 h prior to surgery.
  - Because young children and infants are less tolerant of fasting and because their gastric emptying is faster, preoperative fasting guidelines are often less stringent for them.[3]
  - Centers usually set their own fasting guidelines.

OVERVIEW AND TOOLS

STANDARDS AND MONITORING

- Qualified anesthesia personnel are present throughout the conduction of all general anesthetics, regional anesthetics, and monitored anesthesia care.
- During all anesthetics, the patient's oxygenation, ventilation, circulation, and temperature are continuously monitored (Table 6-2).[4]

TABLE 6-1 Physical Status Classification of the American Society of Anesthesiologists

ASA PHYSICAL STATUS (PS)*	DESCRIPTION	EXAMPLES
PS-1	A healthy patient	
PS-2	A patient with mild systemic disease with no functional limitations	Hypertension Diabetes mellitus Chronic Bronchitis Obesity Extremes of age
PS-3	A patient with severe systemic disease resulting in functional limitations	Poorly controlled hypertension Diabetes mellitus with vascular complications Angina pectoris Prior myocardial infarction Pulmonary disease that limits activity
PS-4	A patient with severe systemic disease that is a constant threat to life	Congestive heart failure Unstable angina Advanced pulmonary, renal, or hepatic dysfunction
PS-5	A moribund patient who is not expected to survive without the operation	Ruptured aortic aneurysm Pulmonary embolus Head injury with increased intracranial pressure
PS-6	A declared brain-dead patient whose organs are being removed for donor purposes	

SOURCE: Reprinted from Stoelting RK, Miller RD. *Basics of Anesthesia*, 2000. Copyright 2000, with permission from Elsevier.

TABLE 6-2 Minimum Requirements for Monitoring During Anesthesia

PARAMETER	MINIMUM CRITERIA	METHOD/EQUIPMENT
Oxygenation	1. Quantitative measurement of the oxygen concentration in the patient breathing circuit	1. Oxygen analyzer with low concentration limit alarm
	2. Quantitative assessment of patient's oxygenation	2. Pulse oximetry
Ventilation	1. Qualitative assessment of adequate ventilation	1. Exhaled CO_2 monitoring
	2. Verification of the correct positioning of an endotracheal tube or a laryngeal mask	2. Clinical assessment at time of insertion or capnography or capnometry
Circulation	1. Electrocardiogram	1. ECG monitor (with automated ST-segment analysis optional)
	2. Blood pressure	2. BP cuff, usually automated
	3. One other assessment of circulatory function	3. Pulse oximetry
Temperature	Continuous monitoring when clinically significant changes in body temperature are intended, anticipated, or suspected	

- In addition to monitoring these vital processes, anesthesiologists sometimes monitor additional parameters as well, depending on the patient and the procedure.
  - Pharmacologic muscle paralysis is monitored using bipolar electrical stimulation of a peripheral motor nerve. Repetitive stimuli (2-Hz muscle "twitch"), four successive stimuli ("train of four" twitches), or 10 s of continuous stimulation ("tetanus" contraction) indicate the amount of remaining neuromuscular blockade.
  - Heart sounds are monitored with an esophageal or chest stethoscope.
    - An esophageal stethoscope can also be used to monitor core temperature.
  - In recent years, pulmonary artery catheters are less frequently used; central venous pressure and intra-arterial catheters are more frequently used to monitor higher-risk patients and higher-risk procedures.
  - Intraoperative transesophageal echocardiography (TEE) is increasingly used in complex and prolonged surgeries.
    - TEE provides information on cardiac ventricular filling, valve function, wall motion, and aortic integrity.
    - It is commonly used in cardiothoracic, trauma, and liver transplantation surgeries.
  - Electroencephalographic (EEG) monitoring is sometimes used during carotid and other surgeries in which cerebral blood flow can be impaired.
    - In about 0.1 percent of surgeries, the patient develops anesthesia awareness; that is, he or she recalls something during some part of the procedure. This is most common during emergent procedures in which deep anesthesia might exacerbate hypotension and impair the perfusion of vital organs, such as multiple trauma surgery and emergent cesarean section. About half of patients with anesthesia awareness report hearing things, half report a feeling of smothering, and one-quarter report pain. Single-lead modified electroencephalographic (EEG) systems have been developed to indicate the depth of anesthesia; however, at this time the value of such "level of consciousness" monitoring remains controversial.
  - Monitoring of somatosensory or motor evoked potentials is sometimes used during spine and other surgeries in which nerve root or spinal cord injury can occur.

AIRWAY MANAGEMENT

- General anesthesia often requires endotracheal intubation to provide efficient ventilation.
  - Endotracheal intubation carries the risks of oral, dental, pharyngeal, and esophageal trauma as well as the potential for misdirected intubation of the esophagus.
  - In order to introduce and maintain the endotracheal tube, the patient is usually anesthetized and paralyzed prior to direct laryngoscopic introduction of the tube.
    - If airway access is anticipated to be difficult or prolonged, the patient is not fully anesthetized so that he or she will continue to breathe.
    - It is not always possible to predict for which patients airway access will be difficult or prolonged.
    - When the patient is not fully anesthetized, sedation and topical anesthesia are often used to make the process less uncomfortable.
  - Some of the alternatives to direct, laryngoscopic intubation include fiberoptic, "blind" nasal, "light-wand"

oral, wire-guided exchange, retrograde wire exchange, and "blind" intubation via a Fastrach laryngeal mask airway.
- An alternative to endotracheal intubation is the laryngeal mask airway (LMA).
  - The LMA is positioned in the hypopharynx and has an inflatable cuff surrounding the glottic opening.
  - The proximal end of the LMA is similar to a traditional endotracheal tube in that it can be attached to the breathing circuit or to a resuscitator bag.
  - Advantages of the LMA include:
    - No need for placement with a laryngoscope.
      - This may be particularly useful in emergencies and for patients who are difficult to intubate.
    - It allows either spontaneous or limited controlled ventilation.
    - The risk of glottic or subglottic injury is less than with endotracheal intubation.
  - The disadvantages of the LMA include the facts that:
    - It may not provide effective ventilation for some patients and some procedures.
    - It does not protect the airway from aspiration of gastric contents.
    - Its use is relatively contraindicated for:
      - procedures requiring higher ventilation pressures.
      - patients at higher risk of gastric reflux and retained gastric contents, including the morbidly obese, those who have hiatal hernia, gastroparesis, or recent food intake, and patients who are in mid- to late pregnancy.
- The ASA has specific guidelines on the management of the "difficult airway."
- Operating rooms should have a "difficult airway cart" (DAC) with appropriate supplies and a fiberoptic intubating bronchoscope.

DEFINITIONS

GENERAL ANESTHESIA

- General anesthesia involves the administration of intravenous and inhaled agents that induce reversible suppression of the central nervous, respiratory, and cardiac systems. These agents can induce sedation, amnesia, unconsciousness, and variable analgesia as well as suppressing autonomic and motor responses to noxious stimuli.

REGIONAL ANESTHESIA

- Regional anesthesia involves the injection of local anesthetics, with or without additives, around peripheral nerves, paraspinal nerve plexuses, or into the subarachnoid or epidural spaces.

INTRAVENOUS REGIONAL ANESTHESIA

- Intravenous regional anesthesia involves the injection of local anesthetic (LA) into a portion of a limb. It is also known as a Bier block. A tourniquet is used to prevent proximal spread of the LA. Duration is usually less than 1 h owing to tourniquet discomfort.

LOCAL ANESTHESIA

- Local anesthesia is achieved by the injection of local anesthetics directly into tissue.

MONITORIED ANESTHESIA CARE

- This is not a specific type of anesthesia; rather, the term means that anesthesia personnel are present to monitor the patient. Intravenous sedation may or may not be used. Sedation may be absent, light, or heavy. Local anesthetic is often used by the surgeon.

ANESTHESIA MACHINE

- The anesthesia machine is a work station that facilitates administration of gases and anesthetic vapors. Oxygen and nitrous oxide may be supplied by piped-in supplies or via on-site tanks. Various monitors, such as ventilation and respiration monitors, are usually included.
  - Inhalation vapors are added to the inspired gas stream via mechanical or electronic vaporizer units.
  - The flow of oxygen, nitrous oxide, air, or helium gas is controlled by calibrated glass or electronic flowmeters.

PHARMACOLOGY

INTRAVENOUS AGENTS[5]

- Medication can be administered intravenously for the induction and maintenance of anesthesia and for sedation.
  - ***Benzodiazepines*** are often used before procedures to provide anxiolysis and amnesia and during procedures to provide sedation.
    - ***Mechanism of action***: stimulation-potentiation of gamma-amino butyric acid (GABA) receptors.
    - ***Midazolam*** (Versed) is the most frequently used intravenous benzodiazepine because of its rapid onset of action, short half-life, and lack of active metabolites.
      - However, midazolam's onset is slightly slower and it is less potent than barbiturates, etomidate, and propofol.

    - ***Flumazenil*** (Romazicon) is a benzodiazepine antagonist that can be used to reverse benzodiazepine-induced sedation.
  - ***Barbiturates*** have historically been the most commonly used induction agents.
    - Barbiturates provide hypnotic effect by stimulating $GABA_A$ receptors.
    - Most barbiturates (except phenobarbital) are metabolized by the liver and excreted by the kidneys.
    - Barbiturates can cause a moderate dose-dependent decrease in blood pressure. This is more pronounced in hypovolemic patients.
    - Barbiturates are contraindicated in patients with porphyria.
    - ***Thiopental and methohexital*** are two of the barbiturates currently used for induction because of their rapid onset and brief duration of action.
  - ***Propofol*** is a milky white emulsion whose mechanism of action may involve potentiation of the $GABA_A$ receptor-induced chloride channels.
    - Propofol can reduce airway reactivity.
    - It has a moderate antiemetic effect.
    - It can instill a sense of well-being.
    - It can significantly decrease blood pressure, especially in hypovolemic patients, by decreasing both cardiac output and systemic vascular resistance.
    - It can cause ventilatory depression and even apnea, especially at higher doses.
    - A poorly understood fatal acidosis syndrome in critically ill patients receiving prolonged propofol infusion has led to restrictions on the duration of propofol infusions in children.
  - ***Ketamine*** is a phencyclidine derivative that acts as an *N*-methyl-D-asparate (NMDA) receptor antagonist to provide a "dissociative" state of hypnosis and analgesia.
    - Ketamine's sympathomimetic action preserves cardiac function.
    - Ketamine has minimal effect on respiration.
    - Ketamine has minimal effect on autonomic reflexes.
    - Ketamine may cause hypersalivation and dysphoria.
  - ***Etomidate*** may be used as an anesthesia induction agent in the elderly and in patients with cardiovascular compromise because it has minimal effect on the cardiovascular and respiratory systems.
    - Etomidate has a rapid onset of action and rapid resolution of effects.
    - Prolonged infusion may result in inhibition of adrenocortical synthesis.
    - Potential adverse effects of etomidate include a burning pain at the injection site, thrombophlebitis, myoclonus, and nausea/vomiting.
  - ***Dexmedetomidine*** is highly selective $alpha_2$ adrenergic agonist that produces sedation, hypnosis, and analgesia with minimal effect on respiration.
    - Although dexmedetomidine can initially raise blood pressure, it causes hypotension and bradycardia and should not be used in patients who are hypotensive, bradycardic, or hypovolemic.

OPIOIDS[6]

- Opioids can modulate the sympathetic response to noxious stimuli including endotracheal intubation and surgery, thereby improving hemodynamic stability and reducing the need for adjuvant anesthetic agents, including inhaled anesthetics.
  - The effects of opioids are mediated via mu opioid receptors located in both the brain and the spinal cord.
  - Table 6-3 shows the classification of opioids and Table 6-4 indicates relative opioid potencies.
  - ***Meperidine*** has greater potential than other opioids for adverse events, but it also has an additional indication—the treatment of postoperative shivering.
    - Meperidine is a synthetic analog of fentanyl, sufentanil, and alfentanil, with analgesic properties similar to those of morphine; however, it is not as potent as morphine and has a shorter duration of action.
    - Meperidine is transformed into a neurotoxic metabolite, normeperidine, which can accumulate after repeated administration in even mild renal insufficiency; therefore, despite its labeled indication, it is not suitable for chronic use.
    - Adverse effects of normeperidine include tremor, myoclonus, and seizures.
    - Meperidine interacts unpredictably with monoamine oxidase (MAO) inhibitors. There are case reports of a symptom cluster including agitation, fever, and seizures that has in some cases progressed to coma, apnea, and death.

TABLE 6-3 Opioids

TYPE	CLASS	EXAMPLES
Naturally occurring		Codeine Morphine
Semisynthetic	Heroin	
	Dihydromorphone	
	Thebaine derivatives	Buprenorphine
Synthetic	Morphinan	Levorphanol, Butorphanol
	Benzomorphan	Pentazocine
	Diphenylpropylamine	Methadone
	Phenylapiperidine	Meperidine Fentanyl Sufentanil Alfentanil Remifentanil

TABLE 6-4 Selected Opioid-Equivalent Dosing

	APPROXIMATE EQUIANALGESIC DOSES (MG)	
OPIOID	PARENTERAL	ORAL
Meperidine	100	300
Morphine	10	30
Hydromorphone	1.5	7.5
Fentanyl	0.1	~ 0.4 (lozenge on a stick)
Sufentanil	0.01–0.02	—
Alfentanil	0.5–1	—
Remifentanil	0.1	—
Oxycodone	—	30
Hydrocodone	—	30

- Meperidine in doses of 25 to 50 mg IV is effective for the prevention or treatment of postanesthesia shivering and rigors due to infusion of medications (e.g., amphotericin) or blood products.

INHALATION ANESTHETICS[7]

- Inhalation anesthetics are grouped into two major classes: vapors and gases.
  - The major vapors are hydrocarbons (e.g., halothane) and ethers (e.g., isoflurane, desflurane, sevoflurane).
  - The only commonly used gas is nitrous oxide, which provides sedation and analgesia but is not an anesthetic by itself.
  - Uptake and distribution of vapors and gases by lungs/blood/tissue compartments is not instantaneous.
    - Cardiac and pulmonary factors strongly influence uptake and distribution.
    - Each agent differs in equilibration time.
    - The degree of metabolism of vapors from the most to the least is as follows: halothane, sevoflurane, isoflurane, desflurane.
  - ***Halothane*** is seldom used for adult anesthesia.
    - In rare instances, repeated exposure to halothane causes hepatic necrosis in adults, likely through an autoimmune reaction.
    - Hepatotoxicity is much less common in children, and halothane is still used in many children's centers because of its acceptable odor, which allows rapid induction through mask inhalation.
    - Halothane can also cause beta adrenergic–mediated arrhythmias.
  - ***Isoflurane*** is commonly used.
    - Isoflurane is minimally metabolized and has no renal or hepatic toxicities.
    - Isoflurane has less effect on blood pressure, heart rate, and cardiac output than halothane.
  - ***Desflurane*** is a highly fluorinated, potent anesthetic.
    - Desflurane's low blood solubility results in a rapid onset of action and rapid pulmonary elimination.
    - High concentrations of desflurane can markedly increase heart rate. Caution is indicated when it is used for patients with heart disease or uncontrolled hypertension.
  - ***Sevoflurane*** also has low blood solubility and is rapidly excreted.
    - Abrupt emergence from anesthesia can cause fear and delirium in children.
    - Sevoflurane is unstable in the presence of dry soda lime, which is used in anesthesia circuits to absorb carbon dioxide.
    - Breakdown of sevoflurane can lead to the accumulation of a toxic metabolite (compound A) that can cause renal dysfunction, although no cases have been reported.

NEUROMUSCULAR BLOCKADE[8]

- The use of neuromuscular blockade for paralysis in anesthesia is guided by several considerations.
  - The need for paralysis is based on characteristics of the surgery, including the anatomic location, intensity, duration, and patient positioning.
  - Neuromuscular blockade can reduce the amount of anesthetic required; however, patients can emerge from anesthesia while still paralyzed—a dysphoric and potentially terrifying experience.
    - Neuromuscular blocking agents do *not* have sedative, anesthetic, or analgesic effects.
    - When neuromuscular blocking agents are used, the effect should usually be monitored with a peripheral nerve stimulator.
  - Two classes of neuromuscular blocking agents are available: depolarizing and nondepolarizing.
    - ***Depolarizing agents*** cause depolarization at the motor endplate.
      - Succinylcholine causes rapid and complete muscle relaxation that is relatively short-lived.
        - Succinylcholine can precipitate malignant hyperthermia in genetically susceptible individuals.
        - Patients with congenital or acquired pseudocholinesterase deficiency have much longer paralysis after succinylcholine and after mivacurium (a nondepolarizing agent).
        - Complications of succinylcholine include postoperative myalgia, transient elevations in serum potassium concentration, and increases in intraocular, intracranial, and intragastric pressures.

TABLE 6-5 Clinical Properties of Nondepolarizing Muscle Relaxants

DURATION CLASS	MUSCLE RELAXANT	ONSET TO MAX ACTION (MIN)	DURATION TO RETURN TO TWITCH >25% (MIN)	SIDE EFFECTS
Long-acting	Pancuronium	3–5	60–90	Tachycardia
Intermediate-acting	Vecuronium	3–5	20–35	None
	Rocuronium	1–2	20–35	None
	Atracurium	3–5	20–30	Histamine Release possible
	Cisatracurium	3–6	20–35	None
Short-acting	Mivacurium	2–3	12–20	Histamine release possible

  - Relative contraindications to succinylcholine include hyperkalemia, penetrating eye injury, and elevated intracranial pressure.
  - Absolute contraindications due to risk of severe hyperkalemia include burns (after 24 h), myopathies, prolonged immobility, stroke, spinal cord injury, active multiple sclerosis or Guillian-Barré syndrome, and other central nervous system diseases.
- ***Nondepolarizing agents*** competitively inhibit acetylcholine at the motor endplate.
  - They are usually classified according to rapidity of onset and duration of action (Table 6-5).

REGIONAL ANESTHESIA AND LOCAL ANESTHETICS

- Local anesthetics can be injected adjacent to the spinal cord, nerve plexuses, nerves, or the operative field to prevent or alleviate perioperative pain.
  - Adjuvants can be added to the anesthetic to intensify and prolong the effects.
    - Adjuvants include epinephrine, phenylephrine, clonidine, ketamine, and opioids.
  - Commonly used types of blocks include, among others, the following:
    - *Neuraxial* (spinal-subarachnoid, epidural, caudal)
    - *Root* (paravertebral)
    - *Plexus* (brachial, interscalene, supraclavicular, infraclavicular, axillary, lumbar-somatic, sympathetic)
    - *Peripheral* (radial, median, ulnar, sciatic, popliteal, ankle)
    - *Intercostal*
    - *Head and neck*
  - Both single injections and continuous catheter infusions are used.
  - Electrostimulation needles and portable ultrasound are sometimes used to locate peripheral neural plexuses or nerves.
  - Neural blocks can be used alone or with sedation or general anesthesia (Table 6-6).
  - There are two different types of local anesthetics:
    - Amino esters: cocaine, procaine, 2-chloroprocaine, benzocaine, and tetracaine

TABLE 6-6 Local Anesthesia Effects and Duration

LOCAL ANESTHETIC	MAX DOSE (MG/KG)	MAX DOSE W/EPI (MG/KG)	SPINAL DURATION (MIN)	EPIDURAL DURATION (MIN)	COMMENTS
Lidocaine	5	7	60–100	80–120	Radicular irritation more common in spinal use
Bupivacaine	2	3	90–150	165–225	
2-Chloprocaine	5–10	—	75	45–60	Spinal use off label
Ropivacaine	2	3	—	165–225	
Mepivacaine	5	7	30–90	60–180	Spinal use off label

- Amino esters account for more than 99 percent of allergic reactions to local anesthetic.
- Tetracaine and benzocaine can cause methemoglobinemia, even when administered topically. Therefore doses of topical tetracaine and benzocaine should be limited in order to avoid symptomatic methemoglobinemia.

- Amino amides: mepivacaine, bupivacaine, ropivacaine, lidocaine, and levobupivacaine
  - Allergies are extremely rare; however, paraben preservatives in amino-amide preparations can cross-react with allergens in amino-ester preparations.
  - Bupivacaine is highly lipid-soluble and strongly protein-bound, giving it a relatively long duration of action.
    - Inadvertent intravenous injection of bupivacaine can cause intractable cardiac arrest from blockade of cardiac sodium channels.
  - Ropivacaine may be less cardiotoxic than bupivacaine.
  - Lidocaine has a rapid onset and predictable duration of action.
    - Injection of lidocaine into tissue is less painful than injection of bupivacaine.

EFFECTS OF ANESTHESIA ON ORGAN SYSTEM FUNCTION

RESPIRATORY

- Anesthesia can impair respiratory function.
  - Inhaled anesthetic induce regular, rapid, shallow breathing.
    - Minute ventilation falls and PCO_2 increases.
    - Ventilatory response to hypercarbia and hypoxemia diminishes.
    - Airway resistance typically falls, but low concentrations can induce airway irritation and laryngospasm.
    - Functional residual capacity decreases and ventilation/ perfusion mismatch increases.
    - Mucociliary clearance can be abolished.
    - Surgical body positions can further impair ventilation.

CARDIOVASCULAR

- Inhaled anesthetics, thiopental, and propofol cause hypotension via a combination of myocardial depression and venoarterial dilatation.
- The magnitude of the effects depends on preanesthetic sympathetic tone, venous capacitance, concomitant medical conditions, the agent, and the dose.
- Altered baroreceptor reactivity may contribute to tachycardia with isoflurane and desflurane.
- Treatment with an angiotensin converting enzyme (ACE) inhibitor or angiotensin receptor blocker (ARB) may exaggerate anesthetic-induced hypotension.

CEREBRAL

- General anesthetics produce dose-dependent changes in cerebral blood flow (CBF), cerebral metabolic rate ($CMRO_2$), and central nervous system electrophysiology.[9]
- In general, modern anesthetic vapors and nitrous oxide increase CBF and decrease $CMRO_2$.
  - Increased CBF can increase intracranial pressure (ICP) in patients with poor intracranial compliance.
- Most intravenous agents except ketamine decrease CBF and $CMRO_2$.
- Anesthetics may be cerebroprotective during focal cerebral ischemia but are not protective during global cerebral ischemia.

HEPATIC

- General anesthetics usually decrease total hepatic blood flow (THBF) to a variable extent.
- This effect is predominantly due to decreased blood pressure and cardiac output.
- Positive-pressure ventilation, surgical manipulation and packing, and vasopressor drugs can have a much greater effect on THBF than anesthetics.
- Modern vapor anesthetics can, in rare instances, produce hepatic injury similar to that due to halothane.

RENAL

- Both general and regional anesthesia temporarily reduce glomerular filtration rate and urine output.
- Surgery-induced increases in sympathetic tone and stress hormones, sepsis, hypovolemia, and positive-pressure ventilation have greater effects on renal perfusion than do anesthetics.
- Sevoflurane-induced nephrotoxicity is theoretically possible but has never been reported, even in patients with impaired renal function.

SPECIAL CONSIDERATIONS

MALIGNANT HYPERTHERMIA[10]

- Malignant hyperthermia (MH) is a life-threatening hypermetabolic state manifest by muscle rigidity,

tachycardia, hypertension, hyperthermia, hypoxemia, hypercarbia, hyperkalemia, and metabolic acidosis.
  - MH occurs in approximately 1 in 50,000 anesthetics for adults and 1 in 12,000 for children.
  - MH can be triggered by all vapor anesthetic agents (e.g., halothane, isoflurane, sevoflurane, and desflurane) but not by nitrous oxide.
  - MH can also be triggered by succinylcholine but not by nondepolarizing neuromuscular blocking agents.
  - The predisposition for MH is inherited and involves variations in sarcoplasmic calcium release.
  - In evaluating a patient prior to general anesthesia, thoroughly screen for a family history of MH, anesthesia-associated deaths, and conditions associated with MH.
    - The only conditions that are agreed to be associated with MH are King-Denborough syndrome, central core disease, and possibly Duchenne muscular dystrophy.
    - Many other conditions have been anecdotally associated with MH without proof of causation.
    - Any inherited myopathy may be a risk factor for MH; however, succinylcholine-induced rhabdomyolysis, with subsequent massive hyperkalemia, can mimic MH.
  - People at risk for MH have increased resting levels of calcium in the sarcoplasmic reticulum of their skeletal muscle. Vapor anesthetics and succinylcholine trigger an excessive release of calcium, causing unabated muscle contraction and the other metabolic abnormalities.
  - The molecular biology and genetics of MH are more complex than single-gene inheritance.
  - The halothane-caffeine contracture test, performed on a fresh muscle biopsy specimen, is available at approximately 10 centers in the United States and might be appropriate for some high-risk patients anticipating general anesthesia.
  - Proceeding to surgery without testing a high-risk patient is also a reasonable option.
    - The entire inhalation circuit should be replaced and flushed and all agents that could induce MH should be removed from the operating theater.
    - Nontriggering agents (such as propotal and nitrous oxide) should be used.
  - Treatment of MH includes:
    - Immediate discontinuation of triggering agents.
      - Dantrolene sodium 2.5 mg/kg with repeated doses up to 10 mg/kg.
      - Treatment of hyperkalemia and of acidosis.
      - Vigorous hyperventilation with 100% oxygen.
      - Induced diuresis.
      - Core and surfacc cooling.
      - Contact with the 24-h hotline of the Malignant Hyperthermia Association of United States (800-644-9737) for expert clinical advice.
      - Patients often relapse after initial response to treatment and must be closely monitored for at least 24 h.

BLOOD COMPONENT TRANSFUSION[8]

- The American Association of Blood Banks has recommendations for the practice of blood component transfusion. See Chap. 30 for additional information.
  - Transfusion of packed red blood cells (PRBCs) is rarely indicated for hemoglobin concentrations above 10 g/dL and is almost always indicated at concentrations below 6 g/dL.
  - Red blood cell "salvage" procedures (e.g., Cell Saver) can reduce the transfusion of allogenic PRBCs; however, other blood components, such as plasma and platelets, are lost in the process.
  - For acute normovolemic hemodilution, whole blood is withdrawn from the patient in the operating room, replaced with crystalloid or colloid, and then transfused back into the patient later in the operation.
  - Patients can also donate blood for themselves in the weeks prior to elective procedures.
  - The transfusion of many units of PRBCs carries the risk of giving the patient excessive amounts of citrate, which is used to prevent coagulation in PRBC units.
    - For patients who have received several units of PRBCs, supplemental intravenous calcium may be needed to bind citrate and prevent bleeding.
    - For some patients and some procedures, it may be appropriate to reduce blood loss with DDAVP (increases release of factor VIII and von Willebrand factor) or with aminocaproic acid (EACA), aprotinin, or tranexamic acid (all three inhibit fibrinolysis).

THE "DO NOT RESUSCITATE" (DNR) PATIENT

- The administration of anesthesia necessarily involves some practices and procedures that might be viewed as "resuscitation" in other settings.
  - Therefore, prior to procedures requiring anesthetic care, clarify existing directives with the patient or the patient's designee and documented in the patient's records.
  - DNR orders are usually suspended temporarily in the immediate perioperative period.
    - Options include:
      - A full attempt at resuscitation.

    - The patient may choose to have full suspension of the existing directive during the anesthetic and the postoperative period.
- Limited attempt at resuscitation during unexpected intraoperative events.
    - The patient may choose to continue certain specific resuscitation procedures while refusing others. For example, a patient may elect for endotracheal intubation and pharmacologic support but not chest compressions or defibrillation.
    - The patient may choose for the anesthesiologist or the surgeon to use clinical judgment in determining the appropriateness of specific resuscitative procedures based on the patient's prognosis and an understanding of the patient's preferences.
- In the ideal situation, the patient's primary care physician and the surgeon should be involved in these discussions with the patient. At a minimum, these discussions and decisions should be thoroughly documented in the medical record.

REFERENCES

1. Guidelines for Patient Care in Anesthesiology. American Society of Anesthesiologists. http://www.asahq.org/publicationsAndServices/standards/13.html. Accessed January 8, 2005.
2. Stoelting RK, Miller RD. *Basics of Anesthesia*. New York: Churchill Livingstone, 2000.
3. Warner MA, Caplan RA, Epstein BS, et al. Practice guidelines for preoperative fasting and the use of pharmacologic agents to reduce the risk of pulmonary aspiration: Application to healthy patients undergoing elective procedures: A Report by the American Society of Anesthesiologists Task Force on Preoperative Fasting. *Anesthesiology* 90:896, 1999.
4. Standards for Basic Anesthetic Monitoring. Amended 2004. American Society of Anesthesiologists. http://www.asahq.org/publicationsAndServices/standards/02.pdf. Accessed January 8, 2005.
5. Reves JG, Glass PS, Lubarsky DA, et al. Intravenous nonopioid anesthestics, in Miller RD et al (eds): *Miller's Anesthesia*, 6th ed. New York: Elsevier, 2005.
6. Fukuda K. Intravenous opioid anesthestics, in Miller RD et al (eds): *Miller's Anesthesia*, 6th ed. New York: Elsevier, 2005.
7. Campagna JA, Miller KW, Forman SA. Mechanisms of actions of inhaled anesthetics. *N Engl J Med* 348:2110, 2003.
8. Wiklund RA, Rosenbaum SH. Anesthesiology. *N Engl J Med* 337:1132, 1997.
9. Patel PM, Drummond JC. Cerebral physiology and the effects of anesthetics and techniques, in Miller RD et al (eds): *Miller's Anesthesia*, 6th ed. New York: Elsevier, 2005.
10. Gronert GA, Pessah IN, Muldoon SM, Tautz TJ. Malignant hyperthermia, in Miller RD et al (eds): *Miller's Anesthesia*, 6th ed. New York: Elsevier, 2005.

7A PERIOPERATIVE MEDICATION MANAGEMENT

Steven L. Cohn and
David S. Macpherson

INTRODUCTION

- Every year millions of patients undergo surgery, and most of them take one or more prescription or over-the-counter medications.
- The medical consultant and surgical team must work with the patient to manage these medications in the perioperative period.
- There are no randomized trials to guide perioperative management of most medications, so there is substantial variation in management from physician to physician.
- Clinical experience has shown that:
    - Certain medications are essential.
    - Most medications can be safely continued perioperatively, although many are unnecessary and therefore optional.
    - A few drugs must be discontinued or continued at a modified dosage in the perioperative period.
- In view of the paucity of randomized trials and the variation in clinical practice, we reviewed the available literature and offer the following recommendations as expert opinion based on available studies, our clinical experience, and theoretical considerations.

PRINCIPLES

- Ask patients about all medications, including prescription drugs, dietary supplements, and over-the-counter products.
- Consider the following principles in your recommendations:
    - Indication and need for the medication
    - Effect on the primary disease of stopping the drug
        - Rebound effect, clinical deterioration, withdrawal symptoms
    - Drug pharmacokinetics and changes in the perioperative setting
        - Absorption, half-life, route of administration, metabolism, and elimination
    - Potential adverse effect of the medication on perioperative risk
        - Bleeding, hypoglycemia
    - Potential benefits of starting a drug prophylactically

    - Prevention of ischemia, thrombosis, infection, aspiration
  - Potential drug interactions with anesthetic agents
- Based on these principles and a risk-benefit analysis, decide whether to continue, discontinue, or modify the regimen for each medication.
- Oral medications that must be continued perioperatively should be given with a sip of water on the morning of surgery.
- Although there may be an order for "NPO after midnight," it should read "NPO except for medications."

RECOMMENDATIONS BY DRUG CLASS

- It is beyond the scope of this chapter to discuss all medications, so we have chosen the medications we think are most important or most common (Table 7A-1). For more detailed information and supporting evidence, the reader is referred to other online references[1–2] and reviews.[3–5]

MEDICATIONS AFFECTING HEMOSTASIS

ANTICOAGULANTS

Warfarin Perioperative management of warfarin therapy is discussed in detail in Chap. 7B. Below are some general guidelines.

- Maintenance of anticoagulation increases the risk of bleeding complications, but discontinuing it places the patient at risk for thromboembolic events. This latter risk is based on the indication for anticoagulation and the periprocedural risk.
- Various regimens have been described for discontinuing warfarin before surgery and for "bridging" therapy with unfractionated or low-molecular-weight heparin if indicated.
- Options include the following recommendations:
  - Continuing anticoagulation for minor procedures where the bleeding risk is low
  - Discontinuing or decreasing the dose of warfarin 3 to 5 days prior to surgery, where the risk of bleeding is higher but the risk of thromboembolism is modest
  - Bridging therapy for patients at high risk for thromboembolism in the absence of anticoagulation
  - Starting warfarin preoperatively on the evening before surgery if indicated for prophylaxis of deep venous thrombosis (DVT) in orthopedic surgery
  - Monitoring the INR

Unfractionated Heparin (UFH)
- ***Recommendations:***
  - Discontinue full-dose anticoagulation 4 to 6 h before surgery. It can be restarted postoperatively as soon as deemed safe by the surgeon (as early as 6 h postoperatively after procedures with secured hemostasis and low risk of bleeding or not before 72 h after craniotomy).
  - Monitor partial thromboplastin time (PTT) and platelet count.
  - Continue or start subcutaneous heparin if indicated for DVT prophylaxis (5000 IU SC q8–12 h depending on level of risk) (see Chap. 46).

Low-Molecular-Weight Heparin (LMWH) Note that these drugs vary in FDA-approved indications and use in special populations (obese, underweight, renally impaired), are given in fixed-dose regimens, do not require monitoring for anticoagulant effect (although anti-Xa levels can be checked if necessary), and are partially reversible with protamine sulfate.

- ***Recommendations:***
  - Discontinue full-dose anticoagulation 24 h preoperatively and restart postoperatively when deemed safe by the surgeon.
  - Continue or start if indicated for DVT prophylaxis (see Chap. 46).
  - Check platelet count after 3 to 5 days.
  - If neuraxial anesthesia is planned, discontinue full-dose LMWH 24 h before and prophylactic-dose LMWH 12 h before spinal or epidural needle insertion. Do not start LMWH until at least 2 h after the needle or epidural catheter has been removed.

Synthetic Pentasaccharides (Fondaparinux) Selectively inhibits factor Xa, has a long half-life (17 h), renal elimination, fixed dose, no monitoring for anticoagulant effect, and is partially reversible with recombinant factor VIIa.

- ***Recommendations:***
  - Start 6 h postoperatively for DVT prophylaxis in orthopedic surgery patients (see Chap. 46).
  - Same caution as LMWH regarding neuraxial anesthesia and epidural catheters.

ANTIPLATELET AGENTS

Aspirin Irreversibly inhibits cyclooxygenase, so the patient will need 5 to 10 days after the last dose to replenish adequate number of platelets.

- If continued, aspirin may increase perioperative blood loss, but it may be beneficial in patients undergoing carotid endarterectomy after a transient ischemic attack (TIA), may improve graft patency after peripheral vascular surgery, decreases mortality if given within 48 hours after coronary artery bypass grafting (CABG) and may decrease perioperative cardiovascular events in patients at high risk.

TABLE 7A-1 Summary of Perioperative Medication Management

MEDICATION CLASS	RECOMMENDATION
Anticoagulants and other drugs affecting hemostasis	Continue for minor surgery.
	Discontinue at appropriate interval before major surgery.
	Consider bridging anticoagulation for patients at high risk of interim thrombosis.
Cardiovascular medications	Continue most agents.
	Initiate beta blockers in patients at high risk of perioperative cardiac morbidity.
	Withhold diuretics on the morning of surgery, especially with signs of volume depletion.
Gastrointestinal agents	Continue.
	Substitute parenteral forms in patients who are NPO for prolonged periods or those at high risk for stress ulceration.
Pulmonary agents	Continue.
Diabetic agents	Withhold oral hypoglycemics on morning of surgery and resume when patient resumes eating.
	For type 1 diabetics, continue some form of insulin (long-acting or intravenous) at all times.
	For type 2 diabetics, decrease dose of morning intermediate insulin depending on anticipated duration of NPO status and time of surgery.
Thyroid agents	Continue thyroid replacement.
	Parenteral substitution needed only if NPO state is prolonged (days).
	Postpone surgery until hyperthyroidism is controlled.
Oral contraceptives, hormone replacement, and SERMs	Discontinue several weeks before surgery in patients at high risk for perioperative venous thromboembolism; otherwise continue.
Lipid-lowering agents	Continue statins.
	Discontinue other agents.
Corticosteroids	Continue chronic corticosteroids. Increase dosage to account for surgical stress.
Psychotropic agents	For most patients, continue SSRIs. Consider holding several weeks before surgery in patients in whom perioperative hemorrhage could be catastrophic (CNS surgery).
	Continue tricyclic antidepressants, benzodiazepines, lithium, and antipsychotics.
	For MAOIs, continue or discontinue depending on anesthesiologist preference.
Chronic opioids	Continue. Substitute equianalgesic or higher doses to manage surgical pain.
Rheumatologic agents	Continue methotrexate.
	Discontinue other DMARDs and anticytokines.
	Continue hypouricemic agents.
Neurologic agents	Continue antiseizure medications.
	Hold antiparkinson agents briefly.
	Continue agents for myasthenia gravis.
Herbal agents	Discontinue all.

CNS = central nervous system; DMARDS = disease-modifying antirheumatic drugs; MAOIs = monoamine oxidase inhibitors; NPO = nil per os (nothing by mouth); SERMs = selective estrogen receptor modulators; SSRIs = selective serotonin reuptake inhibitors.

- Addition of aspirin to an appropriate DVT prophylaxis regimen may decrease postoperative pulmonary embolism in orthopedic patients.
- ***Recommendations:***
  - Consider the indication for therapy and risk of bleeding.
  - Often discontinued 5–7 days before surgery due to fear of increased bleeding.
  - Continue in certain cases (vascular surgery or those at high risk for perioperative vascular events) as noted above, and start postoperatively after CABG.
  - Discuss with surgeon to determine personal preference.

Clopidogrel (and Ticlopidine)

- Irreversibly inhibits ADP-induced platelet aggregation.
- Associated with increased bleeding, especially when combined with aspirin.
- ***Recommendations:***
  - Discontinue clopidogrel 5–10 days prior to surgery (discontinue ticlopidine 10–14 days before surgery).
  - Delay noncardiac surgery for at least 4 weeks after PCI/stenting to allow continuation of aspirin and clopidogrel; then discontinue them approximately 1 week before surgery and restart them as soon as is feasible postoperatively (see Chap. 20).

Dipyridamole

- Reversible platelet adhesion inhibitor, half-life: 10 h.
- ***Recommendations:***
  - Uncertain—minimal data. Need to balance risk of bleeding with any potential benefit of continuing it.

Cilostazol

- Reversible cAMP PDE III inhibitor, half-life: 12 h.
- ***Recommendations:***
  - Discontinue 3 to 5 days before surgery.

Nonsteroidal Anti-Inflammatory Drugs

- Although these drugs may increase the risk of perioperative bleeding and possibly renal insufficiency, they also may decrease postoperative pain and the use of opioid analgesics.
- ***Recommendations:***
  - Controversial. Typically these drugs are discontinued 1 to 3 days before surgery, depending on the half-life of the drug. They can be given postoperatively for analgesia but the timing in this setting is based on the surgeon's preference.

COX-2 INHIBITORS

- Rofecoxib and valdecoxib have been withdrawn.
- Celecoxib had not been shown to affect platelet activity at usual doses (up to 400 mg/day) although theoretical concerns exist for potentiating renal insufficiency.
- ***Recommendations:***
  - Discontinue several days prior to surgery.

CARDIOVASCULAR MEDICATIONS

Beta Blockers

- Beta blockers decrease heart rate and myocardial oxygen demand.
- Several studies and metaanalyses have shown that beta blockers can reduce perioperative myocardial ischemia, myocardial infarction, and cardiac death in patients at high risk for cardiac complications.
- Discontinuation of beta blockers is associated with a withdrawal syndrome, including rebound hypertension or myocardial ischemia.
- ***Recommendations:***
  - Continue beta blockers perioperatively.
  - Consider starting beta blockers prophylactically (ideally at least a week before surgery) in patients with coronary artery disease (CAD) or multiple risk factors for CAD (assuming no contraindications to beta blockers: e.g., bronchospasm, advanced AV block, bradyarrhythmias, pulmonary edema) who are scheduled for intermediate- to high-risk surgery (see Chap. 20).
  - Titrate the dose to a target heart rate between 55 and 65 beats per minute, as blood pressure tolerates, based on protocols used in the studies.

Alpha$_2$ Agonists (Centrally Acting Sympatholytics)

- Clonidine may reduce perioperative myocardial ischemia (and possibly infarction and death) but appears to be less effective than beta blockers in this setting.
- Discontinuation of clonidine is associated with a withdrawal syndrome of rebound hypertension and tachycardia.
- Clonidine may reduce anesthetic requirements.
- ***Recommendations:***
  - Continue perioperatively.
  - Consider starting prophylactically in high-risk cardiac patients who have contraindications to beta blockers.
  - Recognize that clonidine can also cause bradycardia.

Alpha Blockers and Alpha-Beta Blockers

- Alpha blockers (with or without beta blockers) are used to treat pheochromocytomas but are less often used for uncomplicated hypertension. They are most commonly used in patients with benign prostatic hypertrophy.

- Alpha-beta blockers are also used to treat hypertension, pheochromocytomas, and heart failure.
- ***Recommendations:***
  - Continue perioperatively.
  - Start at least 5 days before surgery if treating pheochromocytoma (see Chap. 29).
  - Intravenous labetalol may also be used perioperatively to treat hypertension.

Calcium Channel Antagonists

- Limited data suggest that diltiazem may have beneficial effects in reducing perioperative ischemia. It may also decrease the occurrence of postoperative supraventricular tachyarrhythmias after CABG.
- ***Recommendations:***
  - Continue calcium channel antagonists perioperatively.

Nitrates

- Prophylactic use of nitroglycerin has not been found to reduce perioperative cardiac events.
- ***Recommendations:***
  - Continue nitrates in patients taking them chronically.

Angiotensin Converting Enzyme (ACE) Inhibitors

- By blocking the response of the renin-angiotensin system, these drugs can cause hypotension.
- ACE inhibitors have been associated with an increased incidence of hypotension, requiring pressors intraoperatively; however, there was no significant increase in "hard outcomes." The interaction between the ACE inhibitor and certain anesthetic drugs may be associated with this hypotension.
- ***Recommendations:***
  - Continue ACE inhibitors cautiously, but consider holding them in patients whose baseline blood pressure is low.

Angiotensin II Receptor Blockers (ARBs)

- Like ACE inhibitors, these drugs have been associated with hypotension with induction of anesthesia. These hypotensive episodes were also less responsive to pressors.
- ***Recommendations:***
  - Uncertain, but they are usually continued.

Diuretics

- Diuretics may precipitate hypovolemia and hypokalemia; however, if a patient has been on a diuretic for several weeks, a steady state should have been reached.
- A single dose of a diuretic on the morning of surgery is unlikely to cause hypokalemia or arrhythmias.
- Anesthetic agents may cause hypotension in a volume-depleted patient.
- ***Recommendations:***
  - Diuretics are usually discontinued on the morning of surgery, although this is not universal. If a patient appears markedly volume-depleted, the diuretic should be stopped several days before surgery; conversely, in a patient who is not volume-depleted and has a history of congestive heart failure, the diuretic may be continued on the morning of surgery.
  - Check blood urea nitrogen (BUN), creatinine, and potassium preoperatively.

Antiarrhythmics (Digoxin, Amiodarone, Sotalol)

- ***Recommendations:***
  - In general, these drugs are continued perioperatively.
  - Consider obtaining a preoperative drug level, especially in patients with possible toxicity or noncompliance.

GASTROINTESTINAL MEDICATIONS

- H_2 blockers and proton-pump inhibitors prevent gastric acid production and thereby help prevent stress ulcers. Stress ulcers are more common with prolonged postoperative mechanical ventilation or intensive care unit (ICU) stay.
- ***Recommendations:***
  - Patients taking H_2 blockers or proton-pump inhibitors should remain on these agents throughout the perioperative period.
  - For surgeries in which oral medication absorption is impaired, intravenous forms should be substituted.

PULMONARY MEDICATIONS

- Inhaled bronchodilators and other agents are often used in patients with chronic obstructive pulmonary disease (COPD) or asthma and serve to optimize pulmonary function.
- Optimal pulmonary function is important throughout the perioperative period, especially in patients with underlying obstructive lung disease undergoing thoracic or upper abdominal procedures (see Chaps. 24 and 25).
- ***Recommendations:***
  - Continue inhaled beta agonists and anticholinergics perioperatively via metered-dose inhalers or via nebulizers.
  - There are no studies of theophylline in the perioperative period; hence the drug can be continued or held. If continued, levels should be checked, especially in surgery with major fluid shifts.

- Corticosteroids should be continued throughout the perioperative period, both to optimize pulmonary function and to minimize the risk of adrenal insufficiency (see Chap. 28).
- Leukotriene inhibitors are used for chronic therapy. Despite a short half-life, these agents have continued effect for up to 3 weeks after discontinuation.

ENDOCRINE MEDICATIONS

Diabetic Agents

- Animal studies show that wound healing and white cell chemotaxis are improved when glucose is well controlled.
- CABG patients have fewer wound infections when perioperative glucose levels are low; however, tight glycemic control perioperatively increases the risk of hypoglycemia.
- ***Recommendations:***
  - See Chap. 26 for more detail on perioperative glucose management.
  - Oral hypoglycemics should be held on the morning of surgery and restarted when significant oral intake resumes.
  - Metformin reinitiation should be delayed if the surgery is complicated by renal insufficiency or congestive heart failure.
  - Individualize the management of long-acting insulin (ultralente and insulin glargine) based on the patient and the procedure.
    - For a patient who takes both short- and long-acting insulin and who is undergoing a minor procedure, discontinuing the short-acting but continuing the long-acting insulin may be the best strategy for providing basal insulin without inducing hypoglycemia.
    - Consider reducing evening or bedtime doses of intermediate-duration insulin the evening before surgery, especially in patients who are tightly controlled.
    - The most commonly used method of administering intermediate-acting insulin is to give one-half to two-thirds of the patient's usual dose on the morning of surgery and provide regular insulin coverage perioperatively.
  - For lengthy or complex procedures, continuous insulin infusions should be used to avoid the known perioperative variability in insulin absorption with subcutaneous administration.

Thyroid Agents

- Mild hypothyroidism is not associated with serious perioperative complications.
- Levothyroxine persists in the circulation for many days. Therefore missing several doses of oral thyroid replacement in the perioperative period is inconsequential.
- Postpone elective procedures in patients who are hyperthyroid until the hyperthyroidism is well controlled (see Chap. 27).
- ***Recommendations:***
  - Continue antithyroid medication, including beta blockers, perioperatively.
  - Continue thyroid replacement medication.

Oral Contraceptives, Hormone Replacement Therapy (HRT), and Selective Estrogen Receptor Modulators (SERMs)

- Both low- and high-dose estrogen oral contraceptives, HRT, and SERMs are associated with an increased risk of venous thrombosis.
- The decision to continue oral contraceptives before elective surgery should balance the risk of thrombosis and the risks of discontinuation (unintended pregnancy, estrogen withdrawal symptoms).
- ***Recommendations:***
  - Patients undergoing elective surgery in which the risk of venous thromboembolism is high (see Chap. 46) and in whom alternate contraception is feasible should discontinue these agents several weeks before surgery.
  - Patients undergoing surgeries in which venous thromboembolism risk is not high can continue the medications but should receive DVT prophylaxis perioperatively.
  - If oral contraceptives are discontinued, a pregnancy test should be obtained immediately before surgery and the patient should be counseled that the risk of pregnancy will remain elevated for the first cycle after restarting the oral contraceptive and that barrier methods of contraception should be used in this period.

Lipid-Lowering Agents

HMG-CoA Reductase Inhibitors ("Statins")

- Isolated case reports of rhabdomyolysis related to the use of HMG-CoA reductase inhibitors during surgery led to initial recommendations by the pharmaceutical industry that these agents be held.
- In addition to long-term benefit to prevent atherosclerosis, these agents appear to prevent vascular plaque rupture.
- More recent large observational studies and one small randomized trial have shown that these agents are associated with a mortality benefit, particularly for patients undergoing vascular surgery.
- ***Recommendation:***
  - Continue HMG-CoA reductase inhibitors in the perioperative period.

Other Agents for Lipid Control

- Bile acid sequestrants (cholestyramine, colestipol), fibric acid derivatives (gemfibrozil), niacin, and ezetimibe reduce low-density lipoprotein (LDL) cholesterol levels but have no definite short-term benefit in the perioperative period.
- Bile acid sequestrants can interfere with absorption of other medications.
- ***Recommendations:***
  - Discontinue bile acid sequestrants, niacin, fibric acid derivatives, and ezetimibe the day before surgery and restart them after the perioperative period is complete.

CORTICOSTEROIDS

- Information about the perioperative management of patients on corticosteroids can be found in Chap. 28.
- In general, if steroids have been used at a physiologic dose or greater for several weeks in the previous 6 months, the pituitary-adrenal axis may be suppressed and the patient may not generate the usual adrenocortical response to the stress of surgery.
- ***Recommendations:***
  - Continue or increase the dose of steroids (hydrocortisone or its equivalent) based on the usual dose, duration, and type of surgery.
  - On the day of surgery, a total daily dose of 150 to 200 mg of intravenous hydrocortisone is usually more than adequate.
  - Taper the increased dose as quickly as possible based on the ongoing level of stress and the patient's clinical status.

PSYCHOTROPIC MEDICATIONS

SSRIs

- Selective serotonin reuptake inhibitors (SSRIs) may affect platelet aggregation and have been associated with an increase in gastrointestinal bleeding. One study also showed an increased need for transfusions in patients undergoing orthopedic surgery.
- Stopping SSRIs has been associated with a withdrawal syndrome and may worsen a patient's psychiatric problem.
- ***Recommendation:***
  - Continue SSRIs. There is insufficient evidence to recommend discontinuing these drugs to prevent potential perioperative bleeding; furthermore, the washout period may be several weeks. However, for central nervous system (CNS) surgery where perioperative hemorrhage may have catastrophic consequences, discontinue 3 weeks before surgery.

TRICYCLIC ANTIDEPRESSANTS

- Tricyclic antidepressants inhibit synaptic uptake of norepinephrine and serotonin.
- These agents could increase the potential for perioperative arrhythmia in the presence of some volatile anesthetics or sympathomimetics, but clinical studies supporting this risk have not been published.
- Abrupt withdrawal of these agents can lead to insomnia, headache, nausea, excess salivation, and diaphoresis.
- ***Recommendation:***
  - Continue tricyclic antidepressants in the perioperative period, especially for patients taking high doses.

ANTIANXIETY AGENTS (BENZODIAZEPINES AND BUSPIRONE)

- Benzodiazepines are commonly used in the perioperative period to reduce anxiety.
- Abrupt withdrawal of a benzodiazepine from a patient on chronic therapy can lead to an excitatory state, including delirium and seizures.
- ***Recommendations:***
  - Continue benzodiazepines and buspirone in the perioperative period.
  - Consider substituting parenteral forms for patients unable to take oral medications.

ANTIPSYCHOTIC AGENTS

- Antipsychotics have antiemetic and sedative properties and have been used as part of anesthesia.
- Experience with the newer antipsychotics (olanzapine, quetiapine, risperidone, ziprasidone) during the perioperative period is limited.
- ***Recommendations:***
  - In general, continue antipsychotics perioperatively.
  - If oral agents cannot be given, parenteral forms such as haloperidol are available in both short- and long-acting preparations.

MONOAMINE OXIDASE INHIBITORS (MAOIs)

- In the presence of MAOIs, routine anesthetic care (e.g., the administration of a sympathomimetic agent such as ephedrine), can lead to massive accumulation of norepinephrine in the central and autonomic nervous systems.
- When administered to patients on MAO inhibitors, meperidine and dextromethorphan can cause the serotonin syndrome, manifest agitation, fever, seizures, coma, and even death.
- ***Recommendations:***
  - If the anesthesiologist is familiar with MAO-safe procedures, these agents can be continued throughout the perioperative period.
  - If MAO inhibitors are continued, order a hospital diet that avoids tyramine-containing foods.
  - If the agents are discontinued, allow 2 weeks before surgery for the effects to resolve.

MOOD-STABILIZING AGENTS (LITHIUM, VALPROIC ACID)

- Lithium mimics sodium and therefore decreases release of neurotransmitters. This can prolong the effect of muscle relaxants.
- Impaired concentration of urine is common in patients on lithium. This can lead to volume depletion and hypernatremia when patients' access to free water is limited in the perioperative period.
- Chronic lithium use can cause hypothyroidism and, less commonly, hyperthyroidism.
- There are no reports of valproic acid causing perioperative complications.
- ***Recommendations:***
  - Continue lithium and valproic acid through the perioperative period. There is no parenteral substitute for lithium. Intravenous valproate sodium (Depacon) can be substituted for patients who usually take valproic acid and are NPO.
  - Special attention should be directed to fluid and electrolyte monitoring, as renal concentrating ability is impaired in patients on lithium.
  - If not done recently, thyroid function should be checked before surgery in patients on lithium.

CHRONIC OPIOID THERAPY

- Many patients are on opioids for treatment of chronic pain.
- Abrupt discontinuation of opioids can cause withdrawal and exacerbate chronic pain.
- Higher doses of opioids may be necessary around the time of surgery to treat surgery-related pain.
- ***Recommendations:***
  - Continue chronic opioids in the perioperative period.
  - Intravenous, intramuscular, and topical preparations can be substituted.
  - Equianalgesic doses of parenteral substitutes should be initiated with the realization that higher doses and rapid dose escalation may be needed temporarily to control surgery-related pain.
  - Perioperative pain management is discussed in Chap. 63.

RHEUMATOLOGIC MEDICATIONS

DISEASE-MODIFYING ANTIRHEUMATIC DRUGS (DMARDS)

- DMARDs include methotrexate, hydroxychloroquine, sulfasalazine, azathioprine, and leflunomide.
- Some DMARDs impair the immune system and could increase the risk of perioperative wound infection or impair wound healing.
- One randomized trial in orthopedic patients found no increased rate of infection in patients who continued weekly methotrexate compared to those who held the agent 2 weeks before surgery.
- Withdrawal of DMARDs can lead to flares of rheumatoid arthritis.
- Many DMARDs are excreted through the kidney. Therefore impaired renal function could result in accumulation of excess medication or metabolites that could generate adverse effects, such as bone marrow suppression.
- ***Recommendations:***
  - In the absence of renal insufficiency, continue methotrexate through the perioperative period.
  - Because of its long half-life, stop leflunomide 2 weeks before surgery and resume it shortly after surgery.
  - Continue sulfasalazine and azathioprine.
  - Hydroxychloroquine has few potential side effects and can be continued through surgery.

ANTICYTOKINES

- Anticytokines, also known as biologically active agents, include etanercept, infliximab, adalimumab, anakinra, and rituximab.
- These agents impair the action of tumor necrosis factor alpha or interleukin-1 receptors.
- ***Recommendation:***
  - Consider discontinuing anticytokines 1 to 2 weeks before surgery and restarting them 1 to 2 weeks after surgery; however, infliximab has been shown to be safe if continued perioperatively.

AGENTS FOR GOUT

- Surgery can lead to flares of gout, likely related to fluid and electrolyte shifts that lead to abrupt changes in uric acid concentration.
- ***Recommendations:***
- Uric acid—lowering drugs such as allopurinol, probenecid, and oral colchicine can be continued throughout the perioperative period.
- Perioperative flares of gout can be treated with nonsteroidal anti-inflammatory drugs (NSAIDs) or oral, systemic, or intraarticular corticosteroids.
- Parenteral colchicine should be avoided because of potential skin necrosis with inadvertent intravenous infiltration.

NEUROLOGIC MEDICATIONS (SEE CHAPS. 38 AND 39)

ANTISEIZURE MEDICATIONS

- Certain anesthetic phases, metabolic derangements, ethanol withdrawal, and intracranial procedures can increase the risk of seizures.

- ***Recommendations:***
  - Antiseizure medications should be continued perioperatively, especially in patients with frequent generalized tonic-clonic seizures.
  - If oral antiseizure medication cannot be taken by a patient with motor seizures, intravenous phenytoin, phenobarbital, or valproate can be substituted.

Agents for Parkinson's Disease

- Patients with Parkinson's disease are predisposed to perioperative morbidity related to swallowing difficulty, pulmonary insufficiency, and delirium.
- Withdrawal of antiparkinson agents can increase disease-related symptoms and cause the neuroleptic malignant syndrome.
- Antiparkinson agents can have deleterious hemodynamic effects in the perioperative period.
- ***Recommendations:***
  - Give levodopa/carbidopa the evening before surgery but hold it until the patient can again take oral medications.
  - Hold levodopa/carbidopa/entacapone preparations longer before surgery.
  - Discontinue tolcapone, which prolongs the action of levodopa/carbidopa, 1 day before surgery.
  - Hold bromocriptine and pergolide the evening before surgery and, as long as the patient is hemodynamically stable, restart them when oral medications are resumed.
  - To avoid precipitating the neuroleptic malignant syndrome, have the patient take ropinirole and pramipexole on the morning of surgery and resume them when the patient is taking oral medications.
  - Selegiline is a monamine oxidase inhibitor. Discontinue it several days before surgery.
  - Parenteral anticholinergic agents such as biperiden, benztropine, and diphenhydramine can be used in Parkinson's patients who cannot take oral medications and in whom symptoms flare in the absence of usual therapy.

Agents for Myasthenia Gravis

- Patients with myasthenia gravis can have respiratory insufficiency related to myasthenic crisis during the perioperative period.
- Management of immunosuppressives such as corticosteroids is covered in Chap. 28.
- ***Recommendations:***
  - Pyridostigmine can be held or continued on the morning of surgery.
  - Short-acting pyridostigmine should be substituted for the long-acting preparation the evening before surgery.
  - Parenteral pyridostigmine can be substituted in patients unable to take oral medications for a prolonged period by using 1/10 of the usual dose for intramuscular and 1/30 of the usual dose for intravenous administration or a continuous infusion at 2 mg/h.

Herbal Medications

- Many patients use herbal medications and health supplements.
- Patients may not reveal use of these therapies during usual questioning; therefore it is important to inquire specifically.
- Some herbal preparations have been associated with excessive perioperative sedation (e.g., kava, valerian) and with bleeding complications (e.g., garlic, ginkgo, ginseng).
- ***Recommendation:***
  - Advise patients to discontinue herbal agents and other health supplements 1 week before surgery.

SUMMARY

- Table 7A-1 summarizes the recommendations discussed.
- As noted previously, evidence regarding management of medications in the perioperative period is often scant. As a result, many of these recommendations are based on limited data, expert opinion, and our personal experience.
- Consider a risk-benefit analysis in making any decision to continue, discontinue, or modify the regimen for any medication.

References

1. Cohn SL. Perioperative medication management. http://pier.acponline.org/physicians/diseases/d835/d835.html [Accessed May 20, 2005.] In PIER [online database]. Philadelphia: American College of Physicians, 2005.
2. Muluk V, Macpherson DS. Perioperative medication management, in Rose BD (ed), *UpToDate*. Wellesley, MA: UpToDate, 2005.
3. Kroenke K, Gooby-Toedt D, Jackson JL. Chronic medications in the perioperative period. *South Med J* 91:358–364, 1998.
4. Smith MS, Muir H, Hall R. Perioperative management of drug therapy. *Drugs* 51:238–259, 1996.
5. Cygan R, Waitzkin H. Stopping and restarting medications in the perioperative period. *J Gen Intern Med* 2:270–283, 1987.

7B PERIOPERATIVE MANAGEMENT OF WARFARIN

Amir K. Jaffer, Scott Kaatz, and Daniel J. Brotman

INTRODUCTION

- Approximately 2 million people in North America take warfarin (Coumadin) to prevent arterial or venous thromboembolism.
- Periprocedural management of patients who take warfarin is often problematic.
  - Warfarin must be discontinued or the dose adjusted to avoid excessive bleeding.
  - This places patients at risk for thromboembolism.
  - Some physicians use either unfractionated heparin (UFH) or low-molecular-weight heparin (LMWH) to anticoagulate patients and "bridge" them to and from the procedure.
  - For some minor procedures, warfarin can be continued without alteration in dose (Table 7B-1).

TABLE 7B-1 Procedures That Can Generally Be Performed without Stopping Warfarin

Dental
Restorations
Endodontics
Prosthetics
Uncomplicated extractions
Dental hygiene treatment
Periodontal therapy
Gastrointestinal
Upper endoscopy with or without biopsy
Flexible sigmoidoscopy with or without biopsy
Colonoscopy with or without biopsy
Endoscopic retrograde cholangiopancreatography without spincterotomy
Biliary stent insertion without spincterotomy
Endosonography without fine-needle aspiration
Push enterosocpy of the small bowel
Electroconvulsive therapy (ECT)
Ophthalmologic
Cataract extraction and lens implantation
Trabeculectomy
Dermatologic
Mohs micrographic surgery
Simple excisions and repairs
Orthopedic
Joint aspiration
Soft tissue injection
Minor podiatric procedures

PATIENT-RELATED RISK FACTORS

- The most important initial question to ask is: "Why is this patient on warfarin?"
  1. Patients take warfarin for many different reasons and may have markedly different risks for thrombotic events when not taking warfarin.
  2. For patients with a history of venous thromboembolism (VTE), the time from the most recent thrombotic episode is the most important risk factor for recurrent VTE when not taking warfarin.
     - Estimates of the daily recurrence rate during the first month (first 4 weeks) after an index event range from 0.3 to 1.3 percent.[1]
     - Over the next 2 months (4 to 12 weeks), the rate ranges from 0.03 to 0.2 percent.[1]
     - Beyond 12 weeks from the index event, the rate is less than 0.05 percent.[1]
     - The daily thrombosis rate when warfarin is not taken may be higher for patients with idiopathic VTE as compared with those who have illness-associated VTE.[2,3]
  3. For patients with atrial fibrillation, there are several additional risk factors for thromboembolism[4–6]:
     - Rheumatic heart disease
     - Prior thomboembolic stroke
     - Age above than 75 years
     - Diabetes
     - Hypertension (particularly when poorly controlled)
     - Coronary artery disease
     - Structural heart disease (e.g., congestive heart failure)
     - Possibly female gender
     - Although the average annual stroke rate in untreated patients with atrial fibrillation is 4 to 5 percent, estimated annual stroke rates for individual patients range from 1 to more than 10 percent, depending on the above risk factors.
     - Patients with none of these risk factors (i.e., "lone" atrial fibrillation) should usually not take warfarin, because they have a low risk of thromboembolism, 1 to 2 percent annually, comparable to the risk in aged-matched patients without atrial fibrillation.
     - Patients with major risk factors for stroke—particularly rheumatic heart disease, prior thromboembolic stroke, or three or more of the risks listed above—are at relatively high risk for thromboembolism from atrial fibrillation.
       - For high-risk patients, consider "bridging" anticoagulation with heparin to minimize the risk of periprocedural thromboembolism.

TABLE 7B-2 Preoperative Evaluation and Risk Stratification

High risk: bridging advised
- Venous or arterial thromboembolism within the preceding 3 months
- Mechanical heart valve
  - In the mitral position
  - Any position with placement in the preceding 3 months
  - Older valves (tilting disk, cage ball)
- History of thromboembolism and known hypercoagulable state
  - Antiphospholipid antibody
  - Homozygous factor V Leiden
  - Multiple genetic defects
  - Protein C or S deficiency
- Acute intracardiac thrombus
- Atrial fibrillation
  - With history of stroke, TIA or systemic embolism
  - Associated with rheumatic valve disease
  - With mechanical valve
  - With multiple risk factors for stroke (see text)

Moderate risk: bridging on a case-by-case basis
- Newer mechanical aortic valve (bi-leaflet)
- Atrial fibrillation with risk factors
- Venous thromboembolism
  - Within the past 3-6 months
  - Idiopathic

Low risk: bridging not recommended
- Venous thromboembolism
  - >6 months ago
  - Heterozygous factor V Leiden
- Atrial fibrillation without risk factors

SOURCE: Modified from Jaffer AK. When patients on warfarin need surgery. *CCJM*, 2003.

4. In patients with mechanical heart valves who are not taking warfarin, the risk of stroke is generally higher than it is in patients with atrial fibrillation (Table 7B-2).
   - Patients with mechanical valves in the mitral position have a risk of thromboembolism about twice that of those with valves in the aortic position.[7]
   - Patients with older-model valves (e.g., ball-in-cage) have a higher risk of thromboembolism than do those with newer-model valves (e.g., St. Jude).[7]

SURGERY-RELATED RISK FACTORS

- The type of surgery can be used to stratify the risk of postoperative VTE, but not the risk of thromboembolism.
  - Surgeries associated with moderate to high VTE risk:
    - Knee and hip arthroplasty
    - Surgery for long-bone fractures
    - Major abdominopelvic surgery
    - Intracranial surgery
- The type of surgery is also directly related to the risk of serious postoperative bleeding.
  - The Johns Hopkins Surgical Bleeding Classification[8] categorizes surgeries by risk of bleeding, ranging from category 1 procedures (low risk) to category 5 (high risk).
    - Category 1—minimal risk: minimally invasive, little or no blood loss (e.g., breast biopsy, cystoscopy)
    - Category 2: Minimally to moderately invasive, estimated blood loss less than 500 mL (e.g., arthroscopy, inguinal hernia repair, laparoscopic cholecystectomy)
    - Category 3: Moderately to significantly invasive, blood loss potential 500 to 1000 mL (e.g., thyroidectomy, laminectomy, hip or knee arthroplasty)
    - Category 4: Highly invasive, blood loss about 1500 mL (e.g., major spinal reconstruction, Whipple procedure)
    - Category 5: Highly invasive, blood loss more than 1500 mL (e.g., intracranial surgery, major head and neck procedure, major vascular surgery, major cardiothoracic surgery)
- Generally, use prophylactic as opposed to treatment doses of anticoagulation for 24 to 48 h after procedures with a high risk of postoperative bleeding.
- The type of anesthesia also affects perioperative anticoagulation management.
  - Placement and removal of epidural or spinal catheters should generally be avoided when a patient is fully anticoagulated with warfarin or heparin.

PREOPERATIVE EVALUATION AND RISK STRATIFICATION

- Periprocedural management of anticoagulation must be individualized.
  - There are no randomized clinical trials that determine which patients should receive bridging therapy.
  - Consider the patient's risk of thromboembolism.
    - In general, patients at high and moderate thromboembolic risk should receive perioperative bridging therapy (see Table 7B-2).
    - In general, patients at low thromboembolic risk should not receive bridging therapy.
  - Consider the patient's risk of serious bleeding.
    - Use the Johns Hopkins Surgical Bleeding Classification to estimate the bleeding risk.
    - Consult with the surgeon or proceduralist.
    - In general, patients undergoing procedures with category 3 or greater bleeding risk should not resume full-dose bridging therapy until hemostasis is secured.
      - This is usually 2 to 3 days after surgery.
  - Consider the risk of adverse medication reactions.
  - Consider the patient's preferences.
  - Use VTE prophylaxis based on the patient's risk for periprocedural VTE (see Chap. 46).

WARFARIN DISCONTINUATION

- The target periprocedural international normalized ratio (INR) depends on the type of procedure.
  - Most procedures in otherwise hemostatically normal patients can be performed with minimal risk of serious bleeding at an INR below 1.5.
  - For neurosurgical procedures, cardiac procedures, and some major noncardiac procedures, an INR below 1.2 is preferred.
- The best method to lower the INR depends on the preprocedural steady-state INR and the time available before the procedure.
  - White et al.[9] showed that for almost all patients with a steady-state INR of 2 to 3, the INR falls to below 1.5 within 115 h (4.8 days) after warfarin is discontinued.
  - If the preoperative INR is greater than 3 and/or the patient is elderly, more time may be required for the INR to drop below 1.5.
  - Therefore, if time allows, have patients whose preoperative INR is 2 to 3 stop taking warfarin 5 days (four doses) before the procedure.
  - Have patients whose preoperative INR is above 3 or who are elderly stop taking warfarin 6 days (five doses) before the procedure.
- If the procedure is emergent, use fresh frozen plasma (FFP) and/or vitamin K to lower the INR and reverse the effects of warfarin.
  - FFP works immediately.
    - FFP does not cause resistance to warfarin anticoagulation after the procedure.
    - After FFP administration, monitor the INR at least every few hours to determine the need for additional treatment, because the effects of FFP will dissipate over a few hours.
    - FFP treatment incurs the risks of blood component transfusion.
  - Recombinant activated factor VII (NovoSeven) may become a more specific treatment for the emergent reversal of warfarin effect without the risks of transfusion; however, it is currently not adequately tested. It is also exorbitantly expensive and not the standard of care.
  - Vitamin K can also reverse the effects of warfarin.
    - Reversal usually begins 15 min after intravenous or oral administration and peaks in 4 to 8 h.
    - Do not administer vitamin K intramuscularly; the absorption is erratic and the effects are less reliable than with intravenous or oral administration.
    - Do not administer doses greater than 2 mg intravenously; seizures have been reported.
    - Depending on the preprocedural INR, a large dose of vitamin K (10 mg or more) will usually result in resistance to warfarin for at least several days after the procedure and may prolong hospitalization.

BRIDGING THERAPY

- Both UFH and LMWH can be used for bridging therapy.
  - Use of UFH usually requires at least 2 days of hospitalization prior to the procedure.
    - Standard care is to start with a bolus of 80 U/kg body weight and a continuous intravenous infusion of 18 U/kg body weight/h that is then adjusted hourly to a target partial thromboplastin time (PTT) of 60 to 80 s.
    - Stop the intravenous heparin at least 4 h before the procedure (6 h for patients with renal insufficiency).
  - The predictable pharmacokinetics and the bioavailability of subcutaneous LMWH allow it to be used in the outpatient setting, saving the costs of hospitalization (Table 7B-3).

SPECIAL CONSIDERATIONS WITH NEURAXIAL BLOCAKADE

- Symptomatic epidural hematomas can develop if a spinal or epidural catheter is inserted into or removed from an anticoagulated patient. Therefore anticoagulated patients receiving neuraxial blockade require special considerations both pre- and postoperatively.

TABLE 7B-3 Protocol for Bridging Therapy with Low-Molecular-Weight Heparin

Preprocedure protocol

If INR is 2 to 3, stop warfarin 5 days (four doses) before the procedure.
If the INR is 3 to 4.5, stop warfarin 6 days (five doses) before the procedure.
Start LMWH* 36 h after the last warfarin dose.
Give the last dose of LMWH 24 h before the procedure.
Ensure that the patient is thoroughly educated in self-injection, including providing written instructions and a contact phone number for questions and problems.
Confer with the surgeon and the anesthesiologist to plan treatment.
Check the INR on morning of the procedure.

Postproedure protocol

Restart LMWH* approximately 24 h postprocedure or consider using a thromboprophylaxis dose of LMWH** on postprocedure days 1 to 3 if the patient is at high risk for bleeding.
Confer with the surgeon to make sure that he or she is comfortable with the planned start time for anticoagulant therapy.
On postoperative day 1, restart warfarin at the patient's preoperative dose.
Obtain the PT/INR daily until the patient is discharged.
After discharge, obtain the PT/INR periodically (e.g., Monday, Wednesday, and Friday) until the INR is therapeutic.
Obtain CBC with platelet count periodically (e.g., every third day) while patient is on both warfarin and LMWH.
Discontinue LMWH when the INR is 2 to 3 for 2 consecutive days.

Inclusion criteria

Age above 18 years.
Patient needs LMWH.
Treating physician thinks patient needs bridge therapy.
Medically and hemodynamically stable.
Scheduled for elective procedure or surgery.

Exclusion criteria

Allergy to UFH or LMWH.
Weight more than 150 kg.
Pregnant woman with a mechanical valve.
History of bleeding disorder or intracranial hemorrhage.
GI bleeding within the last 10 days.
Major trauma, or stroke within the previous 2 weeks.
History of HIT or severe thrombocytopenia.
Language barriers.
Potential for medication noncompliance.
Unsuitable home environment to support therapy.
Severe liver disease.

CBC = complete blood count; HIT = heparin-induced thrombocytopenia; INR = international normalized ratio; LMWH = low-molecular-weight heparin; PT = prothrombin time; UFH = unfractionated heparin.
*Enoxaparin 1 mg/kg subcutaneously q12h or 1.5 mg/kg q24h or dalteparin 120 U/kg q12h or dalteparin 200 U/kg q24h.
†For patients with a creatinine clearance below 30 mL/min, consider using unfractionated heparin (UFH) or enoxaparin 1 mg/kg subcutaneously q24h for full-dose LWMH and 30 mg q24h for prophylactic dose.
**Enoxaparin 40 mg SC qd or enoxaparin 30 mg SC q12h or dalteparin 5000 IU SC qd.

The American Society of Regional Anesthesia (ASRA) has specific recommendations, available online at www.asra.com.[10] A few salient points are summarized below.

- Concurrent administration of heparin and warfarin or agents that affect other components of the clotting system—such as antiplatelet agents, oral anticoagulants, and dextran—increases the risk of bleeding complications with neuraxial blockade in an unpredictable fashion and is therefore generally contraindicated.
- UFH
  - Prophylactic subcutaneous UFH (minidose) does not contraindicate neuraxial blockade.
  - The risk of neuraxial bleeding may be reduced by delaying the first heparin injection until after the block.
- LMWH
  - The anti-Xa level is not predictive of bleeding risk and therefore not helpful in managing patients undergoing neuraxial blockade.
  - If there is blood or other evidence of trauma during needle and catheter placement, initiation of LMWH should be delayed for 24 h postoperatively.
  - Preoperative LMWH
    - For patients receiving *thrombophylactic* doses of LMWH, needle placement should occur no sooner than 12 h after the most recent LMWH dose.
    - For patients receiving higher (*treatment*) doses of LMWH (enoxaparin 1 mg/kg every 12 h, enoxaparin 1.5 mg/kg daily, dalteparin 120 U/kg every 12 h, dalteparin 200 U/kg daily, or tinzaparin 175 U/kg daily), needle placement should occur no sooner than 24 h after the most recent LMWH dose.
  - Postoperative LMWH
    - Twice-daily prophylactic dosing regimens may be associated with an increased risk of spinal hematoma. The first dose of LMWH should be administered no sooner than 24 h postoperatively and at least 2 h after neuraxial catheter removal.
    - Single-daily-dosing regimens are apparently safer. Indwelling neuraxial catheters may be safely maintained. The first postoperative LMWH dose should be administered no sooner than 6 h postoperatively. The second postoperative dose should be administered no sooner than 24 h after the first dose. The catheter can be removed 12 h after a dose of LMWH. An LMWH dose can be administered 2h after the catheter is removed.
- Warfarin
  - Early after discontinuation of warfarin, the prothrombin time/international normalized ratio (PT/INR) reflects predominantly factor VII levels and, in spite of acceptable factor VII levels, levels of factors II and X may not be adequate for normal hemostasis. Adequate levels of factors II, VII, IX, and X may not be present until the PT/INR is within normal limits.

- Prior to neuraxial blockade, check the PT/INR of patients who received an initial dose of warfarin more than 24 h prior to surgery.
- Monitor PT/INR daily in patients receiving warfarin during epidural analgesia.
- Try to remove neuraxial catheters before the INR rises above 1.5.
- Continue routine neurologic testing of sensory and motor function for at least 24 h after the neuraxial catheter is removed and longer if the INR was greater than 1.5 at the time of catheter removal.

REFERENCES

1. Kearon C, Hirsh J. Management of anticoagulation before and after elective surgery. *N Engl J Med* 336:1506, 1997.
2. Kearon C, Gent M, Hirsh J, et al. A comparison of three months of anticoagulation with extended anticoagulation for a first episode of idiopathic venous thromboembolism. *N Engl J Med* 340:901, 1999.
3. Pinede L, Cucherat M, Duhaut P, et al. Optimal duration of anticoagulant therapy after an episode of venous thromboembolism. *Blood Coagul Fibrinolysis* 11:701, 2000.
4. Cardiogenic brain embolism. Cerebral Embolism Task Force. *Arch Neurol* 43:71, 1986.
5. Wang TJ, Massaro JM, Levy D, et al. A risk score for predicting stroke or death in individuals with new-onset atrial fibrillation in the community: The Framingham Heart Study. *JAMA* 290:1049, 2003.
6. Gage BF, Waterman AD, Shannon W, et al. Validation of clinical classification schemes for predicting stroke: Results from the National Registry of Atrial Fibrillation. *JAMA* 285:2864, 2001.
7. Cannegieter SC, Rosendaal FR, Briet E. Thromboembolic and bleeding complications in patients with mechanical heart valve prostheses. *Circulation* 89:635, 1994.
8. Pasternak L. Preoperative assessment of the ambulatory and same-day admission patient. *Wellcome Trends Anesthesiol* 9:3, 1991.
9. White RH, McKittrick T, Hutchinson R, et al. Temporary discontinuation of warfarin therapy: Changes in the international normalized ratio. *Ann Intern Med* 122:40, 1995.
10. Horlocker TT, Wedel DJ, Benzon H, et al. Regional anesthesia in the anticoagulated patient: Defining the risks (the second ASRA Consensus Conference on Neuraxial Anesthesia and Anticoagulation). *Reg Anesth Pain Med* 28:172, 2003.

Section II
SURGERY-SPECIFIC RISKS

Harrison G. Weed, MD, Section Editor

8 ABDOMINAL SURGERY

Kenneth Gilbert and Vaishali M. Singh

INTRODUCTION

GENERAL CONSIDERATIONS

- Abdominal surgery is performed for the diagnosis and treatment of many diseases, such as acid-peptic disorders, biliary disease, intestinal disease, cancer, bleeding, obstruction, and trauma.
- One important consideration in abdominal surgery is the type and location of the incision, including transection of muscle and fascia, disruption of nerves, blood loss, and ultimate cosmetic appearance.
  - Improvements in surgical technique, technology, and anesthesia have made it possible to perform many abdominal procedures with minimally invasive techniques using a laparoscope.
  - Advantages of minimally invasive surgeries include more rapid closure, faster postoperative recovery, smaller scars, and decreased adhesion formation.
  - Advantages of open procedures include more rapid entry and fuller exposure of abdominal contents.
  - Open procedures can also often be performed more quickly.

COMPLICATIONS

- The incidence of pulmonary complications is greater after upper abdominal surgeries due to restrictive effects on pulmonary mechanics from pain and splinting.
- Patients undergoing abdominal surgery are at high risk for venous thromboembolism (VTE).
  - Colorectal surgery carries one of the highest risks.
- In this chapter we review patient-related risk factors, procedure-related risk factors, and aspects of preoperative preparation and postoperative management of abdominal surgeries.

PATIENT-RELATED RISK FACTORS

ANEMIA

- Anemia is commonly encountered in patients undergoing abdominal surgery
  - It is more common in patients with cancer, gastrointestinal bleeding, malnutrition, and renal disease.
  - Blood loss during abdominal surgeries can be moderate and can compromise hemodynamic stability.
  - Anemia can exacerbate cardiac disease and impair wound healing (see Chap. 30).

OBESITY

- The mortality rate in obese patients undergoing gastrointestinal surgery is 6.6 percent, compared with 2.6 percent in nonobese patients.
  - Obese patients are more likely to have comorbid conditions, including hypertension, diabetes, gastrointestinal reflux, left ventricular hypertrophy, hypoventilation syndrome, obstructive sleep apnea, pulmonary hypertension, and right ventricular failure.
  - Obesity is a risk factor for venous thromboembolism and for surgical site infection.
    - This might be partly due to inadequate dosing of prophylactic anticoagulants and antimicrobials.
  - Morbid obesity has been identified as a risk factor for surgical site infection, hematoma formation, and dehiscence.
  - A large, protruding panniculus distorts the topography of the abdominal wall, making the usual surface-anatomic reference points unreliable.

- Obese patients are at risk for postoperative pulmonary complications after abdominal surgery; however, after adjusting for comorbid conditions, obesity is not an independent risk factor (see Chaps. 24 and 41).
- Intraoperative pressure and nerve injuries are more common in obese patients, those requiring prolonged operations, and when self-retaining retractors are employed to aid exposure in abdominal procedures.
  - Brachial plexus injury can be caused either by extreme abduction of the arms or by the excessive weight of the patient's outstretched arms.

MALNUTRITION

- Abdominal surgery can cause metabolic and other stresses that can compromise nutrition and exacerbate preexisting malnutrition.
  - Malnutrition compromises immune function, muscle strength, and wound healing, increasing the likelihood of surgical-site infection, sepsis, pneumonia, respiratory failure, and prolonged recovery.
  - Extraordinary nutritional support is appropriate for some patients (see Chap. 49).

PROCEDURE-RELATED RISK FACTORS

LAPAROSCOPY

- Complications of laparoscopy include bowel injury, urologic injury, vascular injury during trocar insertion, biliary/hepatic injury, and prolonged absorption of carbon dioxide gas leading to hypercarbia, acidosis, and respiratory depression.
  - Mortality associated with laparoscopy is low, but it is greater with more extensive procedures.

LAPAROTOMY

- Complications of laparotomy include abdominal wall hematoma, postoperative pain with respiratory splinting, less appealing cosmetic results from large incisions, and abdominal wall/bowel herniation.

PREOPERATIVE PREPARATION

- A successful surgery, whether open or laparoscopic, should begin with proper planning, including defining the anatomy previous to surgery with the use of ultrasound, computed tomography (CT), magnetic resonance imaging (MRI), or other special studies such as fistulograms when appropriate. This is especially true for patients who have undergone previous abdominal surgery in which normal expected anatomy can be altered. However, this is not always possible for patients requiring emergency surgery.
- Preoperative bowel preparation or cleansing is frequently recommended prior to abdominal surgery. Bowel preparation is believed to decrease the morbidity and mortality of colon surgery as well as the incidence of wound infection. Despite a century of surgical dogma that mechanical bowel preparation prior to colon and rectal surgery is essential, a recent meta-analysis failed to demonstrate a consistent benefit of bowel preparation in reducing the incidence of anastomotic leakage, peritonitis, wound infection, reoperation, or mortality.[7]
- Broad-spectrum antibiotics given at the time of surgery help to reduce wound infections rates, but it should also be understood that they can cause antibiotic-associated diarrhea and colitis (see Chap. 48).
- Anticipate surgical blood loss and need for transfusion. Refer appropriate patients for autologous blood banking.
- Proper patient positioning and the use of small, well-padded retractor blades intraoperatively protects against pressure sores and nerve injuries.
- Assess nutritional status. In malnourished patients, total parental nutrition (TPN) given to patients for 7 to 10 days before surgery for GI malignancy was found to reduce postoperative complications by 10 percent (mortality rates remained unchanged). In addition, use of early postoperative TPN in patients who did not receive preoperative TPN also decreased postoperative complications by 10 percent.
- Awareness of associated risk factors and prophylaxis against VTE is essential (see Chap. 46).

ROLE OF ANESTHESIA AND OPERATIVE TECHNIQUE

GENERAL ANESTHESIA

- The vast majority of patients undergoing abdominal surgery will undergo general anesthesia (GA). Neuromuscular blocking agents are frequently employed to relax the abdominal musculature. Thus, intubation and ventilation are integral components of most abdominal surgical procedures, and most of these patients are exposed to the risks associated with GA and paralysis (see Chap. 6).

NEURAXIAL BLOCKADE

- Modern anesthetic technique for abdominal surgery may include neuraxial blockade in addition to GA. Thoracic epidural anesthesia (TEA) in particular provides benefit in terms of improved pain management, reduced need for opioid analgesics, and a reduction in myocardial oxygen demand.

LAPAROSCOPIC VERSUS OPEN PROCEDURES

- Abdominal surgeries that previously required open laparotomy are increasingly being performed laparoscopically. Laparoscopic cholecystectomy is the standard of care for the majority of patients with gallbladder disease requiring surgery. Other procedures now being performed laparoscopically include nephrectomy, adrenalectomy, splenectomy, inguinal hernia repair, colectomy, and a variety of gynecologic procedures.
- Patient recovery times are significantly reduced when open laparotomy can be avoided. However, complications related to laparoscopic surgery may occur, including perforated viscus, bladder trauma, CO_2 retention with respiratory acidosis, or hemorrhage due to vascular injury.
- Some patients may be unsuitable for laparoscopic surgery, including those with marked bowel distention, extensive adhesions due to prior surgery, very large tumor masses, or diaphragmatic hernias. Other procedures must be done with an open laparotomy for technical reasons. Overall patient risk is expected to be greater in these situations.

POSTOPERATIVE MANAGEMENT

USUAL POSTOPERATIVE COURSE

- The majority of abdominal surgeries are uncomplicated and the care of these patients is generally managed entirely by the surgical team. Nonetheless, the consultant should be aware of the expected course of recovery from abdominal surgery, particularly when asked to assess a patient postoperatively.

COMMON COMPLICATIONS

ILEUS

- Postoperative ileus is a common and expected consequence of laparotomy and especially bowel resection. The small intestine generally recovers function within several hours of surgery and the stomach recovers within 24 to 48 h, but the colon is not expected to return to normal function for 3 to 5 days. Impairment of bowel peristalsis lasting longer than this is considered prolonged ileus.
- Some anesthetic agents are associated with impaired bowel motility, and the use of opioid analgesics postoperatively is associated with a prolongation of impaired bowel function in a dose-response relationship.
- The use of TEA has been shown to reduce the degree and duration of ileus. Other treatments, such as early feeding, gut motility–enhancing drugs (e.g., metoclopramide), or early ambulation are often employed but have not been demonstrated to be consistently effective in randomized trials.[8]

PNEUMONIA

- Pneumonia occurs in 0.2 to 15.3 percent of patients undergoing abdominal surgery and is related to the presence of a variety of risk factors, including type of procedure, general anesthesia, advanced patient age, physical dependency, poor nutritional status, alcohol use, smoking, a diagnosis of chronic obstructive pulmonary disease, history of stroke or impaired sensorium, elevated blood urea nitrogen, and preoperative transfusion (see Chaps. 24 and 54).

OTHER INFECTIONS

- Common infections in patients undergoing abdominal surgery include infection of the surgical wound, anastomotic leaks with peritonitis, and infections that may occur with any type of surgery (e.g., venous catheter, urinary tract). For a discussion of surgical wound prophylaxis, see Chap. 28. Postoperative fever is discussed in Chap. 50.

CARDIAC COMPLICATIONS

- Myocardial infarction, arrhythmia, pulmonary edema, and cardiac arrest are relatively more common in patients undergoing major abdominal surgery than in those having most other operations other than cardiovascular procedures. Patients deemed to be at high risk for cardiac events (see Chap. 20) should be observed closely in the postoperative period.

VENOUS THROMBOEMBOLISM

- Abdominal surgery represents a known risk factor for venous thromboembolism; perioperative prophylaxis is generally recommended (see Chap. 46). A detailed discussion of perioperative thromboembolic complications can be found in Chap. 55.

HEMORRHAGE AND TRANSFUSION

- Significant blood loss may occur with major abdominal operations. Although the decision to transfuse blood should depend on clinical symptoms (see Chap. 59), this decision is usually in the hands of the surgical team. Patients may thus receive blood products for a variety of indications and will be at risk for transfusion-related complications such as fever, hemolysis, or infection.

SUMMARY

- Abdominal surgery is performed for a variety of indications.
- Many operations that used to require laparotomy are being performed laparoscopically, with fewer complications and more rapid recovery times.
- Factors influencing perioperative risk include comorbid illness, anemia, nutritional status, and the specific procedure planned.
- Certain complications may be anticipated and prophylactic measures taken to prevent them preoperatively.

REFERENCES

1. Farshad A, Bell R. Assessment and management of the obese patient. *Crit Care Med* 32:S87, 2004.
2. Pettit P, Sevin BU. Intraoperative injury to the gastrointestinal tract and postoperative gastrointestinal emergencies. *Clin Obstet Gynecol* 45(2):469–480, 2002.
3. Bergqvist D. Low molecular weight heparin for the prevention of venous thromboembolism after abdominal surgery. *BMJ* 91:965, 2004.
4. Dillavou ED, Anderson LR, Bernert RA, et al. Lower extremity nerve injury due to compression during intraabdominal surgery. *Am J Surg* 173:504, 1997.
5. Huckleberry Y. Nutritional support and the surgical patient. *Am J Health Syst Pharm* 64:671, 2004.
6. Magrina J. Complications of laparoscopic surgery. *Clin Obstet Gynecol* 45(2):469–480, 2002.
7. Guenaga KF, Matos D, Castro AA, et al. Mechanical bowel preparation for elective colorectal surgery. *Cochrane Database Syst Rev* 2:CD001544, 2003.
8. Baig MK, Wexner SD. Postoperative ileus: A review. *Dis Colon Rectum* 47:516, 2004.

9 THORACIC SURGERY AND LUNG RESECTION

Joann Porter and Gerald W. Smetana

INTRODUCTION

- Patients undergoing thoracic surgery have a high prevalence of cardiac and pulmonary disease, putting them at risk for perioperative medical complications.
- Patient selection is important in order to identify patients with a high likelihood of satisfactory postoperative functional status.

PREOPERATIVE EVALUATION

- Preoperative evaluation of patients for possible lung resection serves two purposes.
  - In the case of resection for suspected non-small cell lung cancer, evaluation serves to exclude patients who have no reasonable likelihood of a surgical cure. This avoids potentially high-risk surgery for those patients in whom surgery would not provide a cure or prolong survival. For example, one would not propose surgery for patients with known metastatic disease.
  - Among patients who may be potentially cured by lung resection, the remainder of the evaluation seeks to determine if the patient is likely to tolerate surgery well and have an acceptable functional status after surgery.
- As the risk of mortality for patients with untreated lung cancer will approach 100 percent over time, one should not deny surgery unless good evidence suggests that the patient will have poor functional status or a high risk of postoperative complications.
- Overall mortality rates for lung resection surgery range from 7 to 11 percent.[1]
- General principles of preoperative assessment, including preoperative cardiac risk stratification (see Chap. 20), apply to all patients preparing for lung resection.
- In addition, a variety of physiologic tests exists to estimate a patient's fitness for surgery, pulmonary reserve, and likelihood of an acceptable postoperative functional status. Clinicians should consider these tests as a series of sequential steps. Patients with acceptable results of initial physiologic tests need no further evaluation. Patients who fail to pass first-line tests should proceed to the next step of evaluation. The potential tests are, in order, spirometry, diffusing capacity, predicted postoperative lung function, and functional capacity testing.

SPIROMETRY

- The forced expiratory capacity in 1 s (FEV_1) has been an important tool to stratify risk for lung resection for decades.
- Screening spirometry is indicated for all candidates for lung resection.
- Patients undergoing pneumonectomy with an FEV_1 >2 L (or >80 percent predicted) or those undergoing lobectomy with an FEV_1 >1.5 L have acceptable levels of perioperative mortality (<5 percent).
- According to a recent evidence-based guideline from the American College of Chest Physicians, patients

who meet these criteria may proceed to lung resection surgery with no further evaluation.[2]

DIFFUSING CAPACITY

- Diffusing capacity (DL_{CO}) provides complementary information to spirometry regarding physiologic fitness for lung resection surgery.
- Not all patients preparing for lung resection require measurement of diffusing capacity. Clinicians should obtain this test for those with interstitial lung disease, demonstrated by chest radiography, or exertional dyspnea that is more than expected based on clinical evaluation.
- If the DL_{CO} and the FEV_1 are both >80 percent predicted, the patient may proceed to surgery with no additional evaluation.

PREDICTED POSTOPERATIVE LUNG FUNCTION

- For patients at higher-than-average risk by virtue of the above tests, the next step is to estimate the predicted postoperative lung function to determine if this falls within an acceptable range.
- The most commonly performed test is a quantitative ventilation/perfusion scan. This test estimates the contribution of each lobe to total lung ventilation. One can estimate the predicted postoperative FEV_1 based on the fraction of total ventilation remaining after the proposed surgery multiplied by preoperative FEV_1.
- Patients whose predicted postoperative FEV_1 is >40 percent have an acceptable degree of risk and can proceed to surgery without further evaluation.[2]

TESTING OF FUNCTIONAL CAPACITY

- Certain patients who fail to meet the above criteria may still be candidates for lung resection. Additional testing for this group of patients seeks to estimate overall fitness as determined by testing of functional capacity. These tests will distinguish between lower- and higher-risk candidates as determined by estimates of predicted postoperative lung function.
- The most commonly employed test is cardiopulmonary stress testing. In this test, patients exercise on a treadmill and their endurance is tested. In contrast to traditional cardiac stress testing, the primary outcome measure is maximal oxygen consumption. Patients who can exercise to obtain a maximum oxygen consumption of >20 mL/kg/min have a low risk of postoperative complications and death.[3] For those with a maximal oxygen consumption of <10 mL/kg/min, the risk is sufficiently high to consider the patient ineligible for surgery.
- Observed stair climbing provides an alternate assessment of fitness for surgery and is an option if cardiopulmonary stress testing is not available in a particular institution. In this test, patients are asked to walk up stairs at a normal pace and to stop based on symptoms. A continuous inverse relationship exists between stair-climbing capacity and risk for postoperative complications. Patients who can climb at least three flights of stairs have a low risk of postoperative complications (positive predictive value 64 percent, negative predictive value 84 percent).[4] Those who cannot walk at least one flight of stairs are at high risk for surgery and are not acceptable candidates for lung resection.

TESTING OF ARTERIAL BLOOD GAS

- Contrary to earlier belief, hypercapnia ($PaCO_2$ >45 mmHg) is not a consistent predictor of risk after lung resection and is not a contraindication to surgery.
- Hypoxemia (O_2 saturation <90 percent) does appear to increase risk for lung resection. These patients should also undergo testing of functional capacity during the preoperative evaluation.[2]

COMMON COMORBID CONDITIONS

CHRONIC OBSTRUCTIVE PULMONARY DISEASE

- Given the shared risk factor of cigarette smoking, chronic obstructive pulmonary disease (COPD) is common among candidates for lung resection.
- COPD is an important contributor to the morbidity and mortality of lung resection surgery. Most patients who fail spirometric or functional capacity criteria for surgery do so by virtue of COPD.
- Cigarette use is an independent risk factor for the development of postoperative pulmonary complications even among those patients without apparent COPD.

OBESITY

- Contrary to common belief, obesity is not a risk factor for postoperative pulmonary complications after lung resection.
- The presence of obesity should not influence patient selection for lung resection.
- Obesity is, however, a risk factor for postoperative venous thromboembolism (VTE) (see Chap. 46).

CORONARY ARTERY DISEASE

- Coronary artery disease (CAD) is common among lung resection candidates due in part to the high incidence of

cigarette use in this cohort. The incidence is approximately 10 percent.
- CAD confers a threefold increase in risk of mortality after lung resection surgery.[5]
- An assessment of perioperative cardiac risk should be part of the evaluation of all candidates for lung resection.

PREOPERATIVE PREPARATION

- Preoperative strategies to reduce pulmonary complications after lung surgery include the well-established interventions described for patients undergoing noncardiothoracic surgery (see Chap. 24). Strategies of particular relevance for the patient undergoing lung resection follow.
- Patients who smoke cigarettes should, when possible, stop smoking at least 8 weeks before surgery. Briefer periods of abstinence may paradoxically increase the risk of postoperative pulmonary complications.
- For patients with COPD or asthma, treat airflow obstruction maximally to bring the patient to his or her optimal baseline level of function. Treatment strategies are the same as those used in the nonoperative setting. See Chaps. 24 and 25 for a detailed discussion of these strategies.
- The indiscriminate use of preoperative antibiotics does not reduce surgical risk. However, if lower respiratory tract infection is present, one should delay elective surgery and treat with antibiotics. The risk of viral respiratory tract infection is unknown and probably small, but the customary practice is to defer elective surgery in this instance.
- Postoperative strategies to reduce risk, such as incentive spirometry, are more effective if patients are instructed in their use before surgery. For high-risk patients, consider outpatient consultation with chest physical therapy before surgery.
- Optimize nutritional status for patients who are malnourished (see Chap. 49).
- As obesity is not a risk factor for pulmonary complications after lung resection and the benefit of weight loss before elective surgery is unknown, clinicians should not recommend weight loss for obese patients in the immediate preoperative period.

ANESTHETIC TECHNIQUE AND OPERATIVE PATHOPHYSIOLOGY

- Notify the anesthesiologist if the patient has a history of asthma or COPD, as this will influence the choice of anesthesia. Surgical manipulation can further increase bronchospasm, and the anesthesiologist can choose a halogenated anesthetic that will reduce airway reactivity.

POSTOPERATIVE MANAGEMENT

- Thoracic surgery carries a high risk of pulmonary complications. Important risk-reduction strategies include lung expansion maneuvers along with adequate pain control and nutrition (see Chaps. 63 and 49).

USUAL POSTOPERATIVE COURSE

- Effective preoperative and postoperative strategies exist to minimize postoperative complications.
- Pulmonary complications are the leading cause of morbidity after thoracic surgery.
- In addition to previous underlying lung disease, other factors that contribute to risk of postoperative complications include positioning during surgery, mismatch of ventilation/perfusion due to surgical manipulation of lung parenchyma and/or vessels, and airway instrumentation. After surgery, decreased cough and inhibition of deep breathing due to pain contribute to risk.

SURGERY-SPECIFIC CONSIDERATIONS

- Mediastinoscopy: Overall complication rates are 1.5 to 3 percent, including hemorrhage, pneumothorax, chylothorax, injury to the recurrent laryngeal nerve, air embolism, and transient hemiparesis.
- Thoracoscopic surgery (including video assisted thoracoscopic surgery, or VATS): Pneumothorax is unavoidable but rarely requires a chest tube.
- Tracheal resection: An arterial line is recommended. Extubate patients as early as possible to reduce pressure from inflated tracheal cuff. Keep the patient's head flexed in order to reduce tension on the suture line. Even though aspiration risk is high, avoid vigorous chest physiotherapy. If secretions are a problem, use bronchoscopy for removal. Bleeding into the airway is a surgical emergency because it indicates erosion into the pulmonary artery or aorta.
- Bullectomy: Reexpansion of the lung may impair hemodynamics and require positive inotropic support. Pneumothorax is common. Patients may require prolonged mechanical ventilation postoperatively; this confers a higher risk for ventilator-associated pneumonia.
- Surgery to reduce lung volume: Monitor patients for positive-pressure air leaks. If possible, avoid intravenous narcotics and use epidural analgesia for pain control. In ventilating the patient, utilize permissive hypercapnia to optimize oxygenation.
- Mediastinal tumor resection: Monitor the airway carefully because of the risk of airway edema and obstruction after surgery.
- Pneumonectomy/lobectomy: Bronchopleural fistula and prolonged air leak are common surgery-specific

complications; however, nosocomial pneumonia is the most important predictor of morbidity and mortality.

COMMON POSTOPERATIVE PROBLEMS AND SOLUTIONS

- Hypoxemia can develop from decreased FiO_2, hypoventilation, V/Q mismatch, shunt, and low cardiac output, especially in presence of intrapulmonary shunt.
- A specific consideration for the postpneumonectomy patient is a right-to-left shunt occurring in a patient with a preexisting asymptomatic atrial septal defect that becomes symptomatic after vascular interruption during surgery. This results from increased right heart pressure that results from a marked decrease in the pulmonary vascular bed.
- Hypoventilation: Keep the patient upright in bed and encourage him or her to get out of bed and ambulate as soon as possible. These strategies can increase functional residual capacity (FRC) by 10 to 20 percent. Encourage patients on narcotics to breathe deeply and cough.
- Atelectasis/pleural effusions: Atelectasis is common after thoracic surgery and is generally well tolerated by patients without impaired lung function. Both narcotics and poorly controlled pain can exacerbate atelectasis.
  - Educate patients before surgery about respiratory therapy protocols.
  - Prescribe incentive spirometry (IS) or deep breathing. Data on chest percussion and drainage are conflicting, but these strategies may be useful in patients with chronic bronchitis who produce a large amount of sputum.
  - Intermittent positive-pressure ventilation is no more effective than IS or deep breathing and can cause barotrauma, especially in patients with bullous emphysema.
  - Use continuous positive airway pressure (CPAP) in patients who do not respond to IS or deep breathing and in those who cannot cooperate with IS.
  - Major lobar atelectasis may actually represent pulmonary infarction or other processes such as mucous plugging. Consider bronchoscopy for refractory cases.
  - For more details about the management of postoperative atelectasis, see Chap. 54.
- Acute respiratory failure is defined as the need for mechanical ventilation for more than 48 h postoperatively. These patients are at higher risk for postoperative complications.
- No studies have evaluated noninvasive positive-pressure ventilation in respiratory failure after thoracotomy, but clinicians may consider this strategy for patients with COPD and for those who have advance directives against intubation.
- Postoperative stridor is a medical emergency that requires immediate anesthesia or consultation with an ear/nose/throat (ENT) specialist to rule out laryngeal edema and establish effective ventilation.
- Noncardiogenic pulmonary edema occurs in 2 to 5 percent of patients who have had a pneumonectomy. It is three times more common in right-sided versus left-sided pneumonectomies.[6] Other causes include upper airway obstruction, reexpansion pulmonary edema, and adult respiratory distress syndrome (ARDS). Noncardiogenic pulmonary edema results from vascular endothelial injury and has a high mortality rate.
  - It usually develops in the first 48 to 72 h after surgery; dyspnea and hypoxemia are presenting findings.
  - The physical examination and chest x-ray are often initially unremarkable but progress rapidly to rales and diffuse pulmonary infiltrates, respectively.
  - Diuretics are not effective in the treatment of noncardiogenic pulmonary edema.
  - Inhaled nitric oxide has been shown to improve gas exchange in case reports (no RCT data are available).
  - Use ventilator settings that minimize barotrauma.
  - Sedate patients adequately while they are on ventilators.
- Nosocomial pneumonia is common after thoracic surgery (see Chap. 54 for more details). COPD, prior antibiotic use, chronic illnesses, mechanical ventilation, and immobilization are additional risk factors.
  - The pathogens are often polymicrobial and include gram-negatives, anaerobes, and staphylococci. The common gram-negatives are *Pseudomonas, Escherichia coli*, and *Klebsiella*.
  - Postoperative pneumonia occurs more commonly after right than after left pneumonectomy.
  - The diagnosis is often confused with atelectasis due to overlapping signs and symptoms that may include a minor elevation in white blood cell count, low-grade fever, and abnormalities on chest x-ray.
  - Delayed treatment can result in progression to respiratory failure.
  - Guide initial antibiotic treatment based on the antimicrobial resistance pattern at the local institution.
- Cardiogenic pulmonary edema: Patients who have received large volumes of intravenous fluids in the perioperative period are at risk for postoperative volume overload and pulmonary edema.
- Bronchospasm is very common postoperatively. Causes include aspiration, allergic response, exacerbation of underlying lung disease, and histamine release secondary to medication (examples include morphine and drugs used during anesthesia, such as tubocurarine and atracurium). The treatment is removal of any offending agent, bronchodilators, and steroids. Corticosteroids do not increase the risk of postoperative infections. See Chap. 25 for the management of COPD and asthma. If wheezing does not respond to routine treatment, consider

increased airway resistance due to mechanical factors such as pulmonary edema or postoperative tissue swelling.

- Embolic phenomena: Administer appropriate VTE prophylaxis for all patients (see Chap. 46).
- Pleural effusions occur more than 80 percent of the time in thoracic surgeries and usually resolve on their own. Benign effusions are small, asymptomatic, and present within 48 h. Perform a thoracentesis for pleural effusions that are symptomatic or that progress. The differential includes pneumonia, empyema, pulmonary embolus, chylothorax, hemothorax, malignant effusions, and congestive heart failure.

INFECTIOUS COMPLICATIONS

EMPYEMA

- Empyema is a purulent infection of the pleural space. Approximately 7 percent of patients undergoing pneumonectomy develop this complication; the mortality rate for patients who develop empyema was 17 percent in one series.[7] Suspect empyema for moderate to large pleural effusions and any size pleural effusion in a febrile patient. In considering this possibility in patients whose chest tube has already been removed, a thoracentesis is mandatory in order to establish or exclude the diagnosis.
- Cavity hematoma, bronchopleural fistula, and wound suppuration are all risk factors for the development of postoperative empyema.
- Gram-positive and gram-negative organisms contribute equally to the microbiology of postoperative empyema.[7]
- Treatment requires antibiotics and collaboration with the thoracic surgeon in order to provide chest tube drainage.

CARDIOVASCULAR COMPLICATIONS

- Atrial fibrillation is the most common dysrhythmia after thoracic surgery; the prevalence is approximately 25 percent.[8] Patients at highest risk are those who are above 70 years of age or have left ventricular dysfunction. The peak timing is 2 to 4 days postoperatively. Pneumonectomy or superior lobectomy also confers higher risk; this is thought to be due to disruption of the pulmonary vein. Prevention and treatment consist of optimal management of any pulmonary disease and electrolyte levels (including magnesium). Anticoagulate if atrial fibrillation lasts longer than 48 h. After discussion with the surgeon, weigh the risk of postoperative hemorrhage against the risk of stroke or other embolic phenomena.
- Multifocal atrial tachycardia (MAT): Elderly patients and those with diabetes are more prone to MAT, characterized by variability in P-wave morphology. MAT is associated with chronic lung disease 60 percent of the time; theophylline also increases the risk. MAT occurs in up to 20 percent of patients with respiratory failure.[6] The primary treatment is to treat the underlying pulmonary disease. Treatment also consists of correcting electrolyte imbalance for patients with low serum potassium or magnesium.
- Right ventricular failure: Patients with right ventricular dysfunction secondary to severe lung disease are unable to increase cardiac output when needed in response to stress. Hypoxemia, by causing pulmonary vasoconstriction, can further reduce right ventricular function. Treatment includes oxygen supplementation as needed and gentle diuresis. Overly aggressive diuresis can lead to intravascular volume depletion, further contributing to decreased cardiac output, and metabolic alkalosis, which can suppress ventilation.
- Hypotension: When postoperative hypotension develops, consider sepsis, myocardial ischemia, cardiac tamponade, volume depletion, adrenal insufficiency, and pulmonary embolus. In patients who have undergone thoracotomy, an additional consideration is acute hemothorax. Management of acute hemothorax is surgical exploration.
- Hypertension: Manage postoperative hypertension routinely, as reviewed in Chap. 51. Many patients with COPD can be managed with beta blockers without adverse effect if they are not actively wheezing.

PAIN CONTROL

- Inadequate postoperative pain control increases the risk of postoperative pulmonary complications.
- Epidural analgesia improves pain control and decreases rates of postoperative pulmonary complications (see Chap. 24). This is the standard of care in most institutions. Potential complications of epidural analgesia include nausea, puritus, motor block, numbness, and hypotension. Respiratory depression is not a common side effect of epidural analgesia.
- Intercostal nerve blocks reduce postoperative pain, but their benefit in reducing postoperative pulmonary complications is less well established.
- NSAIDs are recommended at routine doses in all patients without contraindications after thoracotomy. Be cautious with NSAIDs in patients with asthma. (If contraindicated, they should not be used at all.)
- Cryoanalgesia consists of freezing the intercostal nerves, which causes reversible nerve damage that lasts 1 to 3 months. This results in good pain control in the treated dermatomes and improvement in postoperative pulmonary function. Patients usually have pain only from the chest tubes. This may require use of narcotics unless the chest tube is placed in a treated intercostal area.

MISCELLANEOUS COMPLICATIONS

- Esophageal injury is a rare complication of thoracic surgery. Maintain a high degree of suspicion for this diagnosis. Suspect this possibility in a patient with chest pain and fever. There may be mediastinal widening on chest x-ray along with air in the mediastinum and soft tissues. Antibiotic therapy should cover oral anaerobes; consultation with general surgery is in order.
- Subcutaneous emphysema will usually resolve spontaneously and does not need treatment. However, if the patient is on positive-pressure ventilation, subcutaneous emphysema can indicate pneumothorax over 50 percent of the time.[9] When located in the suprasternal notch, it can indicate postoperative esophageal perforation.

SUMMARY

- Thoracic surgery is a high-risk procedure due to inherent physiologic stresses and the frequent occurrence of major medical comorbidities in surgical candidates, including COPD and coronary artery disease.
- Identify potential surgical candidates through a stepwise series of tests that predict a high likelihood of an acceptable postoperative functional status.
- Employ preoperative and postoperative strategies to reduce risk of morbidity.[10]
- Understand surgery-specific complications (Table 9-1).
- Recognize and effectively treat common postoperative complications.

TABLE 9-1 Surgery-Specific Pointers

TYPE OF SURGERY	PREOPERATIVE POINTERS	POSTOPERATIVE POINTERS
Mediastinoscopy	Relative contraindications: superior vena cava syndrome, severe tracheal deviation, thoracic aortic aneurysm, cerebral vascular disease.*	Complication rate is 1.5 to 3%, including hemorrhage, pneumothorax, chylothorax, recurrent laryngeal nerve injury, air embolism, and transient hemiparesis.
Thorascopic surgery (including VATS)	Obtain preoperative imaging. This helps the surgeon in planning the approach.	Pneumothorax is unavoidable but rarely requires a chest tube.
Tracheal resection	Preoperative PFTs. Severe lung disease is a relative contraindication and flow-volume loops differentiate between extra- and intrathoracic airway obstruction. Inform anesthesiologist of any position-dependent airway obstruction, as this determines positioning during surgery.	Risk of aspiration is high. Arterial line is required. Extubate as early as possible to reduce pressure from inflated tracheal cuff. Flexion positioning of the head reduces tension on suture line. Avoid vigorous chest physiotherapy; if secretions are a problem, use bronchoscopy for removal. Bleeding into the airway is a surgical emergency; indicates erosion into pulmonary artery or aorta.
Bullectomy	Analogous to lung resection; consider radioisotope studies to determine perfusion/function before recommending. PFTs and functional assessment are necessary prior to surgery.	Reexpansion of lung may cause impaired hemodynamics and require positive inotropes. Pneumothorax is common. May require prolonged mechanical ventilation postoperatively.
Lung-volume-reduction surgery	Preoperative PFTs and functional status	Monitor for positive-pressure air leaks. Avoid IV narcotics (epidural best for pain control). Permissive hypercapnia with optimized oxygenation.
Mediastinal tumor resection	Obtain preoperative chest CT, echocardiogram, and PFTs If no life-threatening obstruction of the airways or vasculature is present, then treatment with preoperative radiation/chemotherapy to reduce tumor helps lower risk to pulmonary artery, tracheobronchial tree, aortic arch, and superior vena cava.	Monitor closely for airway obstruction due to tumor edema.
Pneumonectomy/lobectomy	Preoperative PFTs and potentially functional evaluation as per text	Noncardiogenic pulmonary edema can occur; diuretics are not helpful. Bronchopleural fistula and prolonged air leak are the most common complications. Nosocomial pneumonia is the most important predictor of morbidity and mortality.

COPD = chronic obstructive pulmonary disease; PFTs = pulmonary function tests; VATS = video-assisted thoracic surgery.
*Compression of the innominate artery can lead to decreased cerebral blood flow.

REFERENCES

1. Datta D, Lahirit B. Preoperative evaluation of patients undergoing lung resection surgery. *Chest* 123:2096, 2003.
2. Beckles MA, Spiro SG, Colice GL, et al. The physiologic evaluation of patients with lung cancer being considered for resectional lung surgery. *Chest* 123:105S, 2003.
3. Burke JR, Duarte IG, Thourani VH, et al. Preoperative risk assessment for marginal patients requiring pulmonary resection. *Ann Thorac Surg* 76:1767, 2003.
4. Girish M, Trayner E, Dammann O, et al. Symptom-limited stair climbing as a predictor of postoperative cardiopulmonary complications after high-risk surgery. *Chest* 120:1147, 2001.
5. Licker M, de Perrot M, Hohn L, et al. Perioperative mortality and major cardio-pulmonary complications after lung surgery for non-small cell carcinoma. *Eur J Cardiothorac Surg* 15: 314, 1999.
6. Preoperative evaluation for lung resection. UP TO DATE Online 2005-12-03 @*www.utdol.com*
7. Kacprzak G, Marciniak M, Addae-Boateng E, et al. Causes and management of postpneumonectomy empyemas: our experience. *Eur J Cardioth Surg* 26:498, 2004.
8. Rena O, Papalia E, Oliaro A, et al. Supraventricular arrhythmias after resection surgery of the lung. *Eur J Cardiothorac Surg* 20:688, 2001.
9. Murray JF, Nadel JA. *Textbook of Respiratory Medicine,* 3d ed. Philadelphia; Saunders, 2000:2104.
10. Jacobsohn E. The management of the patient after thoracic surgery. http://daccx.bsd.uchicago.edu/manuals/vtmanual/postop-thorej.html 2004-12.

10 VASCULAR SURGERY

Sylvia C. W. McKean and Visala Muluk

INTRODUCTION

- Vascular surgeries range from relatively brief procedures, such as amputation, with minimal morbidity and mortality, to severely stressful procedures, such as emergent aortic aneurysm repair, in which up to half of patients die in the immediate perioperative period.
- Vascular surgery patients are frequently at high risk for perioperative complications because they have a high prevalence of cigarette smoking, diabetes mellitus, and cardiac, pulmonary, and renal disease.
- Patients with peripheral arterial disease are also at increased risk for vascular disease elsewhere, including coronary, renal, and cerebral arteries.
- An endovascular procedure is a lower-risk alternative to some open vascular surgeries; however, long-term outcomes cannot be compared because endovascular procedures have only recently been developed.

PREOPERATIVE EVALUATION

PATIENT-RELATED RISK FACTORS

CORONARY ARTERY DISEASE

- Because peripheral vascular disease (PVD) and coronary artery disease (CAD) share the same risk factors, about half of patients anticipating vascular surgery have at least moderately severe coronary artery disease (50 to 75 percent obstruction of a major coronary vessel).
- CAD is the leading cause of both early and late death after vascular surgery.
- The limitations on exertion imposed by PVD may prevent patients from exerting themselves sufficiently to manifest exertional angina; therefore potentially significant but asymptomatic CAD may go undetected.
- Because of these features plus the higher incidence of postoperative cardiac complications with vascular surgery, both traditional clinical tools and earlier cardiac risk indices may underestimate surgical risk.
- Before vascular surgery, screen patients for CAD with a comprehensive history, physical examination, and electrocardiogram (ECG)[1] (see Chap. 20).
- Reserve prophylactic coronary artery angioplasty or bypass surgery for the highest-risk patients, because for most patients the risks outweigh the benefits.[2,3] (see Chap. 20).

CHRONIC OBSTRUCTIVE PULMONARY DISEASE

- Smoking causes both vascular disease and COPD.
- COPD is a major risk factor for postoperative pulmonary complications (see Chap. 24).

RENAL INSUFFICIENCY

- Many patients with vascular disease have widespread vascular insufficiency, including renal artery stenosis with chronic renal insufficiency (serum creatinine greater than 2 mg/dL).
- Surgery can further exacerbate renal insufficiency (see Chap. 34).
- In addition, vascular procedures often entail perioperative radiologic imaging with intravascular contrast, which can precipitate or exacerbate renal failure.

DIABETES MELLITUS

- Diabetes is a risk factor for vascular disease; therefore many vascular surgery patients have diabetes.

- Furthermore, patients with diabetes undergoing vascular surgery are at greater risk for postoperative complications, including myocardial infarction, stroke, infection, and limb loss (see Chap. 26).

Hypertension

- Vascular surgery patients have a high prevalence of hypertension, either primary or secondary to renal artery stenosis, as well as target end-organ damage (see Chap. 19).

Cerebrovascular Disease

- Patients with peripheral vascular disease often have coexisting cerebrovascular disease.
- A stroke or transient ischemic attack (TIA) in the 2 to 3 months prior to a vascular surgical procedure has been associated with a greater risk of complications; however, an asymptomatic carotid bruit or history of an old stroke does not significantly increase risk of postoperative stroke or necessarily require special testing or intervention (see Chap. 37).

SURGERY-RELATED RISK FACTORS: EVOLVING TECHNOLOGY

- Endovascular procedures are potential lower-risk alternatives to many open vascular surgeries, including aortic aneurysm repair; however, long-term outcomes cannot be compared because endovascular procedures have only recently been developed.[4,5]
  - Endovascular procedures are associated with fewer immediate complications, including less myocardial infarction, congestive heart failure, life-threatening arrhythmia, and death.
  - Endovascular procedures may also result in less reperfusion injury, fewer medical complications, shorter hospital stays, and an earlier return to usual activities.
  - The incidence of postoperative renal failure from radiologic dye is no higher with endovascular procedures.
  - These advantages may allow higher-risk patients to undergo revascularization; however, some complications are more common with or exclusive to endovascular procedures, including endovascular leaks, arterial dissection and rupture, distal embolization, stent migration, and technical failure requiring a second procedure.
  - Endovascular repair of the carotid artery may not be safer than standard carotid endarterectomy.
    - For example, the stroke rate may be greater with carotid stenting than with open carotid endarterectomy.

PREOPERATIVE EVALUATION AND TESTING TO STRATIFY RISK

- Much of the research in perioperative cardiac risk for noncardiac surgery has been done in vascular surgery patients.
  - Before vascular surgery, use standard techniques to evaluate patients' cardiac risk (see Chap. 20).
  - Patients undergoing high-risk elective procedures may warrant noninvasive testing to identify those who may not tolerate an open vascular procedure even with appropriate beta blockade.
    - Early and late survival of patients with vascular disease is related to the number of coronary arteries that are narrowed, the degree of stenosis, and the function of the left ventricle.
      - The number of reversible perfusion defects identified by imaging helps predict future cardiac events (although recent data suggest that prophylactic coronary artery revascularization before elective vascular surgery does not improve long-term survival, at least for those patients who met the inclusion criteria).[3]
      - Abnormalities of left ventricular function may predict patients unable to tolerate open vascular surgery or those who should be evaluated further by cardiac catheterization. However, a normal ejection fraction does not identify low-risk patients, and a cardiac echocardiogram should not be used as an isolated screening test.
- The risk of pulmonary complications is greater after vascular surgeries that require cutting into the thoracic or abdominal cavities, whereas limb surgeries have minimal effect on pulmonary function.
  - Before vascular surgery, use standard techniques to evaluate patients' pulmonary risk (see Chap. 24).
- It is reasonable to use serum testing to screen both for renal failure and for diabetes mellitus prior to major vascular surgery (see Chaps. 5, 26, and 34).
  - Renal insufficiency not only increases the patient's risk of postoperative complications, but also poses challenges to the surgeon owing to large volume shifts and the need for intravascular contrast studies associated with vascular surgery.
  - Catabolic stress from vascular procedures can increase insulin requirements.

PERIOPERATIVE MANAGEMENT TO REDUCE RISK

CARDIAC

- Perioperative cardiac risk reduction includes consideration of preoperative cardiac revascularization in selected high-risk patients as well as aspirin, beta-blockade, and HMG-CoA reductase ("statin") treatment of most patients (see Chap. 20).

- The decision-making process should be individualized depending on the results of testing, the presence of factors independent of the anticipated surgery (such as unstable angina), the type of procedure, and whether an endovascular procedure is an option.
- Although prophylactic cardiac procedures are often performed routinely, the benefit is not clear when the risks of cardiac stenting or cardiac surgery and consequent delays in vascular surgery are factored into the decision analysis.
  - Postoperative management includes screening for clinically silent myocardial ischemia, although there are no trials comparing different methods (ECG, serum cardiac enzymes) or frequencies of screening.
  - Good pain control may minimize postoperative catecholamine-induced cardiac stress (see Chap. 63).
  - Assiduous attention to fluid balance and intravascular fluid volume can reduce the risk of postoperative pulmonary edema.

PULMONARY

- Perioperative pulmonary risk reduction includes smoking cessation, optimal treatment of bronchospasm, and incentive spirometry starting prior to surgery in appropriate patients (see Chap. 24).
  - Postoperatively it is important to avoid excessive sedation and overoxygenating patients who are dependent on oxygen for their respiratory drive.
  - Early mobilization and assiduous pulmonary toilet can also minimize pulmonary complications.

RENAL

- Renal dysfunction after vascular surgery can range from minor abnormalities to acute renal failure (see Chap. 58). Postoperative mortality due to renal failure in vascular surgery patients ranges from 10 to 80 percent.
- Perioperative renal risk reduction includes preoperative hydration and maintenance of optimal blood volume, limiting the period of warm renal ischemia, careful aortic clamping to prevent direct damage to the renal arteries and atheromatous embolization, minimizing potentially nephrotoxic treatments including intravenous contrast, and, possibly, treatment with bicarbonate and/or *N*-acetyl cysteine (see Chap. 34).

DIABETES MELLITUS

✣ Tight control of serum glucose with continuous intravenous insulin infusion may reduce the risk of postoperative sepsis (see Chap. 26).

THROMBOSIS

- Depending on the procedure and the surgeon's preferences, treatments to prevent both arterial and venous thrombosis include glycoprotein (GP) IIb/IIIa receptor antagonists (abciximab, tirofiban, or eptifibatide), ADP receptor antagonists (ticlopidine or clopidogrel), heparinization (usually low-molecular-weight-heparin), and Dextran-40.
- Thromboprophylaxis is started postoperatively in addition to low dose aspirin preoperatively for the majority of patients with vascular disease as started or continued for prevention of stroke and myocardial infarction.

BLEEDING

- Balancing the risks of thrombosis and bleeding is difficult, and bleeding from the surgical site or from other sites, such as the gastrointestinal tract, is common after vascular surgery.
  - Medication to reduce gastric pH may be appropriate in the immediate perioperative period.
  - Reoperation may be needed for surgical site bleeding or to drain a hematoma.

PROSTHETIC VASCULAR GRAFT INFECTION

✣ Graft infection, both early and late, is a serious complication of reconstructive vascular surgery because it is associated with both amputation and death. Preventive measures include:
  - Appropriate prophylactic antibiotics administered within 1 h of the first incision (see Chap. 46).
  - Early recognition and treatment of surgical site infection (see Chap. 50).
  - Prophylactic antibiotics prior to some procedures, such as dental work, for 1 year after surgery (see Chap. 47).

SURGERY-SPECIFIC RISKS

THORACOABDOMINAL ANEURYSM REPAIR

- The morbidity and mortality rates of thoracoabdominal aortic aneurysm (TAAA) repair are among the highest of elective vascular surgeries; however, recently developed techniques, such as selective renal artery perfusion, have decreased risks.[6]
- The most common reasons for reoperation are unsecured small vessel bleeding, leaking anastomoses, and wound disruption.

- Coagulopathy with major hemorrhage is associated with a 25 percent mortality rate.
  - Coagulopathy can be exacerbated by liver ischemia from supraceliac aortic cross-clamping and by high-volume resuscitation and blood transfusion.
- Respiratory failure is common after TAAA repair because of the large chest incisions required.
- Renal dysfunction is more likely after TAAA repair due to the longer duration of suprarenal cross-clamping.
- Spinal cord ischemia can cause lower extremity paresis or paralysis, and it can occur late (even after a patient's initial postoperative neurologic findings are normal).
  - The risk of spinal cord ischemia is proportional to the duration of cross-clamping and to hemodynamic instability.
  - Many surgeons use a lumbar cerebrospinal fluid (CSF) drain to improve cord perfusion; however, this technique has not been validated in controlled trials.

OPEN INFRARENAL AORTIC ANEURYSM REPAIR

- A special concern is lower extremity ischemia due to thromboembolism.
- Other complications include ileus and respiratory insufficiency.
- Late complications include the development of a ventral hernia at the incision site.

ENDOVASCULAR INFRARENAL AORTIC ANEURYSM REPAIR

- The balance of benefits and risks of endovascular versus open infrarenal aortic aneurysm (IAA) repair are under active investigation.[7]
  - A short-term survival advantage for endovascular repair seems greater when its use is limited to patients who are at the highest risk for open surgery.

The most common early complications are those of the groin incision, such as hematoma and lymphocele.

Other early complications include those due to intravenous contrast, including allergic reactions and renal insufficiency.

Later complications include endovascular leaks.
  - Endovascular leaks are diagnosed by screening postoperative CT scans.
    - One common algorithm is to perform CT scans at 1 month, 6 months, 12 months, and then annually.
  - Endoleaks are categorized by type:
    - Type I: Graft attachment site failure at either proximal (aortic) or distal (iliac) attachment sites. These are almost always treated, either by a secondary endovascular procedure or by an open procedure.
    - Type II: Retrograde leakage of blood into the aneurysmal sac, generally from lumbar arteries and/or the inferior mesenteric artery. These are frequently benign and can be observed as long as the sac size is stable.
    - Type III: Failure of the graft-graft junction site. Treatment is mandatory and is usually done endovascularly.
    - Type IV: Endovascular leak due to graft porosity. This is usually transient and is seen only in the first few days after surgery.
  - In endotension there is no demonstrable leak, but the aneurysm sac size increases. The presumed cause is transmission of pressure from an incomplete seal at the proximal attachment site. Management of this situation is controversial, but most authorities recommend intervention.

INFRAINGUINAL BYPASS PROCEDURES

- Graft thrombosis is a concern after infrainguinal bypass.
  - Graft patency is monitored by palpating the distal pulse.
  - If the pulse is not palpable, Doppler ultrasound is used. Duplex interrogation is sometimes necessary to ascertain graft patency, but arteriography is only rarely required.
  - Wound complications are more common after infrainguinal bypass than after other vascular procedures.
  - Leg edema is common after infrainguinal bypass.
  - Treat with leg elevation; avoid compression stockings early after surgery to avoid impairing distal arterial flow.

CAROTID ENDARTERECTOMY

- Early complications include neck hematoma, with the potentially serious consequence of airway compression.
  - Neck hematomas must be promptly explored.
  - Additional procedure-specific morbidities include stroke and cranial nerve injury.
  - These are usually related to technical problems at surgery or to complex anatomy, such as a high carotid bifurcation.
  - Stroke can be caused by plaque emboli, hypotension, poor cerebral protection, and improper flushing.
- Mortality associated with this procedure ranges from 0.5 to 3 percent and is greater in nontertiary hospitals.[8]

CAROTID ARTERY STENTING

- Carotid artery stenting has not yet been fully validated in definitive clinical trials, but there is increasing interest in this modality.[9]
- Procedure-specific morbidities include stroke and stent thrombosis.

TABLE 10-1 Surgery-Specific Postoperative Complications

SURGERY	POSTOPERATIVE COMPLICATIONS
TAAA repair	Postoperative hemorrhage Respiratory failure Renal failure Spinal cord ischemia
Open AAA repair	Leg thromboembolism with ischemia Respiratory failure Descending colon ischemia Ileus Retrograde ejaculation Aortoenteric fistula Ventral hernia
Endovascular infrarenal AAA repair	Lymphocele Groin hematoma Allergy to intravenous contrast or renal insufficiency Endovascular leak Endotension
Infrainguinal bypass surgery	Graft thrombosis Surgical site infection or dehiscence Leg edema
Carotid surgery	Neck hematoma, which may lead to airway compromise Stroke Cranial nerve injury
Carotid stenting	Stent thrombosis Stroke Groin hematoma Pseudoaneurysm
AV fistulas	High-output CHF Hand ischemia Arm edema Later complications, including infection, graft thrombosis, and false aneurysm
Limb amputations	Poor wound healing due to infection and poor perfusion DVT Later complications, including excessive exposure of transected bone due to muscle retraction

AAA = abdominal aortic aneurysm; AV = arteriovenous; CHF = congestive heart failure; DVT = deep venous thrombosis; TAAA = thoracic abdominal aortic aneurysm.

  - Strokes can affect the contralateral hemisphere because they can be caused by plaque dislodged from the aortic arch.
  - Groin hematoma and false aneurysm formation can also occur after carotid stent procedures.

CREATION OF AN ARTERIOVENOUS FISTULA

- Early complications include hand ischemia and arm edema.
- High-output heart failure can be caused by the increased blood flow through the fistula.
- Late complications include infection, graft thrombosis, and false aneurysm formation.

AMPUTATION

- The primary procedure-specific complication after amputation is poor surgical site healing due to poor flap perfusion or infection.
- Late complications include bone protrusion because of muscle retraction.

REFERENCES

1. Abir F, Kakisis I, Sumpio B. Do vascular surgery patients need a cardiology work-up? A review of pre-operative cardiac clearance guidelines in vascular surgery. *Endovasc Surg* 25:110, 2003.
2. Metzler H. Lowering cardiac risk by preoperative interventions. *Minerva Anestesiol* 69:412, 2003.
3. McFalls EO, Ward H, Moritz T, et al. Coronary-artery revascularization before elective major vascular surgery. *N Engl J Med* 351:2795, 2004.
4. Baker B. Anesthesia and endovascular surgery. *Best Pract Res Clin Anaesthesiol* 16:95, 2002.
5. Prinssen M, Verhoeven EL, Buth J, et al. A randomized trial comparing conventional and endovascular repair of abdominal aortic aneurysms. *N Engl J Med* 351:1607, 2004.
6. Wennberg DE, Lucas FL, Birkmeyer JD, et al. Variation in carotid endarterectomy mortality in the Medicare population. *JAMA* 279:1278, 1998.
7. Shapira OM, Aldea GS, Cutter SM, et al. Improved clinical outcomes after operation of the proximal aorta: A 10-year experience. *Ann Thorac Surg* 67:1030, 1999.
8. Prinssen M, Verhoeven EL, Buth J, et al. A randomized trial comparing conventional and endovascular repair of abdominal aortic aneurysms. *N Engl J Med* 351:1607, 2004.
9. Mordecai MM, Crawford CC. Intraoperative management: Endovascular stents. *Anesthesiol Clin North Am* 22:319–332, 2004.

11 ORTHOPEDIC SURGERY

Amir K. Jaffer and Brian F. Mandell

INTRODUCTION

- Approximately, 500,000 hip and knee replacements are done every year in the United States.[1] These surgeries are generally elective and should be performed only after discussion with the patient of the risks, benefits, and alternatives.
- Approximately, 350,000 hip fractures occur annually in the United States. These surgeries are urgent rather than emergent or elective, and only 25 percent of hip fracture patients will make a full recovery. Some 40 percent will require nursing home care; 50 percent

TABLE 11-1 Recommendations to Minimize Risk in Every Orthopedic Patient Undergoing Major Joint Replacement or Hip Fracture Surgery

RISK	RECOMMENDATIONS
Cardiovascular	Optimize underlying cardiac conditions. Consider further stress testing if necessary. Start beta blockers if patients have one of the following: age >65 with history of hypertension, diabetes, chronic renal insufficiency, history of stroke, history of coronary artery disease or Q waves on ECG.
Pulmonary	Optimize underlying pulmonary conditions. Initiate education on lung expansion maneuvers.
Infection	Ensure a careful preop evaluation for occult or obvious wound infection; if present, delay surgery. Initiate prophylactic antibiotics usually within 0 to 2 h of procedure—e.g., first-generation cephalosporin and continue for 24 h. Remove Foley within 24 h of surgery.
Venous Thromboembolism	Initiate pharmacologic prophylaxis—e.g., low-molecular-weight heparin or pentasaccharide (Fondaparinux) postoperatively and continue for minimum of 10 days and up to 28 days for patients with THA and who are still immobile after TKA and hip fracture or with additional risk factors.
Malnutrition	Protein supplementation for all with hip fracture. Nocturnal enteral feeding for those with moderate to severe malnutrition.
Delirium	Check and replete electrolyes. Minimize sedative, anticholinergic medication use. Implement continuous reorientation. Utilize institutional delirium-prevention program (geriatrics consultation). Exclude hypoxia, fat embolism, myocardial infarction, drug withdrawal.
Falls and deconditioning	Ensure early mobilization. Interdisciplinary rehabilitation. Twice-daily physical therapy. Exercise and balance training. Assess risk factors for falls.

THA = total hip arthroplasty.
TKA = total knee arthroplasty.

will need a cane or walker; and 25 percent of those over age 50 will die within 12 months. The rate of hip fracture increases at age 50, doubling every 5 to 6 years. Nearly 50 percent of women who reach age 90 have suffered a hip fracture.[1,2]

PREOPERATIVE MANAGEMENT FOR HIP AND KNEE ARTHROPLASTY

- Preoperative cardiac risk assessment should be done following American College of Cardiology/American Heart Association (ACC/AHA) guidelines, remembering that even though exercise intolerance may be attributed to the underlying joint disease, it must still be considered in evaluating cardiac risk.
- Patients are often taking medications to relieve the pain of their arthritis. As reviewed in Chap. 42 (Table 42-1), traditional nonsteroidal anti-inflammatory drugs (NSAIDs) should be stopped preoperatively. Cyclooxygenase-2 (COX-2)–selective NSAIDs can be continued, since they do not affect platelet function (although they do decrease renal blood flow and their effect on postoperative hypercoagulability is incompletely studied).

STRESS OF SURGERY

- Major orthopedic surgery imposes significant metabolic and cardiovascular stress on the patient. This is magnified by the fact that the majority of patients undergoing spine stabilization, hip and knee arthroplasties, and hip-pinning procedures are elderly. Frequently the activity level of these patients preoperatively is low, limiting the value of the obtained history in recognizing the presence of hemodynamically significant coronary and peripheral vascular disease. The plan for postoperative prophylactic anticoagulation should be expressed at the time of the preoperative assessment.

TOTAL HIP ARTHROPLASTY

- Total hip arthroplasty (THA) is most frequently done emergently for repair of hip fracture and electively for osteoarthritis (OA). OA may be limited to a single hip or generalized. Fracture warrants evaluation for generalized osteoporosis, ideally during the hospital admission, so that it is not forgotten.
- THA often takes 1.5 to 2 h in the operating room.
- General or spinal anesthesia may be used. The inclusion of neuraxial blockade may decrease postoperative complications, including thrombosis, and enhance postoperative rehabilitation. But with the need for aggressive anticoagulation in patients undergoing orthopedic procedures, often with low-molecular-weight heparins (LMWHs), this must be considered preoperatively so as to coordinate the timing of epidural injections and catheter placement with anticoagulant administration.
- Even in the absence of fracture, which may result in a blood loss of approximately 500 mL, THA often necessitates replacement of two units of blood. Thus, autologous blood donation should be considered. Alternatively, a designated donor may be identified by coordinating with the local blood bank.
- Preoperative use of erythropoietin (EPO) may permit autologous donation in anemic patients but may not diminish the need for allogeneic transfusion in all

patients. In patients who are not donating autologous blood, EPO may limit the number of postoperative transfusions.[3]

INTRAOPERATIVE COMPLICATIONS

- Heterotopic ossification complicates THA in up to 50 percent of cases; it is severe in up to 19 percent.[4] Risk factors include prior episodes of heterotopic ossification, hypertrophic OA, ankylosing spondylitis, male gender, and need for trochanteric osteotomy.
  - Effective interventions include use of high-dose NSAIDs in the immediate postoperative setting (these reduce the risk by up to 50 percent) or radiation therapy.
- Postoperative neuropathy complicates THA (femoral) approximately 1 percent of the time.
- Delayed deep postoperative bleeding may occur with pain, with or without associated deep fascial infection.
- Perioperative fracture is an uncommon complication.
- The fat embolism syndrome (FES) is a complication of long bone fractures[5] as well as hip or knee arthroplasty. Sensitive assays have detected fat embolism in 65 percent of 100 patients following bilateral TKA and 46 percent following unilateral TKA.[6] It may be at least as common following hip arthroplasty. The clinical FES is less common.
  - This syndrome, usually presenting within 48 h of long bone trauma or arthroplasty, comprises pulmonary insufficiency, changes in mentation, and central petechial rash. Modest thrombocytopenia is common, as is fever.
  - Neurologic symptoms include delirium, lethargy, headache, and seizures or coma.
  - The diagnosis is generally a clinical one, requiring the exclusion of pulmonary embolism, heparin-induced thrombocytopenia syndrome, drug reaction, and sepsis. There are no currently accepted laboratory criteria for diagnosis.
  - Treatment is supportive.
- Postoperative confusion (delirium), discussed in more detail below, may occur in 24 percent of elderly patients undergoing THA and a higher percentage in those who suffered a hip fracture requiring THA. Hypoxia, myocardial infarction (MI), drug withdrawal, side effects of a new medication, and fat embolism must be excluded as the etiology.
- Postoperative vascular injuries are rare but can occur following THA (or TKA).
- Anemia is common following THA or TKA, but despite the frequent prescription of postoperative iron, the anemia is rarely iron-responsive,[7] and iron contributes to the common problem of postoperative constipation. Although serum ferritin may increase after surgery as part of the acute-phase response, iron deficiency is unlikely unless the serum ferritin is low.

TOTAL KNEE ARTHROPLASTY (TKA)

- Most of the above comments regarding THA also relate to TKA.
- TKA takes approximately 2 to 3 h in the OR and poses similar cardiovascular risk as THA. Transfusion requirement may be less.
- Diabetics have an increased frequency of wound infection. Similar results have been seen in patients undergoing hand surgery. This may be like the situation in coronary artery bypass graft (CABG) surgery, with aggressive perioperative glucose control decreasing the risk for infection; thus a plan for aggressive glucose control should be considered preoperatively for all patients undergoing orthopedic surgery.
- Approximately 15 percent of these patients develop heterotopic ossification, which adversely affects the outcome of surgery less commonly than in THA.[8]
- Peroneal neuropathy complicates the TKA in <1 percent of cases.
- Perioperative fracture may occur in up to 1 percent of cases.
- Postoperative knee warmth, swelling, and capsule tenderness are not unusual. Even in the presence of fever, joint infection is not common, and arthrocentesis is not warranted unless the fever and localized findings persist.

HIP FRACTURE SURGERY

LOCATION OF THE HIP FRACTURE AND TYPE OF REPAIR

- A hip fracture is generally a fracture of the proximal femur. The anatomic location of the fracture (Fig. 11-1) has important implications for healing, because fractures in the femoral neck can disrupt the blood supply and may be associated with an increased incidence of both nonunion and osteonecrosis. These fractures are generally treated with internal fixation with multiple screws or prosthesis replacement. This type of repair is also utilized for patients with minimal displacement and in younger patients with displacement. Fractures in the intertrochanteric region (see Fig. 11-1) do not interfere with the blood supply but are most often associated with malunion and shortening. These type of fractures can also be treated with internal fixation and screws. These two types of fractures comprise 90 percent of hip fractures. Subtrochanteric fractures (see Fig. 11-1) comprise only 10 percent of hip fractures.[2]

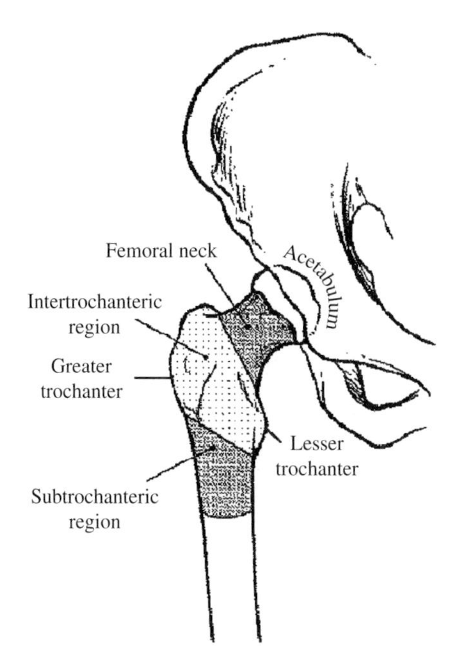

FIG. 11-1 Location of hip fractures. Fractures of the proximal femur are classified on the basis of their location in the femoral neck, intertrochanteric region, or subtrochanteric region. (From Zuckerman,[2] with permission.)

RISK FACTORS FOR HIP FRACTURE

- Falls account for 90 percent of hip fractures. If possible, the underlying reason for the fall should be ascertained at the time of preoperative assessment. An identified reason may affect perio- or postoperative management (impaired mental status, alcohol abuse, arrhythmia, etc.). Osteoporosis is the most commonly identified as well as a reversible risk factor for osteoporosis.

DIAGNOSIS

- Most hip fractures are diagnosed on the basis of clinical findings and standard radiographs. Sometimes a fracture is suspected despite a negative anteroposterior and lateral view on x-ray. These patients require additional rotated radiographs or technetium 99–labeled bone scan or magnetic resonance imaging. The latter study is useful immediately after the injury; however, the bone scan may not be positive until 2 or 3 days after the injury.[2]

TIMING OF SURGICAL INTERVENTION

- The timing of surgical intervention in patients with hip fracture is often determined by the preoperative medical evaluation; however, it ultimately depends on the surgeon.
- If patients have unstable or decompensated medical conditions, they should be optimized as much as possible before surgery. In the presence of a recent MI, surgery may best be delayed until it is deemed safe by a functional stress study indicating that the patient does not have ischemia. However, in general, surgery should occur within 24 to 48 h after admission.[2,9]
- Multiple studies have evaluated the timing of surgery; and the results are mixed and the jury is still out. Most studies found lower mortality rates in patients who underwent surgical repair within 48 h of the injury. However, the largest study to date[10] determined that the time to surgery is more a marker of comorbidity rather than a risk factor for outcomes except for the development of sacral decubiti. A recent observational study again showed that early surgery (within 24 h) decreased length of stay, reduced pain, and reduced major postoperative complications; at 6 months, these patients also had a lower mortality and less need for total assistance.
- Although the results are mixed, more evidence points to early repair of the hip fracture. Therefore our recommendation is to proceed with hip fracture surgery as soon as the patient's medical condition has been optimized.

COMMON PROPYLACTIC INTERVENTIONS FOR MAJOR JOINT REPLACEMENT OR HIP FRACTURE SURGERY

PROPHYLACTIC ANTIBIOTICS

- Considerable evidence from clinical trials supports the use of prophylactic antibiotics (first-generation cephalosporins) in patients with hip fracture because the major pathogen in wound infections is *Staphylococcus aureus*. Antibiotics seem to reduce the risk for deep wound infections by approximately 44 percent, and therapy should probably be continued for 24 h (that is, about three doses should be given). Evidence suggests that antibiotics should be administered 0 to 2 h before surgery.[9]

VENOUS THROMBOEMBOLISM (VTE) PROPHYLAXIS

- VTE is among the leading causes of postoperative morbidity and mortality in patients with hip fractures. In the absence of prophylaxis, the rate of fatal pulmonary embolism (PE) may be as high as 5 percent and the prevalence of venographic deep venous thrombosis (DVT) as high as 60 percent.[9]

- Strong evidence supports the use of LMWH (e.g., enoxaparin or dalteparin) or the pentasaccharide (fondaparinux) as prophylaxis for VTE starting at hospital admission. This last agent is probably slightly more effective but with slightly more bleeding. Aspirin should not be used to prevent VTE but rather for the prevention of arterial disease. Dose-adjusted warfarin can also be used, but the required monitoring of the international normalized ratio (INR) and risk of over- or underanticoagulation are potential drawbacks. This topic is covered in more detail in Chap. 46.
- At present, the use of VTE prophylaxis for 10 days or until the patient is ambulatory is recommended for TKA; however, for patients undergoing hip fracture surgery or THA, in patients with additional risk factors for VTE, such as morbid obesity, prior VTE, or multiple other risk factors for VTE, prolonged prophylaxis (i.e., for up to 28–35 days postoperatively) may be reasonable.

NUTRITIONAL SUPPLEMENTATION

- Malnutrition is associated with increased surgical morbidity and mortality. It is estimated that as many as 20 percent of hip fracture patients are severely malnourished.
- Oral protein supplementation appears to be beneficial in reducing minor postoperative complications, preserving body protein stores, and reducing overall length of stay.
- Patients with evidence of moderate to severe malnutrition may benefit from nocturnal enteral tube feeding if they can tolerate it.

PREVENTION OF URINARY TRACT INFECTIONS

- Indwelling catheters should be removed within 24 h of the surgery; if needed, patients should be managed by straight catheterization.
- If there is bacteriuria ($>1 \times 10^3$/mL) in the absence of any symptoms, the arthroplasty can proceed, but oral antibiotics should be provided postoperatively for 8 to 10 days.
- Based on the low predictive value and the lack of cost-effectiveness associated with urinalysis, we do not recommend routine preoperative urinalysis.

REHABILITATION

- Early mobilization can be done safely. Interdisciplinary rehabilitation is preferred, and patients should receive physical therapy twice daily. Interventions should be directed at the risk factors for falls to help prevent future falls.[9]

POSTOPERATIVE MEDICAL COMPLICATIONS

FEVER

- Fever above 38°C (100.4°F) is common in the first few days after major orthopedic surgery. Most early postoperative fever after orthopedic surgery is caused by the release of inflammatory mediators, not infection. The T_{max} is usually at 48 h postarthroplasty. The erythrocyte sedimentation rate (ESR) and C-reactive protein (CRP) increase as well. The ESR may occasionally rise to as high as 100 mm/h by day 2 postoperatively. The CRP may also rise dramatically but is expected to return to normal by 14 days after surgery. The ESR remains elevated longer.
- Postoperative fever can also be a manifestation of a serious complication such as a surgical site infection (SSI), nosocomial pneumonia, urinary tract infection, drug fever, and VTE.
- For more details on this topic, refer to Chap. 50.

WOUND INFECTION

- Surgical site infections (SSIs) after orthopedic procedures cause significant mortality and morbidity. They increase the total length of hospitalization, double the rate of rehospitalization, and increase total costs.
- The clinical criteria developed by the Centers for Disease Control (CDC) to define a SSI include any of the following:
  - A purulent exudate draining from a surgical site
  - A positive fluid culture obtained from a surgical site that was closed primarily
  - The surgeon's diagnosis of infection
  - A surgical site that requires reopening
- The incidence of SSI after joint replacement is about 0.7 to 1.7 percent.
- The most common organisms are staphylococci.
- The treatment of these nosocomial infections is geared toward the organism isolated, and most prosthetic joint infections require removal of the bioprosthetic parts.
- The treatment requires a stepped process, as follows:
  - The infected prosthesis is removed and the underlying bone and periprosthetic tissues are debrided and cultured.
  - The joint is stabilized with an antibiotic-impregnated spacer.
  - Intravenous antibiotics with activity against the infecting organisms are administered for 6 to 12 weeks.
  - Reimplantation of a prosthesis is usually undertaken following a 6-week course of antimicrobial therapy, with success in approximately 80 to 90 percent of patients.

VENOUS THROMBOEMBOLISM

- Postoperative VTE is common following major surgery; if VTE prophylaxis is not utilized, it occurs, as diagnosed by venography, in over 50 percent of patients undergoing major joint replacement or hip fracture surgery.
- Therefore VTE must be considered, even when signs or symptoms may be related to another diagnosis.
- Prompt diagnosis using duplex ultrasound for DVT and spiral computed tomography are still the first steps, but use of the rules of clinical prediction outlined in Chap. 55 can precede this.
- Prompt institution of anticoagulant therapy, such as unfractionated heparin or LMWH, in conjunction with oral vitamin K antagonists, such as warfarin, are the first steps in treatment. Refer to Chap. 55 for details.
- If anticoagulant therapy is contraindicated due to the high risk of bleeding, inferior vena cava (IVC) filters, either permanent or retrievable, can be considered.

DELIRIUM

- Delirium occurs in over to 60 percent of patients with hip fractures. Delirium in hospitalized patients has been shown to increase length of stay, risk for complications, mortality, and institutionalization. Despite its high prevalence, delirium is often unrecognized or misdiagnosed. Most patients who develop delirium have some persistent symptoms up to 6 months later. Delirium may also affect functional outcome by interfering with rehabilitation and delaying return to weight-bearing activity.[9]
- Modifiable risk factors for delirium include electrolyte and metabolic disorders; psychoactive medications with sedative, hypnotic, and anticholinergic properties; infection; and low cerebral perfusion.[9]
- Environmental and supportive reorientation appears to reduce the incidence of delirium and benefit acutely delirious patients.[9] Patients should receive pain control, but meperidine should be avoided.
- Delirium is discussed in greater detail in Chap. 62.

REFERENCES

1. CDC. Health Care in America, Trends in Utilization. www.cdc.gov/nchs/data/misc/healthcare.pdf, 2004.
2. Zuckerman JD. Hip fracture. *N Engl J Med* 334:1519, 1996.
3. Faris PM, Ritter MA, Abels RI. The effects of recombinant human erythropoietin on perioperative transfusion requirements in patients having a major orthopaedic operation. *J Bone Joint Surg Am* 78:62, 1996.
4. Neal B, Gray H, MacMahon S, et al. Incidence of heterotopic bone formation after major hip surgery. *Aust N Z J Surg* 72:808, 2002.
5. Parisi DM, Koval K, Egol K. Fat embolism syndrome. *Am J Orthop* 31:507, 2002.
6. Kim YH. Incidence of fat embolism syndrome after cemented or cementless bilateral simultaneous and unilateral total knee arthroplasty. *J Arthrop* 16:730, 2001.
7. Sutton PM, Cresswell T, Livesey JP, et al. Treatment of anaemia after joint replacement. A double-blind, randomised, controlled trial of ferrous sulphate versus placebo. *J Bone Joint Surg Br* 86:31, 2004.
8. Dalury DF, Jiranek WA. The incidence of heterotopic ossification after total knee arthroplasty. *J Arthrop* 19:447, 2004.
9. Morrison RS, Chassin MR, Siu AL. The medical consultant's role in caring for patients with hip fracture. *Ann Intern Med* 128:1010, 1998.
10. Grimes JP, Gregory PM, Noveck H, et al. The effects of time-to-surgery on mortality and morbidity in patients following hip fracture. *Am J Med* 112:702, 2002.

12 NEUROSURGERY

James B. Lewis, Jr., and Judi Woolger-Kraft

INTRODUCTION

- Perioperative management of patients undergoing neurosurgery is challenging because assiduous hemostasis is required, the surgery is often critical, and an accurate medical history is often difficult to obtain because of the patient's neurologic deficits.
- Hemostasis is important, particularly in brain and spinal cord surgeries, because any bleeding can cause catastrophic injury; however, no studies have demonstrated a need for routine preoperative hematologic screening.
    - Nonetheless, most neurosurgeons routinely check prothrombin time/international normalized ratio (PT/INR), partial thromboplastin time (PTT), and platelet count prior to surgery. An INR below 1.4 and a platelet count above 50,000/mm^3 are generally considered necessary for surgery.
- Prophylactic antibiotics are used in most neurosurgical procedures (craniotomies and spinal surgeries) despite the low risk of infection (see Chap. 48).
    - Common pathogens are *Staphylococcus aureus* and *Staphylococcus epidermidis*.
    - 1 to 2 g of cefazolin or 1 g of vancomycin is administered within 60 min of the start of the procedure.

- Patients undergoing major neurosurgery are at intermediate risk for perioperative deep venous thrombosis (DVT) and usually require prophylaxis (see Chap. 46).
  - Intermittent pneumatic compression (with or without graded compression stockings), subcutaneous low-dose unfractionated heparin starting preoperatively, and low-molecular-weight-heparin (LMWH) starting within 24 h postoperatively result in a 50 to 70 percent risk reduction.[1]
- Many neurosurgical patients are at risk for stress ulceration.
  - Risk factors include mechanical ventilation, coagulopathy, sepsis, extensive burns, multisystem organ failure, and head injury with increased intracranial pressure (ICP) (see Chap. 36).

SURGICAL PROCEDURES

SPINAL SURGERY

Preoperative Management

- Evaluating the exercise capacity of a patient in need of spinal surgery can be limited by the patient's inability to exercise.
  - Evaluate the patient in a wheelchair on the basis of ability to perform transfers and to push the chair.
  - For patients whose exercise capacity has recently become limited, focus on their historical exercise tolerance in the past year, including prior to their neurologic decline.
  - When no exercise tolerance can be established, assume a minimal cardiac reserve and proceed with any indicated noninvasive testing (see Chap. 20).

Common Comorbidities/Risk Factors

- Most patients undergoing spinal surgery for degenerative conditions are above 50 years of age.
  - Comorbidities in this age range include cardiovascular disease, pulmonary disease, and renal insufficiency.
- Tobacco use is particularly detrimental to wound healing in the spine.
  - Smoking should be stopped before any elective spinal cord surgery.
  - If the patient discontinues smoking at least 8 weeks prior to surgery, there is a greater likelihood of reducing postoperative pulmonary complications (see Chap. 24).
- Rheumatoid arthritis (RA) is a relatively common comorbidity that necessitates surgical intervention to stabilize the spine.
  - In addition to the danger of intubation because of C1 instability, the patient with RA frequently has suppression of the hypothalamic-pituitary axis from chronic steroid use.
    - In patients with erosive joint disease, consider flexion-extension radiography of the cervical spine to check for spinal instability prior to endotracheal intubation (see Chap. 42).
    - Consider perioperative "stress dose" steroid in patients who might have adrenal suppression (see Chap. 28).

Anesthetic Technique and Operative Pathophysiology

- Spinal surgeons prefer to maintain systolic blood pressure above 100 mmHg to avoid spinal cord infarction.
  - Make sure that systolic blood pressure is above 100 mmHg prior to surgery.
- Intraoperative blood loss increases with longer procedures and when a greater number of vertebral levels are exposed.
  - For patients expecting to undergo prolonged procedures or to have surgery on multiple levels, consider banking blood before surgery (see Chap. 30).

Preoperative Preparation/Prophylaxis

- Those undergoing spinal surgeries are at risk for deep venous thrombosis (DVT) and should have sequential compression stockings placed preoperatively and continued until these patients are ambulatory.
  - Heparins can be used, although with caution, as they can pose the risk of bleeding into the spinal cord, which is catastrophic.
  - Consult with the surgeon and tailor DVT prophylaxis for the patient and the procedure (see Chap. 46).

Usual Postoperative Course

- It is difficult to discuss standard postoperative courses in the spinal cord patient because the underlying pathologies and comorbidities can vary so greatly.
- It is important to have a nursing staff that is accustomed to the needs of spinal cord patients and can perform the appropriate neurologic checks required postoperatively.

Common Postoperative Problems/Solutions

- A decline in neurologic function is a warning sign that requires immediate evaluation by the neurosurgical or orthopedic team.
  - It may indicate an epidural hematoma or bleeding.
  - The surgical team must reimage and reexplore the wound site as needed.
- Thromboembolic disease is a potential complication after any surgery (see Chap. 46).
  - Immediately evaluate for pulmonary embolism if the patient develops evidence of hemodynamic compromise, such as unexplained tachycardia, tachypnea, or anxiety.

- Cerebrospinal fluid (CSF) leaks are manifest by recalcitrant headache and/or clear fluid draining from the surgical site.
  - Notify the neurosurgical team immediately.

CRANIOTOMY

- Indications for craniotomy include removal of a primary or metastatic brain tumor, clipping of an aneurysm or arteriovenous malformation, culture and drainage of an abscess, evacuation of a hematoma, elevation of a depressed skull fracture, management of increased intracranial pressure, and management of a refractory seizure disorder.
- Comorbidities include the presence of increased ICP and/or mass effect, cervical or other spinal trauma, and poor wound healing, especially if the patient is receiving chemotherapy, radiation therapy, or corticosteroids.
- Craniotomies and most other neurosurgeries are of intermediate cardiovascular risk, and appropriate evaluation is important (see Chap. 20).
- All patients should receive appropriate DVT and wound prophylaxis.
  - Chronic corticosteroid therapy may require stress dosing of corticosteroids (see Chap. 28).
  - For vasogenic edema, patients are often started on a regimen of 10 mg dexamethasone initially and 6 mg IV every 6 h.
    - It is prudent to monitor glucoses for at least 24 to 48 h on any patient started on high-dose steroids (see Chap. 26).
- Seizure prophylaxis is controversial.
  - Some neurosurgeons will give patients with a cortical incision or injury prophylactic phenytoin for 1 week.
- The postoperative craniotomy patient usually spends 24 h in the intensive care unit (ICU) for observation.
  - Additional ICU stay is dictated by poor respiratory status, deteriorating mental status, seizures, use of ventricular pressure monitoring, and poor blood pressure control.
- Postoperatively, the patient with an abnormal mental status should be monitored closely for aspiration.
  - Loss of the gag reflex is an indication for elective intubation.
  - Bacterial meningitis is commonly caused by staphylococci and aerobic gram-negative bacilli including *Staphylococcus aureus*, coagulase-negative staphylococci, and *Pseudomonas aeruginosa*.
    - Vancomycin plus a third-generation cephalosporin or carbopenem (e.g. ceftazidime, cefepime, or meropenem) is a reasonable empiric antimicrobial regimen pending results of Gram's stain and culture.[2]
- Infection may occur after ventriculoatrial or ventriculoperitoneal shunting or ventriculostomy with external drainage.
  - Shunt infections can present with fever and/or abnormal shunt function with increased ICP.
  - Peritonitis, local scalp pain, or erythema may occur.
  - Diagnose shunt infection by examining CSF obtained via the device or via a lumbar puncture.
  - The infected shunt usually requires removal, some form of external drainage, antibiotic treatment, and sterile CSF before a new shunt is placed.[2]
- Monitor ventriculostomies for infection with serial CSF studies, particularly if an elevated temperature or white blood cell count occurs.
  - For suspected infection, treat empirically with vancomycin plus a third-generation cephalosporin or carbopenem (e.g. ceftazidime, cefepime, or meropenem).
- Increased ICP may be manifest by a change in mental status, nausea and vomiting, or a new neurologic defect.
  - Increased ICP can be caused by a blood clot at the surgical site, obstruction to normal CSF flow (hydrocephalus), or by pneumocephalus.
- Cerebral blood flow depends on cerebral perfusion pressure (CPP), which is mean arterial pressure minus ICP.
  - Normal CPP is above 50 mmHg and ICP is below 20 mmHg.
  - ICP is measured by an external ventricular drain (EVD)/ventriculostomy or by an intraparenchymal pressure monitor.
  - Therapies to reduce ICP and increase CPP include elevating the head of the bed, sedating or paralyzing the patient, controlling body temperature and blood pressure, maintaining normoglycemia, draining CSF, intravenous infusion of a hyperosmolar solution, mild hyperventilation (PCO_2 30 to 35 mmHg), and surgical decompression.
- Hyponatremia is common after craniotomy and is caused by the syndrome of inappropriate antidiuretic hormone (SIADH) and/or by cerebral salt wasting (CSW).
  - Urinary sodium and osmolality are elevated in both.
  - In CSW, the central venous pressure is low, the blood urea nitrogen (BUN)/creatinine ratio is elevated, and there may be clinical dehydration.
    - The treatment for CSW is intravenous normal saline.
- Perioperative stroke may occur.
  - If the stroke is thromboembolic, full-dose anticoagulation may be started 24 to 48 h after surgery irrespective of the size of the stroke.
  - Control of blood pressure is controversial, because lowering of the blood pressure may reduce cerebral perfusion and exacerbate the stroke.
  - Control blood sugar in the postoperative neurosurgical patient (see Chap. 26).

- Management of postoperative seizures is discussed in Chap. 61.
  - Causes include infection, structural abnormalities of the central nervous system (CNS), electrolyte abnormalities, medications, and drug and alcohol withdrawal.
- Neurosurgical patients are predisposed to develop pressure sores from immobility and corticosteroid use.
- Peripheral nerve injury and cord injury can be caused by positioning problems in the operating room.

SUBARACHNOID HEMORRHAGE

- The most common causes of subarachnoid hemorrhage are trauma, ruptured intracranial aneurysms, and ruptured arteriovenous malformations.
  - Prognosis depends on presentation (Table 12-1).
  - Although presentation also determines treatment to some extent, the neurosurgeon also considers factors including the findings of computed tomography (CT) and arteriography, as well as timing.
  - Complications include hypertension, rebleeding, hydrocephalus, vasospasm with neurologic deficits, hyponatremia, deep venous thrombosis (DVT), seizures, and cardiac ischemia and conduction abnormalities.
  - If the patient is stable and not moribund, angiography is usually performed early to determine the source of the bleeding and prepare for prompt surgical correction.
  - The risk of rebleeding is 15 to 20 percent within the first 2 weeks in unoperated patients.
  - Management of hypertension prior to surgery or endovascular aneurysm treatment is controversial, because lowering blood pressure may reduce cerebral perfusion and cause infarction.
    - For a patient with external ventricular drainage (EVD), adjust systemic blood pressure to maintain a cerebral perfusion pressure of 50 to 60 mmHg.
    - An alert patient without EVD likely has normal CPP; maintain a systolic blood pressure of 140 mmHg.
    - In a patient with a depressed level of consciousness, antihypertensive therapy may lower CPP and should be withheld.[3]
    - Table 12-2 lists parenteral antihypertensive agents used in neurosurgical patients.
  - Cardiac manifestations include ECG abnormalities (T-wave changes, QT prolongation, and ST-segment changes) and occasional neurogenic pulmonary edema.
    - Echocardiography may show wall motion abnormalities.
    - Measure serum cardiac enzymes to detect myocardial injury.
  - Use DVT prophylaxis with external pneumatic compression and prophylaxis for surgical site infection with antimicrobials.
  - Seizure prophylaxis may also be used.
  - To reduce the risk of vasospasm, nimodipine 60 mg every 4 h is usually started within 4 days of hemorrhage and continued for 21 days.
  - Hydrocephalus may occur preoperatively or postoperatively because bleeding interferes with CSF flow through the ventricles.
    - Manifestations include impaired consciousness, hypertension, and/or bradycardia.
    - Diagnosis is by CT scanning and treatment by ventriculostomy.

TABLE 12-1 Hunt and Hess Grading System for Subarachnoid Hemorrhage

GRADE	NEUROLOGIC STATUS	PROGNOSIS/COMMENTS
0	Unruptured aneurysm	
1	No symptoms, mild headache	10% mortality/Operate
2	Cranial nerve palsy, moderate to severe headache, stiff neck	25% mortality/Operate
3	Focal deficit, lethargy, confusion	35% mortality/ Medical management
4	Stupor, hemiparesis, early decebrate posture	55% mortality/ Medical management
5	Coma, decebrate posture	95% mortality/ Medical management

SOURCE: Modified from Hunt WE, Hess RM. Surgical risk as related to time of intervention in the repair of intracranial aneurysms. *J Neurosurg* 28:14, 1968.

TABLE 12-2 Parenteral Antihypertensive Agents

MEDICATION	DOSING	SIDE EFFECTS/ COMMENTS
Nitroprusside (vasodilator)	0.25–10 μg/kg/min infusion	Nausea, cyanide toxicity, increased heart rate
Labetalol (alpha,beta blocker)	20–80 mg bolus (every 10 min to 300 mg total) 2 mg/min infusion	Bradycardia, wheeze, CHF
Enalaprilat (ACE inhibitor)	1.25- to 5-mg bolus every 6 h	Variable response
Nicardipine (CCB)	5–15 mg/h infusion	Reflex tachycardia
Nitroglycerin	5–100 μg/min	Headache, tachycardia
Fenoldopam (dopamine agonist)	0.1–1.6 μg/kg/min	Tachycardia, headache, nausea, decreased CBF

ACE = angiotensin converting enzyme; CBF = cerebral blood flow; CCB = calcium channel blocker; CHF = congestive heart failure.

- ◦ Postoperatively, the major complications are vasospasm, hypertension, hyponatremia, and hydrocephalus.
  - ▪ Vasospasm usually occurs within 3 to 12 days following a subarachnoid bleed and may cause neurologic symptoms in 20 to 30 percent of patients.
    - Daily transcranial Doppler ultrasound monitoring is useful for diagnosis.
    - The most commonly used therapy is the "triple-H": hypervolemia, hypertension, and hemodilution.
- ◦ A pulmonary artery catheter or central venous pressure monitor is a useful adjunct in managing hypervolemia.
- ◦ In the operated patient, volume expansion with normal saline and blood (target hematocrit below 40) is done with a CVP target of 8 to 12 mmHg or pulmonary artery wedge pressure target of 18 mmHg.
- ◦ In the unoperated patient, a better CVP and wedge pressure goal is 6 to 10 mmHg and a systolic blood pressure of less than 160 mmHg.
- ◦ Hypertension is induced with dobutamine, dopamine, or phenylephrine to a systolic pressure of 220 mmHg or to reversal of symptoms.
  - ▪ Treatment of hypertension in the postoperative patient is controversial, because an elevated blood pressure may help to prevent vasospasm.
    - After 2 to 3 weeks, hypertension may be managed with usual outpatient goals.
  - ▪ Hyponatremia and hydrocephalus are discussed under "Craniotomy," above. Hydrocephalus is best managed with a ventriculoatrial or ventriculoperitoneal shunt.

TRANSSPHENOIDAL SURGERY

- Indications for transsphenoidal surgery (TSS) are functioning pituitary microadenomas (less than 10 mm) and macroadenomas (more than 10 mm) that cause visual symptoms, hormonal hypersecretion, or hyposecretion.
  - ◦ Some neurosurgeons require the assistance of an otolaryngologist to access the sella.
  - ◦ Prolactinomas are usually managed medically.
  - ◦ Tumors with suprasellar extension occasionally need a transcranial approach, which is associated with greater morbidity.
  - ◦ "Gamma-knife surgery" utilizing treatment with ionizing radiation is often used for recurrent tumors.
  - ◦ Patients requiring TSS may present with pituitary dysfunction and temporal field defects from tumor compression of the optic chiasm.
  - ◦ Patients are at risk for perioperative adrenal crisis because of surgical stress combined with pituitary dysfunction.
  - ◦ They are also at risk for hypothyroidism with delayed anesthetic metabolism (see Chap. 27).
  - ◦ Preoperative evaluation includes radiologic, ophthalmologic, and endocrine assessments.
    - ▪ High-resolution MRI with gadolinium is a better test for pituitary masses and other brain tumors than is contrast CT.
    - ▪ Patients with pituitary macroadenomas require ophthalmologic visual fields assessment and screening for hypopituitarism.
    - ▪ Patients with microadenomas need only be screened for hormone hypersecretion, including thyroid-stimulating hormone (TSH), free T_4, 24-h urine for free cortisol, prolactin, insulin-like growth factor 1, luteinizing hormone (LH), and follicle-stimulating hormone (FSH).
- Stalk compression alone can increase prolactin levels, but to less than 200 ng/mL.
- To screen for hypopituitarism, check cortisol at 8 A.M.
  - ◦ If it is less than 3 μg/dL, a deficiency of adrenocorticotropic hormone (ACTH) is present; more than 18 μg/dL indicates normal function.
  - ◦ Consider an in-hospital metyrapone test for intermediate values.
  - ◦ Check testosterone and estradiol levels as indicated by the patient's gender.
  - ◦ An endocrinology consultation is usually indicated.
- ◦ Patients should receive the recommended DVT and wound prophylaxis (see Chap. 46).
- ◦ Stress-dose steroids should be given to all patients (see Chap. 28).
- ◦ Postoperative complications include diabetes insipidus (DI), CSF rhinorrhea, hypopituitarism, hypothalamic injury with coma (rare), hydrocephalus,

infection, carotid artery rupture (rare), visual loss from optic nerve injury, nasal septal perforation, and sinusitis.

- Diabetes insipidus (DI) is often transient, lasting up to 36 h, but it can occasionally be permanent.
  - Monitor the urine output closely for at least 48 h.
  - Diagnosis is based on a urine osmolality below 150 Osm/L, urine specific gravity less than 1.005, urine output greater than 250 mL/h, serum sodium of 142 mEq/L or higher, and normal adrenal function.
  - Treat mild DI with oral water supplementation.
- Match hourly intake and output in the obtunded patient and closely monitor electrolytes.
- Add desmopressin for moderate to severe DI.
  - Desmopressin may be given orally at 0.1 to 1.2 mg/day or subcutaneously at 2 to 4 μg/day split into two doses.
  - Start at a low dose.
  - Once the patient's nasal packing is removed, give desmopressin as an intranasal dose varying from 10 to 40 μg/day divided into two doses.
- Stop any supplemental steroids at 48 h and measure an A.M. cortisol at 72 h.
  - A morning cortisol greater than 9 μg/dL rules out adrenal insufficiency.
- CSF rhinorrhea increased the risk of meningitis.
  - Treatment is with repeated lumbar puncture or a lumbar drain.
  - Surgical repair may be needed if the leak does not resolve.

CAROTID ENDARTERECTOMY

Preoperative Management

- Atherosclerotic vascular disease, including ischemic heart disease, is common in patients undergoing carotid endarterectomy (see Chap. 20).
- Tobacco abuse is also common (see Chap. 24).

Intraoperative Management

- Some surgeons image the carotid artery during surgery with color-flow duplex ultrasonography or digital subtraction arteriography.

Preoperative Preparation

- DVT prophylaxis is indicated.
  - Mechanical methods of prophylaxis are usually used, because the bleeding risks of anticoagulation outweigh the benefits.

Usual Postoperative Course

- The most common adverse outcomes of carotid endarterectomy are stroke and MI.
  - Therefore postoperative surveillance with serial electrocardiograms, cardiac enzymes, and telemetry monitoring is appropriate.
- Postoperative fluctuations in blood pressure are common; however, keep diastolic blood pressure below 110 mmHg to avoid stroke.
- The hyperperfusion syndrome can arise when there is a sudden increase in blood flow to a region that was previously underperfused because of arterial stenosis.
  - The main symptom is a severe unilateral headache that improves when the patient sits upright.
  - This syndrome can rarely progress to cerebral edema, increased ICP, seizures, and hemorrhage.
  - Control of blood pressure may prevent progression.

References

1. Geerts WH, Pineo GF, Heit JA, et al. Prevention of venous thromboembolism. *Chest* 126:338S–400S, 2004.
2. Tunkel AR, Hartman BJ, Kaplan SL, et al. Practice guidelines for the management of bacterial meningitis. *Clin Infect Dis* 39:1267–1284, 2004.
3. Singer RJ, Ogilvy CS, Rordorf G. Treatment of subarachnoid hemorrhage. *UpToDate* 12:3, 2004.

13 GYNECOLOGIC SURGERY

Joann Porter and
Bruce E. Johnson

INTRODUCTION

- Medical consultants are not asked to see patients undergoing gynecologic procedures as commonly as patients with other surgical conditions. Although many issues bear on this observation, much of the reason is that, with the exception of malignancies, gynecologic patients tend to be younger and the procedures less prolonged. Nonetheless, the consultant should understand common gynecologic operations and be prepared to respond to the more frequent medical complications.
- Of note, this chapter does not address most surgical emergencies in the pregnant woman, nor does it specifically comment on the preparation for and management of therapeutic abortions.

COMMON PREOPERATIVE CONSIDERATIONS

- Age should be no more a barrier to gynecologic surgery than to any other type of surgery.
  - In fact, because many gynecologic procedures involve younger women, one must remain vigilant in search of unidentified or overlooked medical concerns.
    - For example, women with metabolic syndrome might be overrepresented in gynecologic surgery, with investigations related to infertility and dysmenorrhea. Metabolic syndrome carries a higher risk of atherosclerotic heart disease (ASHD).
  - Apply age-specific practices to preoperative evaluation (refer to Chaps. 3 and 5).
- Anesthesia
  - Laparoscopic surgeries often require general anesthesia, with its attendant risks.
  - Regional anesthesia is frequently employed.
  - Local anesthesia—used for minor procedures of the vulva, vagina, and/or cervix—carries a small risk from the effect of lidocaine on cardiac function.
- Infection prophylaxis
  - Such prophylaxis has significantly decreased the likelihood of infection, especially after any procedure involving the vagina (including, of course, hysterectomy).
- Prophylaxis for venous thromboembolism (VTE): see Chap. 46.

COMMON POSTOPERATIVE CONSIDERATIONS

- Blood loss: Patients who have lost over 500 mL of blood during surgery should be held as inpatients and should have their vital signs and urine output monitored every 4 h. Patients who have lost 1 L or more should be monitored more closely. If more than 500 mL of blood has been lost, hemoglobin should be drawn 4 h postoperatively to establish baseline level. If the diagnosis of postoperative hemorrhage is suspected, hemoglobin should be monitored every 1 to 2 h and reexploration considered. Vaginal bleeding after a vaginal hysterectomy can be managed by suturing the bleeding vessel; packing does not usually work in these cases.
- Infection: See Tables 13–1 and 13–2 for common pathogens and infections.
- Thrombophlebitis: Pulmonary embolism accounts for 40 percent of all deaths after gynecologic surgery. Risk factors for deep venousthrombosis (DVT) include malignancy, prior radiation therapy to the pelvis, hormone use [oral contraceptives (OCPs) or hormone replacement therapy (HRT)], obesity, age >40, and pregnancy. Fifty percent of postoperative venous thrombosis occurs in the first 24 h. Prophylaxis with either heparin or pneumatic compression devices should be used in all patients who have no contraindications. Prophylaxis begins in the operating room with the use of pneumatic devices.
  - Factor V Leiden has been associated with hypercoagulability, especially in estrogen replacement. Data at this time do not support changing perioperative care for patients who are known to be factor V-positive, nor do they support screening patients for factor V Leiden preoperatively.
  - A Cochrane Reviews metaanalysis showed that unfractionated heparin (UFH) is equivalent to low-molecular-weight heparin (LMWH) in preventing DVT after major gynecologic surgery.
- Pelvic venous thrombosis is common in patients undergoing gynecologic surgery but difficult to detect. Magnetic resonance angiography is the best available test, but its sensitivity is poor.
  - Septic pelvic vein thrombophlebitis is diagnosed in patients with an associated wound infection. A patient with persistent fevers despite antibiotic therapy should be suspected of septic pelvic vein thrombophlebitis.
  - Ovarian vein thrombophlebitis usually presents 1 week after surgery with unilateral pelvic and flank pain. Fever does not occur in all cases. On examination, a tender rope-like mass may be found.
  - Antibiotics and heparin are used to treat both of these rare syndromes. The heparin prevents septic emboli, which cause most of the morbidity. Pulmonary embolism is not associated with these syndromes.
- Urinary tract injury is a common complication of abdominal gynecologic surgery.
  - If the injury is found intraoperatively and stented at the time of surgery, morbidity is significantly reduced.
  - Bladder injury is usually more evident intraoperatively than ureteral injury. Bladder injury occurs five times more commonly than ureteral.
  - Ureteral injury occurs in 1 in 200 hysterectomies.
  - Simple abdominal hysterectomies account for almost 75 percent of all urinary tract injury in gynecologic surgery.
  - Hematuria is not a reliable sign of ureteral injury.
  - If urinary tract injury is not discovered intraoperatively, patients may present with flank/pelvic pain, pyelonephritis, urinoma (abdominal swelling due to collection of urine), or a fistula. A continuous watery vaginal or wound discharge may indicate a fistula. Creatinine studies can be done on the discharge to evaluate it. Methylene blue dye can be instilled in the bladder; a blue discharge indicates vesicovaginal fistula. Intravenous pyelography (IVP) is used for the diagnosis of ureteral injury.

TABLE 13-1 Pathogens Commonly Isolated from Postoperative Pelvic Infections

Aerobic gram-positive cocci
Viridans and non-group A, B, and D streptococci
Group B streptococci
Enterococcus faecalis
Staphylococcus aureus
Staphylococcus epidermidis
Aerobic gram-negative bacilli
Escherichia coli
Klebsiella species
Proteus mirabilis
Gardnerella vaginalis
Anaerobic organisms
Peptostreptococcus species
Bacteroides fragilis group
Prevotella bivia
Prevotella disiens
Fusobacterium species
Mycoplasmas
Mycoplasma hominis
Ureaplasma urealyticum

SOURCE: From Mandell.[8] Copyright © 2000 Churchill Livingstone, Inc., with permission.

- Bowel dysfunction: The routine use of a nasogastric (NG) tube increases the risk of aspiration. NG tubes should be used only in cases of abdominal bloating and refractory nausea and vomiting, where the aspiration risk increases.
  - Ileus should be managed with NG tube and bowel rest, electrolyte repletion as necessary, and adequate hydration.
  - Postoperative ileus can be differentiated from small bowel obstruction clinically and radiographically. Small bowel obstruction will usually occur after initial return of bowel function, but ileus occurs prior to any return of function. Radiographically, small bowel obstruction will appear as a large amount of air in the small bowel with minimal air in the colon.
  - Small bowel obstruction may not result in abdominal distention. A NG tube should be placed. Nasointestinal intubation has not been shown to be effective. Early postoperative small bowel obstruction can usually be managed conservatively; the adhesions are soft and dissolve easily.
  - Patients who have undergone laparoscopic surgery are the exception to this, as strangulation occurs more often; these patients often require early surgery. They should be monitored for clinical signs of developing leukocytosis, metabolic acidosis, fever, and acute abdomen, as these can indicate strangulation of bowel and need for reoperation.
  - Patients without ileus or obstruction will usually tolerate a liquid or low-residue diet within 6 h of surgery. Patients unable to tolerate nourishment by mouth for any reason, especially those who were malnourished prior to surgery, should be considered for enteral feeding or total parenteral nutrition (TPN) as appropriate.
- Pulmonary: Abdominal surgery leads to a decrease in functional residual capacity; the higher the incision, the greater the impairment. Upper abdominal surgery increases the risk of postoperative pulmonary complications 40 percent more than lower abdominal surgery. Laparoscopic surgery reduces the risk by 30 percent.
  - Nosocomial pneumonia or atelectasis can follow abdominal surgery. Good pain control and early mobilization decrease major pulmonary complications. Incentive spirometry is recommended for all patients who can cooperate.
  - Pulmonary embolus is common in gynecologic surgery. It is important to utilize DVT prophylaxis and to maintain a high level of suspicion for this diagnosis in symptomatic patients.

TABLE 13-2 Gynecologic Surgery: Postoperative Complications

TYPE	PRESENTATION	PHYSICAL EXAM	TREATMENT	NOTES
Pelvic cellulitis	2–3 days postoperatively with fever and pelvic pain	Lower abdominal pain and pain on bimanual exam	Cefotetan, cefoxitin, ampicillin/sulbactam, and ticarcillin/clavulanic acid	Use clindamycin combined with gentamicin in refractory cases
Cuff cellulitis	Fever, vaginal discharge 1–2 weeks postoperatively	Pain only at cuff site, no regional pain	Ampicillin/clauvanate	Follow-up exam in 72 h to rule out cuff abscess
Pelvic abscess	Several weeks postoperatively; ultrasound/CT necessary for diagnosis	Fever, leukocytosis and pelvic pain	Clindamycin combined with gentamicin	Drainage usually not necessary unless refractory to treatment Cover *Bacteroides fragilis*
Osteomyelitis pubis	8 weeks after extensive pelvic surgery, unable to ambulate	Fever, wound drainage, pain on abduction	Prolonged antibiotics covering staphylococci and gram-negative aerobes	Radiographically consistent with osteomyelitis, blood and bone cultures possibly helpful

TABLE 13-3 Postoperative Neuropathies

NERVE	MECHANISM OF INJURY	SYMPTOMS	SIGNS	DIAGNOSIS	TREATMENT
Femoral	Retractor injury	Pain over anterior hip, knee joint instability, numbness over anterior thigh	Absent patellar reflex, unable to raise thigh while supine, decreased sensation in anteromedial thigh and medial leg	Physical exam/EMG	Physical therapy
Sciatic/ peroneal	Stretch/pressure	Lower limb and foot numbness	Unable to evert foot Decreased sensation in lower leg	Physical exam/EMG	Physical therapy
Iliohypogastric	Entrapment	Lower quadrant pain +/– radiation to groin	Point tenderness 3 cm medial to anterosuperior iliac spine	Nerve block	Nerve block or surgical exploration
Obturator	Transection	Decreased sensation in anteromedial thigh	Adductor weakness	EMG/nerve block	Epineural repair if transected

EMG = electromyography.

- Neuropathy
  - See Table 13-3.
- Special issues
  - Hormones (OCPs and HRT) increase the risk of DVT. In women in whom becoming pregnant is an issue, the risk of pregnancy must be weighed against the risk of an embolic event. Low-risk women can continue OCPs. Moderate- and high-risk women should stop OCPs and HRT 6 weeks prior to surgery. These recommendations also apply to women taking selective estrogen receptor modulators (SERMs), such as raloxifene and tamoxifen. In women who are taking tamoxifen for cancer treatment rather than prevention, consultation with the oncologist prior to discontinuing therapy is recommended.

LAPAROSCOPIC PROCEDURES

- Usual procedures
  - Diagnostic, such as anatomic variants, tubal abnormalities, infection, endometriosis.
  - Fertility, including sterilization, tubal repair, and harvesting of eggs.
  - Major procedures including hysterectomy, endometriosis, myomectomy. Laparoscopic hysterectomies carry the highest morbidity rates as compared with vaginal or abdominal hysterectomies.
- Preoperative management including prophylaxis
  - Most of these procedures involve younger patients typically with few confounding medical conditions.
  - Preoperative consultations are relatively infrequent due to the combination of relatively young age and procedures perceived as minor.
- Cardiovascular (CV) risk
  - Apply usual preoperative assessment, including careful questioning for cardiac history, exertion-related symptoms, known valvular disease (including mitral valve prolapse), etc.
  - Recall that women, especially those who are perimenopausal, may have atypical symptoms of ischemia.
    - Symptoms of fatigue, shoulder/neck/jaw pain, and arm (left or right) heaviness are at least as likely as substernal chest pain.
  - At least two valvular conditions, mitral stenosis and mitral valve prolapse, have a somewhat higher prevalence in women.
  - Mitral stenosis, if severe and undetected, can cause major hemodynamic alterations during stress.
  - Mitral valve prolapse is associated with atrial tachyarrhythmias.
  - Apply usual criteria to beta-blocker prophylaxis.
- Pulmonary risk
  - Asthma, smoking, chronic lung disease, and other pulmonary conditions are not managed differently than in other operative situations (see Chap. 24).
  - Important additional concern involves positioning and abdominal distention. The Trendelenburg position is frequently used, with abdominal organs pushing on the diaphragm and lungs. The infusion of large quantities of inert gas can additionally compress the lower lung fields. In patients with relatively less pulmonary reserve, this may result in hypoventilation and hypercapnia.
  - Recall that many autoimmune and inflammatory diseases are more prevalent in women and may be associated with restrictive or interstitial lung disease. This should be evident from the history and physical without necessarily needing pulmonary function testing (PFT).
  - Evidence does not indicate that PFTs change operative outcome.
- Thromboembolism risk

- This is relatively low for most laparoscopic procedures.
- Most procedures are not done for cancer and are relatively brief. Early ambulation is expected, which helps to prevent thromosis.
- A counterissue is the frequent presence of OCP and/or HRT use and surgery performed in the pelvis, close to major venous return.
- For low-risk procedures, OCPs and/or HRT need not be stopped prior to surgery; prophylaxis by compression stockings and early ambulation should suffice.
- For moderate-risk procedures, OCPs and/or HRT may be stopped 6 weeks before surgery. If they are continued, however, this need not change prophylaxis (i.e., with compression stockings +/– LMWH until the patient is ambulatory.
- Few high-risk procedures are done laparoscopically.

- Infectious risk
  - Low unless there has been a operative mistake (e.g., bowel perforation) or a partial vaginal procedure (e.g., vaginal hysterectomy with laparoscopic assistance).
  - Any procedure involving opening of the vagina should be accompanied by antibiotic prophylaxis. Typical prophylaxis is a single dose of a second-generation cephalosporin given 1 to 2 h before surgery; metronidazole and/or clindamycin is recommended for penicillin-allergic patients.
- Common comorbid conditions/risk factors
  - Pain including endometriosis and/or pelvic pain syndromes.
  - Patients should be counseled that they should not expect immediate relief of pain, even after successful endometriosis procedures.
  - Preoperative narcotic use may complicate postoperative management of pain, since tolerance may have developed.
- Anemia
  - This is often a consequence of heavy menstrual bleeding.
  - Iron replacement is the usual treatment, but it may contribute to postoperative delay in bowel function.
- Hormone replacement therapy
  - See above for the role of HRT in postoperative DVT.
  - HRT discontinued close to time of surgery may be the source of hot flashes, which can occasionally confuse evaluation for postoperative fever/sweats.
- Obesity/metabolic syndrome
  - Many women with these states may have dysmenorrhea and/or infertility and may therefore be undergoing diagnostic or therapeutic operations.
  - While obesity is unlikely to pose problems for an otherwise healthy young woman, patients with metabolic syndrome might be marginally more likely to have postoperative issues of glucose management and hypertension.
- Anesthetic technique and operative pathophysiology
  - Most laparoscopic procedures are done under general anesthesia with the patient in the Trendelenburg position.
    - General anesthesia provides a better scope of vision and operative maneuverability than local or regional anesthesia.
  - Ambulatory/surgicenters are frequently used.
  - The attendant risks are those of general anesthesia.
  - Cardiac arrest is reported in only 0.002 percent of cases
  - Cardiac arrhythmias (including sinus tachycardia, ventricular tachycardia, and asystole) can be noted in up to 27 percent of patients during laparoscopies.
  - Cardiac arrhythmias during laparoscopy are generally attributed to rapid peritoneal distention, increased abdominal pressure, or air embolism.
  - An infrequent but not insignificant concern is hypercapnia from two potential sources: obesity and the Trendelenburg position.
    - Trendelenburg position and insufflation combine to compress the diaphragm, potentially compromising diaphragmatic mobility and leading to hypoventilation. Additionally, the inert gas used for insufflation, carbon dioxide, may be absorbed during prolonged procedures.
- Pneumoperitoneum and complications
  - Most air is resorbed within 24 h, though it can be occasionally detected up to 1 week; this is benign and of no consequence.
  - Pneumomediastinum, pneumothorax, and subcutaneous emphysema are attributed to gas that passes through congenital defects in the diaphragm. In general it is benign and not associated with infection. These conditions rarely require intervention; chest tubes are not indicated for small pneumothoraxes.
- Gas embolism
  - This condition is relatively rare (1 in 70,000 cases) but it carries up to 30 percent mortality. Entry occurs by direct inoculation into the venous or arterial circulation during trocar insertion. This usually occurs during insufflation.
  - Carbon dioxide dissolves quickly and is associated with fewer complications than argon, nitrous oxide, or room air.
  - If bradycardia, hypotension, and/or arrhythmias occurs at the time of insufflation, the surgery is stopped and supportive therapy is given.
- Postoperative management
  - Laparoscopic surgery is remarkably safe.
  - Operative complications include bleeding at the site of trocar insertion and/or bleeding from vascular injury,

intestinal injury, or urinary injuries, which infrequently leads to anuria and usually involves urology rather than medical consultation.
- Prolonged hospitalization with medical consultation is more often due to complications of surgery rather than predicted medical diseases and/or lack of prophylaxis.

VAGINAL PROCEDURES

- Usual procedures
  - With the exception of many cervical procedures, these are more likely to be done in older women with more comorbid conditions and for malignant or premalignant disease.
- Preoperative management including prophylaxis (compared to laparoscopic surgery)
  - CV risk
    - Overall higher risk, as women who have these procedures are more likely older, with attendant risks.
    - Usual age-related evaluation as listed in Chap. 20.
    - Follow general recommendations for beta-blocker usage.
    - Many vaginal procedures are done with legs in the lithotomy position, with fluid transfer from legs to the central vasculature; this is a theoretical issue in patients with marginal heart reserve.
  - Pulmonary
    - Few additional concerns
  - Thromboembolism
    - Many nonmalignant vulvar, vaginal, or cervical procedures involve relatively small DVT risk, with no penetration into the pelvis and rare concern about prolonged postoperative hospitalization.
    - Oncologic surgery of the vulva and vagina may be extensive and traumatic; hospitalization may be prolonged.
      - Cancer may predispose to a hypercoagulable state.
      - The prudent course is to use both compression stockings and LMWH as prophylaxis for a few weeks.
  - Infection
    - Antibiotic prophylaxis is routinely used for vaginal surgeries.
    - Multiple studies demonstrate a reduction in postoperative infection from ≥25 percent to <7 or 8 percent.
    - Antibiotic prophylaxis is also routinely used for extensive vulvar surgeries.
    - Consider "routine" bladder culture, especially for cystocoele repair and hysterectomy; if positive, treat.
- Common comorbid conditions/risk factors
  - Bladder dysfunction
    - Frequent causes for surgery are cystocele and hysterectomy.
    - Urinary tract infection is frequent owing to incomplete emptying of the bladder.
    - Treatment is indicated, especially as many of these procedures result in catheterization during the postoperative period.
    - Bladder dysfunction is rarely extensive enough to cause renal impairment.
  - HIV disease
    - Disease of the vagina and cervix is more likely and more extensive.
  - "Failure to thrive" and poor nutrition
    - Many malignancies of the vulva and vagina occur in older and sometimes debilitated women.
    - Assess for conditions of elderly women, including hypertension, cardiac disease, deconditioning, and dementia/delirium.
    - Unfortunately, frequent lack of a specific diagnosis for the failure to thrive leaves little opportunity for effective intervention.
- Anesthetic technique and operative pathophysiology
  - Local, regional, and general anesthesia is used in these procedures.
  - Many procedures done with regional anesthesia (e.g., epidural).
    - There is the advantage of less morbidity when the catheter is left in place for postoperative analgesia.
  - The lithotomy position raises concern over malpositioning and postoperative neuropathies (see Table 13-3).
    - The presence of arthritis of the hip or even the knees can complicate positioning.
- Postoperative management
  - Patient usually should be able to ambulate relatively soon (except with extensive vulvar surgery).
  - Bowel dysfunction is not uncommon with extensive vulvar surgery.
  - Exenteration for vulvar surgery may be accompanied by reconstructive efforts, including extensive use of grafts and flaps. Postoperative care by the surgeon must be careful. Once the patient is ambulating, however, balance may be temporarily difficult (due to altered sensation and the presence of a flap in the perineum).
  - Unfortunately, one of most common complications of vaginal surgery, especially hysterectomy, is ureteral or bladder damage.
    - If such damage is not recognized at the time of operation, the patient may experience complications ranging from urinary collection in abdomen, to abdominal pain, to a decline in renal function.
  - Sexual function
    - Anticipate improvement following hysterectomy and vaginal repair of bladder or rectal prolapse.
    - Vulvar oncologic surgeries may be deforming, leaving a relatively small vaginal introitus.

TABLE 13-4 Surgery-Specific Pointers

TYPE OF SURGERY	PREOPERATIVE POINTERS	POSTOPERATIVE POINTERS
Laparoscopic	Few consistent findings	Rare occurrence of air embolism Small bowel obstruction more likely to result in strangulation; reopening may be necessary. Occasional hypercapnia due to positioning and insufflated air.
Hysterectomy (abdominal or vaginal)	Correct anemia if time permits. Prophylactic antibiotics almost always indicated. For woman on hormones, stop 6 weeks in advance if possible.	Urinary tract injury not rare and may result in fistulas. Risk of DVT high; prophylaxis routinely recommended. Likelihood of infection equal at wound, bladder, lungs.
Vulvar, vaginal	Usually safe unless done for cancer. Patients tend to be older; hence, more concern with CV status. Prophylactic antibiotic use routine, especially with vaginal.	Surgical exenteration associated with high complications, especially infectious, and DVT. Due to prolonged bed rest, prophylactic anticoagulation common.
Malignancies	Often older women with comorbid conditions, such as CV, DM, dementia. Routine consideration of DVT prophylaxis. Preop chemo- or radiotherapy may leave patient anemic or prone to infection.	Ascites, as with ovarian cancer, complicates postop fluid management. Exenterations involve bowel and/or bladder and may lead to prolonged delay in recovery of bowel function.

CV = cardiovascular; DM = diabetes mellitus; DVT = deep venous thrombosis; EMG = electromyography.

ABDOMINAL SURGERIES

PREOPERATIVE MANAGEMENT INCLUDING PROPHYLAXIS

- Malignancies tend to occur in older women. Advanced age should not be a contraindication to surgery. Comorbid conditions and cardiac risk factors are more important predictors of surgical risk. A preoperative electrocardiogram (ECG) should be obtained, but the best predictor of an elderly woman's risk for cardiovascular problems is her preoperative activity level. If a patients has a low level of activity or symptoms such as fatigue, chest pain, or shortness of breath, she should have further cardiac evaluation prior to any elective surgery.
- Age-related changes in renal function: Elderly women can more easily become dehydrated from bowel preparation. In frail women, preoperative admission for close monitoring can be considered.
- Renal clearance should be calculated from serum creatinine and patient age. Medications should be adjusted to the patient's renal clearance.
- Infection prophylaxis: A second-generation cephalosporin should be used, given as a single dose 30 min prior to incision. For patients allergic to cephalosporins, metronidazole can be used.
- Anticoagulation prophylaxis (see Chap. 46).

COMMON COMORBID CONDITIONS/ RISK FACTORS

- Anemia: If patient has been having dysfunctional uterine bleeding or has risk for anemia of chronic disease, a complete blood count (CBC) should be checked preoperatively.
- Malignancy-related issues: Preoperative workup of patients with extensive malignant disease should include expanded preoperative testing.
  - A CBC is indicated in all patients, especially those who have had chemo- or radiation therapy to shrink the tumor preoperatively.
  - Liver (including coagulation factors) and kidney function should be assessed, as tumor bulk may be causing dysfunction.
  - A chest x-ray should be obtained to look for metastatic disease; the surgeon may also want abdominal imaging to help plan the operation.
  - Ascites may be present in extensive disease and can contribute to extensive postoperative fluid shifts that require close monitoring.
  - Patients may be malnourished, and improving nutrition both prior to surgery and postoperatively should be considered if possible.
  - Patients are also at increased risk for DVT; prophylaxis should begin in the OR with pneumatic compression.

Anticoagulation should follow if possible and be continued for 2 to 4 weeks postoperatively.
  - Immune function is probably diminished and can be affected by the cancer itself, chemotherapy, and malnutrition. This will place the patient at higher risk for nosocomial infection.

REFERENCES

1. Tamussino K. Postoperative infection. *Clin Obstet Gynecol* 45:562, 2002.
2. Baker V, Deppe G. *Management of Perioperative Complications in Gynecology*. Philadelphia: Saunders, 1997.
3. Bick RL, Haas S. Thromboprophylaxis and thrombosis in medical, surgical, trauma, and obstetric/gynecologic patients. *Hematol Oncol Clin North Am* 17:217, 2003.
4. Anticoagulant and aspirin prophylaxis for preventing thromboembolism after major gynaecological surgery. *Cochrane Database Syst Rev* 4:CD003679, 2003.
5. Donahue BS. Factor V Leiden and perioperative risk. *Anesth Analg* 98:1623, 2004.
6. Fanning J, Andrews S. Early postoperative feeding after major gynecologic surgery: Evidence-based scientific medicine. *Am J Obstet Gynecol* 185:1, 2001.
7. Magrina JF. Complications of laparoscopic surgery. *Clin Obstet Gynecol* 45:469, 2002.
8. Mandell GL, Bennett JE, Dolin R. *Principles and Practice of Infectious Diseases,* 5th ed. Philadelphia: Churchill Livingstone, 2000:1239–1240.
9. Hullfish HL. Patient centered goals for pelvic floor dysfunction surgery: What is success and is it achieved? *Am J Obstet Gynecol* 187:88, 2002.
10. Preoperative counseling and management, in Stenchever MA, Droegemuller A, et al (eds): *Comprehensive Gynecology,* 4th ed. St. Louis: Mosby, 2001:741.

14 UROLOGIC SURGERY

Joann Porter and Kurt Pfeifer

INTRODUCTION

- Urologic procedures are common.
  - 50 percent of men above 70 years of age will undergo transurethral resection of the prostate (TURP).
  - Operations for prostate disease are the most common urologic procedure in the elderly.
- Many urologic procedures are relatively safe.
  - Mortality from urologic surgery has decreased dramatically in the past 20 years.
  - Many procedures, including kidney retrieval from living donors, can now be done laparoscopically.
- Patients undergoing urologic surgery often have concomitant medical problems.
  - Patients undergoing urologic procedures span a broad spectrum of ages and comorbidities, ranging from otherwise healthy young individuals requiring lithotripsy for nephrolithiasis to octogenarians with several concomitant medical problems requiring radical prostatectomy for locally advanced prostate cancer.
  - 70 percent of patients undergoing surgery for prostatic hypertrophy have at least one concomitant medical problem that affects surgical risk.

PREOPERATIVE EVALUATION AND MANAGEMENT

- Renal insufficiency is common among patients with urologic disorders. Therefore routinely assess renal function in patients anticipating urologic procedures.
  - Further assess patients with impaired renal function for dehydration, hypervolemia, acidemia, hyperkalemia, cardiorespiratory dysfunction, anemia, and dysfunctional hemostasis.
- Routinely obtain a screening urinalysis for bacteriuria prior to many urologic procedures.
  - Some 25 to 80 percent of patients with bacteriuria who undergo a urologic procedure will develop bacteremia. Treat patients at risk for bacteremia with appropriate perioperative prophylactic antimicrobials (see Chaps. 48 and 49).

PROPHYLACTIC ANTIMICROBIALS

- There is some disagreement about which urologic procedures require screening and treatment for asymptomatic bacteriuria.
  - In general, screen and treat for procedures in which bleeding into the genitourinary tract can occur. Recommendations for timing and duration vary depending on the procedure (Table 14-1).[1]
  - Oral therapy with a quinolone is as effective as intravenous therapy.

CARDIAC RISK ASSESSMENT

- Renal insufficiency is consistently correlated with an increased risk of perioperative cardiac complications.
  - A glomerular filtration rate less than 60 mL/min is correlated with an increased risk of coronary artery disease (CAD).[2]

TABLE 14-1 Perioperative Management of Specific Urologic Procedures

PROCEDURE	PREOPERATIVE MANAGEMENT*	INTRAOPERATIVE ISSUES	COMMON POSTOPERATIVE PROBLEMS/MANAGEMENT	RARE POST-OPERATIVE PROBLEMS
Cystoscopy/ureteroscopy	Treat asymptomatic bacteruria in men but not women Treat those with risk factors for UTI with nitrofurantoin†	None	Routine	
Radical cystectomy	Complete cancer staging Check renal/hepatic function to determine candidacy for urinary diversion Check CBC 3 weeks prior to determine need for anemia treatment Discontinue ASA 14 days prior Preoperative antibiotics	Bleeding	Follow serum electrolytes and creatinine Monitor acid/base balance closely Monitor closely for blood loss Ileus	
Lithotripsy	Treat asymptomatic bacteruria	Pacemaker function may be compromised		
Percutaneous nephrosotomy	Treat all with 1.5 g ciprofloxacin			
TURP	Treat all with preoperative antibiotic Prolong treatment postoperatively for those with risk factors‡ Complete cancer staging		Hyponatremia: usually decrease of 8 mmol or less; severe hyponatremia occurs in 4% Follow electrolytes and creatinine	Volume overload Hypoosmolality Glycine toxicity Hemolysis
TURBT	Treat all with prophylactic antibiotic (quinolone or TMP/SMX) 1 h prior to surgery and continue for 3 days Treat with preprocedure enema			
Renal tumor cryosurgery	Complete metastatic workup	None	Monitor renal function	
Stress incontinence	Routine	None	Postoperative voiding difficulty/ urinary retention	
Nephrectomy	Check CBC and renal function	Blood loss Positioning can compromise cardiopulmonary function	Monitor Hgb, renal function, urine output	Neuropathy Atelectasis, pneumothorax
Renovascular surgery	Evaluate for coexistent vascular disease	None	Postoperative monitoring with arterial line Maintain DBP of 90 mmHg using nitroprusside Monitor creatinine Technetium renal scan at 24 h Atheroembolic injury to kidney and lower extremities	Renal artery thrombosis Persistent urinary extravasation (can be a sign of perinephric abscess)

ASA = acetylsalicylic acid; CBC = complete blood count; DBP = diastolic blood pressure; Hgb = hemoglobin; TMP/SMX = trimethoprim/sulfamethoxazole; TURBT = transurethral resection of bladder tumor; TURP = transurethral resection of the prostate; UTI = urinary tract infection.
*Modify antibiotic selection based on hospital resistance patterns.
†Risk factors in cystoscopy are voiding dysfunction, UTI, foreign body, and immunosuppression.
‡Risk factors in TURP: advanced age, procedure lasting more than 70 min, severe bleeding, and surgical skill (resident versus fully trained and in practice).

  - Perioperative morbidity associated with a low glomerular filtration rate (GFR) is primarily cardiac, not renal.
  - See Chaps. 3 and 20 for additional information on risk assessment and ischemic heart disease.

HEMATOLOGIC RISK ASSESSMENT

- Anemia is prevalent in patients undergoing urologic surgery because of advanced age, bleeding, and renal failure.
- Procedures such as radical retropubic prostatectomy, cystectomy, nephrectomy, and postchemotherapy retroperitoneal lymph node dissection present a risk of significant (2000 to 4000 mL) blood loss.
- Prior to surgery, check hemoglobin, discuss the patient's wishes for transfusion, and, if appropriate, obtain blood type and cross match.
- To treat anemia before surgery, consider stimulating erythropoiesis and providing iron supplementation in anemic patients who are anticipating major urologic surgery.

- Depending on the anticipated blood loss, treatment may be appropriate for patients with hemoglobin as high as 14 g/dL.
- Erythropoietin has been used in four weekly doses of 600 IU/kg body weight administered subcutaneously starting 21 days before surgery.[3]

POSTOPERATIVE MANAGEMENT

USUAL POSTOPERATIVE COURSE

Analgesia/Pain Control

- For most minor procedures, pain control can be achieved with the combination of oral acetaminophen and an opioid.
- For major procedures, initial treatment with an injected opioid is usually indicated.
  - Patient-controlled analgesia can achieve better pain control and more rapid weaning to oral pain medications than as-needed (prn) administration of analgesics.
  - Epidural analgesia can provide additional pain control for cystectomy and ileal conduit surgeries.[4]

Nutrition (See Chap. 49)

- Start most patients on oral intake when they have fully wakened from anesthesia.
- Routine use of nasogastric intubation is not indicated for most urologic surgeries.

Physical Activity

- Patients may begin to ambulate within a few hours of minor surgery, but they should wait for approximately 12 to 24 h after major surgery.

Laboratory Tests and Other Monitoring

- Order postoperative laboratory tests based on patient- and surgery-related factors rather than routinely.
  - Most healthy patients recovering from uncomplicated minimally invasive or laparoscopic surgery require no routine postoperative studies.
  - After procedures associated with large intravascular volume shifts or blood loss (prostatectomy, either open or transurethral, cystectomy, nephrectomy and adrenalectomy), test for anemia, electrolyte imbalance, and renal insufficiency.

Special Considerations

- Most patients undergoing urologic procedures will require perioperative bladder catheterization.
  - To minimize risk of iatrogenic urinary tract infection, remove the catheter the day after surgery unless heavy postoperative bleeding or other problems raise the risk of urinary obstruction.
  - After prostatectomy and cystectomy, leave the catheter in place for at least several days to allow adequate time for healing and hemostasis.
  - Use continuous bladder irrigation to prevent clotting of the catheter from postoperative gross hematuria.

Prophylactic Measures

- The risk of venous thromboembolism (VTE) for urologic procedures varies with the extent of the surgery and with the operative approach.
  - Major open procedures (e.g., radical prostatectomy, nephrectomy, and pelvic lymph node dissection) carry a significantly increased risk for VTE, and pulmonary embolism (PE) is the most common cause of postoperative death. Nonetheless, this risk must be balanced with the risk of uncontrolled bleeding.
    - Treat all patients undergoing major open procedures with graded compression stockings (GCS) and/or intermittent pneumatic compression (IPC) devices.
    - Add low-dose (5000 U) unfractionated heparin two to three times daily for patients whose risk for uncontrolled bleeding is not excessive.[5]
  - Laparoscopic (peritoneal, retroperitoneal, and extraperitoneal), transurethral, and percutaneous procedures pose a low risk for VTE.
    - Early postoperative ambulation is usually sufficient for patients undergoing these procedures.[5]

Hospitalization and Disposition

- Otherwise healthy individuals undergoing uncomplicated minimally invasive or diagnostic laparoscopic surgery typically return home the day of surgery.
- Patients undergoing urologic surgery for cancer or requiring an open procedure are usually hospitalized for 2 to 5 days and may require rehabilitation prior to returning home.

Common Postoperative Problems and Solutions

Infection

- Infection is a major cause of postoperative complications in urologic patients.
  - While the genitourinary and gastrointestinal systems are the most common sites of infection, also consider other systems and other causes of postoperative fever (see Chap. 50).

Hemorrhage

- Postoperative hemorrhage is a potential complication of any urologic procedure, but it is particularly common with prostate surgery because the prostate elaborates anticoagulants.

- Evidence of uncontrolled postoperative bleeding includes hematuria, hypotension, persistent bloody drainage, abdominal wall hematoma, and decreasing hemoglobin.
- After abdominal, pelvic, and especially retroperitoneal surgeries, scanning by computed tomography (CT) can be critical for determining the site of bleeding.
- Management of hemorrhage after urologic procedures is similar to that after other procedures (see Chap. 59).
  - Recombinant factor VIIa has been used to treat life-threatening hemorrhage after urologic surgery.[6]
- When bleeding occurs within the urinary collecting system, rapid identification and treatment of its source is necessary to prevent urinary obstruction by clotted blood.
  - Immediately place a urinary catheter (if not already present) and consider continuous bladder irrigation to prevent catheter obstruction.

Urinary Obstruction

- Several different processes can cause urinary tract obstruction after surgery.
  - Focal tissue swelling due to trauma or inflammation
  - Bleeding and clotting within the urinary tract
  - Calculi
  - Nerve damage
  - Medication side effects
  - Preoperative conditions exacerbated by surgery, such as prostatic hypertrophy
- The urinary tract can be obstructed at the level of the urethra, the bladder, or the ureters.
  - Urethral obstruction can be caused by blood clots, traumatic or inflammatory swelling, prostatic enlargement, or combinations of the three.
    - Presenting symptoms and signs of urethral obstruction include suprapubic pain and fullness as well as dullness to percussion above the pubic bone.
    - Ultrasound examination can confirm an overfilled bladder.
    - Bladder catheterization with or without irrigation relieves the obstruction while the cause(s) of obstruction is determined and treated.
  - Obstruction at the level of the bladder is due to a failure of bladder contraction.
    - A common cause is medications with anticholinergic effects, including opioid analgesics, antihistamines, and some antihypertensive agents.
    - Traumatic nerve injury can also cause failure of bladder contraction.
    - This is most likely after surgeries involving extensive mobilization of the bladder or dissection in the pelvis.
    - Symptoms and signs are similar to those of urethral obstruction.
    - Initial treatment is bladder catheterization and discontinuation of medications with anticholinergic effects.
    - Bladder function can recover, depending on the causes.
      - Bladder function usually recovers over hours to days if medication is the primary cause.
      - Bladder function usually recovers over days to weeks if postoperative tissue swelling is the primary cause.
      - Some bladder function may recover over months as nerves regrow if traumatic nerve injury is the cause.
  - Obstruction at the level of the ureters presents differently and is treated differently than obstruction lower in the urinary tract.
    - Ureteral obstruction is not usually associated with decreased urinary output because both ureters are not usually completely obstructed.
    - The primary symptom of ureteral obstruction is flank pain due to hydronephrosis.
    - Pain may not be present; a rising serum creatinine on postoperative screening is often the first indication of ureteral obstruction.
    - Ultrasound of the bladder, ureters, and kidneys or abdominal CT scanning is usually the first step in diagnostic investigation.
    - Ureteral obstruction is commonly caused by calculi, particularly after lithotripsy or lithotomy.
    - Tissue edema due to trauma or inflammation is also a common cause after any surgery of the ureters or adjacent to the ureters.
    - Treatments include surgical relief of the obstruction, ureteral stenting, and percutaneous nephrostomy tube placement to provide a conduit for urine while tissue edema subsides.

Bladder and Ureteral Injuries

- Injuries of the bladder and ureter that are undetected during surgery can occur with any urologic procedure and may be more common after laparoscopic procedures.
  - A high index of suspicion is necessary to identify these complications early and to limit sequelae.
  - The presentation is ureteral obstruction or peritonitis several days after surgery.
  - Cystography reliably identifies significant bladder injuries, while excretory urography, CT, and retrograde ureterography can demonstrate ureteral injuries.

- If detected early, some ureteral injuries may be amenable to percutaneous treatment with stenting, but most bladder and ureteral injuries require open surgical correction.

Gastrointestinal Injuries

- Injuries to the gastrointestinal tract that are undetected during surgery can also occur.
  - Bowel perforation is relatively uncommon but can have devastating consequences.
    - Symptoms and signs of peritonitis may not present for up to a week after surgery.
    - Fever and leukocytosis are not always present.
    - Treatment always requires surgical correction.
- After mobilization of the bowel for ureteral surgery or bowel resection and reanastomosis for urinary diversion, several gastrointestinal tract complications can occur.
  - These include gastrointestinal hemorrhage, anastomotic leak, bowel obstruction, and prolonged ileus.
  - Close monitoring of gastrointestinal function and abdominal radiography can detect these complications.
  - Treatment is with bowel rest, decompression, and sometimes surgical correction.

Electrolyte Abnormalities

- The urologic procedures most commonly associated with electrolyte abnormalities are endoscopic procedures, including transurethral prostate surgery and urinary diversion surgeries.
  - Transurethral prostate surgery and other endoscopic procedures are performed while continuously irrigating with a hypotonic solution.
    - The solution is variably absorbed.
    - Up to 10 percent of patients will develop hyponatremia.
    - If sterile water is used for irrigation, up to 2 percent of patients will develop hemolysis.
      - This is caused by the absorption of water, which leads to intravascular hypoosmolarity.
      - It has been called the transurethral resection syndrome.[7]
      - A variety of osmotic agents—including glycine, mannitol, and sorbitol—are now routinely included in the irrigation solution to minimize the risk of hemolysis.
  - Urinary diversion surgeries can cause electrolyte and metabolic disturbances.
    - In urinary diversion surgeries, a segment of the gastrointestinal tract is cut at both ends and the free ends are anastomosed so that gastrointestinal flow is uninterrupted. The urine flow is diverted into the isolated segment of the gastrointestinal tract and then connected to either the urethra or to a stoma in the abdominal wall.
      - Diversions using segments of ileum and/or colon frequently induce a hyperchloremic metabolic acidosis.
        - Significant potassium wasting can also occur.
        - For these patients, oral sodium bicarbonate and potassium supplements can usually prevent serious metabolic derangement.
        - If oral supplements are insufficient, revision of the anastomosis is sometimes necessary.
    - Diversions using a segment of the stomach frequently induce a hypochloremic hypokalemic metabolic alkalosis.
      - This metabolic disturbance is usually well tolerated except by patients with renal failure.

Laparoscopy-Specific Complications

- ***Hypercarbia:*** In patients with lung disease, the use of carbon dioxide for insufflating the abdomen can cause hypercarbia.
  - Carbon dioxide elimination can be prolonged.
  - Therefore monitor the respiratory status of patients with pulmonary disease for up to 24 h after prolonged laparoscopic surgery.
- ***Oliguria:*** Distention of the abdomen increases intraabdominal pressure, which may result in decreased renal vein blood flow and renal parenchymal compression.
  - This can lead to postoperative oliguria.
  - Most patients recover normal renal function spontaneously.
  - There is no effective treatment for this condition.
  - Intraoperative monitoring of abdominal pressure and adjustment of insufflation pressure can minimize the risk.

SPECIAL CONSIDERATIONS BY SURGERY

TRANSURETHRAL RESECTION OF THE PROSTATE (TURP)

PREOPERATIVE MANAGEMENT

- Thoroughly assess the patient for a bleeding disorder by medical history and physical examination.
  - This is usually straightforward, because most patients undergoing TURP have previously undergone major surgery and any occult, congenital, bleeding disorder would have been revealed.
  - If the patient has never had major surgery, dental extraction, or traumatic injury, ask about any bleeding disorders in the family, specifically ask about hemophilia, Christmas disease, and von Willebrand's disease.

- Also assess for acquired bleeding disorders by examining the patient's mouth and feet for any evidence of bruising.
- Discontinue aspirin and other antiplatelet agents at least 7 days before surgery to minimize the risk of bleeding.

Anesthetic Technique and Operative Pathophysiology

- Spinal anesthesia is usually used.
- Positioning is usually in the lithotomy position with Trendelenburg.
  - This can lead to decreased lung volumes.
  - Carefully monitor patients with preexisting pulmonary disease.

Postoperative Management

- Every TURP results in the absorption of some irrigation fluid due to the vascularity of the prostate.
  - Excessive absorption of isotonic solutions can cause hyponatremia and/or volume overload, with hypertension or even pulmonary edema.
  - Treatment consists of fluid restriction and loop diuretics, with cardiac support as indicated.
  - Other complications, depending on the solute used, include hyperglycemia, negative inotropy, hypotension, dysrhythmias, and retinal problems.
- Bladder perforation can occur.
  - It is usually diagnosed during surgery.
  - Delayed diagnosis often presents as periumbilical, suprapubic, or inguinal pain.
- Postoperative bacteremia is common and is usually asymptomatic, but about 7 percent of cases leads to sepsis.[8]
- Blood loss is common owing to the release of prostatic stores of plasmin and thromboplastin.
  - Management of hemorrhage is described further in Chap. 59.

TRANSURETHRAL RESECTION OF BLADDER TUMOR (TURBT)

Preoperative Management

- Ensure that patients have been fully evaluated for extent of disease.
- Measure baseline serum electrolytes, blood urea nitrogen (BUN), and creatinine, because metabolic abnormalities and azotemia are common after surgery.
- Ensure that all patients receive prophylactic antimicrobials.
- Discontinue aspirin and other antiplatelet agents at least 7 days before surgery so as to minimize the risk of bleeding.

Anesthetic Technique and Operative Pathophysiology

- General endotracheal anesthesia (GETA) is preferred so as to minimize bladder spasm.
- Hypotonic solutions are instilled into the bladder while a cystoscope is used to inspect the mucosal surface of the bladder and the ureteral ostia.
- Bladder lesions are resected by electrocautery.

Postoperative Management

  - Postoperative bleeding is common and often requires bladder catheterization and continuous irrigation to prevent urinary obstruction.

OPEN RADICAL NEPHRECTOMY

Preoperative Management

- The procedure is extensive, protracted, and associated with significant blood loss.
- Discontinue aspirin at least 7 days before surgery to minimize the risk of bleeding.
- Obtain a complete blood count (CBC) and type and screen.
- Optimize cardiac and pulmonary function.
- Screen and treat for urinary tract infection (UTI).
  - Treat with antimicrobials for at least 48 h prior to surgery.

Anesthetic Technique and Operative Pathophysiology

- Operative positioning can cause hypotension if the inferior vena cava is compressed, thus decreasing venous return.
- For patients with a large tumor load, cardiopulmonary bypass is used to prevent embolization of tumor to the lungs.
- Operative positioning can also compromise diaphragmatic excursion, thus impairing ventilation.

Postoperative Management

- Closely monitor urine output, renal function, and serum electrolytes.
- Consider using an arterial line to closely monitor hemodynamics.
- Follow for any evidence of tumor embolization.

RADICAL CYSTECTOMY

Preoperative Management

- Fully evaluate the patient for evidence of locally advanced or metastatic bladder cancer.
- Obtain hemoglobin, platelets, type and cross match, and serum electrolytes and creatinine because of the risk of substantial blood loss, metabolic abnormalities, and azotemia.

- Discontinue aspirin and other antiplatelet agents at least 7 days before surgery so as to minimize the risk of bleeding.
- Consider autologous blood donation and preoperative oral iron supplementation.
- Determine the patient's renal and hepatic function to help guide decisions regarding the type of urinary diversion that can be used.
  - If glomerular filtration rate (GFR) is less than 60 mL/min or hepatic function is abnormal, the patient may not tolerate the reabsorption of metabolites and urinary constituents that occurs with continent urinary diversions.[9]
- Give prophylactic antibiotics.

Anesthetic Technique and Operative Pathophysiology

- Following anesthesia induction, the patient is placed in the Trendelenburg position with the table flexed, so that the legs are parallel to the floor.
- The peritoneal cavity is first explored for evidence of metastatic disease; then bilateral pelvic lymphadenectomy is performed.
- After removal of the bladder, the urinary diversion is created. If there is no evidence of prostatic or urethral tumor involvement, a continent urinary diversion through the prostatic urethra can be created. Otherwise other forms of urinary diversion will have to be employed.[10]

Postoperative Management

- Closely monitor renal function and urine output.
- Closely monitor serum electrolytes and bicarbonate.
- Use electrolyte supplements aggressively.

RENOVASCULAR SURGERY

Preoperative Management

- Surgical revascularization of renal artery occlusion can provide excellent results for patients with renal artery aneurysms or ostial lesions or those who have failed percutaneous angioplasty.
  - However, the causal relationship between azotemia and/or hypertension and renal artery stenosis must be clearly established prior to surgery and the risks and benefits of revascularization carefully weighed.
- The most common cause of renovascular stenosis is atherosclerosis, and concomitant coronary artery disease is common in this population.
  - Myocardial infarction is the most common cause of postoperative death in patients with atherosclerotic renovascular occlusion.
  - Therefore perform a thorough preoperative evaluation for cardiac and other vascular disease.
- Intravenous fluids and mannitol are typically started before surgery and maintained through the immediate postoperative period to optimize renal perfusion and diuresis.
- Check serum potassium and other electrolytes before surgery and follow them closely through the perioperative period.
  - Electrolyte abnormalities are common, because renal artery occlusion can induce hyperaldosteronism.

Anesthetic Technique and Operative Pathophysiology

- GETA is preferred.
- Invasive arterial blood pressure and central venous pressure monitoring are routine.
- Wide variations in blood pressure are common and managed with intravenous fluids and nitroprusside.
- The most common surgical exposure is transperitoneal laparotomy; in most cases, revascularization is accomplished through an aortorenal bypass using an autologous saphenous vein or hypogastric artery.

Postoperative Management

- Monitor central venous pressure and arterial blood pressure in an intensive care unit for 48 h after surgery.
- After surgery, maintain diastolic blood pressure at 90 mmHg to assure adequate renal perfusion.
- Use nitroprusside as needed to treat hypertension.
- Renal artery thrombosis is uncommon (<5 percent) and occurs within a few days of surgery.
  - Renal artery thrombosis usually manifests as acute, recalcitrant hypertension and renal insufficiency.
- Acute renal failure can occur; closely monitor urine output, BUN, and creatinine.
- A technetium renal scan is typically performed 24 h after surgery to assess renal perfusion.

ADRENALECTOMY

Preoperative Management

- Most patients undergo adrenalectomy for resection of tumors including pheochromocytomas, adenomas, and metastatic cancers.
  - Prior to invasive manipulation of any adrenal tumor, measure 24-h urinary catecholamines to identify pheochromocytoma (see Chap. 29).
    - If the results of these tests are abnormal, measurement of plasma catecholamines and other assays may be indicated.
    - Patients with a suspected or confirmed pheochromocytoma require preparation, which may take up to 2 weeks, prior to surgery.
      - Phenoxybenzamine (an alpha blocker) is started at 10 mg PO twice daily and titrated by 10 mg

every other day until blood pressure and symptoms are adequately controlled.
  - Metyrosine (a catecholamine synthesis inhibitor) is sometimes used in addition to phenoxybenzamine.
  - Once adequate alpha blockade is achieved, a beta blocker can be added for additional control of heart rate.
- Thoroughly assess the risk of ischemic heart disease prior to surgery (see Chap. 20).

Anesthetic Technique and Operative Pathophysiology

- GETA is the preferred mode of anesthesia.
- Invasive blood pressure monitoring is recommended for all adrenalectomy patients, especially those with pheochromocytoma.
  - Intraoperative hypertension is common and is treated with phentolamine or nitroprusside.
  - The effects of adrenal hormones on insulin metabolism can also precipitate hyper- and hypoglycemia.
- Several different surgical approaches are used, including retroperitoneal laparoscopic, intraperitoneal laparoscopic, posterior laparotomy, anterior laparotomy, and thoracoabdominal laparotomy.
  - The surgical approach is based on the tumor's size, location, malignancy, and other considerations.
  - Though somewhat controversial, laparoscopic adrenalectomy has been used for almost all indications, including cancer and pheochromocytoma.

Postoperative Management

- Follow the patient in an intensive care unit so as to rapidly detect and treat labile blood pressure and blood glucose.
- Postoperative hypotension is common.
  - Treat it with aggressive intravascular fluid replacement.
  - Treat hypotension unresponsive to fluid with corticosteroid supplementation for adrenal insufficiency.
- Treat hypertension with intravenous nitroprusside or phentolamine.

References

1. Nicolle LE. Asymptomatic bacteriuria: When to screen and when to treat. *Infect Dis Clin North Am* 17:367, 2001.
2. Anavekar NS, McMurray JJ, Velazquez EJ. Relation between renal dysfunction and cardiovascular outcomes after myocardial infarction. *N Engl J Med* 351:1285, 2004.
3. Gilbert WB, Smith J. Blood use strategies in urologic surgery. *Urology* 55:461, 1999.
4. Conacher I, Soomro N, Rix D. Anaesthesia for laparoscopic urological surgery. *Br J Anaesth* 93:859, 2004.
5. Michalska-Krzanowska G, Sajdak R, Stasiak-Pikula E. Effects of recombinant factor VIIa in haemorrhagic complications of urological operations. *Acta Haematol* 109:158, 2003.
6. Mills RD, Studer UE. Metabolic consequences of continent urinary diversion. *J Urol* 161:1057, 1999.
7. Geerts WH, Pineo GF, Heit JA, et al. Prevention of venous thromboembolism: The seventh ACCP conference on antithrombotic and thrombolytic therapy. *Chest* 126:338S, 2004.
8. Miller R. *Miller's Anesthesia,* 6th ed. Philadelphia: Elsevier, 2005:2192–2209.
9. Walsh PC (ed). *Campbell's Urology,* 8th ed. Philadelphia: Saunders, 2002.
10. Inman B, Harel F, Tiguert R, et al. Routine nasogastric tubes are not required following cystectomy with urinary diversion: A comparative analysis of 430 patients. *J Urol* 170:1888, 2003.

15 OPHTHALMIC SURGERY

Brent G. Petty and Bruce E. Johnson

INTRODUCTION

- The perioperative risk of ophthalmologic surgery is low, and most ophthalmologic surgery is conducted in the outpatient setting.
- If problems occur, they are usually related to the patient's underlying medical conditions, such as advanced age, hypertension, diabetes, and atherosclerotic cardiovascular disease.
- Because most ophthalmologic surgery is performed with local anesthesia and/or moderate sedation, systemic complications from the anesthetic are uncommon.
- General anesthesia is used for pediatric ophthalmic surgery, oculoplastic procedures, and more extensive surgeries such as enucleation or repair of oculofacial trauma.

PROCEDURES

- The most common ophthalmologic surgery in the United States is cataract extraction; about 1.5 million such procedures are performed annually.
  - Nearly all are performed under local/regional anesthesia in the outpatient setting.
  - Trabeculectomy for glaucoma and vitreoretinal procedures are also usually performed under local/regional anesthesia.

- General anesthesia is required for patients who are unable to comprehend instructions or who might resist while under moderate sedation.

PREOPERATIVE MANAGEMENT

PREOPERATIVE TESTING

- Most or all "routine" preoperative laboratory testing can be omitted prior to cataract surgery without adversely affecting outcome.[1]
  - It is sufficient that the patient have a screening history and physical examination plus any laboratory testing needed to assess or address any discovered problems.
  - Prothrombin time/international normalized ratio (PT/INR) and partial thromboplastin time (aPTT) should not be obtained routinely before ophthalmologic surgery.[2,3]
- Screening laboratory testing might benefit patients who have not been receiving primary medical care.

COMMON COMORBID CONDITIONS AND RISK FACTORS

- Because of the advanced age of patients undergoing cataract extractions, the most common comorbidities are atherosclerotic cardiovascular disease and hypertension.
- Diabetes predisposes to cataract formation and may be more common in patients undergoing cataract extraction than in age-matched controls.
- The use of systemic steroids and ocular trauma also predispose to cataract formation; they may also be more common in patients undergoing cataract surgery.

ANESTHETIC TECHNIQUE

- Local anesthesia is usually adequate for most ophthalmologic procedures.
- Retrobulbar or periorbital blocks are used for some procedures.

PREOPERATIVE PREPARATION

- Most patients fast on the day of surgery, but they should take necessary medications with enough water to wash them down.
- Among the most common mistakes in the management of patients undergoing ophthalmologic surgery is to discontinue anticoagulant medications.
  - Cataract extractions, vitrectomy, and retinal detachment repair have been performed safely while patients remain therapeutically anticoagulated with warfarin for atrial fibrillation, prosthetic heart valves, or other indications.[4–6]
  - Inhibitors of platelet function should usually be continued through cataract extraction, especially in the setting of recent interventional vascular procedures such as angioplasty or vascular stent placement.[5–7]
    - Even the continued use of a potent platelet inhibitor, such as ticlopidine or clopidogrel, does not sufficiently increase the perioperative bleeding risk of ophthalmologic surgery to justify increasing the patient's risk of stroke and myocardial infarction by stopping them. For example, small sclerocorneal or corneal incisions for cataract surgery enable patients to continue ticlopidine without increasing bleeding risk.[8]
  - Perioperative management of anticoagulants and antiplatelet agents should be based on the risks and benefits for the individual patient.
  - Make management decisions collaboratively and include the ophthalmologist, the prescriber of the medication, and the perioperative management team.
  - Most patients undergoing ophthalmologic surgery should continue anticoagulant and antiplatelet medications; stopping these medications puts the patient at unnecessary risk for serious complications. Exceptions might be limited to the more extensive surgeries requiring general anesthesia.

POSTOPERATIVE MANAGEMENT

USUAL POSTOPERATIVE COURSE

- Most patients undergoing outpatient ophthalmologic surgery recover uneventfully.
- They commonly return to the surgeon's office in the first week after surgery; thereafter, they return infrequently unless they encounter unexpected problems or complications.
- Systemic perioperative prophylactic antibiotics are not used for ophthalmologic surgery unless there is a potential for bacterial soiling of the surgical site—for example, after traumatic eye injury.
- Prophylactic topical antibiotic drops are often used in ophthalmologic surgery; however, there is no good evidence supporting this practice.

COMMON PERIOPERATIVE PROBLEMS AND SOLUTIONS

- Hypertension
  - Postoperative hypertension, particularly immediately after surgery, is among the most common reasons for consultation with an internist.

- Often, the patients did not take their usual medications on the day of surgery.
- If there is evidence of acute end-organ injury, such as chest pain or neurologic dysfunction, admission for management of hypertensive urgency is probably appropriate.
- Also, there are ophthalmologic procedures in which hypertension jeopardizes the success of surgery (e.g., retinal laser surgery).
  - For these procedures, the surgeon may request assistance in managing hypertension in order to increase the chance of obtaining the desired outcome.
- In the absence of extenuating circumstances, having patients take their usual antihypertensive medications before being discharged is usually sufficient.

SUMMARY

- In general, ophthalmologic surgery poses little risk and, after any urgent problems identified by a history and physical examination are addressed, patients can safely undergo ophthalmologic procedures.
- No laboratory testing is indicated routinely before ophthalmologic surgery.
- Continue patients' usual medications without interruption in the perioperative period, including antiplatelet agents and anticoagulants.

REFERENCES

1. Schein OS, Katz J, Bass EB, et al. The value of routine preoperative medical testing before cataract surgery. *N Engl J Med* 342:168–175, 2000.
2. Smetana RW, Macpherson DS. The case against routine preoperative laboratory testing. *Med Clin North Am* 87:7–40, 2003.
3. Armas-Loughran B, Kaha R, Carson JL. Evaluation and management of anemia and bleeding disorders in surgical patients. *Med Clin North Am* 87:229–242, 2003.
4. Morris A, Elder MJ. Warfarin therapy and cataract surgery. *Clin Exp Ophthalmol* 28:419–422, 2003.
5. Norendran N, Williamson TH. The effects of aspirin and warfarin therapy on haemorrhage in vitreoretinal surgery. *Acta Ophthalmol Scand* 81:38–40, 2003.
6. Katz J, Feldman MA, Bass EB, et al. Risks and benefits of anticoagulant and antiplatelet medication use before cataract surgery. *Ophthalmology* 110:1784–1788, 2003.
7. Assia EI, Rasin T, Kaiserman I, et al. Effects of aspirin intake on bleeding during cataract surgery. *J Cataract Refract Surg* 24:1243–1246, 1998.
8. Saitoh AK, Saitoh A, Tamiguchi H, Amemiya T. Anticoagulation therapy and ocular surgery. *Ophthalm Surg Lasers* 29:909–915, 1998.

16 OTOLARYNGOLOGY

Harrison G. Weed

INTRODUCTION

- Most of the perioperative medical issues associated with otolaryngologic surgery arise in patients undergoing major surgery for cancer of the head and neck.
  - Most endoscopic and minor prcedures involving the ear and sinus are low-risk, outpatient procedures that do not require medical consultation.
  - Noncancer procedures that require general anesthesia and sometimes involve medical consultants include anterior maxillary artery ligation for intractable epistaxis, open sinus exploration (Caldwell-Luc), mastoidectomy, tympanoplasty, resection of acoustic neuroma, and thyroidectomy.

COMMON MEDICAL ISSUES

CARDIAC RISKS

- Patients with squamous cell cancer of the head and neck often have risk factors for cardiac complications such as older age, male gender, and a history of cigarette smoking.
- Apply standard methods of assessing cardiac risk (see Chap. 20).
- Recognize that, because patients with stage IV or recurrent cancer are at high risk for dying of the cancer in the following year, they are unlikely to benefit from invasive cardiac testing or treatment and will therefore be subjected only to the risks.
  - Therefore it is only occasionally indicated to postpone surgery for advanced head and neck cancer in order to allow time for invasive cardiac intervention.
  - For most patients, assiduous perioperative antianginal therapy with a beta blocker is preferred over stress testing.

PULMONARY RISKS

- Procedures involving the airway pose a higher risk of aspiration because of disordered swallowing.
  - Standard precautions are indicated; they include keeping the head of the hospital bed elevated above 30 degrees and maintaining assiduous pulmonary toilet.
- Mucous plugging is common after tracheotomy because airway clearance of mucus is compromised.

- It is more frequent in patients with emphysema and chronic bronchitis, both of which are common in patients undergoing major surgery for cancer of the head and neck, because of the association with cigarette smoking.
- The critical preventive intervention is frequent thorough suctioning.
  - Capable postoperative pulmonary care and good education of postdischarge caregivers about tracheostomy care are essential for patients with tracheostomies.

DEEP VENOUS THROMBOSIS

- Deep venous thrombosis (DVT) and pulmonary embolism (PE) are less common in patients with cancer of the head and neck than in those with other types of cancer.
  - Nonetheless, standard DVT prophylaxis is indicated for patients over 40 years of age who undergo major surgery.
  - Use pneumatic compression hose or low-dose unfractionated heparin (5000 U SC twice daily) starting prior to surgery and continuing until the patient is ambulating well.
  - Use more potent chemical prophylaxis for patients at higher risk for DVT (see Chap. 46).

METASTATIC STAGING

- Clinically detectable distant metastatic cancer is uncommon at the time of presentation of squamous cell cancer of the head and neck.
  - Most practitioners do not perform an extensive search for distant metastases prior to surgery for most patients; however, whole-body positron-emission-tomography (PET) is being increasingly used to detect distant metastases in patients with stage IV cancer.
  - In addition to the history and physical examination, standard screening includes chest radiography and computed tomography (CT) of the neck.

CACHEXIA

- Cachexia is common in patients with major cancer of the head and neck because the cancer often compromises chewing and/or swallowing.
  - Routine screening of serum albumin concentration is not indicated; however, it is appropriate to test patients who appear cachectic or who have lost more than 10 percent of their premorbid body weight.
  - One week of intensive enteral nutritional support prior to surgery is appropriate for severely malnourished (serum albumin below 2.5 g/dL) patients, but additional delay prior to surgery is usually not indicated (see Chap. 49).

ALCOHOLISM

- Because alcohol use is a major risk factor for squamous cell cancer of the head and neck, alcoholism is common in patients undergoing resection of these cancers.
  - History and physical examination screening for alcohol use and hepatic cirrhosis is appropriate for all patients; counseling and support for preoperative abstinence and prophylactic treatment for alcohol withdrawal are appropriate for selected patients (see Chap. 43).

HYPERCALCEMIA

- Squamous cell cancers of the head and neck sometimes cause hypercalcemia through the production of parathyroid hormone–like peptides.
  - Although it is reasonable to test symptomatic patients, a preoperative screening serum calcium test in an asymptomatic patient is usually unhelpful because the findings are unlikely to affect care.
  - In a symptomatic patient, preoperative treatment with hydration-diuresis and bisphosphonate may be indicated (see Chap. 56).

HYPOCALCEMIA

- Transient, asymptomatic hypocalcemia is common after thyroid surgery or radical neck dissection because of disruption of blood flow to the parathyroid glands.
  - If sufficient parathyroid tissue remains intact, whether in situ or transplanted, parathyroid function usually returns within a week or two after surgery.
  - It is appropriate to clinically screen all patients after surgeries that may disrupt parathyroid blood flow. Observe for latent tetany—Chvostek's or Trouseau's signs.
  - Routine screening of the serum calcium concentration is not necessary unless, in consideration of the specifics of the procedure and any previous neck radiation therapy, parathyroid ablation is possible.
  - Initially treat hypocalcemia-induced tetany with continuous intravenous calcium infusion.
    - Subsequently treat with supplemental dietary calcium (500 to 1000 mg thrice daily), plus vitamin D_3 (calcitriol 0.25 to 1 μg/day).
  - Patients who require calcitriol at discharge may subsequently recover parathyroid function and develop hypercalcemia.

- Therefore periodically test the serum calcium concentration of patients who are receiving calcitriol and might recover parathyroid function.

HYPOTHYROIDISM

- Primary hypothyroidism is common after radiation therapy of the neck.
  - It is detectable as early as 4 months after treatment and occurs in over half of patients after 3 years.
  - Prior to surgery, obtain a screening serum TSH on all patients who have undergone neck radiation more than 6 months previously and who are not already being treated for hypothyroidism.
- Hypothyroidism secondary to hypopituitarism is common after radiation therapy of the skull base.
  - Prior to surgery, obtain a screening serum free T_4 on all patients who have undergone radiation of the skull base more than 6 months previously and who are not already being treated for hypopituitarism.
  - Also screen such patients for adrenal insufficiency (see Chap. 28).

CONSIDERATIONS FOR DIFFERENT SURGERIES

CRANIOFACIAL RESECTION OF ETHMOID CANCERS

- These surgeries are often done in collaboration with a neurosurgeon.
- Surgery usually lasts from 5 to 10 h.
- Depending on the extent of resection, blood loss can range from 1000 to 3000 mL.
- Complications include bleeding, cerebrospinal fluid (CSF) leak, meningitis, and vision problems.
  - Lumbar spinal drainage, supine position, and blood pressure control are used to minimize CSF pressure and allow healing of the leak.
  - Reoperation for closure is required for recalcitrant leaks.
- Meningitis is more common in patients who develop CSF leak.
  - Diagnosis includes lumbar puncture for CSF.
  - Empiric treatment should cover *Staphylococcus aureus* and gram-negative rods (e.g., vancomycin plus cefepime) (see Chap. 50).
- Nasal sinus packing typically remains in place for 10 days to allow time for healing; however, this warm, serum-soaked environment is well-suited to bacterial growth.
  - Prophylactic antibiotics are often continued during this period.
  - Follow temperature and symptoms closely. If there is evidence of infection, such as fever and/or tachycardia, consider obtaining blood cultures.

ENDOSCOPIC SINUS SURGERY

- This is usually a relatively minor procedure performed in an outpatient setting, with an estimated blood loss of less than 200 mL.
- Nasal polyposis can be associated with aspirin-inducible asthma (see Chap. 25).
- Serious complications are uncommon but include bleeding, anosmia (usually unilateral), CSF leak, meningitis, and orbital damage with vision problems including diplopia and blindness.

PEDICLE FLAPS (SUCH AS PECTORALIS, DELTOPECTORAL, AND STRAP MUSCLES)

- Flaps are used in the course of cancer resection, fistula repair, or any reconstruction requiring additional soft tissue.
  - The purpose is to bring healthy tissue with a good blood supply to the surgical site to improve healing.
  - The pedicle includes the artery supplying and the vein draining the muscle.
- Surgical stress is minimal to moderate.
- Blood loss is less than 200 mL, depending on the flap.
- Complications include surgical site infection and bleeding or hematoma.
- Also, if the flap does not receive adequate arterial perfusion, it will die.
- Inadequate perfusion can be caused by arterial obstruction, vasospasm, or venous obstruction.
  - Avoid inadvertently compressing the graft with lines, hoses, equipment, bandages, or circumferential dressings.
  - Avoid medications that might induce vasospasm, such as nicotine and alpha-adrenergic agonists.
  - Initially assess flap perfusion hourly.
  - A flap with inadequate arterial inflow is usually pale; a flap with inadequate venous outflow is usually dusky.
  - Arterial blood flow to the flap can also be assessed by Doppler and capillary flow by pinprick for bleeding.
  - A flap that is initially congested and edematous due to inadequate venous outflow can grow new venous drainage over several days.

FREE FLAPS (SUCH AS RADIAL AND FIBULAR FLAPS)

- The purpose of a free flap is the same as that of the pedicle flap described above.

- The difference is that free flaps are completely disconnected from the donor site, and their arteries and veins are reconnected at the receptor site.
  - A fibular free flap also includes a section of bone to provide form and scaffolding for a resected section of mandible.
- The surgical stress is usually comparable to that of a pedicle flap, as is the blood loss (about 200 mL).
- Complications are similar to those for a pedicle flap except that there are two surgical sites, creating two sites of possible infection and/or bleeding.
- In addition, if the flap includes bone, the donor-site bone is weakened and more easily fractured.
  - Patients with fibular free flaps can usually resume careful ambulation on postoperative day 6, but they must avoid excessively stressing the lower leg until it is well healed, usually after 6 to 8 weeks.

GLOSSOMANDIBULOPHARYNGECTOMY WITH TRACHEOTOMY, NECK DISSECTION, AND FLAP REPAIR

- These procedures are done to resect cancer.
- The surgery takes 4 to 10 h, depending on the extent of the neck dissection (e.g., unilateral or bilateral) and any flap repair.
- Blood loss ranges from 500 to over 2000 mL, depending on the extent of the surgery.
- Surgical stress is severe with extensive procedures.
- 24 h of monitoring in an intensive care unit (ICU) is appropriate for patients with concomitant unstable medical problems.
- Patients can often begin ambulation on postoperative day 1 or 2.
- Enteric tube feeding is started on postoperative day 1 if there are no contraindications.
- To minimize the risk of fistula formation and aspiration, oral feeding may not be started for several weeks, or until healing is well advanced.
- Hospital stay is usually 10 to 14 days.
- Complications are those of tracheotomy, plus the following:
  - Pneumonia
  - Surgical site infection
    - The risk of surgical site infection is substantially greater when the surgical site penetrates the oral cavity.
  - Nerve injury: this may involve the mandibular, hypoglossal, vagus, or phrenic nerves as well as the brachial plexus.
    - Phrenic nerve injury may become manifest as unilateral elevated hemidiaphragm with associated atelectasis.
    - Nerve injuries can improve over days, weeks, months, or never, depending on whether the nerve was only stunned by traction or compression or has been transected or resected.
  - Another potential complication is the formation of a chylous fistula due to inadvertent injury to the thoracic duct.
    - Healing is promoted by minimizing chyle flow with an extended period of a strictly fat-free diet or of fasting with parenteral feeding only.
    - A pressure dressing is applied to the region of the thoracic duct.
    - Reexploration of the surgical site and ligation of the thoracic duct may be required.
- Pharyngocutaneous fistula is more common in patients with prior radiation therapy of the neck.
- Carotid blowout is rupture of the carotid artery with exsanguination.
  - This complication can be horrific and fatal within minutes.
  - Patients are usually at risk because of friable carotid tissue, often invaded by cancer.
  - Patients and their families should be educated on the possibility, the sentinel signs, and how to prepare and respond.
    - Sentinel signs include choking, neck swelling, and any oral bleeding.
    - Preparation may include an emergency response plan.
    - Response can vary from emergently contacting the surgeon for a hospitalized patient to comfort care only for a patient with cancer that is recalcitrant to treatment.

LARYNGECTOMY WITH OR WITHOUT RADICAL NECK DISSECTION

- This is usually done to resect cancer.
  - It can also be done to treat intractable aspiration with recurrent pneumonia, often due to prior hemilaryngectomy to resect cancer.
- It results in a permanent tracheal stoma.
  - Some 3 to 6 weeks after surgery or sometimes at the time of the surgery, vocal restoration can be achieved by placing a prosthesis through a tracheoesophageal puncture. The patient can then speak normally by temporarily blocking the tracheal stoma with a thumb.
- The procedure takes 3 to 7 h depending on the extent of the tumor, whether neck dissection is unilateral or bilateral, and any flap repair (e.g., pectoral, deltopectoral).
- Blood loss varies from 300 to over 1000 mL, depending on the extent of the surgery.

- Surgical stress is moderate to severe, depending on the extent of the surgery and on surgical site characteristics, such as damage due to radiation therapy.
- 24 h of ICU monitoring is appropriate for patients with concomitant unstable medical problems.
- Patients can often begin ambulating on postoperative day 1.
- Tube feeding is started on postoperative day 1 if there are no contraindications.
- Oral liquids are usually started on about postoperative day 7 if healing has progressed normally.
  - Patients with previous neck radiation usually do not start oral liquids for several weeks so as to minimize the risk of fistula formation.
- Hospital stay is usually 7 to 14 days.
- The risk of complications depends on the extent of the surgery.
  - Complications are much more frequent and more often severe in patients who have previously received neck radiation.
- The types of complications are the same as those for glossomandibulopharyngectomy, described above.
- In addition, total thyroidectomy is sometimes required.

LARYNGOSCOPY WITH BIOPSY OR LASER SURGERY

- These procedures are usually relatively minor and brief (1 h) with minimal blood loss.
- One day of observation is appropriate after procedures that can lead to laryngeal edema and airway obstruction.
- Airway obstruction is the major potential complication.
- After partial or hemilaryngectomy, recurrent aspiration is common.
- Other potential complications include dental or oral cavity trauma from the scope and temporary or permanent hoarseness.

MASTOIDECTOMY

- Mastoidectomy can be done for a variety of reasons including drainage of chronic mastoiditis unresponsive to antibiotics, drainage of otogenic brain abscess, resection of cholesteotoma, and as part of the approach to the resection of an acoustic neuroma.
- Surgical stress is moderate.
- Mastoidectomy usually takes 2 to 4 h.
- Resection of an acoustic neuroma more commonly takes 7 to 8 h but may last much longer and may be done in collaboration with a neurosurgeon.
- Intraoperative monitoring of the facial nerve is sometimes used.
- In addition to facial nerve damage, complications include CSF leak, hearing loss, and vertigo with nausea (see "Craniofacial Resection," above).
- If the vestibular nerve is injured or resected, then, depending on the size of the tumor and preoperative nerve function, the patient may have vertigo and nausea, often with vomiting, because of the sudden change in vestibular input.
  - Antiemetics are not used so as to avoid inhibiting the vestibular input and the brain's natural adaptation, a process that usually takes a few days.
- Steroids used to minimize nerve swelling can cause insulin resistance and exacerbate or precipitate diabetes mellitus.
- Patients are sometimes treated prophylactically with acyclovir with the goal of reducing the recrudescence of herpes simplex and varicella zoster viruses.
- Chronic complications include hearing loss and chronic ear drainage.

PARATHYROIDECTOMY

- This procedure is done to cure hyperparathyroidism. Thyroidectomy or hemithyroidectomy is usually performed for resection of a parathyroid carcinoma.
- The surgery lasts for 1 to 4 h, depending on the need for and difficulty of identifying all four parathyroid glands.
- Stress is usually less than that for thyroidectomy and recovery is usually more rapid.
- Complications are the same as those for thyroidectomy except that there is no risk of hypothyroidism.
- Postoperative monitoring should include examination for hypocalcemia (see "Hypocalcemia," above).

PAROTIDECTOMY

- Parotidectomy is done to resect parotid tumors or skin cancers metastatic to the parotid gland.
- The procedure usually lasts for 3 to 4 h.
- The anticipated blood loss is less than 200 mL.
- The primary concern for complication is injury to the facial nerve.
- Extensive resections of large tumors are sometimes complicated by injury to the temporomandibular joint (TMJ).
- The risk of surgical site infection is substantially less than that of head and neck surgeries that enter the oral cavity.

SINUS SURGERY, OPEN: MAXILLECTOMY, ETHMOIDECTOMY

- The extent of these procedures depends on the indication.

  - Treatment of chronic sinusitis unresponsive to medical treatment is generally a less extensive procedure than is resection of a cancer.
  - Resections of maxillary tumors or repair of fractures that impinge on the orbit may be done in collaboration with an ophthalmologist.
  - Resections of the floor of the maxilla may be done in collaboration with a dentist/prosthodontist.
- Complications of operations on the ethmoid sinuses and the roof of the maxilla include damage to the eye or orbit, with consequent vision problems, CSF leak, and meningitis (see "Craniofacial Resection," above).
- Complications of the maxillary floor include damage to maxillary teeth.

THYROIDECTOMY, HEMITHYROIDECTOMY

- These procedures are done to resect a cancer, a goiter impinging on the airway, an autonomous hyperfunctioning nodule, a hyperfunctioning thyroid (e.g., Graves' disease) that has failed medical therapy, or for cosmetic reasons.
- Anticipated blood loss is less than 200 mL, but it can be more than 2000 mL with difficult resections.
- The patient is usually ambulating on postoperative day 1, eating on postoperative day 2, and discharged on postoperative day 3 to 5.
- Complications include recurrent laryngeal nerve injury, thyrotoxicosis, hypocalcemia, and postoperative bleeding with hematoma formation and the possibility of tracheal compression (see "Parathyroidectomy," above).
- Potential long-term consequences are hypothyroidism and hypoparathyroidism.

TONSILLECTOMY

- This is a relatively minor procedure, usually with minimal blood loss.
- Postoperative stay is as needed to ensure that the patient can swallow adequately to maintain hydration.
- The most common complication is bleeding.

TRACHEOTOMY

- A tracheotomy is usually done to relieve or avoid upper airway obstruction, often as part of resection of a pharyngeal or laryngeal cancer.
- It is a relatively minor procedure, lasting less than 1 h and with minimal blood loss.
- Complications include bleeding, subcutaneous emphysema which can track into the mediastinum, and surgical site infection.
- The most common serious postoperative complication is obstruction of the tracheotomy tube with respiratory arrest.
  - The critical prophylactic intervention is assiduous pulmonary toilet, including frequent suctioning.
- The tube can also become displaced.
- Long-term complications include erosion of the trachea, including erosion into a blood vessel with hemorrhage; nonclosure of the tracheotomy after tube removal, with fistula formation; and tracheomalacia, requiring tracheal reconstruction.

TYMPANOPLASTY/OSSICULOPLASTY

- Middle ear surgeries are performed to drain infection or repair the tympanum or ear bones so as to improve the conduction phase of hearing in patients with inherited or traumatic conductive hearing loss.
- Surgeries usually last from 1 to 3 h.
- Surgical stress and blood loss are minimal and the surgery is usually performed in an outpatient setting.
- Acute complications include seventh nerve injury with facial weakness, bleeding with hematoma, and vertigo with nausea and vomiting.
- Subacute and chronic complications include infection, tinnitus, facial palsy, and persistent vertigo.

UVULOPALATOPHARYNGOPLASTY

- This procedure is usually done in obese patients to treat sleep apnea.
- It is a moderately stressful surgery lasting about 2 h with an estimated blood loss of less than 200 mL.
- Overnight ICU monitoring of the airway, bleeding, and cardiac rhythm is standard at some institutions.
- The postoperative hospital stay is usually about 3 days, or until the patient can swallow adequately to maintain hydration.
- Complications include bleeding and dehydration.
- Sleep apnea causes chronic cardiac damage that can become manifest in the perioperative period as pulmonary edema from systolic and/or diastolic dysfunction and from dysrhythmia, often atrial fibrillation.

SUMMARY

- Otolaryngologic surgery spans a range of procedures from those performed endoscopically, quickly, and with minimal or no sedation to major cancer resections lasting half a day or longer and requiring collaboration with other surgical and medical specialties to minimize the substantial risks.

17 BARIATRIC SURGERY

Donna L. Mercado and
Judi Woolger-Kraft

INTRODUCTION

- Surgical treatment of obesity, or bariatric surgery (from the Greek *baros,* "weight," and *iatrikos,* "the art of healing"), is the most rapidly growing area of surgical practice today. Because it is the most effective method of weight loss, it will likely remain a cornerstone of treatment for morbid obesity in the foreseeable future. Jejunocolic bypass was performed for weight loss in the 1960s and 1970s, but it has now been abandoned because it had severe side effects, including diarrhea, electrolyte imbalances, and liver failure. The Roux-en-Y procedure for weight loss developed in the 1990s. It has less severe side effects and, combined with the epidemic of obesity, its development has led to the rapidly increasing popularity of weight-reduction surgery. Furthermore, there is evidence that adding bariatric surgery to the treatment of morbid obesity reduces the mortality rate by two-thirds, compared to medical treatment alone.[1]

OBESITY

- Worldwide, about 1.7 billion people are either overweight or obese.[2] In the United States, about 6 million people have a body mass index (BMI) that qualifies them for bariatric surgery.[3]
  - Obesity causes or exacerbates many diseases, including diabetes mellitus, hypertension, dyslipidemia, heart disease, stroke, arthritis, steatohepatitis, gastroesophageal reflux, and sleep apnea.
  - Counseling about eating and exercising is relatively ineffective, and anorexogenic medications often carry more risk than benefit. Nonsurgical weight loss methods have success rates of approximately 5 percent, whereas surgical interventions have a success rate of approximately 70 percent.[4]
  - Nonetheless, prior to bariatric surgery, all patients should undergo at least 6 months of a multidisciplinary effort at weight loss. This effort should include education and counseling to develop an understanding of nutrition, exercise, and health and to build up the skills for healthy eating and exercising. Even if the patient cannot lose sufficient weight without surgery, these skills will be important to the long-term success of the surgery.

BARIATRIC PROCEDURES

- Bariatric procedures are commonly divided into three categories: malabsorptive, restrictive, and combined malabsorptive-restrictive.
  - In malabsorptive procedures, the small intestine is partly bypassed. As a result, food is poorly digested and rapidly transits to the large intestine. This reduces calorie absorption. Types of malabsorptive procedures include jejunoileal bypass and biliopancreatic bypass. Because of their severe side effects, including diarrhea, electrolyte imbalances, and liver failure, these procedures are now rarely used.
  - In restrictive procedures, stomach size and emptying rate are reduced, with the intention of producing satiety with smaller meal sizes. Restrictive procedures have fewer adverse effects than malabsorptive procedures; however, they are also less effective. Types of restrictive procedures include gastric banding, adjustable gastric banding, vertical-banded gastroplasty (VBG), and gastric stapling. All can be performed laparoscopically.
  - Combined restrictive-malabsorptive surgery is more effective and has fewer adverse effects than either alone. The degree of malabsorption can be varied by the surgeon. Combined procedures include Roux-en-Y gastric bypass and partial biliopancreatic diversion. Combined procedures are more difficult to perform than restrictive procedures and, because there is some malabsorption, chronic deficiencies of specific nutrients remains a problem.[5]
- Contraindications to bypass procedures include:
  - Biventricular heart failure
  - Severe pulmonary hypertension
  - Nephrogenic diabetes insipidus
  - Uncontrolled psychiatric illness, including:
    - Untreated psychiatric illness
    - Noncompliance with psychiatric treatment
    - Psychosis

PREOPERATIVE ASSESSMENT AND MANAGEMENT

CARDIOVASCULAR

- Cardiovascular disease is common in morbidly obese people, and assessment is made more difficult by the obesity.
  - Coronary artery disease (CAD) is common in morbidly obese patients because they often have potent risk factors for CAD, including hypertension, hyperlipidemia, and diabetes mellitus.
    - The independent contribution of obesity to cardiovascular risk seems to be relatively modest.

- Obtain noninvasive stress testing for CAD as directed by standard guidelines (see Chap. 20).
- Treat patients at risk for CAD with beta blockers as directed by standard guidelines (see Chap. 20).
- Treat and control the risk factors for CAD (see Chap. 19).
  - There is evidence that treatment of hyperlipidemia with HMG-CoA reductase inhibitors ("statins") can reduce the perioperative morbidity and mortality from CAD (see Chap. 20).
- Cardiomyopathy of obesity is thought to be due to chronic high cardiac output as the body provides circulation to excess adipose tissue.
  - It is characterized by pulmonary and systemic vascular congestion, ventricular volume overload, and eccentric left ventricular hypertrophy.[6]
  - It should be suspected in the presence of unexplained dyspnea, orthopnea, and peripheral edema.
  - Echocardiography can be diagnostic, and determining left ventricular ejection fraction can be important for guiding treatment in the perioperative period.
  - Treat as for congestive heart failure (see Chap. 22).
  - Cardiac assessment is more difficult in morbidly obese patients.
    - Assessment of functional capacity is limited by the patient's ponderousness and deconditioning, physical findings are obscured by adipose tissue, weight limits on diagnostic machines can preclude some studies, and studies can be difficult to interpret because images are obscured by adipose tissue.

PULMONARY/RESPIRATORY

- All morbidly obese patients suffer some degree of respiratory compromise.
  - Obesity-associated restrictive lung disease is thought to have many causes.
    - The mass of adipose tissue in the chest wall and abdomen increases the work of breathing and decreases functional residual capacity.
    - Adipose tissue protruding into the upper airways can increase airflow resistance and further increase the work of breathing.
    - Chronic hypoventilation can lead to pulmonary atelectasis, hypoxemia, fibrosis, and decreased lung compliance.
  - Upper airway obstruction can also contribute to sleep apnea.
    - Hypoxemia due to sleep apnea causes fibrosis of the pulmonary vasculature, leading to pulmonary hypertension.[6]
    - It also causes fibrosis of the heart leading to diastolic dysfunction and heart failure.
  - Pulmonary dysfuction is exacerbated during and after surgery for several reasons.
    - A recumbent position increases the work of breathing.
    - Anesthetics and postoperative pain medications decrease respiratory drive and reduce muscle tone in the chest and neck.
  - There are several actions that may reduce the risk of postoperative pulmonary complications (see Chaps. 24 and 25).
    - Begin incentive spirometry and deep breathing exercises for all patients before bariatric surgery and continue these after surgery.
    - Use continuous pulse oximetry to monitor patients in the immediate postoperative period.
    - Recognize that supplemental inhaled oxygen can mask hypoventilation, and emergently obtain a blood gas to detect hypercarbia on any patient with unexplained confusion or somnolence after surgery.
    - Use inhaled bronchodilators in patients with evidence of bronchospasm.
    - Have patients with sleep apnea bring their CPAP (continuous positive airway pressure) masks to the hospital and use them after surgery.
    - Obtain sleep studies in any patient suspected of having sleep apnea.

THROMBOEMBOLISM

- Deep venous thrombosis and pulmonary embolism are common complications of surgery in morbidly obese patients.
  - Dose prophylactic anticoagulants adequately for the patient's body size (see Chap. 46).

INFECTION

- Dose prophylactic antimicrobials adequately for the patient's body size (see Chap. 48).

ENDOCRINE/METABOLIC

- Endocrine abnormalities are common in morbidly obese patients.
  - Diabetes mellitus is an obesity-related disease, and elevated blood sugar is associated with poor wound healing.
    - Optimize control of diabetes prior to surgery (see Chap. 26).
  - Hypothyroidism is common in morbidly obese patients.

- Check serum TSH prior to bariatric surgery (see Chap. 27).
- Nephrogenic diabetes insipidus (DI) is rare, but is a contraindication to bariatric surgery, because the patient cannot ingest and absorb an adequate volume of fluid to maintain fluid balance after surgery.
  - Poorly controlled central DI is also a contraindication for the same reason.[7]
- Gallstones form in the setting of rapid weight loss.
  - Therefore it has become routine to screen for cholelithiasis prior to bariatric surgery, and prophylactic cholecystectomy is often done along with the bariatric procedure.[8]

PSYCHIATRIC

- Psychiatric illnesses and eating disorders are common in morbidly obese patients.
  - Ensure that patients obtain appropriate psychiatric evaluation and treatment before bariatric surgery.

ANESTHETIC TECHNIQUE AND OPERATIVE PATHOPHYSIOLOGY

- Anesthetic techniques are similar to those used in other abdominal surgeries.
- Nitrous oxide is usually avoided in laparoscopic procedures because it diffuses into gas-filled organs, dilating them and obstructing laparoscopic views.
- A fiberoptic laryngoscope is available in the operating room because endotracheal intubation is more likely to be difficult in morbidly obese patients.

POSTOPERATIVE MANAGEMENT

- Patients should begin ambulation as soon as feasible after surgery to optimize pulmonary function and minimize the risk of thromboembolism.
- The patient's diet should be advanced gradually after surgery. Schedules vary; an example of one schedule follows:
  - Initially limit oral intake to clear liquids.
  - Open or crush all capsules and tablets larger than the "head of a thumbtack."
  - On the fifth day, advance the diet to pureed foods and blended soft foods.
  - On the sixth day, advance the diet to soft foods such as baked white fish, canned fruits, and heavily cooked vegetables. No hard meats such as beef, pork, or chicken.
  - In the second week, try a regular diet. Add no more than one type of food at a time. Try adding whole capsules and tablets.
  - Patients must learn to eat significantly smaller portions than most people consider normal, to eat slowly, and to chew food thoroughly.
  - Low-carbohydrate foods are preferred because they minimize bacterial overgrowth and bowel gas.

COMPLICATIONS

- Infective peritonitis is a potentially fatal postoperative complication.
  - Leakage of bowel contents can occur from inadvertent nicks or, more commonly, from an anastomosis.[9]
  - Symptoms include fatigue, anorexia, and abdominal pain.
  - Signs include fever, tachycardia, tachypnea, and abdominal tenderness; however, clinical suspicion for this complication must remain high, because physical findings are sometimes within normal parameters until a sepsis syndrome ensues.
  - A meglumine diatrizoate (Gastrografin) swallow test or abdominal computed tomography scan can aid in the diagnosis and should be obtained at a relatively low threshold; however, abdominal exploration may be required to make the diagnosis. There is no substitute for the judgment of an experienced surgeon.
- Intestinal obstruction can occur; however, simply eating too fast or too much or not chewing food thoroughly can also cause reflux symptoms and/or vomiting.
- Insulin requirements typically decrease dramatically after surgery, and diabetes may resolve.
  - The patient and doctor must monitor blood glucose and adjust diabetes treatments frequently in the days, weeks, and months after surgery.

LONG-TERM COMPLICATIONS AND MANAGEMENT

- Long-term management includes medical, surgical, and psychological support.
  - A consistent exercise plan that includes walking at least 1 mile a day should be part of postoperative recovery and long-term hygiene.
  - Have the patient avoid heavy lifting for 3 to 6 weeks after surgery, as advised by the surgeon.
  - Lifelong dietary supplementation with a multivitamin, thiamine, vitamin B_{12} (cyanocobalamin), calcium, and iron is usually indicated.[5]

- Patients in whom longer segments of the small intestine have been bypassed may benefit from the measurement of serum carotenes (vitamin A) to check for malabsorption.
- With significant weight loss, sleep apnea may resolve.
  - Consider sleep studies for patients with sleep apnea who lose significant weight after bariatric surgery.
- With significant weight loss, sagging skin and skin folds may cause cosmetic, hygienic, and infectious problems. Surgery can be beneficial for these.
- Short and long-term psychological care can be critical.
  - For the surgery to be successful, the patient must develop and maintain new habits of eating and exercise.
  - Furthermore, patients who lose substantial weight often develop new habits, hobbies, friends, and a new self-image.
  - These changes present a myriad of psychological issues that can be difficult and even frightening.
  - Some patients become anorectic after bariatric surgery.
  - Group and individual counseling can be extremely important in helping the patient to deal effectively with the issues.

REFERENCES

1. MacDonald KG, Long DS, Swanson MD, et al. The gastric bypass operation reduces the progression and mortality of non-insulin dependent diabetes mellitus. *J Gastrointest Surg* 1:213, 1997.
2. Buchwald H, Avidor Y, Braunwald E, et al. Bariatric surgery: A systemic review and meta-analysis. *JAMA* 292:1724, 2004.
3. Flegal KM, Carroll MD, Ogden CL, et al. Prevalence and trends in obesity among US adults, 1999–2000. *JAMA* 288:1723, 2002.
4. MacGregor AM. The patient factor. *Obes Surg* 6:325, 1996.
5. Mattison R, Jensen MD. Bariatric surgery. *Postgrad Med* 115:49, 2004.
6. Herrera MF, Lozano-Salazar RR, Rull JA. Diseases and problems secondary to massive obesity, in Deitel M, Cowan GSM (eds): *Update: Surgery for the Morbidly Obese Patient*. Toronto: FD-Communication (Mothersill Printing), 2000:55,56.
7. Mercado DL, Liew PY. Diabetes insipidus complicating gastric bypass surgery. *J Gen Intern Med* 19(suppl):45, 2004.
8. Colquitt J, Clegg A, Sidhu M, et al. Surgery for morbid obesity. *Cochrane Database Syst Rev* 4, 2004.
9. Marshall JS, Srivastava A, Gupta SA, et al. Roux-en-Y gastric bypass leak complications. *Arch Surg* 138:520, 2003.

18 ELECTROCONVULSIVE THERAPY

Anjala V. Tess and Jeffrey R. Allen

INTRODUCTION

- Electroconvulsive therapy (ECT) is commonly used to treat psychiatric disorders by inducing seizure activity with an external electrical current while the patient is under general anesthesia.
- Following observations in the 1930s that schizophrenia transiently improved after spontaneous seizures, a technique was developed to use external current to induce seizures. ECT treatment of schizophrenia was first described in 1938.
- The most common indication for ECT is major depression with features of psychosis, severe suicidality, catatonia, or pregnancy where a rapid response is required. It is often used for patients whose depression has been refractory to antidepressant medications or who do not tolerate medication side effects. Success rates as high as 80 percent are reported, and one metaanalysis has suggested that ECT can be more effective than antidepressant medications.
- According to the American Psychiatric Association (APA), other potential indications for ECT include schizophrenia, bipolar disorder, organic delusional disorder, organic mood disorder, obsessive compulsive disorder, neuroleptic malignant syndrome, neuroleptic-induced parkinsonism, and tardive dyskinesias.
- The mortality of ECT is estimated to be 4 deaths per 100,000 treatments.[1] Morbidity is limited but includes cardiovascular, central nervous system (CNS), and somatic symptoms.

PREOPERATIVE MANAGEMENT

- Because of the lifesaving potential of ECT and low risk of adverse effects, there are no absolute contraindications; however the APA lists several conditions that may increase risk:[2]
  - Unstable or severe cardiovascular disease
  - Space-occupying intracranial lesion with increased intracranial pressure
  - Recent cerebral hemorrhage or stroke
  - Bleeding or unstable vascular aneursym
  - Severe pulmonary dysfunction
  - American Society of Anesthesiologists (ASA) class 4 or 5 (Table 18-1)

TABLE 18-1 ECT Pointers

PREOPERATIVE POINTERS	POSTOPERATIVE POINTERS
Focus preoperative evaluation on the cardiac, pulmonary, and neurologic systems. With stable/controlled disease, most patients can safely undergo ECT.	Monitor all patients with oximetry and frequent measures of vital signs while they are in the recovery phase of anesthesia (approximately 2 h post-ECT)
Patients with stable/controlled cardiac disease (including CAD, CHF, arrhythmias, and pacemakers/defibrillators) can safely undergo ECT.	Use continuous ECG monitoring in patients at higher cardiac risk.
Continue usual medications for CAD, congestive heart failure, or arrhythmia.	CNS effects are common but usually self-limited. If findings such as disorientation or headache persist beyond 24 h, further neurologic evaluation is probably indicated.
Initiating treatment with beta blockers or anticholinergics may be appropriate in high-risk cardiac patients.	Asystole, arrhythmias, or ischemic symptoms may occur and should be stabilized and evaluated before continuing with treatment.
In patients with persistent neurologic symptoms, evaluation for increased intracranial pressure and recent stroke is indicated.	Routine testing is not indicated either before or after ECT. Tests such as ECG, chest x-ray, head CT, etc., should be obtained only for patient-specific indications.
Pre-ECT laboratory tests (including serum electrolytes, pregnancy testing, and ECG) are indicated for specific patient populations.	

CAD = coronary artery disease; CHF = congestive heart failure; CNS = central nervous system; ECG = electrocardiogram; ECT = electroconvulsive therapy.

CONCOMITANT CONDITIONS AND RISK

Cardiac Disease

- Studies evaluating the cardiac morbidity of ECT suggest that the incidence of serious events is low. They are more likely to occur in older patients and in those with known cardiovascular disease, including hypertension, coronary artery disease, congestive heart failure, and arrhythmias.
  - In one early retrospective study of 42 patients undergoing ECT, 28 percent had at least one complication. Transient "arrhythmia" was the most frequent event (atrial or ventricular premature complexes, atrial or ventricular bigeminy, or atrial tachycardia). Four patients had major complications including chest pain, subendocardial ischemia, pulmonary edema, and cardiopulmonary arrest (cause of death not elucidated by autopsy). Seventy percent of the complications occurred in patients with cardiovascular disease, and every patient was above 50 years of age.[3]
  - A later study found a 55 percent incidence of complications among patients with cardiac disease. Of these complications, two-thirds were minor, such as transient ST-segment changes or atrial or ventricular premature complexes and atrial or ventricular bigeminy. Few patients had major complications such as asystole, persistent arrhythmias, or ST changes. The overall complication rate of 55 percent compared with a rate of 7.5 percent among patients without cardiac disease, where all events were minor. Most patients went on to complete treatment regardless of preexisting cardiac disease.[4]
- Use the American Heart Association/American College of Cardiology guidelines for noncardiac surgery to assess patients anticipating ECT (see Chap. 20). ECT is a low-cardiac-risk procedure. Except for patients with uncontrolled heart disease (unstable angina, severe valvular disease, unstable arrhythmias, or decompensated heart failure), most of those with cardiac disease do well with appropriate medical management.
  - Patients with hypertension can safely undergo ECT.
    - Because of the risk of postprocedure hypertension, make sure that blood pressure is well controlled prior to ECT.
    - Have patients continue their usual blood pressure medications.
  - Patients with stable ischemic heart disease can safely undergo ECT.
    - Continue antianginal medications, including aspirin, nitrates, and beta blockers.
  - Patients with compensated heart failure can safely undergo ECT.
    - Postpone ECT if the patient has decompensated heart failure.
    - Continue vasodilators and diuretics.
    - For patients with a history of heart failure that has not been characterized, consider obtaining an echocardiogram to assess left ventricular function, because this can help to guide perioperative treatment.
  - Patients with controlled arrhythmias, pacemakers, and defibrillators can safely undergo ECT.

- Continue usual antiarrhythmic medications.
- Be prepared to deactivate pacemakers with a magnet should there be problems. Deactivate defibrillators immediately prior to ECT. Monitor patients with continuous electrocardiogaphy (ECG) through treatment and in the posttreatment phase.
- Make sure that appropriate equipment is available and that personnel in the ECT suite and recovery area are trained for cardiopulmonary resuscitation.

  ◦ Have available and consider prophylactic use of atropine or glycopyrrolate in patients who are at risk of heart block because of underlying conductive heart disease and/or medications, including beta blockers and calcium channel antagonists.

Anticoagulation

- Patients who are anticoagulated can be safely treated with ECT if the international normalized ratio (INR) is less than 3.5.
  - ◦ One recent retrospective study evaluated 300 ECT treatments administered to patients receiving warfarin. Indications for warfarin included thromboembolic and cardiovascular disease. Some 3 percent of patients had an INR greater than 3.5. There were no adverse events related to warfarin.[5]

Chronic Obstructive Pulmonary Disease (COPD)

- No specific studies address the risk of ECT among patients with COPD.
  - ◦ Optimize pulmonary function with bronchodilators and inhaled steroid prior to ECT (see Chap. 24).
  - ◦ Postpone ECT if COPD is uncontrolled.
  - ◦ Theophylline increases the risk of status epilepticus with ECT. If feasible, discontinue theophylline and allow adequate time for it to be metabolized before ECT.

Diabetes Mellitus (DM)

- Patients with DM can generally receive ECT without complication. There are no randomized controlled trials that explicitly address this issue; however, anecdotal data do not show specific problems attributable to hyperglycemia.
  - ◦ Attempt to normalize blood glucose prior to ECT; however, there is no known reason to postpone ECT in asymptomatic hyperglycemic patients.
  - ◦ Because hypoglycemia compromises brain function, make sure that patients are not hypoglycemic before, during, or after ECT.
  - ◦ Adjust diabetes medications, because patients will not be eating before or for a few hours after ECT (see Chap. 26).

Stroke

- Depression occurs in about one-third of patients within 2 years after a stroke. ECT and oral antidepressant therapy can treat these patients successfully.[6]
  - ◦ There are no randomized controlled trials of ECT in poststroke patients: the published data are from case reports and retrospective studies.
  - ◦ A retrospective cohort study of ECT for poststroke depression showed a 95 percent rate of improvement.[7]
  - ◦ ECT has been performed safely after patients have recovered from lacunar infarctions, hemorrhagic infarctions, and in the setting of structural brain changes including cortical atrophy and ventricular enlargement.
    - ▪ There is a case report of a patient with a frontal lobe infarct having nonconvulsive status epilepticus after ECT.
  - ◦ Published data show that ECT can be performed safely more than 1 month after stroke.
  - ◦ Avoid ECT within 1 month of a stroke.
    - ▪ There is at least one case report of successful ECT in the acute poststroke period.[6]
  - ◦ Prior to poststroke ECT, obtain magnetic resonance imaging (MRI) or computed tomography (CT) of the brain to rule out intracranial mass, vascular malformation, or acute hemorrhage.

Dementia

- Major depression afflicts between 25 and 80 percent of patients with dementia.[8] There are no recent randomized, controlled trials of ECT in patients with dementia and depression; however, observational evidence indicates that ECT can improve depressive symptoms in about two-thirds of these patients. ECT can also be effective in treating agitation, aggression, and other behavioral symptoms that often accompany dementia.
  - ◦ ECT is helpful in treating depression and behavioral symptoms in Alzheimer's disease, vascular dementia, and Lewy body dementia.
  - ◦ Both patients with mild and advanced dementia are at low risk for major complications after ECT.
  - ◦ The most common post-ECT minor complications are confusion, somnolence, and memory impairment, but these are usually self-limited.
  - ◦ Acetylcholinesterase inhibitors may decrease post-ECT adverse cognitive effects.

Seizure Disorders

- Depression occurs in 29 to 48 percent of adult patients with epilepsy and is associated with a high risk of suicide.[9] Because many antidepressant medications lower the seizure threshold, ECT can be a safer alternative.

- Continue the patient's anticonvulsant medications through ECT. Although the ECT-induced seizure threshold will be higher, ECT is still effective.
- Spontaneous epileptic seizures after ECT are rare if patients have maintained therapeutic anticonvulsant levels.
- ECT has even been used to treat refractory status epilepticus.

Intracranial Space-Occupying Lesions

- Depression is common in patients with intracranial space-occupying lesions such as tumors, aneurysms, and abscesses; however, ECT is usually not appropriate for these patients because of the risks of hemorrhage and increased intracranial pressure.
  - For severe, refractory depression, ECT is sometimes undertaken with extreme caution.
    - ECT is contraindicated if there is evidence of increased intracranial pressure on clinical examination (e.g., papilledema, headache, or an abnormal neurologic examination) or on brain imaging.
    - When ECT is planned for patients with intracranial space-occupying lesions, involve colleagues from neurology or neurosurgery.
    - Assiduously maintain control of blood pressure and heart rate throughout ECT in these patients.
      - For example, use a short-acting beta blockers such as esmolol or metoprolol.
    - Consider using glucocorticoids to minimize brain swelling and intracranial pressure.

ANESTHETIC TECHNIQUE AND OPERATIVE PATHOPHYSIOLOGY

- ECT is typically delivered two or three times a week for up to 12 treatments.
- To induce a seizure that is effective (usually lasting 30 to 60 s), electrodes are placed either unilaterally or bilaterally on the scalp and either a pulse or sine-wave current is applied.
- The seizure usually has two phases: a tonic phase followed by a clonic phase.
- The procedure is performed under general anesthesia with short-acting agents, most often propofol or methohexital.
- Paralytic agents such as succinylcholine are delivered to prevent musculoskeletal injury during the seizure.
  - If a patient is unable to receive succinylcholine due to pseudocholinesterase deficiency, atracurium is often used.
- Patients may also receive atropine or glycopyrrolate to minimize salivation and decrease aspiration as well as to prevent bradycardia.
- Airway management usually involves a bite block and mask ventilation.
- Cardiovascular effects include an initial 15- to 20-s parasympathetic discharge as patients are in the tonic phase of the seizure.
  - This can lead to bradyarrhythmias and even asystole.
- Once the patient enters the clonic phase, a sympathetic discharge results in a catecholamine surge that causes tachyarrhythmias and hypertension.
  - These hemodynamic changes persist into the post-procedure phase and usually resolve in 15 to 20 min.
- ECT can also transiently change the ejection fraction of patients undergoing treatment. These changes are generally well tolerated.
- ECT-induced neurohumeral discharges increase cerebral blood flow and intracranial pressure and may increase the permeability of the blood brain barrier.

PREOPERATIVE PREPARATION AND PROPHYLAXIS

HISTORY AND PHYSICAL

- Obtain a thorough history and physical examination, including assessment for cardiac, pulmonary, and neurologic compromise.
  - Include a mental status examination and a funduscopic examination for evidence of elevated intracranial pressure.

PREPROCEDURAL LABORATORY EVALUATION

- The preprocedural laboratory evaluation should be based on the patient's medical comorbidities and medications (see Chap. 5).
  - Check electrolytes and renal function for patients taking diuretics, angiotensin-converting enzyme (ACE) inhibitors, or angiotensin-receptor blockers (ARBs) and in the setting of uncontrolled hypertension or heart failure.
  - Obtain a pregnancy test in women of childbearing potential.
  - Check prothrombin time (PT)/INR in patients taking warfarin.
  - Because the neurohumoral surges of ECT subject patients to brief but significant cardiac stress, obtain a screening preprocedural electrocardiogram (ECG) in all patients who have or are at risk for heart disease.
  - Procedural noninvasive cardiac studies are generally not indicated.
- Correct electrolyte abnormalities prior to ECT.

- Attempt to normalize blood glucose prior to ECT; however, there is no known reason to postpone ECT in asymptomatic hyperglycemic patients.
- Make sure that operators and post-ECT-care personnel know whether the patient has any compromise in renal function so that medications can be adjusted appropriately.
- Use continuous ECG monitoring through ECT for all patients.

MEDICATIONS

BETA BLOCKERS

- Short-acting intravenous beta blockers including labetalol and esmolol can be used to manage severe hypertension or tachycardia.
  - Labetalol is a potent alpha and beta blocker but also blocks beta-2 receptors and can exacerbate or induce bronchospasm.
- The role of prophylactic beta blockers in ECT is unknown.
  - The cardiac stress is relatively brief.
  - Beta blockers theoretically increase the risk of severe bradycardia and asystole during the parasympathetic phase of ECT.
  - The APA has not made specific recommendations regarding the prophylactic use of beta blockers for ECT.

ANTICHOLINERGIC DRUGS

- Atropine or glycopyrrolate is often used by the anesthesiologist to decrease salivation and reduce the risk of aspiration.
  - These drugs also help to reduce the risk of asystole and should be used for patients who are taking medications that inhibit the AV node, such as beta blockers and the calcium channel antagonists verapamil and diltiazem.
  - In one small study, elderly patients who developed asystole during ECT were subsequently pretreated with atropine and none had recurrent asystole.[10]

POSTPROCEDURAL MANAGEMENT

- Monitor blood pressure, heart rate, and pulse oximetry for 2 h after ECT.
  - Accepted goals are to keep systolic blood pressure at 120 to 160 mmHg and diastolic blood pressure below 90 mmHg.
  - Pulse oximetry can help to detect early pulmonary edema, nonconvulsive seizures, and oversedation.
    - Do not rely solely on oximetry to monitor patients receiving supplemental inhaled oxygen, because oxygen saturation can remain high even when the patient is hypoventilating and developing hypercarbia.
  - Use only continuous ECG monitoring after ECT for patients at high risk for cardiac complications.

COMMON POSTOPERATIVE PROBLEMS AND SOLUTIONS

CNS EFFECTS

- Headache, somnolence, short-term memory impairment, and confusion, similar to a postictal state, are common after ECT. These usually resolve over the following 24 h. Evaluation of persistent symptoms should focus on ruling out other possible causes, such as stroke, pulmonary edema, cardiac ischemia, metabolic abnormalities, and medication side effects.
  - Simple headaches can be treated with analgesics (e.g., acetaminophen, nonsteroidal anti-inflammatory drugs).
  - Transient short-term memory impairment is common, as is loss of memory of the procedure, both anterograde and retrograde. The memory loss is likely to be permanent; however, it often becomes less with subsequent procedures.
  - If symptoms persist beyond 24 h or if there are abnormal physical findings, additional evaluation is warranted.
    - Consider stroke in a patient with uncontrolled blood pressure, either high or low, either during or after the procedure.
    - Consider medication side effects.
    - Reserve brain imaging for patients with specific indications.

CARDIAC COMPLICATIONS

- Asystole can occur at any time during ECT.
  - Atropine is the treatment.
  - Patients can usually safely continue ECT therapy with prophylactic atropine premedication.
- Arrhythmias are common and are usually transient and self-limited.
  - If persistent, they can be managed with appropriate medications, such as beta blockers or antiarrhythmic agents.
  - Address any angina or CHF before proceeding with ECT treatment.

REFERENCES

1. American Psychiatric Association. *The Practice of Electroconvulsive Therapy: Recommendations for Treatment, Training,*

and Privileging, 2nd ed. Washington DC: American Psychiatric Association, 2001.

2. American Psychiatric Association. Practice guideline for the treatment of patients with major depressive disorder. *Am J Psychiatry* 157:1, 2000.
3. Gerring JP, Shields HM. The identification and management of patients with a high risk for cardiac arrhythmias during modified ECT. *J Clin Psychiatry* 43:140, 1982.
4. Zielinski RJ, Roose SP, Devanand DP, et al. Cardiovascular complications of ECT in depressed patients with cardiac disease. *Am J Psychiatry* 150:904, 1993.
5. Mehta V, Mueler P, Gonzalez-Arriaza H, et al. Safety of electroconvulsive therapy in patients receiving long-term warfarin therapy. *Mayo Clin Proc* 79:1396, 2004.
6. Weintraub D, Lippmann SB. ECT in the acute poststroke period. *J ECT* 16:415, 2000.
7. Cole MG, Elie LM, McCusker J, et al. Feasibility and effectiveness of treatments for post-stroke depression in elderly inpatients: Systematic review. *J Geriatr Psychiatr Neurol* 14:37, 2001.
8. Rao V, Lyketsos CG. The benefits and risks of ECT for patients with primary dementia who also suffer from depression. *Int J Geriatr Psychiatry* 16:919, 2001.
9. Harden CL, Goldstein MA. Mood disorders in patients with epilepsy: Epidemiology and management. *CNS Drugs* 16:291, 2002.
10. Burd J, Kettl P. Incidence of asystole in electroconvulsive therapy in elderly patients. *Am J Geriatr Psychiatry* 6:203, 1998.

Section III
PREOPERATIVE EVALUATION AND MANAGEMENT WITH COEXISTING DISEASES

Steven L. Cohn, MD, Section Editor

19 HYPERTENSION

Tariq Shafi and Steven L. Cohn

INTRODUCTION

- The prevalence of hypertension in the United States is increasing;[1] it is the most common reason for physicians' ambulatory office visits.
- Hypertension is a major risk factor for cardiovascular disease. Perioperative management of hypertensive patients involves not only the management of their blood pressure (BP) levels but also close attention to other comorbid conditions.[2]
- This review focuses on the management of hypertension in the preoperative period. Postoperative hypertension is discussed in Chap. 51.

PATIENT-RELATED RISK FACTORS

ELEVATED CARDIOVASCULAR RISK PROFILE

- Hypertension is a major risk factor for left ventricular hypertrophy, coronary artery disease, congestive heart failure, renal disease, and cerebrovascular disease.[1] It is also closely associated with obesity and diabetes.

PROPENSITY FOR MYOCARDIAL ISCHEMIA

- Hypertension, left ventricular hypertrophy, diabetes mellitus, and coronary artery disease are preoperative predictors of postoperative myocardial ischemia.
- Each 10-mmHg increase in admission systolic BP above 140 mmHg is associated with a 20 percent increased risk of postoperative silent myocardial ischemia.[3]

COMPENSATORY MECHANISMS WITH UNCONTROLLED HYPERTENSION

- Patients with long-standing uncontrolled hypertension adapt to high pressures with hypertrophy of the arterioles. This allows them to tolerate markedly elevated levels of BP that in normotensive individuals can lead to encephalopathy. This phenomenon is well described in the cerebral circulation but is also observed in other vascular beds.
- Sudden acute lowering of BP in these uncontrolled hypertensive individuals can lead to adverse outcomes.

MULTIPLE ANTIHYPERTENSIVE MEDICATIONS

- More than two-thirds of all hypertensive individuals require multiple medications for adequate BP control.[1] These agents increase the risk of drug interactions with anesthesia as well as that of withdrawal syndromes in the postoperative period.

HISTORY OF SEVERE HYPERTENSION

- A past history of severe elevations in BP predicts postoperative uncontrolled hypertension.[4]

SECONDARY HYPERTENSION

- Patients with undiagnosed secondary causes of hypertension are potentially at increased risk for perioperative complications. Patients with pheochromocytoma can develop severe elevations of BP, and and those who remain untreated have a high mortality.

SURGERY-RELATED RISK FACTORS

CARDIOVASCULAR LABILITY

- Hypertension is associated with elevated peripheral resistance, sympathetic nervous system hyperactivity, and baroreceptor dysfunction.
- During induction of anesthesia, BP can rise acutely due to sympathetic activation.[5]
- On the other hand, anesthetic agents lead to systemic vasodilatation, which reduces peripheral resistance and decreases blood pressure.
- Remarkably, both normotensive and hypertensive patients eventually reach a similar intraoperative blood pressure nadir.[4,5] Uncontrolled hypertensive patients with high preoperative BP levels are likely to have a greater absolute decline in BP with induction of anesthesia.

INTRAOPERATIVE HYPOTENSION

- Several studies have demonstrated that the major determinant of adverse clinical outcomes in patients with hypertension is not the level of BP prior to surgery but the degree of decline in the BP in the intraoperative period.
- In one study, 5 of 7 patients with untreated severe hypertension (average BP 204/102 mmHg before induction of anesthesia) had transient electrocardiographic evidence of myocardial ischemia during surgery. All of these episodes were associated with an approximately 50 percent decrease in BP (average BP 106/57 mmHg during surgery).[5]
- Goldman and Caldera noted that treated and untreated hypertensive patients had increased postoperative cardiac complications with marked hypotension (decrease in BP to less than 50 percent of preoperative levels or greater than 33 percent for more than 10 min).[4] In their study, five patients had a diastolic BP greater than 111 mmHg.
- Charlson and colleagues demonstrated that mean arterial pressure greater than 110 mmHg, poor functional capacity, and volume depletion prior to surgery are predictive of BP lability, with both hypotension and hypertension intraoperatively.[6] They also noticed that a change of more than 20 percent (either increase or decrease) in mean arterial pressure compared to preoperative levels was associated with postoperative cardiac or renal complications.[7]
- These studies form the basis of the guidelines (supported by the American College of Cardiology, the American Heart Association, and the Seventh Report of the Joint National Committee on Prevention, Detection, Evaluation, and Treatment of High Blood Pressure) recommending that a BP greater than 180/110 mmHg be controlled prior to elective surgery.[1]

PREOPERATIVE EVALUATION

Preoperative evaluation of the hypertensive patient should focus on the following:

- Careful history and examination (Table 19-1):

TABLE 19-1 Preoperative Evaluation of Patients with Hypertension

FINDINGS	PATHOLOGY	PERIOPERATIVE SIGNIFICANCE
Spells of headache, palpitations, hypertensive crisis	Pheochromocytoma	Severe hypertension
Obesity, short neck, history of snoring	Associated with sleep apnea, which can lead to resistant hypertension	Airway problems Risk of postoperative hypertension
Abdominal striae, buffalo hump	Cushing's syndrome	Metabolic abnormalities Resistant hypertension
Orthostatic hypotension	Baroreceptor dysfunction, volume depletion, pheochromocytoma	Perioperative hypertension and hypotension
White-coat effect	Unknown	Elevated perioperative BP readings
Hypertensive retinopathy	Long-standing hypertension	Risk of postoperative hypertension
Sustained apex beat, S_4	Left ventricular hypertrophy	Postoperative myocardial ischemia
Bruits	Atherosclerosis causing stenosis of renal, coronary, and carotid arteries	Postoperative myocardial ischemia Severe hypertension Flash pulmonary edema
Diminished peripheral pulses	Peripheral arterial disease	Indicative of coronary artery disease Poor functional capacity
Hypokalemia	Primary hyperaldosteronism, diuretic therapy	Risk of cardiac arrhythmias with anesthesia

- Detailed history of hypertension, including the duration, severity, highest recorded BP, and level of control.
- Assessment of target-organ damage.
- Detection of clues to secondary causes of hypertension.
- Review of antihypertensive medication regimen and the use of over-the-counter medications or herbal products.
- Evaluation of functional capacity to assess cardiovascular risk.
- Obtaining records of outpatient BP measurement from the primary care provider's office.
- Further evaluation of target organ damage as indicated.

PERIOPERATIVE MANAGEMENT

ASSESSMENT OF CARDIOVASCULAR RISK

- A history of hypertension should serve as a reminder to assess carefully for occult coronary artery disease and congestive heart failure.

MANAGEMENT OF CHRONIC ANTIHYPERTENSIVE MEDICATIONS (TABLE 19-2)

- Oral antihypertensive medications should be continued up to the time of surgery. Discontinuation of medications in difficult-to-treat hypertensive patients will lead to severe elevation of BP preoperatively.
- Abrupt discontinuation of beta blockers and centrally acting sympatholytic drugs such as clonidine is associated with rebound hypertension.
- Continue beta blockers throughout the perioperative period, switching to parenteral formulations if oral intake is delayed. Patients taking clonidine can be switched to a transdermal patch in preparation for surgery. However, transdermal clonidine takes 48 to 72 h to become effective.

ELEVATED BP BEFORE SURGERY

- Medical consultants are often asked to evaluate patients with elevated BP before surgery and to decide whether to proceed or cancel the procedure. There are a number of causes of preoperative elevation of BP. A suggested approach to determining the cause of elevated BP is depicted in Fig. 19-1.

MANAGEMENT OF PREOPERATIVE ELEVATED BP

BP <180/110 mmHg

- Despite the fact that patients in this category often have surgery postponed or canceled arbitrarily, it appears that, with careful perioperative management, patients with BP <180/110 mmHg can safely proceed to surgery.[8]

BP >180/110 mmHg

- Patients with persistent elevation of BP >180/110 mmHg pose a challenge in management. Recommendations to delay surgery[1,9] result in an incremental cost of operating room time, distress to the patient, and delay in a required procedure.[2] Proceeding with surgery at this BP level may be associated with increased postoperative cardiac complications along with increased cost of intraoperative and postoperative intensive monitoring.

TABLE 19-2 Perioperative Management of Antihypertensive Medications

DRUG CLASS	PERIOPERATIVE CONCERNS	SUGGESTED APPROACH
Diuretics	Hypokalemia	1. Provide potassium supplementation. 2. Consider holding for 24 h prior to surgery if BP is well controlled. 3. Check electrolytes prior to induction of anesthesia.
Aldosterone antagonists	Hyperkalemia	Check electrolytes.
Beta blockers	Abrupt discontinuation is associated with rebound hypertension and ischemia.	1. Continue in the perioperative period. 2. Use IV formulations.
Centrally acting sympatholytics (clonidine)	Abrupt discontinuation is associated with rebound hypertension.	Taper and discontinue preoperatively or switch to transdermal patch.
Calcium channel blockers	These increase postoperative blood loss and transfusion requirements after surgery for hip trauma.	Benefits outweigh potential risks; continue for BP control.
Angiotensin-converting enzyme inhibitors and angiotensin II receptor blockers	Some reports of hypotension with induction of anesthesia; others report no change in BP.	1. Benefits outweigh potential risks; continue for BP control. 2. If BP is well controlled, can hold dose on the morning of surgery.

SOURCE: Adapted with permission from Shafi T. Perioperative management of hypertension, in *Perioperative Medicine, A Special Supplement to The Hospitalist*. January 2005, with permission.

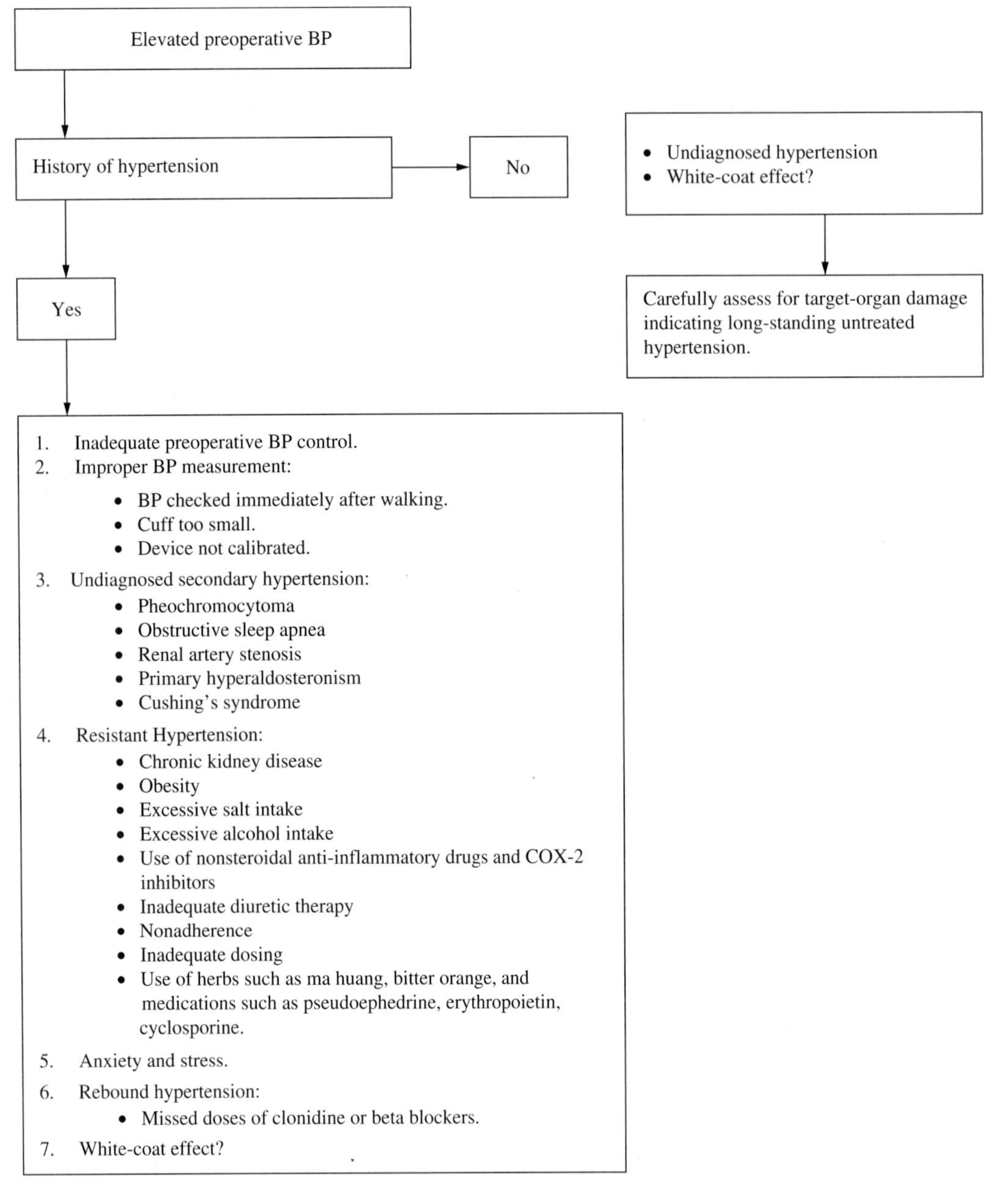

FIG. 19-1 Preoperative approach to the patient with elevated blood pressure.

Recommendations for the management of these patients are based on observational and retrospective studies.

- Weksler and colleagues recently reported their 9-year experience with patients with previously controlled blood pressure (control not defined) and elevated BP at the time of presentation for surgery.[10] Although the study has been criticized for its methodologic weakness,[11] it does suggest that, at least in a very select group of patients with severe hypertension and no other comorbidities (left ventricular hypertrophy, chronic renal failure, coronary artery disease, cardiac conduction, or valvular abnormalities), it may be safe to proceed with surgery.
- Howell and colleagues, based on an extensive review of literature, recommend proceeding with surgery if a careful evaluation does not reveal any evidence of target-organ damage or coronary artery disease and the only factor of concern is an elevated BP level.[11]

A SUGGESTED APPROACH FOR SEVERE PREOPERATIVE HYPERTENSION

- There are no randomized controlled trials addressing the problem of preoperative severe hypertension. Based on the available observational studies, the following approach is suggested (Fig. 19-2):

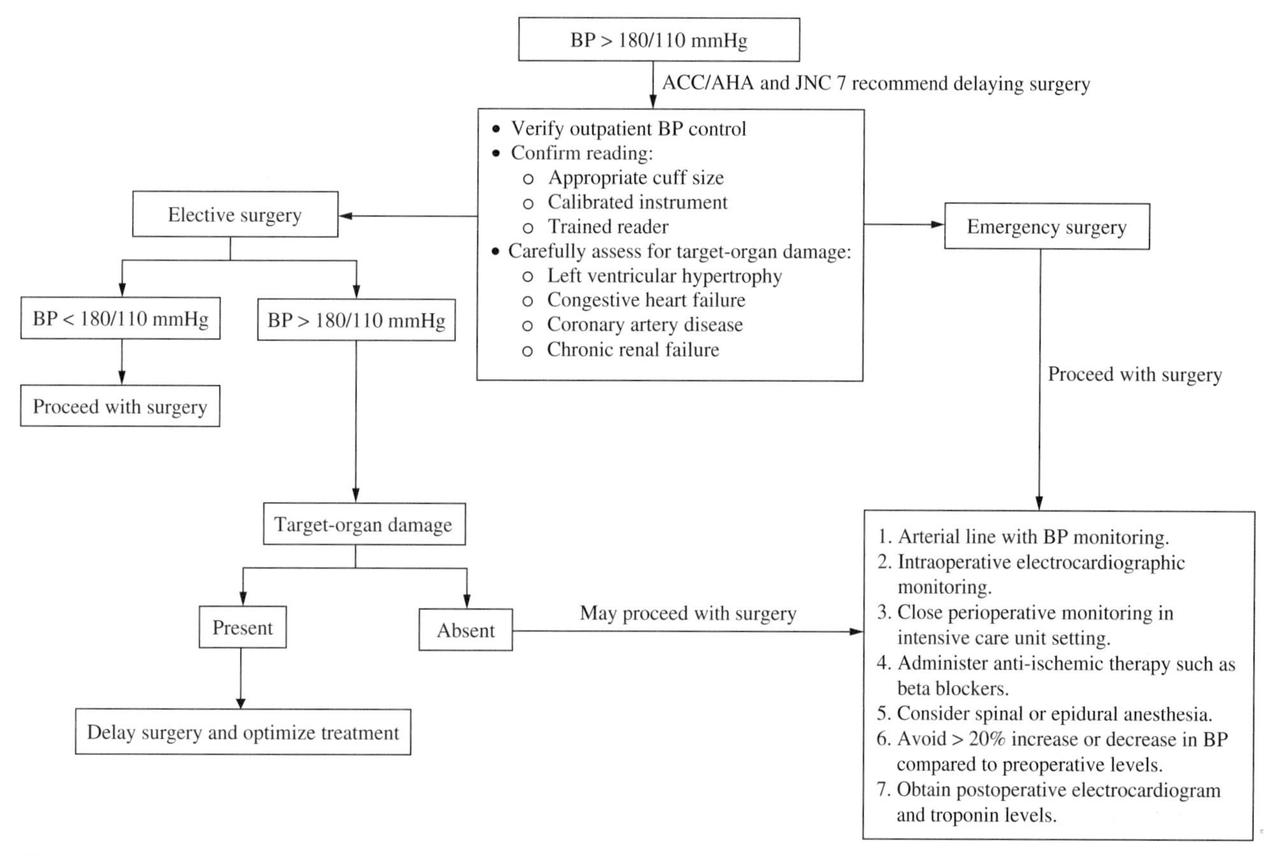

FIG. 19-2 Preoperative management of patients with elevated blood pressure. (Adapted from Shafi T. Perioperative management of hypertension, in *Perioperative Medicine, A Special Supplement to The Hospitalist*. January 2005, with permission.)

- Verify elevated BP reading:
  1. Measure BP using proper technique with the patient at rest, using a cuff of appropriate size.
  2. Try to obtain outpatient records of BP recordings and level of control from the primary care provider's office.
- Determine the presence of hypertension-related target-organ damage that can adversely affect surgical outcome (left ventricular hypertrophy, coronary artery disease, chronic renal failure, or congestive heart failure).
- Proceed with surgery if the preoperative evaluation does not find any factor other than elevated BP level associated with postoperative cardiac complications.
- Perioperative management includes:
  - Placement of arterial line and monitoring of arterial BP intra- and postoperatively.
  - Administration of anti-ischemic therapy. Intravenous esmolol is a short-acting, parenteral and titratable beta blocker, making it uniquely suitable in this situation.
  - Use of neuraxial block with spinal or epidural anesthesia if possible. Neuraxial block is associated with a reduction in postoperative mortality and may reduce perioperative myocardial injury.
  - Active intraoperative management of BP to maintain a mean BP within 20 percent of baseline.
  - Close monitoring of BP in the postoperative period in a critical care setting.

REFERENCES

1. Chobanian AV, Bakris GL, Black HR, et al. Seventh Report of the Joint National Committee on Prevention, Detection, Evaluation, and Treatment of High Blood Pressure. *Hypertension* 42(6):1206–1252, 2003.
2. Spahn DR, Priebe HJ. Editorial II: Preoperative hypertension: Remain wary? "Yes"—Cancel surgery? "No." *Br J Anaesth* 92(4):461–464, 2004.
3. Howell SJ, Hemming AE, Allman KG, et al. Predictors of postoperative myocardial ischaemia. The role of intercurrent arterial hypertension and other cardiovascular risk factors. *Anaesthesia* 52(2):107–111, 1997.
4. Goldman L, Caldera DL. Risks of general anesthesia and elective operation in the hypertensive patient. *Anesthesiology* 50(4):285–292, 1979.
5. Prys-Roberts C, Meloche R, Foex P. Studies of anaesthesia in relation to hypertension. I. Cardiovascular responses of treated and untreated patients. *Br J Anaesth* 43(2):122–137, 1971.
6. Charlson ME, MacKenzie CR, Gold JP, et al. Preoperative characteristics predicting intraoperative hypotension and

hypertension among hypertensives and diabetics undergoing noncardiac surgery. *Ann Surg* 212(1):66–81, 1990.
7. Charlson ME, MacKenzie CR, Gold JP, et al. Intraoperative blood pressure. What patterns identify patients at risk for postoperative complications? *Ann Surg* 212(5):567–580, 1990.
8. Eagle KA, Berger PB, Calkins H, et al. ACC/AHA guideline update for perioperative cardiovascular evaluation for noncardiac surgery—executive summary: A report of The American College of Cardiology/American Heart Association Task Force on Practice Guidelines (Committee to Update the 1986 Guidelines on Perioperative Cardiovascular Evaluation for Noncardiac Surgery). *J Am Coll Cardiol* 39:542, 2002.
9. Fleisher LA. Preoperative evaluation of the patient with hypertension. *JAMA* 287(16):2043–2046, 2002.
10. Weksler N, Klein M, Szendro G, et al. The dilemma of immediate preoperative hypertension: To treat and operate, or to postpone surgery? *J Clin Anesth* 15(3):179–183, 2003.
11. Howell SJ, Sear JW, Foex P. Hypertension, hypertensive heart disease and perioperative cardiac risk. *Br J Anaesth* 92(4):570–583, 2004.

20 CORONARY ARTERY DISEASE

Steven L. Cohn and Kenneth Gilbert

INTRODUCTION

- In 2002, over 25 million patients underwent noncardiac surgery. Millions of these patients had either known coronary artery disease (CAD) or risk factors for CAD.
- Perioperative cardiac morbidity is the leading cause of death following anesthesia and surgery. This chapter reviews preoperative evaluation and perioperative management of the cardiac patient undergoing noncardiac surgery.

PATIENT-RELATED RISK FACTORS

HISTORY

- Age
  - Age >70 is a risk factor in various risk indices but is a minor clinical predictor in the guidelines of the American College of Cardiology (ACC).
  - Age probably represents a marker for decreased cardiac reserve, silent cardiac disease, and increasing comorbidity rather than being a risk factor in itself.
- Prior cardiac disease
  - ***Previous myocardial infarction (MI):*** The time interval between a prior MI and the planned noncardiac surgery influences risk.
    - A recent MI is a major risk predictor that mandates further investigation prior to elective surgery. The definition of "recent" has changed from <6 months (Goldman[1] and Detsky[2]) to <3 months (Larsen) to <1 month (ACC). In the past, time selected out high-risk patients; now most patients with an acute MI undergo primary angioplasty or have noninvasive testing done and are identified as high-risk on that basis or are treated.
    - An "old MI" (>30 days) is an intermediate clinical predictor (ACC).
  - ***Angina:*** Ascertain severity and stability of angina.
    - Unstable angina and New York Heart Association (NYHA) class III to IV angina carry a risk similar to that of a recent MI.
    - Mild stable angina (class I to II) is an intermediate clinical predictor (ACC) but did not predict major postoperative cardiac complications in the indices of Goldman[1] and Detsky[2].
  - ***CHF:***
    - Heart failure [S_3, jugular venous distention (JVD), rales, and symptoms] is a major clinical predictor of postoperative complications that requires treatment before elective surgery.
    - Compensated congestive heart failure (CHF) or a previous history of CHF is an intermediate predictor.
  - ***Arrhythmias:*** Hemodynamically significant arrhythmias [ventricular tachycardia, supraventricular tachycardia (SVT), symptomatic bradyarrhythmias, advanced heart block] are major clinical predictors of risk and should be controlled prior to surgery (see Chap. 23).
  - ***Valvular heart disease:*** Severe aortic stenosis is the valvular lesion that most commonly increases the risk of postoperative cardiac complications. Important associated symptoms include chest pain, dyspnea, or syncope; signs include decreased and delayed carotid pulses and a late-peaking systolic ejection murmur at the base of the heart, especially when right carotid radiation is present (see Chap. 22).
- Prior cardiac intervention
  - ***Coronary artery bypass grafting (CABG):*** Prior revascularization with CABG may be protective for up to 5 years if no new (or worsening) symptoms are present.
  - ***Percutaneous coronary intervention (PCI) [percutaneous transluminal angioplasty (PTCA) or stent]:*** Prior PCI may also be somewhat protective in the absence of new symptoms.
- Prior cardiac evaluation
  - ***Noninvasive tests (NITs):*** Obtain detailed results of prior cardiac tests.

- For electrocardiographic (ECG) exercise tests, note the peak heart rate, systolic blood pressure, and rate pressure product along with the number of metabolic equivalents (METs) achieved, percent of target heart rate attained, symptoms or ECG abnormalities, and the reason the test was stopped.
- For nuclear tests, the presence, number, and severity of reperfusion abnormalities are important. Fixed defects are less predictive of short-term risk.
- For echocardiograms, note the presence and extent of systolic wall motion abnormalities and the left ventricular ejection fraction (LVEF) (in addition to any valvular pathology).

◦ ***Coronary angiography:*** Left main or three-vessel CAD is associated with increased risk and should be corrected if time permits, as they are indications for revascularization independent of the need for noncardiac surgery.

- Risk factors for CAD
  - ***Hypertension (HTN):*** HTN itself is not a risk factor unless diastolic blood pressure (BP) is >110 (and possibly systolic BP >180 to 200). However, its etiology (especially pheochromocytoma) and evidence of organ damage are more important predictors.
  - ***Diabetes mellitus(DM):*** Diabetes (requiring insulin) is a risk factor in the Lee Revised Cardiac Risk Index and the ACC guidelines. It is considered as a coronary disease equivalent.
  - ***Dyslipidemia:*** Hyperlipidemia may suggest the presence of silent underlying coronary disease; however, it is not an independent risk factor for postoperative cardiac complications.
  - ***Cigarette smoking:*** Although smokers are at higher risk for underlying CAD and pulmonary disease, cigarette use is not an independent risk factor for postoperative cardiac complications.
- Associated comorbid diseases
  - ***Peripheral vascular disease (PVD) and cerebrovascular accident (CVA):*** PVD and stroke are coronary equivalents that often coexist with CAD.
  - ***Chronic kidney disease (CKD):*** Renal insufficiency (creatinine >2.0 or 2.5 mg/dL) was an independent risk predictor in all of the published cardiac risk indices.
  - ***Chronic obstructive pulmonary disease (COPD):*** Concomitant pulmonary disease may be associated with increased cardiac complications.
- Current clinical status (symptoms)
  - ***Chest pain and dyspnea:*** Note the presence, severity, and stability of these symptoms as well as related symptoms (orthopnea and paroxysmal nocturnal dyspnea).
  - ***Functional status/exercise capacity:*** Inquire about the patient's usual activities of daily life.
    - The inability to walk two to four blocks or climb one or two flights of stairs, regardless of the reason, increases the risk of postoperative complications.
- Medications
  - Obtain a list of all current medications, both prescription and over-the-counter, and note whether or not the patient is compliant with the regimen.

PHYSICAL EXAMINATION (TO CORROBORATE HISTORY OR ELICIT/ASSESS RISK FACTORS)

- Vital signs: Assess BP control, heart rate, irregular pulse (arrhythmias), and respiratory status (tachypnea).
- Vascular system: Look for evidence of CHF/left ventricilar (LV) dysfunction (S_3, JVD, rales, edema), valvular disease (murmurs), peripheral vascular disease (pulses, bruits, neurologic deficit).

SURGERY-RELATED RISK FACTORS

TYPE OF SURGERY

- High-risk procedures:
  - ***Emergent major operations:*** Emergency surgery increases the risk for cardiac complications due to increased emotional and physiologic stress and resultant increased levels of epinephrine and cortisol. The lack of time to perform a detailed cardiac evaluation also contributes to risk.
  - ***Major vascular surgery:*** Aortic aneurysm repair and infrainguinal arterial bypass surgery are the highest-risk procedures for perioperative cardiac events. Patients undergoing these procedures frequently have underlying CAD.
  - ***Prolonged procedures with significant blood loss or fluid shifts:*** Major operations, such as Whipple's procedure, debulking of intraabdominal tumor masses, or major head and neck resections may be associated with marked blood loss, transfusion requirements, and significant fluid shifts, which pose an increased risk to patients with CAD.
- Intermediate-risk procedures:
  - ***Intraperitoneal or intrathoracic surgery:*** Significant hemodynamic changes occur with major abdominal and thoracic surgery. Intrathoracic operations alter the normal pressure gradients in the thoracic cavity while potentially limiting blood oxygenation, both of which can lead to increased myocardial oxygen demand and ischemia.
  - ***Carotid endarterectomy:*** Cardiac risk with carotid endarterectomy is lower than with other vascular surgeries. Nonetheless, many patients with cerebrovascular disease also have significant CAD and may be at risk for cardiac complications.
  - ***Major orthopedic procedures:*** Patients undergoing these procedures are often elderly and have comorbid

illnesses, including known or suspected CAD. Many of these patients have been unable to exercise due to their joint disease, and it is difficult to gauge their functional status.
  - ***Major head and neck surgery:*** These procedures are often prolonged and may require up to 12 h of general anesthesia. Most patients with head and neck malignancies have significant smoking histories and are thus at increased risk of having significant underlying coronary disease.
- Low-risk procedures:
  - Superficial and minor operations on the skin, breast, or eyes (e.g., cataract) or endoscopic procedures usually portend minimal risk for patients with stable coronary disease.

TYPE OF ANESTHESIA

- The belief that neuraxial (spinal or epidural) anesthesia is safer than general anesthesia remained unsubstantiated until recently. Although earlier research suggested no clear morbidity or mortality benefit of either modality, a recent metaanalysis by Rodgers and colleagues, including 9559 patients, indicated a lower risk for overall mortality [odds ratio (OR) 0.7] and a reduced frequency of deep vein thrombosis, pulmonary embolism, transfusion requirements, pneumonia, and respiratory depression with neuraxial blockade.[3] Risk of MI and renal failure was also reduced. A practical advantage to neuraxial anesthesia is that, in the awake patient, cardiac ischemia may elicit symptoms that can alert the anesthesiologist to the need for further evaluation. However, the decision as to the type of anesthesia is still best left to the anesthesiologist.
- For minor procedures performed with local anesthesia, the expected risk of coronary ischemia is minimal. Although patient anxiety may be a factor, this can often be alleviated with small doses of perioperative anxiolytics.

PREOPERATIVE EVALUATION

CARDIAC RISK INDICES (TABLE 20-1)

Since the late 1970s, a number of multivariate cardiac risk indices have facilitated risk stratification for perioperative cardiac complications including MI, unstable angina, acute pulmonary edema, and cardiac death.

- **Goldman's original cardiac risk index (CRI)**
  - Goldman's multivariate cardiac risk index was the first major attempt to determine and quantify the independent variables predictive of cardiac risk.[1] This index is easy to use, is widely employed, has been repeatedly validated, and provides a reasonable indication of patients' cardiac risk.
- **Detsky's modified cardiac risk index**
  - In 1986, Detsky and colleagues published a modified version of the cardiac risk index via a Bayesian approach of adjusting pretest probabilities using likelihood ratios.[2] To use this index, one must determine site-specific pretest probabilities for various surgical procedures.
- **American College of Physicians (ACP) Guidelines (Fig. 20-1)**
  - These guidelines, published in 1997, advocate the use of Detsky's modified cardiac risk index to determine whether a patient falls into a low risk category, or the moderate to high risk category, based upon the number of points scored.[4] For patients at low risk, further stratification using low-risk variables is recommended (e.g., age over 70, history of angina, DM, Q-waves on the ECG, history of ventricular ectopy). Overall, the ACP guidelines suggest a conservative approach to cardiac testing, recommending this primarily for intermediate-risk patients undergoing vascular surgery and for high-risk patients with known coronary disease.
- **American College of Cardiology (ACC) guidelines**
  - The 2002 ACC/AHA guideline provides a stepwise approach to preoperative cardiac risk assessment.[5]
    - For patients requiring emergency surgery, those who had coronary revascularization in the preceding 5 years without recurrent symptoms or those with a recent coronary evaluation (within 2 years) with favorable results, the recommendation is to proceed to surgery without further workup.
    - For all other patients, clinicians sequentially consider clinical predictors, functional status, and surgery-specific risk. The guidelines recommend noninvasive testing for certain intermediate-risk patients (Fig. 20-2). The application of this guideline leads to a greater proportion of patients that undergo cardiac testing than would be the case under the ACP guidelines.
    - Although this approach may lead to a greater degree of comfort for the patient and physician, the evidence to support it is inconclusive. For example, a recent randomized controlled trial of coronary revascularization prior to vascular surgery failed to demonstrate a significant mortality benefit from an aggressive strategy.[6]
- **Revised Cardiac Risk Index**
- Lee and colleagues published a new cardiac risk index composed of six variables, each given equal weight: high-risk type of surgery (intrathoracic, intraabdominal, suprainguinal, vascular), ischemic heart disease (not revascularized), history of CHF, history of cerebrovascular disease, insulin therapy for diabetes, and serum

TABLE 20-1 Comparison of Cardiac Risk Indices

RISK FACTOR	GOLDMAN	NUMBER OF POINTS	DETSKY	NUMBER OF POINTS	LARSEN	NUMBER OF POINTS	LEE	NUMBER OF POINTS	ACC/AHA	LEVEL OF RISK
Ischemic heart disease										
MI	<6 months	10	<6 months	10	<3 months	11	Hx of ischemic heart disease (nonrevascularized)	1	Unstable coronary syndromes (MI <1 month, class III–IV or unstable angina)	Major
			>6 months	5	>3 months or angina	3			Prior MI (>1 month), mild stable angina (class I–II)	Intermediate
Angina			CCS class III	10						
			CCS class IV	20						
			Unstable	10						
CHF	S_3/JVD	11	Pulmonary edema < 1 week	10	Persistent pulmonary congestion	12	CHF	1	Decompensated CHF	Major
			Pulmonary edema ever	5	No congestion but previous pulmonary edema	8			Compensated or prior CHF	Intermediate
					Neither, but previous heart failure	4				
Cardiac rhythm	Other than sinus or APCs on last ECG	7	Other than sinus or APCs on last ECG	5	-----		-----		Hemodynamically significant arrhythmias	Major
	>5 PVCs/min at any time	7	>5 PVCs/min at any time	5					Abnormal ECG, nonsinus rhythm	Minor
Valvular heart disease	Important AS	3	Suspected critical AS	20	-----		-----		Severe valvular disease	Major
CVA	-----		-----		-----		CVA	1	CVA	Minor
Diabetes mellitus	-----		-----		DM	3	DM requiring insulin	1	DM	Intermediate
General medical status	Po_2 <60, Pco_2 >50, K <3, bicarb <20, BUN>50, Cr >3, abnormal AST, chronic liver disease, bedridden patient	3	Po_2 <60, Pco_2 <50, K <3, bicarb <20, BUN>50, Cr >3. abnormal AST, chronic liver disease, bedridden patient	5	Cr >1.5	2	Cr >2	1	Cr >2; low functional capacity, uncontrolled systemic hypertension	Intermediate, minor
Age	>70 years	5	>70 years	5	-----		-----		Advanced age	Minor
Type of surgery	Intraperitoneal, intrathoracic, aortic	3	Procedure considered separately		Aortic	5	High-risk surgery	1	Procedure considered separately	High, intermediate, low risk
					Other intraperitoneal or pleural	3				
Emergency operation	Yes	4	Yes	10	Yes	3	-----		Yes	Go to OR

APC = atrial premature contractions; AS = aortic stenosis; AST = aspartate transaminase; bicarb = bicarbonate; BUN = blood urea nitrogen; CCS = Canadian Cardiovascular Society; CHF = congestive heart failure; CVA = cerebrovascular accident; DM = diabetes mellitus; Hx = history; JVD = jugular venous distention; K = potassium; MI = myocardial infarction.

SOURCE: From Cohn and Goldman,[8] with permission from Elsevier.

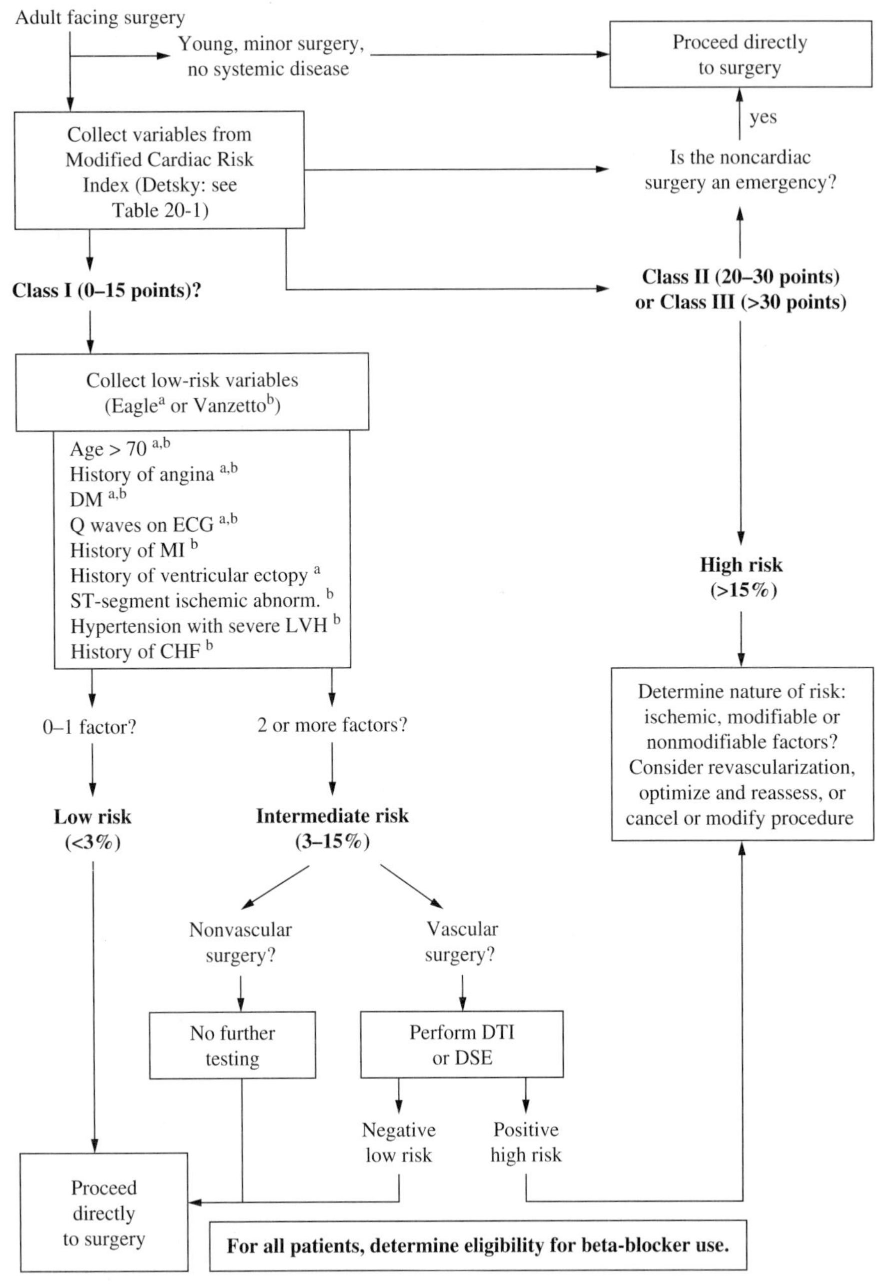

FIG. 20-1 American College of Physicians (ACP) algorithm. (Adapted from Palda VA, Detsky AS. *Ann Intern Med* 127:309–312, 1997, with permission.)

creatinine >2.0 mg/dL.[7] The frequency of major cardiac complications (MI, pulmonary edema, ventricular fibrillation, primary cardiac arrest, or complete heart block) increased with the number of risk factors present in both the derivation and validation patient cohorts (0.4 to 1.3 percent with 0 to 1 factor, 4 to 7 percent with 2 factors, and 9 to 11 percent with 3 or more factors).

- Figure 20-3 presents a modified, stepwise approach to cardiac risk assessment that incorporates the revised cardiac risk index and current recommendations for treatment.[8]

SUMMARY OF RISK INDICES

- Given the variety of cardiac risk-assessment methods currently in existence, it may be difficult for the clinician to select a given method over any of the others. Indeed, there is no evidence to conclusively guide practice. Generally, one should select a method with which one is comfortable, that is easily implemented and, most importantly, that represents a reminder of the important features of the history that must be elicited preoperatively.

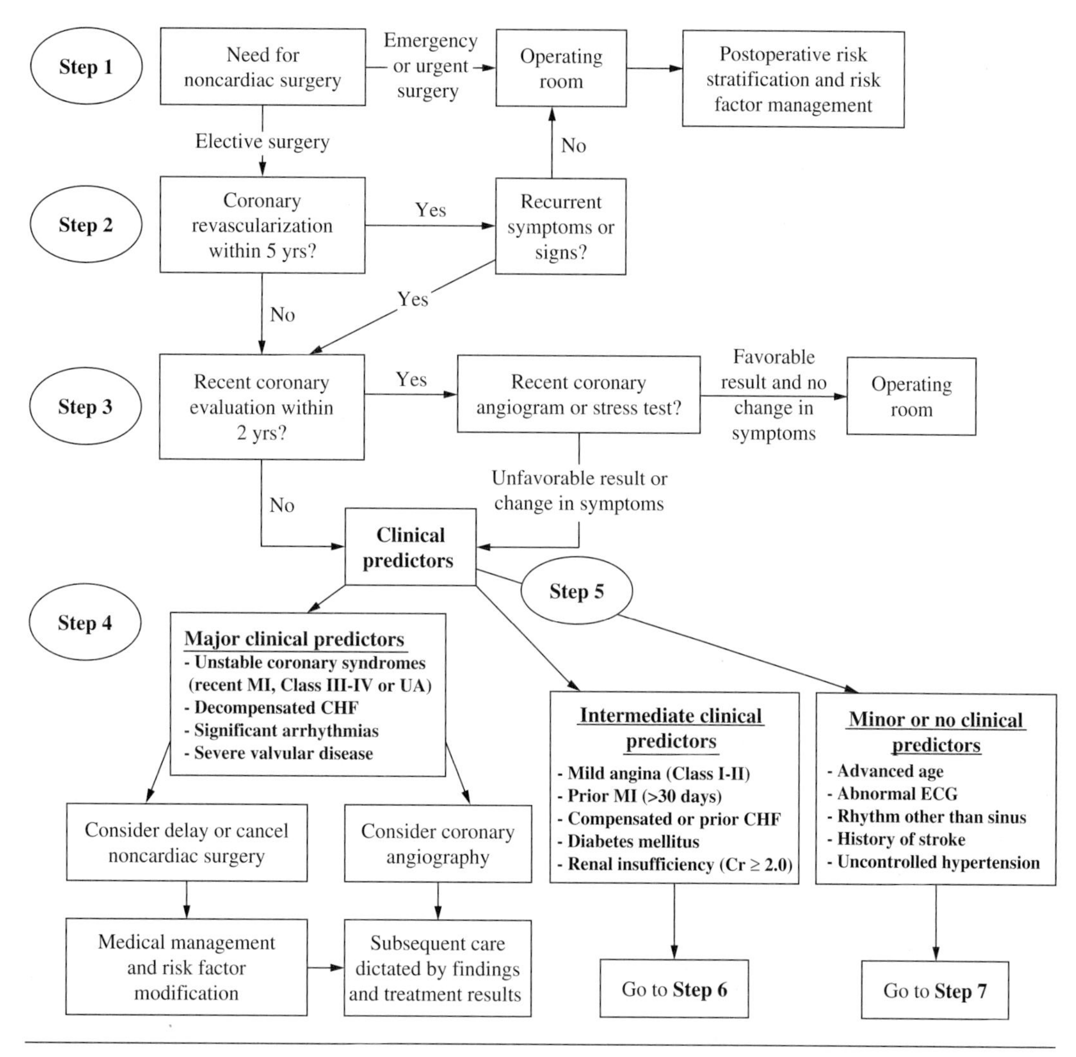

FIG. 20-2 Stepwise approach to preoperative cardiac assessment (ACC/AHA). (From Cohn and Goldman,[8] ©2003, with permission from Elsevier.) (Adapted from Eagle et al.,[5] with permission.)

DIAGNOSTIC TESTS

Resting Tests

- ***Electrocardiogram:*** The ECG remains a standard, inexpensive preoperative screening tool for patients with or at risk for CAD. It allows an immediate assessment of cardiac rate and rhythm and identification of new arrhythmias or conduction blocks. The presence of pathologic Q waves may alert the clinician to previously undetected CAD or new infarction, and new ST-segment changes associated with ongoing ischemia may be identified. It is unknown whether routine or selective use of preoperative ECGs improves perioperative cardiac outcomes.
- ***Echocardiogram:*** No evidence supports routine resting echocardiography in the preoperative setting. However, this test may provide essential information for patients with known or suspected significant valvular heart disease or left ventricular dysfunction (see Chaps. 21 and 24).

DYNAMIC NONINVASIVE TESTS

Exercise Testing

- Although exercise stress testing is not routinely recommended, information about recently performed stress tests may be useful, particularly if functional nuclear imaging was performed concurrently. A patient with a negative stress test of good quality has a low risk of significant perioperative ischemia. However, for patients with limited exercise capacity,

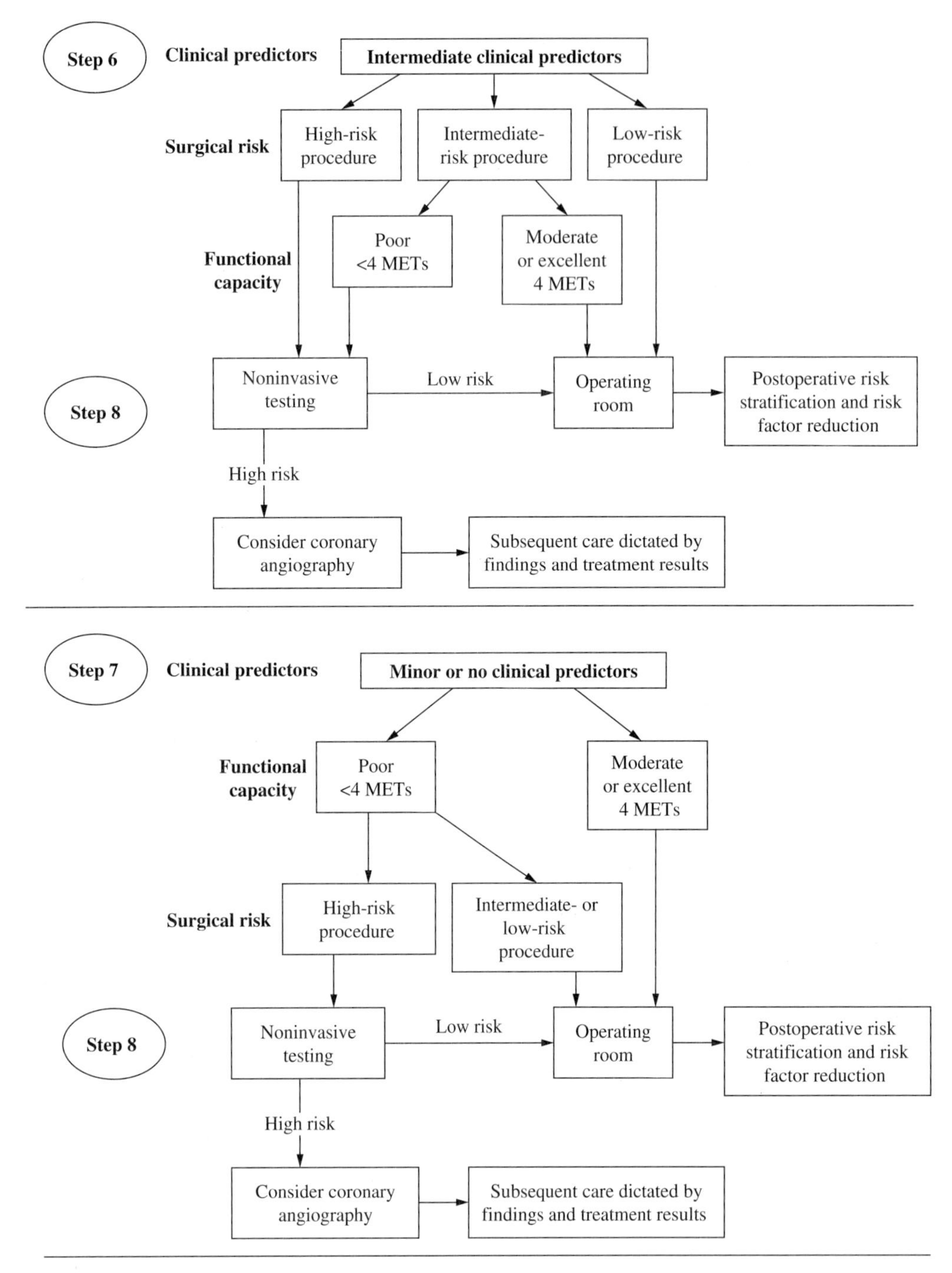

FIG. 20-2 *(Continued)*

such as those undergoing major joint replacement or peripheral vascular bypass, treadmill exercise testing is likely to be a futile endeavor.

Pharmacologic Stress Testing

- ***Dipyridamole stress testing*** with nuclear imaging (technetium or thallium) is indicated for selected patients with limited exercise capacity. Although the positive predictive value (PPV) of such testing is limited (PPV 15 to 25 percent), a negative test confers a low likelihood of cardiac complications [negative predictive value (NPV) >95 percent]. Additionally, the degree of abnormal stress perfusion predicts the likelihood of subsequent cardiac events. Fixed defects or small reperfusion abnormalities confer lower perioperative cardiac risk. The presence of ventricular dilation or a significant drop in ejection fraction with stress suggests more significant underlying ischemia.

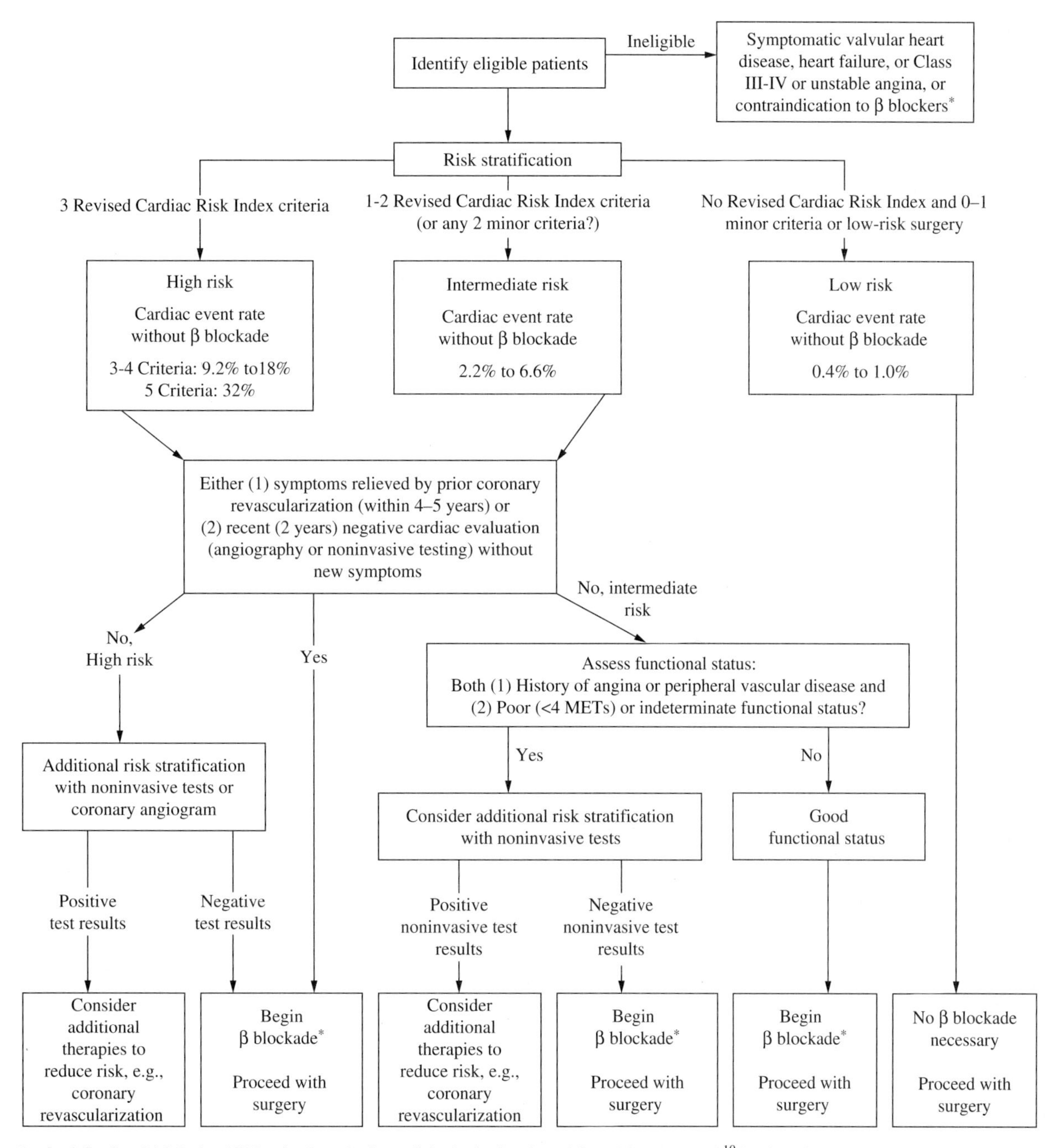

Revised Cardiac Risk Index (CRI) criteria and minor clinical criteria adapted from Mangano et al.[10] Revised CRI criteria exclude patients with CHF because the safety and efficacy of perioperative beta blockers has not been proven in these patients. Cardiac event rates without beta blockade are ranges based on rates from Lee et al.[7] for cardiovascular complications observed in the validation set and on estimates from Poldermans et al.[11] Options for noninvasive testing for further risk stratification include dipyridamole thallium scintigraphy, stress echocardiography, exercise electrocardiography, or cardiac catheterization in appropriate patients. Examples of activities that expend about 4 METs (metabolic equivalent tasks) include climbing 1 flight of stairs, being able to walk on level ground at 4 mph, or being able to climb a short hill without difficulty.

*Assumes no contraindications (COPD/asthma, hypotension, bradycardia, heart block, or acute CHF/pulmonary edema) to using beta blockers.

FIG. 20-3 Perioperative beta blockers for elective surgery: Patient selection and preoperative risk stratification. (From Cohn and Goldman,[8] © 2003, with permission from Elsevier.) (Modified from Auerbach AD, Goldman L. Beta-blockers and reduction of cardiac events in noncardiac surgery: A scientific review. *JAMA* 287:1435–1444, 2002.)

- ***Dobutamine stress echocardiography (DSE)*** is another noninvasive testing option. The number and degree of cardiac wall motion abnormalities detected with this method is associated with short- and long-term outcome. The PPVs and NPVs of DSE are similar to those of nuclear imaging techniques.

INVASIVE TESTING

- ***Coronary angiography*** is the definitive method of evaluating coronary anatomy. For patients assessed in the preoperative clinic, referral for angiography would generally follow obtaining a strongly positive result with a noninvasive test. Coronary revascularization should never be used to "get a patient through" a noncardiac procedure. Determine the need for angiography independent of the planned noncardiac operation.

PERIOPERATIVE MANAGEMENT

For high-risk patients, the consultant considers various interventions to lower that risk. Options include CABG, PCI, medical therapy, invasive monitoring, a lesser surgical procedure, or canceling surgery. The question arises as to whether or not these interventions decrease surgical risk, how long their protection lasts, the optimal time to perform noncardiac surgery after these procedures, and which patients are likely to benefit. However, there are few randomized controlled trials to evaluate these choices.

PREOPERATIVE INTERVENTION

- CABG
  - Among patients in the Coronary Artery Surgery Study (CASS) who subsequently underwent major noncardiac surgery, those randomly assigned to CABG had a lower risk of death (1.7 versus 3.3 percent) and nonfatal MI (0.8 versus 2.7 percent) than patients who were treated medically. There was no benefit if the surgery was a lower-risk procedure.[9]
  - This "protective" effect was felt to last for 4 to 6 years after CABG.
  - Another study found that patients undergoing major vascular surgery who survived preliminary CABG had a lower surgical mortality after the vascular procedure; however, taking the CABG mortality into account, there was no difference for the overall combined surgical mortality for the group.
  - Data from the Coronary Artery Revascularization Prophylaxis (CARP) trial failed to demonstrate either a short-term benefit (no reduction in perioperative MI or death, although underpowered) or improved long-term survival (22 to 23 percent mortality at 2.7 years in both groups) after CABG or PCI in patients with stable cardiac symptoms scheduled for elective vascular surgery.[6] However, both groups received intensive perioperative medical therapy.
  - The ACC guidelines state that the indication for CABG in the preoperative period is the same as for the nonsurgical patient and that CABG should not be performed solely to get the patient through noncardiac surgery.
  - Regarding the timing of subsequent noncardiac surgery, several studies have demonstrated an increased surgical risk if the noncardiac surgery was performed within 30 days of the CABG.
- PCI
  - PTCA
    - Several studies revealed perioperative morbidity and mortality to be less than expected in patients who had undergone balloon angioplasty before noncardiac surgery.
    - Conflicting results exist as to the optimal timing of the noncardiac surgery, with all except one study showing no increase in risk if performed within 90 days of PTCA (many averaged around 10 days).
  - Stents
    - A study of 40 patients undergoing stent placement within 6 weeks of noncardiac surgery reported very high rates of postoperative MI, major bleeding, and death. The majority of these events occurred in patients subjected to noncardiac surgery less than 14 days after stenting.
    - The recommendation was to delay noncardiac surgery for at least 2 and preferably 4 weeks.
    - A subsequent publication of 207 patients who underwent surgery within 2 months of stent placement reported that only eight patients either died or had an MI or stent thrombosis; all eight of these events occurred within 6 weeks of stent placement.
    - The authors recommended delaying elective surgery for at least 6 weeks after stent placement.
    - It has been suggested that noncardiac surgery be delayed even longer after placement of drug-eluting stents to allow more time for endothelialization while antiplatelet agents are continued.
    - If revascularization is indicated and the planned noncardiac surgery cannot be delayed for at least 4 weeks, consider PTCA without stenting.
- Medications
  - ***Beta blockers:*** Several randomized clinical trials have demonstrated lower rates of perioperative ischemia, MI, and cardiac death in patients with or at risk for CAD who received perioperative beta blockers.
    - Atenolol started immediately before surgery and continued up to 7 days postoperatively reduced

perioperative ischemia and subsequent 2-year mortality.[10]

- Bisoprolol started at least 7 days before surgery and continued for at least 30 days after surgery significantly reduced perioperative MI and cardiac death in a group of high-risk patients (abnormal dobutamine echocardiogram) undergoing elective vascular surgery.[11] It also reduced cardiac events over the next 2 years.
- Beta blockers will probably not significantly reduce the likelihood of perioperative cardiac complications in low-risk patients or those undergoing low-risk procedures. In moderate-risk patients (with one or two modified CRI criteria), beta blockers may be beneficial and may obviate the need for noninvasive testing (NIT). In high-risk patients (with three or more revised CRI criteria), NIT may be helpful in defining a subset of very high risk patients with multiple abnormalities on testing who would not benefit from beta blockers and who warrant coronary angiography and possible revascularization.
- Metaanalyses demonstrated these beneficial effects of beta blockers; however, the confidence intervals for MI and death approached or included 1. A large-scale randomized trial (POISE) is currently under way to evaluate the patients and operations in which beta blockers may be beneficial.
- Clinicians should start beta blockers preoperatively (preferably at least 3 to 7 days before) and titrate to achieve a heart rate of 55 to 65. A team approach and a specific protocol improve optimal use of perioperative beta blockers. In studies of clinical practice, the average heart rate is often >70, which may not be protective.

◦ ***Alpha agonists:*** Several studies and metaanalyses demonstrated lower rates of perioperative cardiac events in patients treated with various $alpha_2$ agonists. This benefit occurred primarily in patients undergoing vascular surgery who were given mivazerol (which is not FDA-approved).
- Clonidine has been shown to have potentially beneficial effects in small studies; however, this effect may not be as great as for patients given beta blockers.
- In high-risk patients undergoing moderate- to high-risk surgical procedures, consider using prophylactic clonidine for those patients with contraindications to beta blockers.

◦ ***Calcium channel blockers:*** There are insufficient data regarding the use of calcium channel blockers to prevent cardiac complications after noncardiac surgery.
- Diltiazem has been shown to have some benefit in reducing perioperative ischemia and supraventricular tachycardia (SVT), primarily in patients undergoing CABG.

◦ ***Nitrates:*** The limited data on the prophylactic use of nitrates demonstrate no significant beneficial effect for noncardiac surgery; however, a patient requiring nitrates for control of angina should continue them perioperatively.

◦ ***"Statins":*** Several studies (most retrospective) demonstrate a beneficial effect of statins on improving perioperative outcome (usually lower mortality). It is unclear whether the statins should be started prophylactically, either preoperatively or soon after surgery.

INTRAOPERATIVE MONITORING

- Monitoring of the patient once he or she enters the operating room falls under the purview of the anesthesiologist. The consultant should communicate information pertaining to the patient's cardiac status in a clear and focused manner. Include the results of any recent cardiac investigations on the patient's chart. Document any newly prescribed medications (e.g., beta blockers, statins).
- Standard intraoperative monitoring includes heart rate and rhythm, BP (noninvasive or arterial-line), respiratory rate, pulse oximetry, and temperature. Additional modalities may include pulmonary artery catheters or ST-segment monitors. There is no evidence that the latter two confer any consistent morbidity or mortality benefit despite a number of attempts to validate these tools.

POSTOPERATIVE MANAGEMENT

- A substantial proportion of patients with perioperative ischemia and infarction are asymptomatic. Since silent ischemia predicts future cardiac events, its detection is important. Patients with asymptomatic rises in cardiac enzymes postoperatively are at increased risk for long-term cardiac sequelae and should be investigated after they recover from surgery. Manage patients with unstable angina or definite infarction in the coronary care unit, as per standard practice, and obtain postevent risk stratification. The diagnosis and management of postoperative ischemia is discussed in Chap. 52.

PAIN MANAGEMENT

- The surgical team and anesthesiologist are generally responsible for pain management postoperatively; rarely will the internist be directly involved in this aspect of postoperative care. Poorly controlled pain increases rates of cardiac ischemia due to increased sympathetic tone (tachycardia, hypertension). Alert the surgical team to assess the patient's pain control if this appears to be inadequate to the consultant.

CONTINUATION OF MEDICAL THERAPY

- Continue anti-ischemic medications throughout the perioperative period. This is especially true for beta blockers or centrally acting alpha agonists, as there is a known rebound phenomenon associated with abrupt discontinuation of these drugs. Continue other cardiac medications postoperatively unless specifically contraindicated (e.g., septic shock, acute renal failure). See Chap. 7 for a detailed discussion of perioperative medication management.

SUMMARY

Preoperative assessment of the patient with CAD should include a focused history and physical based upon established guidelines. Selected patients will require noninvasive cardiac investigation and/or angiography. Employ risk-reduction strategies, including beta blockers, for intermediate- and high-risk patients. With the application of these methods, the consultant may improve the likelihood that a patient with CAD will be able to undergo noncardiac surgery with a good outcome.

REFERENCES

1. Goldman L, Caldera DL, Nussbaum SR, et al. Multifactorial index of cardiac risk in noncardiac surgical procedures. *N Engl J Med* 297:845–850, 1977.
2. Detsky AS, Abrams HB, McLaughlin JR, et al. Predicting cardiac complications in patients undergoing non-cardiac surgery. *J Gen Intern Med* 1:211–219, 1986.
3. Rodgers A, Walker N, Schug S, et al. Reduction of postoperative mortality and morbidity with epidural or spinal anaesthesia: Results from overview of randomised trials. *BMJ* 321(7275):1493, 2000.
4. American College of Physicians. Guidelines for assessing and managing the perioperative risk from coronary artery disease associated with major noncardiac surgery. *Ann Intern Med* 127:309–312, 1997.
5. Eagle KA, Berger PB, Calkins H, et al. ACC/AHA guideline update for perioperative cardiovascular evaluation for noncardiac surgery—executive summary: A report of the American College of Cardiology/American Heart Association Task Force on Practice Guidelines (Committee to Update the 1996 Guidelines on Perioperative Cardiovascular Evaluation for Noncardiac Surgery). *J Am Coll Cardiol* 39:542, 2002.
6. McFalls EO, Ward HB, Moritz TE, et al. Coronary-artery revascularization before elective major vascular surgery. *N Engl J Med* 351:2795–2804, 2004.
7. Lee TH, Marcantonio ER, Mangione CM, et al. Derivation and prospective validation of a simple index for prediction of cardiac risk of major noncardiac surgery. *Circulation* 100: 1043–1049, 1999.
8. Cohn SL, Goldman L. Preoperative risk evaluation and perioperative management of patients with coronary artery disease. *Med Clin North Am* 87(1):111–136, 2003.
9. Eagle KA, Rihal CS, Mickel MC, et al. Cardiac risk of noncardiac surgery: Influence of coronary disease and type of surgery in 3368 operations. CASS Investigators and University of Michigan Heart Care Program. Coronary Artery Surgery Study. *Circulation* 96(6):1882–1887, 1997.
10. Mangano DT, Layug EL, Wallace A, Tateo I. Effect of atenolol on mortality and cardiovascular morbidity after noncardiac surgery. *N Engl J Med* 335:1713–1720, 1996.
11. Poldermans D, Boersma E, Bax JJ, et al. The effect of bisoprolol on perioperative mortality and myocardial infarction in high-risk patients undergoing vascular surgery. *N Engl J Med* 341:1798–1794, 1999.

21 CONGESTIVE HEART FAILURE

William A. Ghali and Nadia A. Khan

INTRODUCTION

- Congestive heart failure (CHF) is a common condition, with epidemiologic trends indicating that its incidence and prevalence may be increasing as population demographics shift toward an older population.
- As a result, the medical consultant is frequently asked to assess patients with CHF before noncardiac surgery.
- This chapter covers issues that the medical consultant must consider in assessing patients with CHF. Beyond the initial consideration of whether the underlying etiology of the CHF is ischemic or nonischemic, the consultant must also consider the prognostic relevance of CHF in relation to postoperative outcomes, the need for special preoperative diagnostic testing for CHF, and issues relating to the perioperative management of CHF.[1]

PROGNOSTIC RELEVANCE OF CHF AS A PREOPERATIVE RISK FACTOR

- The survival prognosis of patients with CHF is generally quite poor even in the absence of surgery, with studies suggesting that only about one-third of patients survive beyond 5 years.

- Surgical procedures bring additional risk by introducing physiologic stress, which can compromise the clinical status of patients with CHF and precipitate adverse events.
- Cardiac risk indices consistently identify CHF to be a significant predictor of postoperative cardiovascular events and mortality (Table 21-1).
  - In the original cardiac risk index developed by Goldman and colleagues,[2] a number of preoperative clinical variables were empirically assessed for their independent associations with postoperative cardiac complications. Among variables assessed in a multivariable analysis, CHF (defined based on the presence of either an S_3 gallop or jugular venous distention) was the strongest single predictor of adverse cardiac events after surgery: 20 percent of CHF patients died of cardiac causes and another 14 percent had nonfatal cardiac complications. As a result, CHF was assigned the highest weight of all variables in the Goldman risk scale.
  - In the modified cardiac risk index developed in the mid-1980s by Detsky and colleagues,[3] CHF was again heavily weighted as an important prognostic factor, with an assigned score of 10 points for the presence of alveolar edema within 1 week and a score of 5 points for the presence of alveolar edema at any time in the past. Unlike the original risk score developed by Goldman and colleagues, however, the scoring algorithm derived by Detsky and colleagues was derived on the basis of clinical experts' ratings of how individual clinical variables should be prognostically weighted.
  - Both the Goldman and Detsky risk indices identified aortic stenosis as an important risk factor for adverse cardiac events.[2,3] CHF associated with aortic stenosis therefore represents a particularly high-risk clinical state for surgery.
  - More recently, Lee and colleagues[4] have described a revised cardiac index for which a more contemporary cohort of surgical patients in a Boston teaching hospital was followed from the preoperative period, when information on clinical status was gathered, through to the postoperative period for ascertainment of outcomes. CHF is loosely defined in this new index as any prior history of CHF or current presence of findings for CHF on either chest x-ray and/or physical examination. On multivariable analysis in the study's validation cohort, CHF emerged as the single strongest predictor of cardiac risk, with more than fourfold higher odds of adverse cardiac events.

TABLE 21-1 Summary Of Prognostic Relevance of CHF According to Three Preoperative Cardiac Risk Indices

RISK SCORING METHOD	BOTTOM LINE
Original cardiac risk index (Goldman et al.[2])	CHF was one of only nine variables to emerge as an independent predictor of adverse events and carried the highest prognostic weight in the final scoring algorithm.
Modified cardiac risk index (Detsky et al.[3])	CHF was considered to be an important risk factor, especially if recent, by the panel of clinicians who rated the importance of specific variables.
Revised cardiac risk index (Lee et al.[4])	CHF was one of only six variables to emerge as an independent predictor of adverse cardiac events and had the highest odds ratio (4.3) in the validation cohort.

PATIENT-SPECIFIC RISK FACTORS

- Based on the risk indices discussed, the pertinent patient risk factors that increase the risk of perioperative cardiac complications include:
  - History of CHF
  - Current CHF based on symptoms, signs (S_3, jugular venous distention, rales), or abnormalities on chest radiography
  - Presence of aortic stenosis
- Most experts agree that acutely decompensated CHF is a particularly concerning preoperative state. This view is captured in the Detsky index[3] through the greater prognostic weighting of recent CHF relative to the weighting assigned to the presence of CHF at any time in the more distant past.

SURGERY-SPECIFIC RISK FACTORS

- The surgery-specific risk factors predisposing to increased risk in the context of CHF are less well studied, though "major" procedures (i.e., major thoracic and abdominal procedures) are identified to pose a risk for adverse cardiac events in the Goldman and Lee indices.[2,4] This may relate to the often significant fluid shifts (i.e., "third-spacing") and fluid requirements associated with such procedures.
- According to the Goldman and Detsky indices, emergency procedures, regardless of type, also carry increased risk.[2,3]
- Vascular surgical procedures are also associated with a higher risk for adverse cardiac events, though this may relate more to the patient-specific risk factor of generalized vascular disease than to the procedures per se.
- General anesthesia may be associated with myocardial depression, though there is no firm evidence to support

a recommendation for preferential use of regional anesthesia, when possible, in patients with CHF.

PREOPERATIVE DIAGNOSTIC EVALUATION FOR CHF

- The prognostic data summarized in the preceding section underline the importance of detecting the presence of CHF, as it is clearly an indicator of increased risk.
- The available diagnostic "tools" for detecting the presence of CHF include clinical assessment, chest radiography, echocardiography, other strategies for the measurement of ejection fraction,, measurement of brain natriuretic peptide (BNP), and other diagnostic testing to determine whether the CHF is ischemic or nonischemic.
- Our focus is on the value of each of these approaches in the context of preoperative medical consultation.

CLINICAL ASSESSMENT

- A careful history and physical examination are central elements of the assessment of patients with possible CHF. Either a history of CHF reported by patients or the physical findings of an S_3, elevated jugular venous pressure, or bilateral rales on auscultation of the chest were used as indicators of increased risk in the various risk indices described earlier. Accordingly, the medical consultant must ascertain the presence or absence of these factors.

CHEST RADIOGRAPHY

- A chest x-ray is generally not recommended as a routine test for "all comers" having surgery,[5] but it should be considered in patients where there is clinical suspicion based on history and/or examination that CHF may be present. The presence of radiographic features of CHF can be used as a criterion for determining presence of CHF as a preoperative risk factor.

ECHOCARDIOGRAPHY

- A two-dimensional echocardiogram is generally not recommended for use as a routine test for purposes of preoperative risk stratification.[6] However, if the underlying diagnosis of CHF is unknown (i.e., ischemic versus valvular versus other etiologies) or if significant valvular disease (and especially aortic stenosis) is clinically suspected but not well characterized, echocardiography can be of value.

OTHER METHODS FOR MEASURING EJECTION FRACTION

- We do not recommend the routine use of multiple gated acquisition (MUGA) scanning or ventriculography. The combination of the cost of such tests, their frequent lack of availability, and the general lack of close links between test results and specific preoperative management decisions make their routine use unwarranted.

BRAIN NATRIURETIC PEPTIDE

- Blood testing for BNP can shed light on the presence or absence of CHF in certain clinical situations.[7] In particular, BNP can be useful for differentiating dyspnea associated with chronic lung disease from dyspnea related to CHF. Considering the rather different therapeutic strategies required for perioperative management of CHF as opposed to the management of chronic lung disease, selective use of BNP testing is a reasonable strategy for distinguishing these conditions when the source of dyspnea is not clear.

DIAGNOSTIC TESTING FOR CORONARY ARTERY DISEASE

- If cardiac ischemia is suspected in association with CHF, the physician may consider further diagnostic testing for coronary artery disease (CAD). See Chap. 20 for more information on the preoperative assessment of patients with suspected CAD.
- The preceding discussion may leave readers with the impression that accurate preoperative diagnosis of CHF makes a difference to patients' postoperative outcomes. We acknowledge, however, that there is no published evidence in the context of perioperative medical care to indicate that this is actually the case. Nevertheless, attempts at accurate preoperative diagnosis of CHF should be made, as a better-informed medical team can make better perioperative medical management decisions in relation to CHF, which in turn *could* positively influence patient outcomes.

PERIOPERATIVE CHF MANAGEMENT

- There are a number of specific management issues that need attention in the perioperative care of patients with CHF. These include the possibility of postponing surgery for unstable CHF, the monitoring of fluid and electrolyte status, consideration for right heart catheterization and beta-blocker use, and perioperative medication orders.

POSTPONING SURGERY

- Surgery should, when possible, be postponed for patients with unstable and/or decompensated CHF in order to permit attempts at stabilization. In the case of surgical emergencies, however, this may not possible, in which case the medical consultant can only attempt to enhance CHF control as much as possible before surgery.

FLUID AND ELECTROLYTE STATUS

- Carefully assess fluid and electrolyte status preoperatively, and follow up at least daily for most patients in the early postoperative period. The use of intravenous solutions and blood transfusions as well as fluid shifts and increased production of antidiuretic hormone can all deregulate fluid balance. Various CHF medications can also contribute to disturbances of sodium levels, potassium levels, and volume status. Renal function should also be assessed preoperatively and rechecked postoperatively, as CHF therapies can also compromise renal function through a variety of mechanisms.

RIGHT HEART CATHETERIZATION

- Right heart catheterization for determination of central hemodynamic measurements can theoretically provide useful data to guide perioperative volume management and medication decisions for selected patients. Right heart catheterization cannot, however, be recommended for widespread use, as a recent multicenter trial[8] has shown no evidence of benefit from routine right heart catheterization for high-risk surgical patients. This does not necessarily mean that the procedure should *never* be used but that it should be reserved for only a limited number of patients where there is a perception of strong need for central hemodynamic measurements to guide management decisions (e.g., in patients with a combination of alveolar edema with associated azotemia from "forward" renal hypoperfusion—a scenario for which it is difficult to know what to do in the absence of central hemodynamic measurements).

BETA BLOCKERS

- Although there are established long-term survival benefits from the use of beta blockers in patients with CHF, the safety and efficacy of new preoperative beta blockade in patients with CHF is not known. Patients who are stable and using a beta blocker chronically should generally continue their beta blocker perioperatively. It is more difficult, meanwhile, to make firm recommendations regarding the possible addition of beta blockers in CHF patients who are not taking beta blockers preoperatively. Most would agree that beta blockers should generally *not* be added preoperatively in the case of decompensated or poorly controlled CHF, as there is potential for acute deterioration in such cases. For more stable CHF patients not on a beta blocker, however, consideration could be given to adding such an agent preoperatively provided that there is sufficient time to observe the patient's clinical status preoperatively to ensure that he or she is tolerating the new therapy and stable for surgery. Such a strategy of selectively considering the addition of beta blockers preoperatively in stable CHF patients is unproven but has the potential to provide perioperative risk reduction, particularly if patients have associated ischemic heart disease.

PERIOPERATIVE MEDICATION ORDERS

- ***Angiotensin-converting enzyme (ACE) inhibitors and angiotensin-receptor blockers (ARBs):*** Patients with CHF commonly use these drugs given their proven long-term benefits. Accordingly, they should generally be taken as usual on the days before and after planned surgical procedures. There is, however, some controversy surrounding the administration of ACE inhibitors and ARBs on the actual day of surgery, as patients on these agents have been found to be more likely to experience intraoperative hypotension.[9] Whether intraoperative hypotension is a meaningful surrogate outcome for more notable adverse outcomes such as postoperative myocardial infarction, arrhythmia, or death is not entirely clear, though most experts would agree that intraoperative hypotension is to be avoided whenever possible. This may be particularly important in patients with aortic stenosis, carotid stenosis, or severe coronary disease, where intraoperative hypotension has the potential to be particularly problematic.
- The studies linking ACE inhibitors and ARBs to intraoperative hypotension unfortunately do not provide firm guidance as to how to approach the decision of continuing versus discontinuing these drugs in patients already taking these agents. In the absence of firm evidence to guide decisions around these medications, we recommend an approach of administering the agents as usual on the day of surgery if preoperative blood pressure readings are at least above 120 systolic. If, on the other hand, preoperative blood pressure readings are "on the low side," as is sometimes the case in patients with end-stage CHF, it may be best to withhold

TABLE 21-2 Summary of Perioperative CHF Management Considerations

ISSUE	BOTTOM LINE
Fluid and electrolyte status	CHF patients are quite susceptible to fluid and electrolyte disturbances. Electrolytes and renal function should be checked preoperatively in all patients and postoperatively in most.
Right heart catheterization	Not recommended for routine use based on a recent negative clinical trial but still may have a role in selected patients.
Beta blockers	Recommended if CHF is related to active ischemia. Role in nonischemic CHF is less clear, though beta blockers are still likely to be beneficial given demonstrated benefit in nonsurgical CHF cases.
Angiotensin-converting enzyme inhibitors and angiotensin-receptor blockers	May cause intraoperative hypotension, so these drugs should be held in circumstances where the risk of intraoperative hypotension is perceived to be high.
Diuretics	Controversial. Some experts recommend holding diuretics like furosemide on the day of surgery, though evidence to support this is limited.
Spironolactone	Risk of hyperkalemia.
Digoxin	Need to follow potassium levels to ensure that patient is not hypokalemic with digoxin therapy. Also should consider measuring a digoxin level if there is any clinical evidence to suggest toxicity.

ACE inhibitors and ARBs on the day of surgery so as to reduce the likelihood of intraoperative hypotension. We emphasize, however, that this recommendation is not based on clinical trial evidence.

- ***Diuretics:*** Similar controversy and uncertainty surround the use of diuretics such as furosemide—specifically what to do about furosemide dosing on the day of surgery. Citing concerns in relation to volume depletion and intraoperative hypotension, some experts have recommended that furosemide and other potent diuretics be held on the day of surgery.[10] Weighing against such a recommendation, however, is the concern that holding diuretics in stable CHF patients can result in undesirable volume overload on the day of surgery. Given the lack of data to support either argument and the lack of data to firmly associate diuretics with intraoperative hypotension, we cannot make any specific recommendations regarding administration of diuretics on the day of surgery; more definitive recommendations on this issue will have to await the results of currently ongoing research into the administration of furosemide on the day of surgery.
- ***Spironolactone:*** This has recently been added to the armamentarium of survival-modifying CHF therapies. However, patients taking spironolactone should have their potassium levels monitored regularly, given the increased risk of dangerous hyperkalemia on this medication.
- ***Digoxin:*** The use of digoxin has declined somewhat in recent years as other new proven therapies for CHF have emerged. The drug continues to be used, however, and recognizing this, providers must be aware of two perioperative issues in relation to digoxin therapy. The first concern is that normokalemia should be diligently maintained when patients are on digoxin so as to reduce the risk of arrhythmias due to hypokalemia. A second consideration is the risk of digoxin toxicity. While not all patients on digoxin need to have their preoperative digoxin levels measured, we do recommend that such a measurement be considered where there is suspicion that the digoxin levels may be high (e.g., clinical evidence on history or ECG to suggest digoxin toxicity or digoxin therapy in the presence of renal insufficiency).
- The many management considerations discussed above are summarized in Table 21-2.

CONCLUSIONS

- This chapter provides information on several prognostic, diagnostic, and therapeutic issues to be considered in the approach to the patient with CHF who is planning to undergo surgery.
- CHF is certainly a notable adverse prognostic factor; therefore its accurate diagnosis in the preoperative setting is an important first objective. A careful history and physical examination forms the basis of the diagnostic approach, with or without the use of additional testing such as chest radiography and occasional use of BNP assays.
- The management issues discussed in the preceding section involve considerations unique to the patient with CHF, and the recommendations that we have provided are largely based on opinion and pathophysiologic reasoning rather than firm clinical trial data to support the approaches proposed. In this regard, we look forward to the appearance of future research assessing many of the unique dilemmas in the medication management of patients with CHF.

REFERENCES

1. Hernandez AF, Newby LK, O'Connor CM. Preoperative evaluation for major noncardiac surgery: Focusing on heart failure. *Arch Intern Med* 164:1729, 2004.
2. Goldman L, Calder DL, Nussbaum SR, et al. Multifactorial index of cardiac risk in noncardiac surgical procedures. *N Engl J Med* 297:845, 1977.

3. Detsky AS, Abrams HB, McLaughlin JR, et al. Predicting cardiac complications in patients undergoing non-cardiac surgery. *J Gen Intern Med* 1:211, 1986.
4. Lee TH, Marcantonio ER, Mangione CM, et al. Derivation and prospective validation of a simple index for prediction of cardiac risk of major noncardiac surgery. *Circulation* 100:1043, 1999.
5. Smetana GW, Macpherson DS. The case against routine preoperative laboratory testing. *Med Clin North Am* 87:7, 2003.
6. Halm EA, Browner WS, Tubau JF, et al. Echocardiography for assessing cardiac risk in patients having noncardiac surgery. *Ann Intern Med* 125:433, 1996.
7. Maisel AS, Krishnaswamy P, Nowak RM, et al. Rapid measurement of B-type natriuretic peptide in the emergency diagnosis of heart failure. *N Engl J Med* 347:161, 2002.
8. Sandham JD, Hull RD, Brant RF, et al. A randomized, controlled trial of the use of pulmonary-artery catheters in high-risk surgical patients. *N Engl J Med* 348:5, 2003.
9. Bertrand M, Godet G, Meersschaert K, et al. Should the angiotensin II antagonists be discontinued before surgery? *Anesth Analg* 92:26, 2001.
10. Jarnberg PO. Acute effects of furosemide and mannitol on central haemodynamics in the early postoperative period. *Acta Anaesth Scand* 22:184, 1978.

22 VALVULAR HEART DISEASE

Michelle V. Conde
and Valerie A. Lawrence

INTRODUCTION

- The American College of Cardiology/American Heart Association guidelines identify severe valvular heart disease, particularly aortic stenosis, as a major clinical predictor for increased postoperative cardiac complications following noncardiac surgery.[1]
- Recognition of coexisting valvular heart disease is important in selecting and tailoring anesthetic techniques, perioperative medications, and surgical procedures with respect to the hemodynamic changes associated with the valvular disease.
- In the absence of symptomatic congestive heart failure, patients with chronic regurgitant valvular heart disease tolerate noncardiac procedures well.
- Coexisting valvular heart disease may also require assessments for endocarditis prophylaxis and perioperative management of anticoagulation (see Chaps. 7A and 47).

AORTIC STENOSIS

PATIENT-RELATED RISK FACTORS

- History
  - Calcific aortic stenosis is a common cause of aortic stenosis; other causes include leaflet disease (e.g., bicuspid aortic valve) and underlying systemic disorders (e.g., rheumatic fever and, rarely, rheumatoid arthritis).
  - Careful inquiry for chest discomfort, syncope, and congestive heart failure symptoms, which occur late in the course of aortic stenosis, is mandatory.
  - Many patients, especially those who are sedentary, with hemodynamically significant aortic stenosis remain asymptomatic or have subtle symptoms, such as infrequent episodes of paroxysmal nocturnal dyspnea.
- Physical examination findings
  - A late peak intensity of the systolic murmur and paradoxical splitting of S_2 predict severe aortic stenosis.
  - In a prospectively evaluated bedside clinical prediction rule, general internal medicine staff and residents found that a combination of either three or four of the following physical findings sufficiently ruled in moderate or severe aortic stenosis: reduced carotid artery volume, slow carotid artery upstroke, reduced intensity of S_2, or maximal murmur intensity at the second right intercostal space and parasternal area.[2] Echocardiographic moderate or severe aortic stenosis was defined as a valve area of ≤ 1.2 cm^2 or a peak instantaneous gradient of ≥ 25 mmHg. In this prediction rule, absence of a murmur over the right clavicle ruled out aortic stenosis.

SURGERY-RELATED RISK FACTORS

- Poorly tolerated hemodynamic changes include (1) a sudden reduction in preload, (2) a sudden reduction in systemic vascular resistance, and (3) atrial fibrillation with a rapid ventricular response.[9,10]
- Procedures
  - Procedures significantly altering hemodynamics include aortic cross-clamping and unclamping and long abdominal procedures with large fluid shifts. Aortic cross-clamping at or above the diaphragm can result in dramatic increases in arterial blood pressure; consequently, aortic unclamping can result in dramatic decreases in arterial blood pressure and venous return, which are poorly tolerated in the setting of significant aortic stenosis.
  - Case series have demonstrated that minor procedures (e.g., ophthalmologic surgery and oral surgery with local anesthesia and intravenous sedation under strict hemodynamic control) are associated with minimal

postoperative cardiac complications.[3] Preoperative recognition of severe aortic stenosis was established in all cases, potentially affecting management.

- Type of anesthesia and anesthesia agents
  - Induction of anesthesia can result in profound hypotension and left ventricular dysfunction in patients with severe aortic stenosis.
  - Neuraxial blockade (spinal or epidural anesthesia) induces a sympathetic blockade below the level of the dermatomal block, with the onset of sympathetic blockade more rapid with spinal technique than epidural technique. Neuraxial blockade may produce dramatic reductions in systemic vascular resistance or vasodilation, setting off an ischemic cascade.[9,10]
  - Compared with opioid-based anesthesia, volatile inhaled agents (e.g., halothane) have myocardial depressant properties and a predisposition to junctional rhythms due to depression of sinoatrial node automaticity.[9,10]

PREOPERATIVE EVALUATION

- Assessing severity of aortic stenosis (Table 22-1)
  - The bedside physical examination can identify moderate to severe aortic stenosis and should prompt further evaluation with transthoracic echocardiography.
  - Echocardiographic predictors of postoperative cardiac complications following noncardiac surgery include:
    - Peak instantaneous aortic gradient ≥40 mmHg, which is associated with an odds ratio of 6.8 (95 percent CI 1.3 to 31) in predicting postoperative cardiac complications.[4]
    - Moderate aortic stenosis, defined as an aortic valve area between 0.7 and 1 cm^2 or a mean gradient between 25 and 49 mmHg.
    - Severe aortic stenosis, defined as an aortic valve area <0.7 cm^2 or a mean gradient ≥50 mmHg.[5]
    - Clinical studies:
      - In a retrospective study matching 108 surgical patients with moderate or severe aortic stenosis to 2 control subjects, patients with aortic stenosis had a 14 percent incidence of perioperative mortality and nonfatal myocardial infarction versus 2 percent incidence for the control subjects. The associated odds ratio was 5.2 (95 percent CI 1.6 to 17.0). The rate of complications was 31 percent in patients with severe aortic stenosis versus 11 percent in those with moderate aortic stenosis.[5]
      - In the same study, patients (n = 18) with a revised cardiac index of zero (one point for each of the following: high-risk surgery, history of ischemic heart disease, history of congestive heart failure, history of cerebrovascular disease, insulin treatment for diabetes mellitus, and preoperative serum creatinine >2 mg/dL) had no adverse outcomes.[5,6]

TABLE 22-1 Preoperative Risk Assessment

VALVE DISEASE	RISK CHARACTERISTICS
Aortic stenosis	Symptoms: angina, syncope, congestive heart failure (CHF) Physical examination: reduced carotid artery volume, slow carotid artery upstroke, late peaking murmur, and paradoxical splitting of S_2 suggesting severe aortic stenosis Transthoracic echocardiography findings: peak instantaneous gradient ≥40 mmHg; moderate aortic stenosis (aortic valve area 0.7–1 cm^2 or mean gradient 25–49 mmHg); severe aortic stenosis (aortic valve area <0.7 cm^2 or mean gradient ≥50 mmHg)
Mitral stenosis	Symptoms: CHF, hoarseness, hemoptysis, chest discomfort Physical examination: low-pitched diastolic rumbling murmur heard best over the apex in left lateral decubitus position
Chronic mitral regurgitation	Symptoms: decreased exercise tolerance, CHF Physical examination: holosystolic apical murmur radiating to left axilla
Chronic aortic regurgitation	Symptoms: decreased exercise tolerance, CHF Physical examination: high-pitched diastolic murmur heard best in end-expiration with patient sitting up and leaning forward

PERIOPERATIVE MANAGEMENT/ RISK REDUCTION (TABLE 22-2)

- Aortic valve replacement
  - Cancel noncardiac surgery in patients with symptoms of angina, syncope, and congestive heart failure and consider aortic valve replacement prior to any elective noncardiac surgery.[1]
- Aortic valvotomy
  - Aortic valvotomy is a temporizing measure for high-risk patients undergoing moderate to high-risk noncardiac surgery. The definitive treatment for severe aortic stenosis remains aortic valve replacement.
    - Complications of balloon aortic valvotomy include cerebrovascular events, acute aortic regurgitation, myocardial infarction, and left ventricular perforation.
- Hemodynamic considerations
  - Sudden reduction in preload, sudden reduction in systemic vascular resistance, and atrial fibrillation with a rapid ventricular response are poorly tolerated.
  - Studies describing patients with severe aortic stenosis undergoing noncardiac surgery and for whom corrective aortic valve replacement was not feasible

TABLE 22-2 Perioperative Risk-Reduction Strategies*

Aortic stenosis (AS)	Cancel or delay elective noncardiac surgery for symptomatic AS and pursue corrective valve replacement if feasible. Communicate diagnosis of moderate to severe AS to anesthesiologist. Sudden reductions in preload or systemic vascular resistance or atrial fibrillation with a rapid ventricular response are poorly tolerated.
Mitral stenosis (MS)	Cancel or delay elective noncardiac surgery for symptomatic MS and pursue mitral valvotomy or mitral valve replacement if feasible. Control ventricular response with an AV-nodal blocking agent. Alert anesthesiologist to presence of MS. Sudden reductions in systemic vascular resistance, tachycardia, and marked increases in central blood volume are poorly tolerated.
Chronic mitral regurgitation (MR)and chronic aortic regurgitation (AR)	Treat and medically optimize congestive heart failure signs and symptoms prior to noncardiac surgery. Communicate diagnosis of severe MR or AR to the anesthesiologist. Increases in systemic vascular resistance diminish forward left ventricular volume flow, increasing the risk for pulmonary edema. Bradycardia decreases forward left ventricular volume flow in patients with AR.

*See Chaps. 7A and 47 for assessments for endocarditis prophylaxis and perioperative management of anticoagulation.

preoperatively reported close hemodynamic monitoring with central venous monitoring, intraarterial monitoring, or pulmonary artery catheterization and an increased use of opioid-based general anesthesia. Patients with preserved left ventricular function had minimal postoperative cardiac complications.[7]

- Phenylephrine, an alpha-agonist with no chronotropic properties, can be used to aggressively treat hypotension following induction of anesthesia, particularly in patients with no significant coronary artery disease and normal left ventricular function.

GENERAL CONCLUSIONS

- Postpone elective surgery in patients with symptomatic aortic stenosis and evaluate them for possible aortic valve replacement prior to noncardiac surgery.
- Alert the anesthesiologist to the diagnosis and severity of aortic stenosis prior to surgery.
- Asymptomatic patients with severe aortic stenosis undergoing minor noncardiac surgical procedures have a favorable risk profile.
- With careful hemodynamic monitoring, asymptomatic patients with moderate to severe aortic stenosis who have good exercise tolerance and a revised cardiac index of zero have a favorable risk profile for most noncardiac surgical procedures.

MITRAL STENOSIS

PATIENT-RELATED RISK FACTORS

- History
  - Rheumatic heart disease is the most common cause of mitral stenosis in adults. While still common in developing countries, rheumatic heart disease is uncommon in the United States.
  - Symptoms include dyspnea, hemoptysis, hoarseness, orthopnea, chest discomfort, paroxysmal nocturnal dyspnea, or thromboembolic events.
- Physical examination findings
  - The murmur of mitral stenosis is a low-pitched diastolic rumbling heard best over the apex with the stethoscope bell and the patient in the left lateral decubitus position.
  - Atrial fibrillation and right-sided heart failure signs portend a poor prognosis.

SURGERY-RELATED RISK FACTORS

- Poorly tolerated hemodynamic changes include (1) a sudden reduction in systemic vascular resistance; (2) tachycardia; and (3) a marked increase in central blood volume, which can precipitate pulmonary edema.[9,10]
- Procedures
  - Procedures significantly altering hemodynamics include aortic cross-clamping and unclamping and long abdominal procedures with large fluid shifts. Aortic cross-clamping at or above the diaphragm can result in dramatic increases in arterial blood pressure; consequently, aortic unclamping can result in dramatic decreases in arterial blood pressure and venous return, which are poorly tolerated in the setting of mitral stenosis.
  - Postoperative atrial fibrillation with a rapid ventricular response leads to reduced cardiac output by impairing ventricular filling.
  - The Trendelenburg position markedly increases pulmonary blood flow and can precipitate pulmonary edema.
- Type of anesthesia and anesthesia agents
  - Anesthesia management includes ensuring minimal changes in heart rate and systemic and pulmonary vascular resistance.[9,10]

PREOPERATIVE EVALUATION

- Assess for symptoms of dyspnea, thromboembolic events, pulmonary edema, right-sided congestive heart failure, and the presence of atrial fibrillation.
- If the patient is symptomatic or undergoing moderate- to high-risk noncardiac surgery, assess the severity of mitral stenosis on transthoracic echocardiography.

PERIOPERATIVE MANAGEMENT/ RISK REDUCTION

- Mitral valvotomy/mitral valve replacement
  - If feasible, cancel elective surgery in patients with symptomatic mitral stenosis and evaluate them for mitral valvotomy or mitral valve replacement prior to noncardiac surgery.
- Perioperative hemodynamic considerations
  - Use atrioventricular-nodal blocking agents to control ventricular rate in patients with atrial fibrillation.
  - Diuretics can diminish pulmonary edema.
  - Invasive hemodynamic monitoring may be necessary to monitor pulmonary and systemic vascular resistance and cardiac output.

GENERAL CONCLUSIONS

- Alert the anesthesiologist to the diagnosis and severity of mitral stenosis prior to noncardiac surgery.
- Cancel elective surgery in patients with symptomatic mitral stenosis and consider mitral valvotomy or mitral valve replacement prior to noncardiac surgery.

CHRONIC MITRAL REGURGITATION

PATIENT-RELATED RISK FACTORS

- History
  - Causes of chronic mitral regurgitation involve damage to the leaflet (e.g., endocarditis, connective tissue disorders, myxomatous degeneration, rheumatic fever), chordae tendineae (e.g., endocarditis, myxomatous degeneration, ischemia, rheumatic fever), papillary muscles (e.g., ischemia, dilated cardiomyopathy), and mitral annulus (e.g., calcification, connective tissue disorder, rheumatic fever, chronic renal failure).
  - Many patients with chronic mitral regurgitation are asymptomatic.
  - Ascertain symptoms of decreased exercise tolerance, dyspnea, orthopnea, paroxysmal nocturnal dyspnea, or lower extremity edema.
- Physical examination findings
  - The mitral regurgitation murmur is a holosystolic apical murmur that radiates to the left axilla. It is best heard with the bell of the stethoscope over the apex, ideally with the patient in the left lateral decubitus position.

SURGERY-RELATED RISK FACTORS

- Procedures
  - Increases in systemic vascular resistance, as in aortic cross-clamping, diminish forward left ventricular volume. Patients with chronic mitral regurgitation are at an increased risk for pulmonary edema.[9,10]
- Type of anesthesia and anesthesia agents
  - Anesthesia management includes minimizing increases in systemic vascular resistance.[9,10]

PREOPERATIVE EVALUATION

- Clinical assessment
  - Identify symptoms of decreased exercise tolerance and congestive heart failure.
  - Identify signs of volume overload and/or left ventricular enlargement on physical examination.
  - Patients with mitral valve prolapse and a murmur of mitral regurgitation but no congestive heart failure symptoms are low risk and require only an assessment for endocarditis prophylaxis.
- Transthoracic echocardiography
  - If the patient is symptomatic or undergoing moderate- to high-risk noncardiac surgery, assess severity of mitral regurgitation on transthoracic echocardiography.
  - Clinical studies: significant valvular heart disease (defined as significant aortic and mitral valvular dysfunction on the preoperative transthoracic echocardiogram) was shown to be a risk factor for perioperative myocardial infarction following major vascular surgery in a case-control study (OR 2.07, 95 percent CI 1.09 to 3.94).[8]

PERIOPERATIVE MANAGEMENT/ RISK REDUCTION

- Mitral valve repair or replacement
  - Little evidence is available on the timing of mitral valve repair or replacement in patients with severe symptomatic mitral regurgitation who require noncardiac surgery.
- Perioperative hemodyamic considerations
  - Minimize congestive heart failure symptoms with diuretics and afterload-reducing agents [e.g., angiotensin-converting enzyme (ACE) inhibitors].

- Invasive hemodynamic monitoring may help minimize increases in systemic vascular resistance, which diminish forward flow.

GENERAL CONCLUSIONS

- Asymptomatic patients with chronic mitral regurgitation tolerate minor procedures well.
- Treat and medically optimize patients with signs or symptoms of congestive heart failure prior to major elective surgery.
- In major elective surgery, invasive hemodynamic monitoring may be helpful in perioperative management.

CHRONIC AORTIC REGURGITATION

PATIENT-RELATED RISK FACTORS

- History
  - Causes of chronic aortic regurgitation in adults include disorders affecting the aortic root or ascending aorta (e.g., hypertension, Ehlers-Danlos syndrome, ankylosing spondylitis, inflammatory bowel disease, Reiter's syndrome, or other systemic disorders) or leaflet abnormalities (e.g., rheumatic heart disease, endocarditis, bicuspid aortic valve, fenfluramine-phentermine, Marfan's syndrome, myxomatous degeneration, rheumatoid arthritis, ankylosing spondylitis, or other systemic disorders).
  - Many patients with chronic aortic regurgitation are asymptomatic.
  - Ascertain symptoms of decreased exercise tolerance, dyspnea, orthopnea, paroxysmal nocturnal dyspnea, or lower extremity edema preoperatively.
- Physical examination findings
  - The murmur of chronic aortic regurgitation is a high-pitched diastolic murmur heard best at end-expiration along the left sternal border (primary aortic valvular disease) or right sternal border and apex (aortic root dilatation) with the patient sitting up and leaning forward.

SURGERY-RELATED RISK FACTORS

- Procedures
  - Increases in systemic vascular resistance, as in aortic cross-clamping, diminish forward left ventricular volume. Patients with chronic aortic regurgitation are at increased risk for pulmonary edema.[9,10]
- Type of anesthesia and anesthesia agents
  - Anesthesia management includes minimizing increases in systemic vascular resistance and bradycardia, which diminish forward flow. [9,10]

PREOPERATIVE EVALUATION

- Identify symptoms of decreased exercise tolerance and congestive heart failure.
- Identify signs of volume overload and/or left ventricular enlargement on physical examination.
- If the patient is symptomatic or undergoing moderate- to high-risk noncardiac surgery, assess the severity of aortic regurgitation on transthoracic echocardiography.

PERIOPERATIVE MANAGEMENT/ RISK REDUCTION

- Aortic valve replacement
  - Little evidence is available on the timing of aortic valve replacement in patients with severe symptomatic aortic regurgitation who require noncardiac surgery.
- Perioperative hemodynamic considerations
  - Minimize congestive heart failure symptoms with diuretics and afterload-reducing agents (e.g., ACE inhibitors).
  - Invasive hemodynamic monitoring may help minimize increases in systemic vascular resistance and bradycardia, which diminish forward flow.

GENERAL CONCLUSIONS

- Asymptomatic patients with chronic aortic regurgitation tolerate minor procedures well.
- Treat and medically optimize patients with signs or symptoms of congestive heart failure prior to major elective surgery.
- In major noncardiac surgery, invasive hemodynamic monitoring may be of assistance in perioperative management.

REFERENCES

1. Eagle KA, Berger PB, Calkins H, et al. ACC/AHA guideline update for perioperative cardiovascular evaluation for noncardiac surgery—executive summary: A report of the American College of Cardiology/American Heart Association Task Force on Practice Guidelines (Committee to Update the 1996 Guidelines on Perioperative Cardiovascular Evaluation for Noncardiac Surgery). *J Am Coll Cardiol* 39:542, 2002.
2. Etchells E, Glenns V, Shadowitz S, et al. A bedside clinical prediction rule for detecting moderate or severe aortic stenosis. *J Gen Intern Med* 13:699, 1998.
3. O'Keefe JH Jr, Shub C, Rettke SR. Risk of noncardiac surgical procedures in patients with aortic stenosis. *Mayo Clin Proc* 64:400, 1989.

4. Rohde LE, Polanczyk CA, Goldman L, et al. Usefulness of transthoracic echocardiography as a tool for risk stratification of patients undergoing major noncardiac surgery. *Am J Cardiol* 87:505, 2001.
5. Kertai MD, Bountioukos M, Boersma E, et al. Aortic stenosis: An underestimated risk factor for perioperative complications in patients undergoing noncardiac surgery. *Am J Med* 116:8, 2004.
6. Lee TH, Marcantonio ER, Mangione CM, et al. Derivation and prospective validation of a simple index for prediction of cardiac risk of major noncardiac surgery. *Circulation* 100:1043, 1999.
7. Raymer K, Yang H. Patients with aortic stenosis: Cardiac complications in non-cardiac surgery. *Can J Anaesth* 45:855, 1998.
8. Sprung J, Abdelmalak B, Gottlieb A, et al. Analysis of risk factors for myocardial infarction and cardiac mortality after major vascular surgery. *Anaesthesiology* 93:129, 2000.
9. Conde MC, Henderson MC, Kumar R. Perioperative valvular disease risk assessment. *http://pier.acponline.org/physicians/diseases/periopr875/risk/periopr875-s1.html.* [Date accessed: 2005 Feb 17] In: PIER [online database]. Philadelphia: American College of Physicians, 2005.
10. Roizen MF, Fleisher LA: Anesthetic implications of concurrent diseases, in Miller RD (ed): *Miller's Anesthesia,* 6th ed. Philadelphia: Churchill Livingstone, 2005:1077–1083.

23 ARRHYTHMIAS/ CONDUCTION DEFECTS

Seth McClennen and Peter J. Zimetbaum

INTRODUCTION

- Preoperative evaluation of patients undergoing surgical procedures should include an assessment of arrhythmia risk as well as the initiation of a formal plan for management of any previously recognized arrhythmias.
- The intraoperative and (most importantly) the postoperative periods are well-recognized times for arrhythmic complications.
- Anticipation of possible arrhythmias as well as appropriate medical management of chronic cardiac arrhythmias can minimize dangerous sequelae of postoperative arrhythmic complications.
- Risk of cardiac arrhythmias depends heavily on patient-related risk factors (only some of which are modifiable) and the type of procedure. Specifically, open cardiac surgery carries an exponentially higher risk of intraoperative and postoperative arrhythmias.
- Recognition and appropriate intervention for modifiable patient-related risk factors may reduce perioperative arrhythmic complications.
- This chapter addresses patient-related risk factors, surgical procedure-related risk factors, appropriate preoperative testing, and perioperative interventions to prevent new cardiac arrhythmias as well as complications of chronic arrhythmias.
- Specific postoperative arrhythmias and their management are discussed separately (see Chap. 53).

PATIENT-RELATED RISK FACTORS (TABLE 23-1)

AGE

- Advancing age is the most important risk factor in the development of postoperative arrhythmias.
  - Many studies have consistently shown an age-related increase in perioperative arrhythmia complications. One series of 5807 consecutive patients undergoing coronary artery bypass grafting (CABG) demonstrated that the incidence of postoperative atrial fibrillation (AF) and/or atrial flutter was 3.7 percent in patients under the age of 40 years but 27.7 percent in patients over the age of 70.[1]
  - Postoperative bradyarrhythmias are also found with increasing frequency in older patients. A large prospective observational study of more than 10,000 patients undergoing open cardiac procedures showed that patients 75 years of age and older were significantly more likely to require implantation of a permanent pacemaker in the postoperative period (OR 3.0, CI 2.0 to 4.4).[2]

TABLE 23-1 Patient- and Surgery-Related Risk Factors for Perioperative Arrhythmias

PATIENT-RELATED RISK FACTORS	PROCEDURE-RELATED RISK FACTORS
Older age	Cardiac surgery (valvular > nonvalvular)
Presence of congestive heart failure	Surgical techniques involving vagal stimulation (see text)
Baseline electrocardiographic abnormalities	Planned non-low-risk procedure
Baseline electrolyte abnormalities	
Presence of atrial fibrillation	
History of paroxysmal arrhythmias	
Previously implanted cardiac device	

- Postoperative arrhythmias have also been demonstrated to occur with increased frequency in older patients undergoing major nonemergent noncardiac procedures.

CONGESTIVE HEART FAILURE (CHF)

- Patients with active CHF at the time of surgery have an increased risk for developing postoperative arrhythmias.
  - In an observational cohort of over 4181 patients undergoing major nonemergent noncardiac procedures, the presence of preoperative CHF was independently correlated with the development of postoperative supraventricular arrhythmias (OR 1.7, CI 1.1 to 2.7).[3]
  - In a prospectively collected case-control study of over 4400 patients undergoing CABG, the incidence of postoperative ventricular tachyarrhythmias was 1.6 percent, and moderately impaired or poor ejection fraction significantly increased the risk of these arrhythmias.[4]
- Diastolic heart failure (left ventricular end-diastolic pressure over 20 mmHg) has also been independently associated with an increased risk of postoperative supraventricular arrhythmia.
- The presence of history or physical signs and symptoms of CHF should prompt medical adjustments and reevaluation prior to any elective or semielective surgical procedures.

BASELINE ELECTROCARDIOGRAPHIC (ECG) ABNORMALITIES

- Some baseline ECG abnormalities are associated with an increased risk of perioperative arrhythmias. Recognition of these abnormalities prior to surgery can allow for prompt recognition and treatment of new perioperative arrhythmias.
- Atrial conduction defects (e.g., left atrial enlargement) and atrial premature beats on baseline sinus rhythm ECG are associated with an increased risk of postoperative AF.
- Asymptomatic bifascicular block (left anterior or posterior fascicular block plus right bundle-branch block) has not been consistently associated with an increased risk of postoperative bradyarrhythmias such as complete heart block. Preoperative left bundle-branch block is an independent but weak risk factor in the development of post-CABG complete heart block (incidence of 0.8 percent).[5]
- Preoperative left bundle-branch block is associated with a risk of transient complete heart block during pulmonary arterial catheterization or placement of permanent or temporary transvenous right ventricular pacing electrodes. Heart block due to mechanical injury to the right bundle can occur in these circumstances; however, it is usually reversible if the mechanical pressure on the right bundle is relieved by removing the causative catheter or electrode.

ELECTROLYTE ABNORMALITIES

- A serum potassium level of less than 3.5 μmol/L was associated with a more than twofold increase in the risk of perioperative arrhythmias in patients undergoing cardiac surgery.[6] This risk may be attenuated in patients undergoing noncardiac surgery.
- Hypomagnesemia and hypocalcemia are associated with prolongation of the QT interval and may put patients at risk for torsades de pointes in the operative environment.

ATRIAL FIBRILLATION

- The presence of paroxysmal or chronic AF dictates an increased complexity in preoperative medication management. A history of these arrhythmias also increases risk for postoperative arrhythmic complications. Evaluation should include a management plan for perioperative anticoagulation, rate-controlling agents, and rhythm-controlling agents if applicable.
- Most patients with AF are on warfarin to prevent thromboembolic complications. Specific management of warfarin in the perioperative period is addressed in Chap. 7A.
- Rate control of chronic or persistent AF may be difficult in the postoperative period due to high adrenergic levels as well as limitations on oral medications. Preoperative and perioperative continuation of all atrioventricular (AV)-nodal agents is recommended
- Patients on chronic antiarrhythmic agents should have these medications continued throughout the perioperative period in an effort to suppress recurrent AF. Recurrent paroxysmal AF is commonly noted in the postoperative period even in otherwise suppressed patients due to high levels of circulating catecholamine.

OTHER PAROXYSMAL ARRHYTHMIAS

- Patients with a history of other paroxysmal supraventricular tachycardias (SVTs) have an increased risk of recurrent SVT in the perioperative period mediated by high levels of circulating catecholamine. This risk is minimized with the administration of perioperative AV-nodal agents. Appropriate arrhythmia-specific interventions are reviewed in Chap. 53.

IMPLANTED DEVICES (PACEMAKERS AND IMPLANTABLE CARDIOVERTER/DEFIBRILLATORS)

- Patients with preexisting pacemakers or implantable cardioverter/defibrillators (ICDs) should be seen in conjunction with a health care professional qualified and experienced in their management.
- Both ICDs and pacemakers can malfunction during surgery as a result of electrocautery-induced electromagnetic interference. Electromagnetic interference can be interpreted as intracardiac activity, leading to inappropriate inhibition of pacing and/or attempts at tachycardia therapy (overdrive pacing or defibrillation) from an ICD.
- The American College of Cardiology/American Heart Association (ACC/AHA) guidelines currently recommend preoperative and postoperative assessment (interrogation) of pacemakers and ICDs by qualified individuals.[7]
- Magnet use usually will temporarily revert a pacemaker to a nonsensing mode (DOO or VOO) or temporarily suspend detection of tachyarrhythmic events in ICDs. Upon removal of the magnet, the ICD usually reverts to detection mode. Older devices may not behave in this characteristic fashion, and some older ICDs will remain inactivated after magnet use.

SURGERY-RELATED RISK FACTORS (TABLE 23-1)

CARDIAC VERSUS NONCARDIAC SURGERY

- The risks of procedure-related arrhythmias can be subdivided by cardiac and noncardiac planned surgical procedures. In open cardiac procedures, a perioperative arrhythmia incidence of 25 to 50 percent can be expected, as compared to an 8 to 13 percent incidence in patients undergoing noncardiac surgery.
- Cardiac procedures can be further subdivided in arrhythmia risk on the basis of valvular intervention. The likelihood of perioperative arrhythmias (most commonly AF and heart block) after open cardiac surgery is approximately 30 percent in patients without valvular intervention but up to 50 percent in patients undergoing valvular surgery.
- A large prospective observational study of more than 10,000 patients undergoing both CABG and valvular heart surgery showed the following OR and CI for the risk of receiving a permanent pacemaker during the index hospitalization for each of the following valve replacements[2]:

  Aortic: OR 5.8, CI 3.9 to 8.7
  Mitral: OR 4.9, CI 3.1 to 7.8
  Tricuspid: OR 8.0, CI 5.5 to 11.9
  Double: OR 8.9, CI 5.5 to 14.6
  Triple: OR 7.5, CI 2.9 to 19.3

VAGALLY MEDIATED BRADYARRHYTHMIAS

- Numerous surgical techniques involve vagal stimulation and the risk of vagally mediated heart block, including:
  - Spinal/epidural anesthesia (inhibition of cardiac-innervating preganglionic sympathetic fibers)
  - Procedural narcotic use
  - Mesenteric traction during intraabdominal surgery
  - Intrascalene block
  - Ophthalmologic surgery

LOW-RISK SURGERY

- Some minimally invasive procedures have such a low risk of perioperative arrhythmic complications that preoperative testing is unnecessary.
- Current ACC/AHA guidelines do not support the use of preoperative electrocardiography (ECG) for asymptomatic individuals without comorbid conditions or symptoms prior to low-risk procedures.[7]

PREOPERATIVE EVALUATION AND TESTING TO STRATIFY FOR PERIOPERATIVE ARRHYTHMIA RISK

- Clinical evaluation
  - The patient should be evaluated for evidence of CHF, ischemic heart disease, or valvular abnormalities which may be associated with arrhythmias.
- Baseline ECG: A routine preoperative ECG should be done in all patients with:
  - History of arrhythmia
  - Planned cardiac or major noncardiac surgery
  - Symptoms suggestive of paroxysmal arrhythmia
  - Preexisting implantable cardiac device (pacemaker or defibrillator)
  - Patients with history of ischemic cardiovascular disease, peripheral vascular disease, or symptoms to suggest these conditions or patients with risk factors for atherosclerotic vascular disease
- Baseline electrolyte panel
  - Preoperative hypokalemia is associated with an increased risk of perioperative arrhythmia.[6]
  - Preoperative electrolytes may not be indicated prior to minimally invasive/low-risk procedures.[8]
- Evaluation of pacemaker or defibrillator
  - Preoperative interrogation of a previously implanted pacemaker or cardiac defibrillator should be performed

or at the least its function should be evaluated by qualified personnel.[7]

PERIOPERATIVE MANAGEMENT TO REDUCE RISK OF POSTOPERATIVE ARRHYTHMIA (TABLE 23-2)

PREOPERATIVE INTERVENTIONS

- Beta-adrenergic blockade
  - In absence of contraindications, preoperative beta blockade is indicated for all patients undergoing open cardiac procedures or high-risk noncardiac procedures. This reduces risk of ischemic cardiac complications (see Chap. 20) as well as the risk of postoperative atrial and ventricular tachyarrhythmias.
  - A metaanalysis of 24 studies including patients undergoing CABG showed that preoperative prophylactic beta blockade was associated with significantly reduced incidence of postoperative AF (OR 0.28).[9]
  - The most recent ACC/AHA consensus guideline supports the use of prophylactic beta blockade in any patient at increased risk for perioperative arrhythmias.[7]
- Amiodarone
  - Oral amiodarone is a safe antiarrhythmic drug with a high efficacy in preventing AF. Multiple studies have evaluated the efficacy of preoperative amiodarone (oral or intravenous) in the prevention of postoperative AF. Although most trials suggest that amiodarone has a preventive effect, many do not require all enrolled patients to be on concurrent beta-adrenergic blocking medications.
  - In 124 patients in a double-blind randomized study of amiodarone for the prevention of post-coronary bypass AF, patients taking 600 mg of amiodarone daily for the 7 days preceding surgery had a significantly reduced risk of postoperative AF compared with control (25 versus 53 percent). An unexpectedly high incidence (53 percent) of atrial tachyarrhythmias was noted in the control group, however, and beta-blocker use in both the amiodarone and control groups was low (26 and 18 percent, respectively).[10]
- Rate/rhythm control for AF:
  - Preoperative and perioperative continuation of all AV-nodal agents is recommended, with conversion to intravenous agents when oral agents are contraindicated from a surgical perspective. Commonly prescribed AV-nodal agents such as beta blockers and calcium channel blockers (and, to a lesser extent, digoxin) are available in both intravenous and oral formulations.
  - Antiarrhythmic agents should be administered throughout the perioperative period in an effort to suppress recurrent AF. Some antiarrhythmics lack safe intravenous alternatives and should be held while patients are taking nothing by mouth because of surgical issues.

INTRAOPERATIVE INTERVENTIONS

- Open cardiac procedures: Anticipation of postoperative arrhythmias has led to preventive interventions during the intraoperative period.
  - Placement of epicardial pacing wires: After open cardiac procedures, overdrive atrial pacing (pacing the atrium at a rate higher than the intrinsic normal sinus rate) has been shown to reduce the incidence of postoperative AF. It remains unclear whether this effect is superior to standard medical therapy.[11,12]
  - The placement of epicardial wires during surgery also allows for the possible therapeutic option of overdrive antitachycardia pacing of the atrium to terminate postoperative atrial flutter.
  - During open cardiac procedures, removal of the left-atrial appendage should be considered, as most left atrial clot originates from this thrombogenic vestigial structure.
  - Aortic cross-clamp time during open cardiac procedures is associated with a higher risk of postoperative AF and should be minimized as much possible.

TABLE 23-2 Preoperative, Intraoperative, and Postoperative Prevention of Arrhythmias

PREOPERATIVE INTERVENTIONS	INTRAOPERATIVE INTERVENTIONS	POSTOPERATIVE INTERVENTIONS
Beta-adrenergic blockade	Epicardial wires	Beta-adrenergic blockade
Amiodarone for patients at high risk for postoperative atrial fibrillation	Consider intraoperative magnesium	Amiodarone in patients at high risk for postoperative atrial fibrillation
	Anticipate and respond appropriately to vagally mediated hypotension and bradyarrhythmias	Telemetry
		Overdrive pacing of the atrium

- Intravenous magnesium: Administered along with intraoperative beta blockade, intraoperative intravenous magnesium may be associated with an independent lower risk of postoperative tachyarrhythmia.[13]
- Intraoperative vagal stimulation should be anticipated during ophthalmologic procedures, operations involving mesenteric traction, and other procedures with possible vagally mediated bradyarrhythmias, as noted previously. If these are encountered, treatment with intraveous atropine is the most typical appropriate response.

POSTOPERATIVE INTERVENTIONS

- Postoperative telemetry
  - The peak incidence of post-CABG AF is on postoperative days 2 to 4.
  - Postoperative arrhythmia monitoring (telemetry) is recommended by the ACC for at least 3 days after cardiothoracic surgery.[14] Longer monitoring periods may be necessary in patients with clinically important arrhythmias, conduction defects, or shock.
  - Postoperative cardiac monitoring is not recommended for patients at low risk for postoperative arrhythmias, including young patients after low-risk operations not involving cardiopulmonary bypass.[14]
- Overdrive atrial pacing in the immediate post-CABG period is associated with a lower risk of postoperative AF.[12]
- Beta blockade and possibly amiodarone should be considered in the postoperative period.
  - The morbidity and mortality of postoperative AF is high; thus prevention of AF may reduce in-hospital mortality and patient-related costs. The most cost-effective use of these medications is in the patients at highest risk for arrhythmias: the post-CABG patients.
  - Perioperative beta-adrenergic blockade is also associated with an overall reduction in the risk of postoperative cardiac events, including myocardial infarction and congestive heart failure (see Chap. 20).
  - A multicenter prospective observational study of 4657 patients undergoing CABG showed a reduced risk of AF in patients who were given beta-blocking drugs in the postoperative period (OR 0.32, 95 percent CI 0.22 to 0.46).[15]
  - A metaanalysis of 24 randomized controlled trials comprising patients after CABG revealed an OR of 0.28 for those developing postoperative AF while receiving beta-adrenergic blocking medications.[9]
  - A placebo-controlled randomized trial comparing amiodarone (intravenous for 24 h, then oral for 4 days, $n = 77$) versus placebo ($n = 83$) in patients who had undergone cardiothoracic surgery showed the risk of AF to be reduced significantly in the group receiving amiodarone (22 versus 39 percent, $p = 0.037$). In both groups, over 80 percent of the patients were receiving beta-blocking medications.[11]
  - Multiple other antiarrhythmic medications—including sotalol, verapamil, digoxin, procainamide, propafenone, and diltiazem—have been evaluated for postoperative prevention of arrhythmias in patients after cardiothoracic surgery. None have been shown to be superior to placebo and/or beta-blocking medications.

REFERENCES

1. Leitch JW, Thomson D, Baird DK, et al. The importance of age as a predictor of atrial fibrillation and flutter after coronary artery bypass grafting. *J Thorac Cardiovasc Surg* 100:338, 1990.
2. Gordon RS, Ivanov J, Cohen G, et al. Permanent cardiac pacing after a cardiac operation: Predicting the use of permanent pacemakers. *Ann Thorac Surg* 66:1698, 1998.
3. Polanczyk CA, Goldman L, Marcantonio ER, et al. Supraventricular arrhythmia in patients having noncardiac surgery: Clinical correlates and effect on length of stay. *Ann Intern Med* 129:279, 1998.
4. Ascione R, Reeves BC, Santo K, et al. Predictors of new malignant ventricular arrhythmias after coronary surgery: A case-control study. *J Am Coll Cardiol* 43:1630, 2004.
5. Emlein G, Huang SK, Pires LA, et al. Prolonged bradyarrhythmias after isolated coronary artery bypass graft surgery. *Am Heart J* 126:1084, 1993.
6. Wahr JA, Parks R, Boisvert D, et al. Preoperative serum potassium levels and perioperative outcomes in cardiac surgery patients. Multicenter Study of Perioperative Ischemia Research Group. *JAMA* 281:2203, 1999.
7. Eagle KA, Berger PB, Calkins H, et al. ACC/AHA guideline update for perioperative cardiovascular evaluation for noncardiac surgery—executive summary: A report of the American College of Cardiology/American Heart Association Task Force on Practice Guidelines (Committee to Update the 1996 Guidelines on Perioperative Cardiovascular Evaluation for Noncardiac Surgery). *J Am Coll Cardiol* 39:542, 2002.
8. Schein OD, Katz J, Bass EB, et al. The value of routine preoperative medical testing before cataract surgery. Study of Medical Testing for Cataract Surgery. *N Engl J Med* 342:168, 2000.
9. Andrews TC, Reimold SC, Berlin JA, et al. Prevention of supraventricular arrhythmias after coronary artery bypass surgery. A meta-analysis of randomized controlled trials. Circulation 84:III236, 1991.
10. Daoud EG, Strickberger SA, Man CK, et al. Preoperative amiodarone as prophylaxis against atrial fibrillation after heart surgery. *N Engl J Med* 337:1785, 1997.
11. White CM, Caron MF, Kalus JS, et al. Intravenous plus oral amiodarone, atrial septal pacing, or both strategies to prevent post-cardiothoracic surgery atrial fibrillation: The Atrial Fibrillation Suppression Trial II (AFIST II). *Circulation* 108(suppl II):II-200, 2003

12. Crystal E, Connolly SJ, Sleik K, et al. Interventions on prevention of postoperative atrial fibrillation in patients undergoing heart surgery: A meta-analysis. *Circulation* 106:75, 2002.
13. Maslow AD, Regan MM, Heindle S, et al. Postoperative atrial tachyarrhythmias in patients undergoing coronary artery bypass graft surgery without cardiopulmonary bypass: A role for intraoperative magnesium supplementation. *J Cardiothorac Vasc Anesth* 14:524, 2000.
14. Emergency Cardiac Care Committee Members. Recommended guidelines for in-hospital cardiac monitoring of adults for detection of arrhythmia. *J Am Coll Cardiol* 18:1431, 1991.
15. Mathew JP, Fontes ML, Tudor IC, et al. A multicenter risk index for atrial fibrillation after cardiac surgery. *JAMA* 291:1720, 2004.

24 PULMONARY EVALUATION

Gerald W. Smetana
and Michelle V. Conde

INTRODUCTION

- Postoperative pulmonary complications (PPCs) are a major source of morbidity among patients undergoing surgery. The incidence is similar to that of cardiac complications in most series. Patients who sustain a PPC are more likely to have a prolonged hospital stay than those who sustain a cardiac complication.
- Major PPCs that affect length of stay, morbidity, and mortality include pneumonia, atelectasis, respiratory failure, exacerbation of chronic obstructive pulmonary disease (COPD), and bronchospasm.
- The primary mechanism for PPCs is a reduction in lung volumes after surgery and anesthesia. This increases the risk for atelectasis and other PPCs.
- PPC risk factors are not intuitive and differ from those for other common major postoperative complications, including those for venous thromboembolism and cardiac complications. For example, procedure-related risk factors predominate for PPCs; this differs from preoperative cardiac evaluation, where patient-related risk factors are more important.
- Due to the morbidity and frequency of PPCs, all requests for preoperative medical evaluation should include an assessment of pulmonary risk.
- This chapter considers patient-related risk factors, procedure-related risk factors, laboratory testing, and interventions to reduce PPC risk in high-risk patients.
- Preoperative evaluation and management of the patient with COPD and asthma (Chap. 25) and management of postoperative atelectasis and pneumonia (Chap. 54) are discussed separately.

PATIENT-RELATED RISK FACTORS

AGE

- The impact of age on the risk of PPCs has been controversial. Many studies suggesting age as a risk factor did not control for the impact of comorbidities, which are more common with advancing age. With adjustment for such comorbidities, the impact of age decreases.
    - For example, in a study of 4315 patients undergoing noncardiac surgery, rates of postoperative pneumonia or respiratory failure climbed from 2.0 percent for patients 50 to 59 years of age to 6.0 percent for patients ≥80 years of age.[1] After multivariate adjustment for comorbidities, age ≥80 was still a risk factor, but the odds ratio (OR) compared to patients 50 to 59 years of age was only 2.0. This is similar to odds ratios determined by other published multivariate analyses; age cutoffs to define elderly ranged from 70 to 80.
- Advanced age is a modest risk factor for PPCs and confers an approximately twofold increase in risk. By itself, the risk is not prohibitive. and one should not deny surgery due to concern for PPCs based on advanced age alone in the absence of other important risk factors.

CIGARETTE SMOKING

- Cigarette smoking increases the risk of PPCs, even for patients without COPD. The basis for the risk is an increase in bronchial secretions and airway reactivity.
    - In a recent systematic review, the pooled odds ratios for current cigarette use was 1.9.[2] However, among multivariate studies that adjusted for the presence of COPD and other comorbidities, only 6 of 17 studies found cigarette smoking to be an independent risk factor.
- Elicit a smoking history from all patients before surgery, as current cigarette use is a modest risk factor for the development of PPCs.

CHRONIC OBSTRUCTIVE PULMONARY DISEASE

- COPD is a major risk factor and is one of the strongest risk factors for PPCs. The magnitude of the increase in risk is approximately threefold.
- Asthma is not a risk factor for PPCs.
- Each of these risk factors is discussed in more detail separately (Chap. 25).

FUNCTIONAL STATUS

- Various measures of overall health and functional status predict PPC rates in addition to overall perioperative mortality.
  - The classification of the American Association of Anesthesiologists (ASA) was derived to predict perioperative mortality. In addition, it predicts PPC rates. ASA class >2 confers a sevenfold increase in risk of PPCs.[2]
  - Both self-reported and directly observed exercise capacity identify patients at higher risk of PPCs. Self-reported inability to climb at least two flights of stairs or walk at least four blocks on level ground confers a modest increase in PPC rate (OR 1.4).[3]
  - Directly observed stair climbing also predicts risk for patients undergoing high-risk surgeries. Patients who can climb at least four flights of stairs without resting have a low risk of PPCs. The positive predictive value is 52 percent and the negative predictive value 89 percent, which confirms a low risk for patients with good exercise capacity.[3a]
- Inquire about exercise capacity as part of the routine preoperative evaluation. In selected patients undergoing high-risk surgeries (pulmonary, cardiac, upper abdominal), it is reasonable to directly observe stair climbing during preoperative evaluation.

OBESITY

- Obesity is not a risk factor for PPCs. This holds true even for morbid obesity. This is one of the most misunderstood areas in preoperative pulmonary risk assessment as it runs contrary to intuition and the physiology of PPCs (reduction in lung volumes).
- In a systematic review, PPC rates for obese and nonobese patients were 6.3 and 7.0 percent, respectively.[2] Obesity was a risk factor in only 1 of 8 studies that used multivariate analysis to identify PPC risk factors.
- Among patients undergoing gastric bypass surgery for obesity, PPC rates are similar to those of nonobese patients. PPC rates also do not differ among gastric bypass patients when stratified by body mass index. Even the heaviest patients referred for gastric bypass surgery have no greater PPC risk than patients with lesser degrees of obesity.

OBSTRUCTIVE SLEEP APNEA

- Although obesity itself is not a PPC risk factor, obstructive sleep apnea (OSA) may increase risk. The risk exists even for patients whose condition has not been previously diagnosed. Of importance to anesthesiologists is the higher incidence of airway management problems in the immediate postoperative period, such as hypoxia, hypercarbia, and the need for reintubation.
- Traditional PPCs, such as pneumonia and atelectasis, may also be more common among patients with OSA, but this is less well established.
- Until further information is available, consider OSA to be a modest risk factor for PPCs and inquire about symptoms of OSA in obese patients preparing for surgery.

SURGERY-RELATED RISK FACTORS

SURGICAL SITE

- The surgical site is the single most important risk factor for the development of PPCs. PPCs are rare for low-risk procedures, even for high-risk patients.
- PPCs are more common as the incision approaches the diaphragm. Esophageal, thoracic, and upper abdominal surgeries carry the highest risk. The risk is due to splinting of the abdominal muscles and diaphragmatic dysfunction, which contribute to a decrease in postoperative lung volumes. Low-risk procedures include hip, gynecologic, urologic, and other lower abdominal surgeries.
- Estimates of PPC rates for different procedures follow[2]:

Esophageal	35 percent
Thoracic	30 percent
Upper abdominal	24 percent
Aortic	21 percent
Head and neck	16 percent
Lower abdominal	5 percent
Hip	4 percent
GU or GYN	<1 percent

- The most important consideration in stratifying PPC risk is to determine the planned procedure and surgical site.

TYPE OF ANESTHESIA

- Whether a particular anesthetic technique influences overall morbidity or PPC rates remains controversial. In particular, there has been much discussion about the relative risks in comparing general anesthesia to either spinal or epidural anesthesia (collectively referred to as neuraxial blockade). If a difference in PPC risk existed, then medical consultants would have a justification for offering advice about anesthetic type as part of the preoperative evaluation.
  - In the largest metaanalysis to date of randomized controlled trials of anesthetic technique, neuraxial blockade conferred lower rates of PPCs than general anesthesia.[4] The odds ratios were 0.61 for pneumonia and 0.41 for respiratory failure.
- General anesthesia confers a higher risk of PPCs than neuraxial blockade. Therefore the use of neuraxial

blockade is a potential risk-reduction strategy in high-risk patients. The nuances of anesthetic selection go beyond the expertise of medical consultants, and factors other than PPC risk enter into this decision. Therefore medical consultants should collaborate with anesthesiologists to determine the optimal strategy for a given patient.

NEUROMUSCULAR BLOCKERS

- Long-acting neuromuscular blockers, such as pancuronium, lead to more residual neuromuscular blockade after surgery.
  - Conceivably, this residual neuromuscular blockade could lead to postoperative hypoventilation and an increased risk of PPCs.
- In fact, patients who receive pancuronium do have a higher incidence of residual neuromuscular blockade than those who receive shorter-acting agents such as vecuronium or atracurium. Among patients with residual blockade, there is a threefold increase in PPC rates.
- The use of pancuronium increases PPC rates. This suggests a strategy to reduce risk among high-risk patients.

SURGICAL TECHNIQUE

- There is no difference in PPC rates between midline and transverse incisions for patients undergoing abdominal surgery.
- Laparoscopic surgery may confer a lower risk for PPCs than open abdominal surgery, but the evidence is conflicting. Other reasons for choosing laparoscopic techniques often exist, including less postoperative pain, quicker return to normal functioning, and a less conspicuous scar.
- Perioperative use of pulmonary artery catheters does not reduce the risk of mortality or postoperative pneumonia.
- Surgeries lasting longer than 3 or 4 h are associated with higher PPC rates than briefer operations.
- Emergency surgery is a moderate risk factor for the development of PPCs. In a multivariate study of the risk for postoperative respiratory failure, the relative risk was 3.81 and was second only to surgical site as predictor of PPCs.[5]

PREOPERATIVE EVALUATION AND TESTING TO STRATIFY RISK

HISTORY AND PHYSICAL EXAMINATION

- Table 24-1 summarizes elements of the clinical examination pertinent to risk stratification.

TABLE 24-1 Patient- and Surgery-Related Risk Factors for Postoperative Pulmonary Complications*

PATIENT-RELATED RISK FACTORS	PROCEDURE-RELATED RISK FACTORS
Chronic obstructive pulmonary disease	Esophageal surgery
ASA class >2	Thoracic surgery
Poor exercise capacity	Upper abdominal surgery
Cigarette use	Aortic surgery
Age >70	Head and neck surgery
Obstructive sleep apnea	Pancuronium as neuromuscular blocker
	General anesthesia
	Surgery lasting >3 h
	Emergency surgery

*Ranked by relative importance, with the most important factors listed first.

CHEST RADIOGRAPHY

- Routine preoperative chest radiography in healthy individuals rarely adds useful information to the preoperative evaluation, nor does it predict PPCs or change perioperative management.
  - A metaanalysis of the value of routine preoperative testing showed that abnormalities were found in 10 percent of 14,390 preoperative chest radiographs reviewed; only 1.3 percent of the abnormalities were unexpected.[6] This resulted in a change in perioperative management in only 0.1 percent cases.
- Obtain chest radiographs in patients to further evaluate unexplained dyspnea or better characterize underlying cardiac or pulmonary disease that is not at baseline.

LABORATORY TESTING

- Selected laboratory abnormalities are risk factors for the development of PPCs.
- Hypoalbuminemia (albumin <3.0 g/dL) and blood urea nitrogen (BUN) >30 mg/dL were associated with odds ratios of 2.53 and 2.29, respectively, for the development of postoperative respiratory failure in a large veteran population surgical cohort.[5] Low BUN (<8 mg/dL) and high BUN (>22 mg/dL) increased the risk for the development of postoperative pneumonia.[7]
- Obtain serum albumin and BUN in patients at high risk for PPCs due either to patient-related risk factors or a planned high-risk procedure.

ARTERIAL BLOOD GAS ANALYSIS

- Older studies concluded that hypercarbia ($Paco_2$ >45 mmHg) was helpful in predicting PPCs; however, these patients had clinical evidence of severe obstruction and probably would have been identified as at high risk for developing PPCs simply from the clinical history and physical examination alone.

- Similarly, other retrospective studies concluded that hypoxemia predicted PPCs, but they did not compare hypoxemia to other relevant clinical information gathered from the history and physical examination.
- Avoid ordering routine arterial blood gas analysis to assist in predicting PPCs following noncardiothoracic surgery. Arterial blood gas analysis, however, can be helpful in the perioperative management of patients with severe lung disease who require home oxygen supplementation or in those with chronic CO_2 retention.

PULMONARY FUNCTION TESTING (SPIROMETRY)

- Spirometric testing (FEV_1 and FEV_1/FVC) is helpful in predicting PPCs following lung resection and is part of the standard preoperative evaluation for this procedure. This is discussed in detail in Chap. 9.
- Whether routine spirometry accurately predicts the development of PPCs following noncardiothoracic surgery has been the subject of much debate. There is also concern that clinicians overuse spirometry as part of the preoperative pulmonary evaluation process.
    - Few studies have compared the relative value of clinical findings and spirometry results in predicting PPC risk. In general, spirometry adds little to the risk estimate established by clinical evaluation. Clinicians may identify most high-risk patients by history and physical examination and by consideration of the patient- and procedure-related risk factors discussed above.
    - In one case-control study of patients undergoing elective abdominal surgery, abnormal results of lung examination (which included decreased breath sounds, prolonged expiration, rales, wheezes, or rhonchi), abnormal chest radiograph (including hyperinflation, pulmonary hypertension, vascular redistribution, atelectasis, effusion, and parenchymal abnormalities), cardiac morbidity, and overall comorbidity each predicted PPCs.[8] In contrast, spirometric results did not predict PPC rates.
- The bulk of the literature fails to support routine spirometry as an independent predictor of PPCs following noncardiothoracic surgery, even among patients with severe COPD.[2]
- As no prohibitive cutoff levels exist for FEV_1 and FVC, do not order routine spirometry as part of the preoperative evaluation in patients awaiting noncardiothoracic surgery. Consider preoperative spirometry for the evaluation of dyspnea that remains unexplained after clinical evaluation. It may also be helpful for a patient with asthma or COPD if it is uncertain whether the patient is at his or her optimal baseline before surgery.

RISK INDICES

- Two risk indices, developed and validated across a large number of Veterans Affairs Medical Centers, identified patients at risk for postoperative pneumonia and respiratory failure[5,7] (see Tables 24-2 and 24-3).
- These risk indices confirmed previously established risk factors for the development of PPCs, including surgical site, tobacco use, COPD, functional status, and age. The authors also identified additional risk factors that had not previously been well defined in the literature. These included other surgical sites (e.g., neck, neurosurgery, and vascular procedures), blood transfusion, additional comorbidities (e.g., cerebrovascular disease and low or elevated BUN), and other markers of general health status, including weight loss, steroid use, and alcohol intake.
- The risk indices did not evaluate the role of spirometry or elevated body mass index in predicting PPCs.
- Whether these risk indices can be generalized to other segments of the population is unknown. Until further studies seek to verify these results, we recommend the use of these indices as a tool to stratify risk of PPCs. Unfortunately, most of the risk factors in these indices cannot be modified.

PERIOPERATIVE MANAGEMENT TO REDUCE RISK

- Table 24-4 provides a summary of risk-reduction strategies.

PREOPERATIVE INTERVENTIONS

- Delay elective surgery to treat any significant acute illness.
- Consider delaying elective surgery in a patient with an acute viral upper respiratory infection, especially one of recent onset or with worsening symptoms. The available information is from the pediatric literature, which suggests that there may be an increased incidence of laryngospasm, bronchospasm, and oxygen desaturation; however, the associated morbidity may be minimal.
- Optimize existing treatment for airflow limitation for patients with COPD or asthma (see Chap. 25 for more detail).
- Encourage smoking cessation for at least 8 weeks prior to elective surgery, if possible, to achieve maximum benefit in reducing PPCs.[9,10]

TABLE 24-2 Comparison of the Risk Factors Included in the Postoperative Pneumonia and Respiratory Failure Risk Indices

RISK FACTORS	POSTOPERATIVE PNEUMONIA RISK INDEX POINT VALUE	POSTOPERATIVE RESPIRATORY FAILURE RISK INDEX POINT VALUE
Type of surgery		
AAA repair	15	27
Thoracic	14	21
Upper abdominal	10	14
Neck	8	11
Neurosurgery	8	14
Vascular	3	14
Emergency surgery	3	11
General anesthesia	4	—
Age		
≥80 years	17	—
70–79 years	13	—
60–69 years	9	—
50–59 years	4	—
>70 years	—	6
60–69 years	—	4
Functional status		
Totally dependent	10	7
Partially dependent	6	7
Albumin		
<3.0 g/dL	—	9
Weight loss >10% (within 6 months)	7	—
Chronic steroid use	3	—
Alcohol >2 drinks per day (Within 2 weeks)	2	—
History of COPD	5	6
Current smoker		
Within 1 year	3	—
Impaired sensorium	4	—
History of CVA	4	—
Blood urea nitrogen		
<8 mg/dL	4	—
8–21 mg/dL	referent	referent
22–30 mg/dL	2	—
>30 mg/dL	3	8
Preoperative transfusion (>4 U)	3	—

AAA = abdominal aortic aneurysm; COPD = chronic obstructive pulmonary disease; CVA = cerebrovascular accident.
SOURCE: Adapted from Arozullah et al.,[5,7] with permission.

- ○ Smoking cessation initiated less than 8 weeks prior to surgery may paradoxically increase PPC rates[9]; however, existing studies were small and limited in methodology. This observation should not dissuade physicians from encouraging lifelong smoking cessation.
- Begin patient education on lung-expansion maneuvers.

INTRAOPERATIVE INTERVENTIONS

- Anesthesiologists and surgeons direct intraoperative risk-reduction strategies; however, a working knowledge of procedure-related risk factors can help the internist to communicate effectively with the different teams.

TABLE 24-3 Risk-Class Assignment in the Risk Indices for Postoperative Pneumonia and Respiratory Failure

RISK CLASS	POSTOPERATIVE PNEUMONIA RISK INDEX (POINT TOTAL)	PREDICTED PROBABILITY OF PNEUMONIA	RESPIRATORY FAILURE RISK INDEX (POINT TOTAL)	PREDICTED PROBABILITY OF RESPIRATORY FAILURE
1	0–15	0.2%	0–10	0.5%
2	16–25	1.2%	11–19	2.2%
3	26–40	4.0%	20–27	5.0%
4	41–55	9.4%	28–40	11.6%
5	>55	15.3%	>40	30.5%

SOURCE: Adapted from Arozullah AM, Conde MV, Lawrence VA. Preoperative evaluation for postoperative pulmonary complications, *Med Clin North Am* 87:153–173, 2003, with permission from Elsevier, and from Arozullah et al.,[5,7] with permission.

- If the risk of PPCs is deemed prohibitive, then consider cancellation of surgery or a lower-risk procedure (e.g., laparoscopic surgery) if available.
- Other intraoperative risk-reduction interventions in the domain of anesthesiologists and surgeons include minimizing the duration of surgery, the use of neuraxial blockade instead of general anesthesia, and avoiding long-acting muscle relaxants (e.g., pancuronium).

POSTOPERATIVE INTERVENTIONS

LUNG-EXPANSION MANEUVERS

- Lung-expansion maneuvers—which include deep breathing exercises with chest physiotherapy, incentive spirometry, intermittent positive-pressure breathing, and continuous positive airway pressure (CPAP)—can maximize alveolar inflation.
- In high-risk patients, particularly following upper abdominal surgery, lung-expansion maneuvers can decrease PPCs by 50 percent.[11]
  - One recommended deep breathing regimen (with or without an incentive spirometer) is 8 to 10 breaths with a 3- to 5-s inspiratory hold every 1 to 2 h while awake followed by forced expirations and coughing. Another regimen is 10 breaths over 15 min with an incentive spirometer four times a day postoperatively.
  - Initiate lung-expansion maneuvers postoperatively in high-risk patients, either with incentive spirometry or deep breathing exercises. Despite limitations in methodology, studies support that the two methods are equal in efficacy.[11]
- There is no advantage to intermittent positive-pressure breathing (IPPB) versus incentive spirometry or deep breathing exercises. IPPB is associated with abdominal distention.
- Use CPAP in patients who find it difficult to perform deep breathing exercises or use an incentive spirometer.
- Continue CPAP postoperatively in patients with obstructive sleep apnea who use home CPAP.

POSTOPERATIVE PAIN CONTROL

- Postoperative chest and abdominal discomfort results in decreased lung volumes and atelectasis by interfering with deep breathing and coughing.
- Postoperative pain control with parenteral narcotic analgesia is a double-edged sword. With effective pain management, deep breathing will improve; however, the therapeutic window may be narrow in some patients and its use may blunt respiratory drive, thus contributing to PPCs.
- Postoperative epidural analgesia provides superior pain relief versus parenteral narcotic analgesia and can reduce PPCs, notably respiratory failure.

TABLE 24-4 Risk-Reduction Strategies

PREOPERATIVE	INTRAOPERATIVE	POSTOPERATIVE
Communicate with anesthesiologists and surgeons to make decisions regarding surgical site, technique, and type of anesthesia with adequate information.	Minimize duration of surgery. Choose spinal or epidural anesthesia instead of general anesthesia in high-risk patients	Initiate lung expansion maneuvers. Continue CPAP in patients with OSA Use epidural analgesia instead of parenteral analgesia
Treat acute illness and delay surgery. Optimize existing airflow limitation.	Perform laparoscopic procedure versus an open procedure if possible.	
Initiate smoking cessation 8 weeks prior to surgery. Initiate education on lung expansion maneuvers.	Avoid long-acting muscle relaxant, pancuronium.	

- For example, 915 high-risk patients undergoing major abdominal surgery were randomized to (1) combined general anesthesia with intraoperative epidural anesthesia and postoperative epidural analgesia or (2) general anesthesia and postoperative parenteral narcotics. The incidence of respiratory failure was 23 versus 30 percent, respectively.[12]
- Manage postoperative pain following high-risk procedures with postoperative epidural analgesia when feasible.

Postoperative Placement of a Nasogastric Tube

- Impairment of cough reflex and oropharyngeal aspiration due to postoperative nasogastric tube placement contributes to the development of PPCs.
- In a systematic review of blinded studies evaluating risk factors for PPCs, postoperative nasogastric tube placement was identified in more than one study and in multivariate analysis as a risk factor.[13] Postoperative nasogastric tube placement, however, is not a firm risk factor for the development of PPCs. Studies finding a positive correlation were small and await validation in other settings.

References

1. Polanczyk CA, Marcantonio E, Goldman L, et al. Impact of age on perioperative complications and length of stay in patients undergoing noncardiac surgery. *Ann Intern Med* 134:637, 2001.
2. Smetana GW, Lawrence VA, Cornell JE. Preoperative pulmonary risk stratification for non-cardiothoracic surgery: A background review for an American College of Physicians guideline. *Ann Intern Med* 2006. In press.
3. Reilly DF, McNeely MJ, Doerner D, et al. Self-reported exercise tolerance and the risk of serious perioperative complications. *Arch Intern Med* 159:2185, 1999.

3a. Girish M, Trayner E, Dammann O, et al. Symptom-limited stair climbing as a predictor of postoperative cardiopulmonary complications after high-risk surgery. *Chest* 120:1147, 2001.

4. Rodgers A, Walker N, Schug S, et al. Reduction of postoperative mortality and morbidity with epidural or spinal anaesthesia: Results from overview of randomised trials. *BMJ* 321:1493, 2000.
5. Arozullah AM, Daley J, Henderson WG, Khuri SF. Multifactorial risk index for predicting postoperative respiratory failure in men after major noncardiac surgery. The National Veterans Administration Surgical Quality Improvement Program. *Ann Surg* 232:242, 2000.
6. Archer C, Levy AR, McGregor M. Value of routine preoperative chest x-rays: A meta-analysis. *Can J Anaesth* 40:1022, 1993.
7. Arozullah AM, Khuri SF, Henderson WG, et al. Development and validation of a multifactorial risk index for predicting postoperative pneumonia after major noncardiac surgery. *Ann Intern Med* 135:847, 2001.
8. Lawrence VA, Dhanda R, Hilsenbeck SG, Page CP. Risk of pulmonary complications after elective abdominal surgery. *Chest* 110:744, 1996.
9. Warner MA, Offord KP, Warner ME, et al. Role of preoperative cessation of smoking and other factors in postoperative pulmonary complications: A blinded prospective study of coronary artery bypass patients. *Mayo Clin Proc* 64:609, 1989.
10. Moller AM, Villebro N, Pedersen P, Tonnesen H. Effect of preoperative smoking intervention on postoperative complications: A randomized clinical trial. *Lancet* 359:114, 2002.
11. Thomas JA, McIntosh JM. Are incentive spirometry, intermittent positive pressure breathing, and deep breathing exercises effective in the prevention of postoperative pulmonary complications after upper abdominal surgery? A systematic overview and meta-analysis. *Phys Ther* 74:3, 1994.
12. Rigg JR, Jamrozik K, Myles PS, et al. Epidural anaesthesia and analgesia and outcome of major surgery: A randomised trial. *Lancet* 359:1276, 2002.
13. Fisher BW, Majumdar SR, McAlister FA. Predicting pulmonary complications after nonthoracic surgery: A systematic review of blinded studies. *Am J Med* 112:219, 2002.

25 ASTHMA AND COPD

Ahsan M. Arozullah and Valerie A. Lawrence

INTRODUCTION

- Several chronic diseases, including obstructive lung diseases such as asthma and chronic obstructive pulmonary disease (COPD), place patients at increased risk for postoperative mortality and morbidity.
- Patients with COPD are at increased risk for postoperative complications, particularly postoperative pulmonary complications (PPCs). Clinically important PPCs include pneumonia, respiratory failure, and prolonged mechanical ventilation.[1] Atelectasis, bronchitis, bronchospasm, and hypoxemia may or may not evolve into clinically important complications.
- Although patients with asthma have not been shown to be at high risk for PPCs, poorly controlled asthma may predispose to poor postoperative outcomes.[2]
- Asthma is characterized by reversible airway obstruction and airway inflammation. Pulmonary function

tests usually reveal mild obstructive deficits that are reversible with bronchodilators.

- Although airway obstruction in asthma was traditionally thought to be completely reversible, recent evidence suggests that over time, patients with asthma have diminished pulmonary function that is irreversible.
- COPD is characterized by airflow limitation that is not fully reversible. An estimated 10.5 million U.S. adults had COPD in the year 2000, with approximately 24 million adults having impaired lung function suggesting underdiagnosis. During 2000, COPD was responsible for 726,000 hospitalizations and was the fourth leading cause of death in the United States, with 119,000 deaths.[3]
- COPD includes emphysema and chronic bronchitis. Emphysema is a pathologic diagnosis made when there is significant destruction of lung parenchyma, enlargement of air spaces resulting in loss of lung elasticity, and closure of small airways. Chronic bronchitis involves inflammation and obstruction of small airways and is characterized by a productive cough for greater than 3 months in 2 or more successive years.
- Nearly 90 percent of patients with COPD have a history of tobacco use, typically reporting greater than 20 pack-years of smoking. Other risk factors for COPD include $alpha_1$-antitrypsin deficiency and occupational exposures to coal dust, crystalline silica, cotton dust, and cadmium.
- Pulmonary function tests typically reveal FEV_1 (forced expiratory volume in 1 s) less than 70 percent predicted and FEV_1/FVC (forced vital capacity) less than 70 percent predicted.
- General preoperative pulmonary risk assessment, including two risk indices that identify patients at risk for postoperative pneumonia and respiratory failure, was discussed previously (see Chap. 24). Whether these risk indices can be generalized to patients with COPD is unknown; however, the study populations had a high prevalence of COPD (nearly 40 percent), making the use of these indices reasonable in COPD patients. Asthma was not formally assessed in these studies.[1,5]
- This chapter focuses on the preoperative evaluation and management of patients with asthma and COPD. Patient- and surgery-related risk factors specific to patients with obstructive lung disease are discussed in addition to the role of preoperative testing. The final section of this chapter focuses on perioperative interventions aimed at reducing risk.

PATIENT-RELATED RISK FACTORS

ASTHMA

- Although asthma has not been shown to be an independent risk factor for postoperative mortality or morbidity, there are special considerations for asthmatic patients undergoing surgical procedures.
- Preoperative history for asthmatic patients should include detailed history for asthma-related factors that increase risk of PPC, including frequency, duration, and inciting factors; recent antiasthma drug use; recent hospital treatment of asthma symptoms, including emergency room visits and hospital admissions; and any prior intubations.[4]
- History of cough, along with fever and sputum production, should be specifically assessed to ensure that the patient does not have any underlying pulmonary infections that could further exacerbate asthma.
- Physical examination should focus on evidence of an acute asthma exacerbation, including labored breathing, wheezing or distant lung sounds, high respiratory rate, and tachycardia. Evidence of acute infections, such as bronchitis or pneumonia, should be sought, including fever, increased respiratory rate, wheezes, or rhonchi on lung examination.
- Other commons causes of wheezing that should be considered include pulmonary edema, pneumothorax, drug reactions, aspiration, carinal irritation, and endobronchial intubation.

CHRONIC OBSTRUCTIVE PULMONARY DISEASE

- COPD is a major independent risk factor for PPCs, with an increased risk of approximately threefold compared to patients without COPD. However, few studies have examined risk factors for postoperative mortality and morbidity specifically among patients with COPD.
- Stable patients with COPD may become unstable in the perioperative period because of the detrimental respiratory effects of surgery and anesthesia. Patients with COPD typically have chronically fatigued respiratory muscles that are particularly sensitive to additional stress such as surgery.[5] Patients who demonstrate increased respiratory muscle strength after muscle training have fewer PPCs than those who do not increase their respiratory muscle strength. Determination of exercise capacity may also help to assess risk.
- Although COPD has been shown to have an independent association with PPCs, patients with COPD may be at increased risk for postoperative mortality and morbidity because of poor functional status, which is also independently associated with PPCs.[1,5]
- Poor nutritional status in these patients may affect wound healing and recovery. Poor nutrition combined with decreased respiratory muscle strength makes patients with severe COPD particularly susceptible to PPCs.
  - Nearly 50 percent of patients with emphysema undergoing surgery for lung-volume reduction were

found to have deficient nutritional status as assessed by body mass index (BMI). This impaired nutritional status was associated with increased postoperative morbidity.[6]

- The preoperative history of patients with COPD should focus on recent history of exacerbations and current symptoms or signs indicating acute bronchitis or pneumonia. Preoperative sputum production and pneumonia are risk factors for postoperative respiratory failure. Dyspnea, at rest or on minimal exertion, is a risk factor for respiratory failure.[5]
- Physical examination should include assessment for fever, increased respiratory rate, wheezes, or rhonchi on lung examination that may indicate acute bronchitis or pneumonia.

CIGARETTE SMOKING

- As noted in Chap. 24, cigarette smoking increases the risk of PPCs even for patients without COPD.
- Patients who have been active smokers within 2 weeks of noncardiac surgery are at increased risk for respiratory failure. Active smokers within 1 year prior to noncardiac surgery are at increased risk for pneumonia.[1,5] For patients with COPD who are chronic smokers, the evidence supporting preoperative smoking cessation is inconclusive.
- There is also evidence to suggest that smoking cessation less than 8 weeks prior to surgery may increase risk of PPCs.[5] A compensatory short-term increase in sputum production after smoking cessation may explain this paradoxical finding. Increased sputum production may be particularly detrimental to patients with COPD manifesting as chronic bronchitis.
- For patients with acute asthma or COPD exacerbations preoperatively, smoking cessation can facilitate faster recovery.
- In stable COPD patients, undergoing surgery may provide an ideal context for smoking cessation interventions. Establishing a smoking quit date 8 weeks before elective surgery or in the immediate postoperative period may be effective.

OBSTRUCTIVE SLEEP APNEA

- In some patients, COPD may coexist with obstructive sleep apnea (OSA). OSA is characterized by nocturnal snoring, daytime somnolence, hypertension, and abnormal waking patterns during monitored sleep studies.
- OSA is associated with an increased risk of PPCs. This risk exists even in previously undiagnosed patients, thus making the preoperative assessment of OSA symptoms worthwhile.[5]
- Patients with OSA have a higher incidence of hypoxemia, hypercarbia, and respiratory failure in the immediate postoperative period. These risks are probably even higher in patients with the combination of OSA and COPD or asthma, where postoperative bronchospasm may also be a contributing factor.

SURGERY-RELATED RISK FACTORS

- As noted in Chap. 24, the surgical site is the single most important risk factor for the development of PPCs. Although esophageal, thoracic, and upper abdominal surgeries carry the highest risk, this section focuses on surgeries in which outcomes for COPD patients have been studied specifically.
- Laparoscopic surgery usually results in less postoperative pain and spirometric compromise than open abdominal surgery. However, it is unclear whether laparoscopic techniques confer a lower risk of PPCs.[7]
- Since the vast majority of patients with COPD have long-standing smoking histories, they are also at increased risk for developing lung cancer.
- Patients with COPD undergoing lung-resection surgery should be evaluated to ensure that adequate pulmonary function will exist following resection. This is usually evaluated through preoperative regional pulmonary function tests.
  - In one series of 266 patients undergoing lung-resection surgeries, 25 percent developed PPCs. The independent risk factors included an American Society of Anesthesia (ASA) score greater than or equal to 3 (OR 2.1, 95 percent CI 1.1 to 4.2), operating time greater than 80 min (OR 2.1, 95 percent CI 1.1 to 4.0), and the need for postoperative mechanical ventilation >48 h (OR 2.0, 95 percent CI 1.0 to 3.8).[8]
  - Detailed preoperative pulmonary function tests did not contribute to the identification of high-risk patients.[8]
- Evidence suggests that COPD may increase the risk of postoperative mortality and supraventricular arrhythmias following lung resection for non-small cell lung cancer.[9]
  - In a retrospective analysis of 244 patients who underwent lung-resection surgery, 32 percent had COPD by pulmonary function test criteria.[9]
  - The incidence of supraventricular arrhythmias was significantly higher in the COPD group compared to the non-COPD group (59 versus 27 percent, $p < 0.001$).
  - The incidence of supraventricular arrhythmias refractory to initial treatment with digoxin was also significantly higher in patients with COPD.
  - The overall postoperative mortality rate was significantly higher in the COPD group compared to the non-COPD group (14.1 versus 3.0 percent, $p < 0.004$).

- Patients with COPD undergoing coronary artery bypass grafting (CABG) have also been studied.
  - In one series, 191 patients with COPD, defined by pulmonary function test criteria, underwent CABG surgery.[10]
  - The overall hospital mortality rate was 7 percent and the morbidity rate was 50 percent. However, patients receiving steroids who were above 75 years of age had a hospital mortality of 50 percent.
  - PPCs and atrial fibrillation were significantly more frequent in the COPD patients compared to non-COPD patients.

ANESTHESIA-RELATED RISK FACTORS

- Bronchospasm can occur in any patient during anesthesia, but patients with asthma are particularly susceptible because of their hyperreactive airways.
- The type of anesthesia (general versus spinal) has not been demonstrated to be an independent risk factor for PPCs among patients with asthma. However, regional anesthesia should be considered in patients with poorly controlled asthma so as to avoid the additional bronchospasm that may occur during intubation of the airway.
  - Warner's study of over 1500 patients with asthma found that complication rates for general and regional anesthesia were similar.[11]
  - The risk of bronchospasm in the perioperative period was low in stable asthmatic patients and was not usually associated with serious morbidity.
- Anesthetic agents
  - Propofol, which is associated with reductions in wheezing during induction, is useful in patients with bronchospasm.[4]
  - Lidocaine and a $beta_2$ aerosol, used in combination, have synergistic effects in attenuating the airway response to bronchoconstriction.[4]
  - Long-acting neuromuscular blocking agents such as pancuronium are associated with a threefold increase in PPC rates compared with shorter-acting agents such as vecuronium or atracurium. They should be especially avoided in patients with obstructive lung disease.[5]

PREOPERATIVE EVALUATION AND TESTING

CLINICAL ASSESSMENT

- Preoperative history for asthmatic patients should include frequency, duration, and inciting factors; history of cough as well as fever and sputum production; recent use of antiasthma drugs; recent hospital treatment of asthma symptoms, including emergency room visits and hospital admissions; and any prior intubations.[4]
- Preoperative history of patients with COPD should include recent exacerbations, dyspnea, and symptoms indicating acute bronchitis or pneumonia, such as a change in sputum production.
- Physical examination of patients with COPD and asthma should include assessment for fever, increased respiratory rate, wheezes, or rhonchi on lung examination that may indicate acute bronchitis or pneumonia.

PREOPERATIVE TESTING

There are two distinct, but often overlapping reasons for performing preoperative testing:

- Risk stratification: For example, obtaining a preoperative albumin level will enhance risk assessment because albumin <3.0 g/dL has been shown, in a large veteran population surgical cohort, to be a significant risk factor for the development of postoperative respiratory failure.[5]
- Risk reduction and management: For example, preoperative pulmonary function tests may help guide perioperative ventilator management, although pulmonary function test results do not enhance risk assessment beyond clinical factors.
- Although details of preoperative testing and the evidence supporting their use are reviewed in Chap. 24, this section focuses on the use of preoperative tests in patients with COPD or asthma.

CHEST RADIOGRAPHY

- Routine preoperative chest radiography in patients with COPD or asthma rarely adds useful information to the preoperative evaluation.
- Potential indications for a chest radiograph in these patients include increased cough, sputum production, dyspnea, fever, and abnormalities on lung examination suggestive of underlying pulmonary infection.
  - Patients with asthma or COPD undergoing surgery may have acute exacerbations in the perioperative period if preoperative bronchitis or pneumonia is present.

LABORATORY TESTING

- Abnormal levels of albumin and blood urea nitrogen (BUN) are known risk factors for the development of PPCs. Therefore risk assessment will be aided if these tests are obtained preoperatively.[1,5]

- For patients with COPD or asthma who present with worsening respiratory complaints and fever, a white blood cell count may assist in ruling out an active infection.

ARTERIAL BLOOD GAS ANALYSIS

- Among patients with severe obstructive lung disease, hypercarbia ($Paco_2$ >45 mmHg) and hypoxemia appear to be risk factors for PPCs. However, it remains unclear whether arterial blood gas results add significantly to preoperative risk assessment using only clinical factors.
    - Most patients with severe abnormalities on arterial blood gas analysis are detected during routine preoperative evaluations.
- Arterial blood gas analysis may guide the perioperative management of patients with severe lung disease.
    - Among COPD patients requiring home oxygen supplementation, baseline oxygenation status can be useful in titrating oxygen use in the perioperative period. Supplementing these patients with high oxygen levels may diminish respiratory drive if they are chronic CO_2 retainers.
    - Conversely, in asthma patients requiring ventilation postoperatively, permissive hypercapnia (allowing $Paco_2$ to rise above normal levels) can avoid high airway pressures. Preoperative arterial blood gas analysis in these patients may be helpful for establishing baseline $Paco_2$.

PULMONARY FUNCTION TESTING (SPIROMETRY)

- As discussed in Chap. 9, preoperative spirometric testing (FEV_1 and FEV_1/FVC) is routinely performed in patients undergoing lung resection.
- However, routine spirometry does not appear to predict the development of PPCs following noncardiothoracic surgery. Several studies found that routine spirometry did not contribute significantly to predicting PPCs, even among patients with severe COPD.[2]
- Preoperative spirometry may be helpful in determining whether undiagnosed patients with related symptoms actually have asthma or COPD.
- Spirometry can also assess the severity of asthma and COPD in patients with established diagnoses.
- Peak flow testing, an inexpensive bedside alternative to formal pulmonary function tests, can establish baseline pulmonary function in asthma patients. Preoperative peak flow results can be used as a benchmark for determining respiratory distress postoperatively.

OTHER RELATED TESTS

- A sleep study for diagnosing OSA should be considered in patients who report nocturnal snoring and daytime somnolence. Since OSA appears to be a risk factor for PPCs, it may be of value to establish this diagnosis prior to surgery in COPD and asthma patients.
- Preoperative pulmonary exercise testing may be helpful in determining the severity of COPD in patients undergoing surgery. Patients with COPD can have chronically fatigued respiratory muscles that are particularly sensitive to additional stresses such as surgery.
    - Pulmonary exercise testing may detect patients who will benefit from preoperative muscle training. Patients with increased respiratory muscle strength after muscle training had fewer PPCs than those who did not increase their respiratory muscle strength.

PERIOPERATIVE MANAGEMENT TO REDUCE RISK

PREOPERATIVE INTERVENTIONS

There are several preoperative interventions that may be useful for decreasing postoperative morbidity and mortality among patients with COPD and asthma.

- For patients with active bronchospasm, treatment with $beta_2$-adrenergic agents and corticosteroids is effective in attenuating bronchospasm.[4] In patients with COPD, ipratropium (Atrovent) treatment should also be considered.
    - Steroid treatment should begin 24 to 48 h before surgery because its beneficial effects on airway reactivity occur over a period of hours.
    - Although there is limited evidence regarding specific preoperative steroid regimens, steroids can be administered orally (e.g., prednisone 40 to 60 mg per day) or intravenously (e.g., methylprednisolone 60 to 80 mg every 8 h) in patients unable to swallow. Inhaled steroids can be considered for milder exacerbations.
    - Severe exacerbations of asthma can result in persistent airway hyperreactivity lasting for several weeks. Elective surgeries should be postponed until airway hyperreactivity improves and peak flow rates return to baseline.
    - In the absence of bronchospasm, short-term steroids started prophylactically before surgery can be discontinued postoperatively without tapering doses.
    - There is no evidence that short-term perioperative steroid use increases wound infections or causes poor wound healing.
- In patients with asthma or COPD, acute bronchitis or pneumonia should be treated completely with appropriate antibiotics prior to surgery (Tables 25-1 and 25-2).

TABLE 25-1 Asthma Severity Classification

SEVERITY CLASSIFICATION	SYMPTOMS
Mild intermittent asthma	Symptoms occur less than weekly with normal or near-normal lung function
Mild persistent asthma	Symptoms occur more than weekly but less than daily with normal or near-normal lung function
Moderate persistent asthma	Daily symptoms with mild to moderate variable airflow obstruction
Severe asthma	Daily symptoms, frequent night symptoms, and moderate to severe variable airflow obstruction

- Delaying elective surgery in patients with asthma or COPD who are suffering from acute viral upper respiratory infections may be prudent. Although the evidence for this recommendation comes primarily from studies in children, these patients may experience increased rates of laryngospasm, bronchospasm, and oxygen desaturation related to anesthesia induction and airway instrumentation.
- Smoking cessation at least 8 weeks prior to elective surgery should be encouraged.[7]
- Lung-expansion maneuvers (e.g., incentive spirometry) clearly prevent PPCs and should be used aggressively. No one modality is clearly superior.[7]
- Patient education on lung-expansion maneuvers has been shown to improve the use of incentive spirometers postoperatively.
    - Typically, patients do not receive any formal preoperative instruction about why incentive spirometers are useful and how they should be used.
    - Postoperatively, when they are semiconscious, patients are often unable to understand instructions about using incentive spirometers.
    - Therefore the educational process should begin preoperatively and may be particularly beneficial in high-risk patients, such as those with COPD.

TABLE 25-2 Global Initiative for Chronic Obstructive Lung Disease Staging Criteria for COPD

STAGE	FEV_1, % PREDICTED	SYMPTOMS
0 (at risk)	>80%	No symptoms
1 (mild)	>80%	Variable symptoms
2 (moderate)	50–79	Mild-to-moderate symptoms
3 (severe)	30–49	Symptoms that limit exertion
4 (very severe)	<30	Symptoms that limit daily activities

FEV_1 = forced expiratory volume in 1 s, given as percentage of predicted normal value.

INTRAOPERATIVE INTERVENTIONS

- Regional anesthesia should be considered in patients with poorly controlled COPD or asthma so as to avoid bronchospasm, which may occur during airway intubation.
- For patients who require general anesthesia, laryngeal mask airways cause less airway reaction than endotracheal tubes. These laryngeal mask airways may be particularly useful in patients with asthma and reactive airway disease.[4]
- Although laparoscopic surgery may cause less postoperative pain and spirometric compromise than open abdominal surgery, the evidence is not clear that these effects result in clinically important reductions in the incidence of PPCs.[7]

POSTOPERATIVE INTERVENTIONS

- As noted in Chap. 24, lung-expansion maneuvers such as incentive spirometry, intermittent positive-pressure breathing, and continuous positive airway pressure (CPAP), can maximize alveolar inflation and minimize postoperative atelectasis.
- These maneuvers may be particularly beneficial in patients with COPD or asthma who are already experiencing diminished pulmonary function postoperatively.
- Early postoperative ambulation may be beneficial in patients with COPD or asthma.
- The management of postoperative pain in patients with COPD or asthma requires a delicate balance between adequate pain control and the blunting of respiratory drive. Narcotics should be used with caution, particularly in patients with COPD and hypercarbia.
- Selective rather than routine nasogastric tube use after abdominal surgery reduces PPC. However, in patients with asthma that is exacerbated with gastroesophageal reflux, nasogastric tube drainage may be beneficial.[7]

REFERENCES

1. Arozullah AM, Khuri SF, Henderson WG, et al. Development and validation of a multifactorial risk index for predicting postoperative pneumonia after major noncardiac surgery. *Ann Intern Med* 135:847–857, 2001.
2. Smetana GW, Lawrence VA, Cornell JE. Preoperative pulmonary risk stratification for non-cardiothoracic surgery: A systematic review. *Ann Intern Med* 2005. In press.
3. Mannino DM, Homa DM, Akinbami et al. Chronic obstructive pulmonary disease surveillance—United States, 1971–2000. *MMWR Surv Summ* 51(SS06):1–16, 2002.

4. Rock P, Passannante A. Preoperative assessment: Pulmonary. *Anesth Clin North Am* 22:77–91, 2004.
5. Arozullah AM, Conde M, Lawrence VA. Preoperative evaluation for postoperative pulmonary complications. *Med Clin North Am* 87:153–173, 2003.
6. Mazolewski P, Turner JF, Baker M, et al. The impact of nutritional status on the outcome of lung volume reduction surgery: A prospective study. *Chest* 116:693–696, 1999.
7. Lawrence VA, Cornell JE, Smetana GW. Strategies to reduce postoperative pulmonary complications after noncardiothoracic surgery: A systemic review. *Ann Intern Med* 2005. In press.
8. Stephan F, Boucheseiche S, Hollande J, et al. Pulmonary complications following lung resection: A comprehensive analysis of incidence and possible risk factors. *Chest* 118(5):1263–1270, 2000.
9. Sekine Y, Kesler K, Behnia M, et al. COPD may increase the incidence of refractory supraventricular arrhythmias following pulmonary resection for non-small cell lung cancer. *Chest* 120:1783–1790, 2001.
10. Samuels LE, Kaufman MS, Morris RJ, et al. Coronary artery bypass grafting in patients with COPD. *Chest* 113:878–882, 1998.
11. Warner DO, Warner MA, Barnes RD, et al. Perioperative respiratory complications in patients with asthma. *Anesthesiology* 85:460–467, 1996.

26 DIABETES MELLITUS

Nadia A. Khan, Jennifer C. Kerns, and William A. Ghali

INTRODUCTION

- Patients with diabetes mellitus (DM) constitute a high-risk population for postoperative death, myocardial infarction, stroke, and infectious complications.
- The achievement and maintenance of good perioperative glycemic control is often challenging, depending on the type of surgery that patients are undergoing as well as their preoperative drug regimen and degree of control. Yet most agree that we should attempt to achieve perioperative euglycemia, given that there is some evidence to suggest that tighter glucose control may mitigate adverse outcomes such as wound infections, vascular complications, and even death.
- In this chapter, we discuss the patient and procedure-related risk factors for developing perioperative complications; the preoperative evaluation, including laboratory testing to stratify risk; and pre- and postoperative management strategies to improve glucose management.

PATIENT-RELATED RISK FACTORS

CARDIOVASCULAR RISK

- In general, patients with DM have a substantially higher cardiovascular risk and mortality than patients without DM.
- The presence of insulin-dependent DM is one of the six major prognostic factors associated with postoperative major cardiac events (OR 1.8 to 3.0) in the Lee Revised Cardiac Index.[1]
- The presence of DM is also one of the major prognostic markers for postoperative mortality or cardiac event in the Eagle criteria for vascular surgery. In Eagle's study, with the presence of DM alone, the incidence of these postoperative complications was 15.5 percent (95 percent CI 7 to 21 percent).[2]
- As DM is a major prognostic factor for postoperative cardiovascular events, all patients with DM require a thorough cardiac risk assessment. Detailed descriptions of the general cardiovascular risk assessment indices and associated management strategies are discussed separately (see Chap. 20).

RISK OF DEVELOPING HYPER/ HYPOGLYCEMIA

- Surgery and anesthesia stimulate the production of counterregulatory hormones—such as glucagon, epinephrine, and corticotropin—and decrease endogenous insulin production. In addition to these factors driving hyperglycemia, increased lipolysis and ketogenesis during surgery combined with poor caloric intake can cause significant derangements in the overall glycemic control. Additional postoperative factors such as sepsis, hyperalimentation, and emesis can also lead to labile blood glucose levels. The complex interplay of these factors can make it challenging to predict and control postoperative hyper- and hypoglycemia.
- Patients with insulin-dependent DM require insulin even when their glucose levels are in the normal range. Inadequate insulin therapy may result in the development of diabetic ketoacidosis or a nonketotic hyperosmolar state, conditions that can lead to death.
- Hypoglycemia may result from overly aggressive glucose reduction therapy, insufficient glucose intake, or increased glucose utilization perioperatively and can lead to seizures, coma, and death.
- The anticipation and prevention of marked hyperglycemia and hypoglycemia are among the major goals in managing the surgical patient with DM.

RISK OF DEVELOPING INFECTIOUS COMPLICATIONS

- Rates of postoperative wound and urinary tract infections are much higher in patients with DM than in those without.
- Many observational studies report that rates of mediastinitis are also higher among patients with DM compared with nondiabetic patients.

SURGERY-RELATED RISK FACTORS

TYPE OF SURGERY AND ANESTHESIA

- The more prolonged, invasive, and complicated the type of surgery, the greater the degree of hyperglycemia.
  - In a prospective cohort study, 150 patients undergoing either anesthesia without surgery, surface surgery, thoracic surgery, or intraabdominal surgery had serial blood glucose levels measured. The largest rises in blood glucose were found in the patients undergoing intraabdominal procedures, followed by those having thoracic procedures. Body-surface surgery and anesthesia without surgery had the smallest changes in glucose levels.[3]
  - Minor surgeries are typically of short duration, with minimal fluid shifts or tissue dissection (e.g., laparoscopic procedures, hernia repair, or mastectomy).
  - Major surgical procedures are long and technically complex, often including major fluid shifts or tissue dissection (e.g., intraabdominal and intrathoracic procedures, major vascular surgery, multiple-trauma surgery, neurosurgery, cardiac or transplantation surgery).
- DM patients undergoing cardiac procedures such as coronary artery bypass grafting (CABG) are also at higher risk of developing deep wound infections and mediastinitis.[4]
- Physiologic studies also suggest that epidural anesthesia has less impact on glucoregulatory hormones than does general anesthesia.
- The type of surgery also affects perioperative management strategies.
  - Because the type of major surgery is associated with increased postoperative hyperglycemia and glucose targets are different for the different types of surgery, the medical consultant must consider this factor in determining the perioperative drug management strategy.
  - Several interventional studies demonstrate the beneficial effects of tight glucose control among individuals undergoing major surgery.

PREOPERATIVE EVALUATION AND TESTING TO STRATIFY RISK

PREOPERATIVE EVALUATION

- Preoperative evaluation should begin with a general health assessment and assessment of cardiovascular risks.
- Risk indices for cardiovascular risk stratification and management are presented in Chap. 20.
- To stratify risk for the development of wound infections and postoperative hyper- or hypoglycemia, the medical consultant must consider the type of surgery planned and the patient's outpatient medication and glucose control.

LABORATORY TESTING

Selected laboratory tests aid in risk stratification and management of the patient with DM.

ECG

- ECG abnormalities—such as abnormal Q waves indicating previous MI, ventricular ectopy, or atrial ectopy—predict postoperative cardiovascular outcomes from cardiac risk indices for noncardiac surgery, such as the Lee Revised Cardiac Index[1] and the Eagle criteria for vascular surgery.[2] (See Chap. 20 for details on these risk indices.)
- Patients with DM are more likely to have coexisting ischemic heart disease and an abnormal ECG than patients without DM. Furthermore, patients with DM may have atypical or silent symptoms of ischemia, only detected only by the ECG.

BLOOD GLUCOSE

- Obtain serum glucose levels (before a meal or fasting) prior to surgery to aid in stratifying risk for postoperative wound and urinary tract infections.
  - In a case-control study of patients undergoing coronary artery bypass surgery, patients with deep sternal wound infections were more likely to have preoperative glucose levels >200 mg/dL (>11 mmol/L) than those who did not have wound infections (OR 10.2, 95 percent CI 2.4 to 43, $p = 0.003$).[4]
- Consider postponing surgery if glucose levels are very high (for example, >360 mg/dL or >20 mmol/L) or if patients have signs or symptoms of dehydration due to hyperglycemia. Surgery may be rescheduled once glucose levels are normalized and symptoms of hyperglycemia have resolved.

SERUM CREATININE

- Obtain a serum creatinine level prior to surgery to aid in cardiac risk stratification.
  - In a validated prospective cohort study of 4315 patients undergoing elective noncardiac surgery, renal dysfunction (creatinine >2.0 mg/dL or 177 mmol/L) was found to be an independent risk factor for major postoperative cardiac complication both in univariate and multivariate analyses. (univariate testing in the Lee Revised Cardiac Risk Index: OR 5.2, 95 percent CI 2.6 to 10.3).[1]

URINALYSIS

- Do not order routine urinalysis for asymptomatic patients with DM.
  The costs of preoperative screening for urinary tract infection far outweigh the costs of treating additional cases of postoperative wound infection.[5]

A1C LEVEL

- Although there is some suggestion that elevated levels of A1C (>8 percent) may also predict a higher risk of wound infection, there is currently not enough evidence to support routine measurement of these levels to aid in stratifying risk for postoperative wound infections.
- An underpowered cohort study of 1000 cardiothoracic surgery patients reported an odds ratio of 2.0 for wound infection when A1C was >8 percent. This finding was not, however, statistically significant given lack of power, and the corresponding confidence interval was very wide (95 percent CI 0.8 to 5.0, $p = 0.15$).[6]

OTHER CARDIOVASCULAR TESTS

- Because patients with DM have a two to four times higher risk of coronary artery disease than those without DM, further cardiac risk stratification may be warranted. (Refer to Chap. 20 for further details on noninvasive testing for cardiac risk stratification.)

MANAGEMENT OF GLUCOSE LEVELS

- There are many potential approaches to managing diabetes medications perioperatively and little published evidence to suggest the superiority of any one approach over others. The current literature is generally restricted to cardiac surgery patients or patients admitted to a surgical intensive care unit (ICU); most studies evaluate glucose levels rather than major cardiovascular endpoints, and those studies that do examine cardiovascular outcomes test glycemic targets rather than the route of insulin administration. As a result, there is no consensus on the optimal strategy for managing and controlling perioperative glycemic levels. The specific strategies for pre- and postoperative drug management presented in this chapter are largely derived from the review of Jacober and Sowers,[7] as it reflects a sensible and practical approach to managing the patient with DM.

PREOPERATIVE MANAGEMENT OF GLUCOSE LEVELS

- Advise patients to monitor their glucose levels prior to surgery and to use diet, exercise, and drug therapy if necessary to maintain glucose levels below 200 mg/dL (<11 mmol/L).
- Although often not in the control of the medical consultant, recommend that elective surgery take place as early in the morning as possible so as to minimize disruption in the patient's diet and medication regimen.

MANAGEMENT OF DIABETIC MEDICATIONS

- ***Diet-Controlled:*** Diabetic patients who are only diet-controlled can proceed to surgery with or without a dextrose-containing intravenous solution.
- ***Oral hypoglycemic agents (OHAs) only:*** Patients should hold all oral hypoglycemic agents on the morning of surgery.
  - Historically, biguanides (metformin) were discontinued 48 h prior to surgery because of overstated concerns regarding lactic acidosis, but current practice is to discontinue them only on the day of surgery.
  - For patients taking sulfonylureas, intravenous solutions given prior to surgery should contain dextrose.
- ***Insulin ± OHA:*** Patients should hold all oral hypoglycemic agents on the morning of surgery. Patients using insulin still require basal insulin to meet their metabolic needs, but at a lower amount to allow for the decreased caloric intake. The fraction of outpatient insulin dosage that the patient takes on the day of surgery depends on the timing of the surgery, the type of surgery (minor or major surgical procedure), and the patient's outpatient medication regimen.
  - For those using a very long acting insulin such as Ultralente, switch to an intermediate-acting insulin 1 or 2 days prior to surgery.
  - If the surgical procedure is very short and early in the morning, so that breakfast may only be delayed, hold insulin until the delayed breakfast and resume it after breakfast if the patient is eating well.
  - If the surgical procedure is short but breakfast will likely be missed altogether, administer a fraction of

the patient's usual morning insulin in the form of intermediate-acting insulin (e.g., Humulin N or NPH) on the morning of surgery:
  - For those who take insulin only in the morning, give two-thirds of their morning dose
  - For those who take insulin more than once a day, give one-half of their total morning insulin
- If the surgical procedure will likely cause the patient to miss at least both breakfast and lunch or for procedures scheduled later in the day, administer a fraction of the usual morning insulin in the form of intermediate-acting insulin on the morning of surgery:
  - For those who take insulin only once per day in the morning, give half of their morning dose
  - For those who take insulin twice a day only, give one-third of their total morning dose of insulin on the morning of surgery.
  - For patients using only short-acting insulin taken before meals multiple times per day, give one-third of the usual premeal short-acting insulin at the usual premeal times even though they are not eating.
  - For patients using continuous insulin infusion pumps, continue their usual basal infusion rate without boluses.
  - For patients on peakless long-acting insulin (e.g., glargine), continue their usual dosage on the morning of surgery but hold any boluses of short-acting insulin entirely on the day of surgery.

MONITORING/GLUCOSE TARGETS

- Measure glucose levels on the morning of surgery and every 2 to 4 h prior to surgery. The glucose levels should be maintained between 75 to 200 mg/dL (4.0 to 11.0 mmol/L). This recommendation is based on the association of preoperative glucose levels >200 mg/dL (>11.0 mmol/L) with postoperative wound infections.[4]

POSTOPERATIVE MANAGEMENT OF GLUCOSE LEVELS

MANAGEMENT OF DIABETIC MEDICATIONS

- For patients who are diet-controlled, on oral hypoglycemic agents alone, or well-controlled (and nonketosis-prone) on insulin, consider providing supplemental short-acting insulin (e.g., regular or lispro) on a sliding scale (see Table 26-1 for development of sliding scale). Intravenous solutions infused at 100 to 150 mL/h may or may not contain dextrose, depending on the duration of the procedure.
- For patients on insulin who are ketosis-prone or who are undergoing major surgical procedures such as CABG or surgery requiring postoperative ICU care, consider using an intravenous insulin infusion (see Figs. 26-1 and 26-2 for intravenous insulin infusions). This recommendation is based on observational studies evaluating the optimal route of insulin administration rather than randomized controlled trial (RCT) evidence. As well, RCT data demonstrating lower mortality with tight glycemic control generally employ insulin infusions in the ICU setting.
  - In a prospective cohort study of 2402 patients undergoing coronary artery bypass surgery, 968 patients received treatment with sliding-scale insulin for the first 2 days postoperatively and 1499 patients received a continuous intraveous insulin infusion. There was a significant reduction in the incidence of deep sternal wound infections in the group that received the insulin infusion (0.8 versus 2.0 percent).[8]
  - In a large observational study of patients with diabetes undergoing CABG (n = 3554), patients were treated aggressively with either subcutaneous insulin (1987 to 1991) or a continuous insulin infusion (1992 to 2001). Mortality with the continuous insulin infusion (2.5 percent, n = 65/2612) was significantly lower than with

TABLE 26-1 Example Calculation for a Subcutaneous Short-Acting Sliding Scale

BLOOD GLUCOSE, mg/dl (mmol/L)	INCREMENT FORMULA*	CALCULATION†	SHORT-ACTING INSULIN, UNITS
0–200 (0–11)	0	0	0
201–250 (11.1–14.0)	1 × (TDI/30)	1 × (60/30)	2
251–300 (14.1–17.0)	2 × (TDI/30)	2 × (60/30)	4
301–350 (17.1–20.0)	3 × (TDI/30)	3 × (60/30)	6
351–400 (20.1–23.0)	4 × (TDI/30)	4 × (60/30)	8

*TDI refers to total daily insulin (i.e., the total sum of the number of units of insulin taken during a 24-h period).
†In this example, the patient uses 60 U of insulin per day. If the patient uses less than 30 U or even no insulin, the default TDI/30 ratio would be 1.
SOURCE: From Jacober and Sowers,[7] with permission.

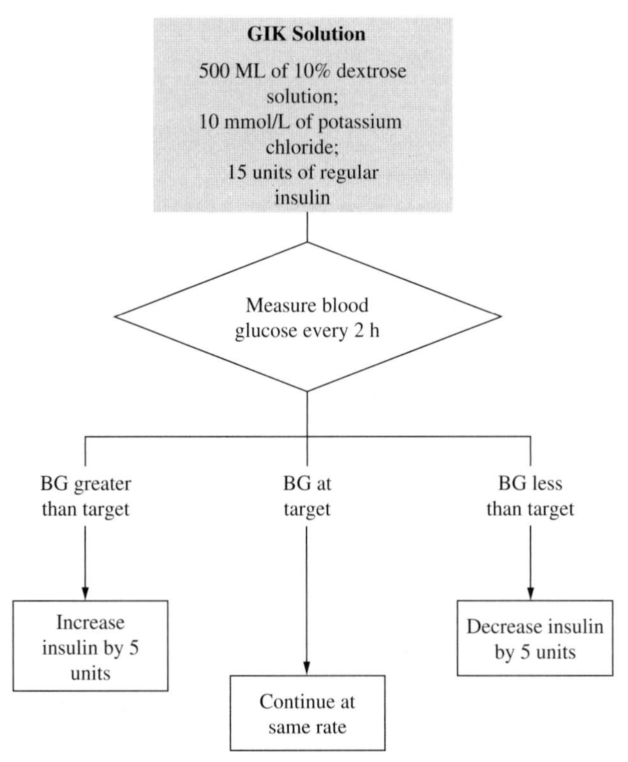

FIG. 26-1 Management algorithm for glucose-potassium-insulin (GIK) infusion. (From Jacober and Sowers,[7] with permission.)

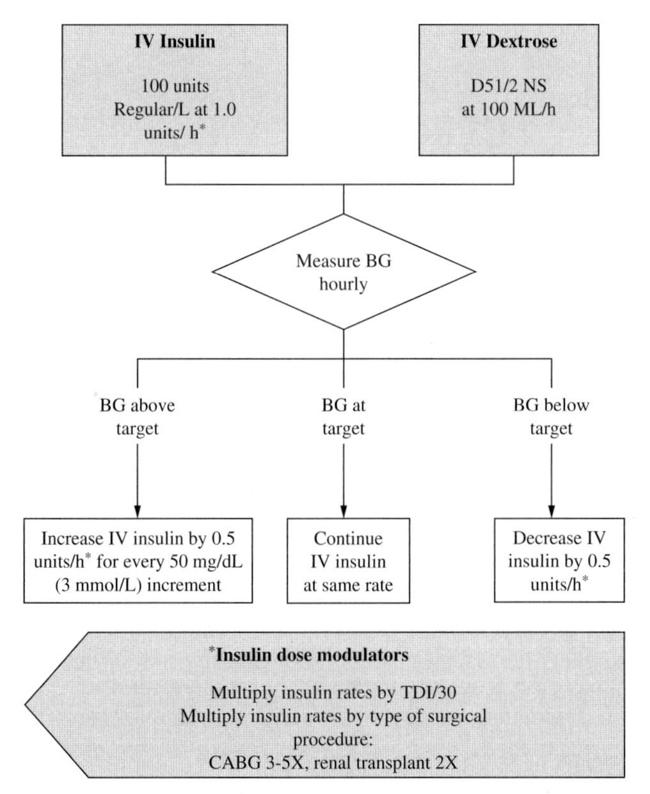

FIG. 26-2 Management algorithm for separate glucose and insulin intravenous infusion. (From Jacober and Sowers,[7] with permission.)

subcutaneous insulin (5.3 percent, $n = 50/942$, $p < 0.001$). Likewise, glucose control was significantly better with the continuous insulin infusion (177 ± 30 mg/dL or 9.8 ± 1.6 mmol/L versus 213 ± 41 mg/dL or 11.8 ± 2.3 mmol/L, $p < 0.001$). Multivariate analysis showed that continuous insulin infusion was independently protective against death (odds ratio 0.43, $p = 0.001$).[9]

- Whether the recommendation to use insulin infusion can be generalized to other major surgical procedures (e.g., noncardiac or not requiring postoperative ICU care) is unclear. The administration of an insulin infusion is more labor-intensive than that of subcutaneous insulin and the infusion may carry a higher risk of hypoglycemia. In a multivariable analysis of ICU patients, lower blood glucose levels were associated with decreased mortality while increased exogenous insulin administration was not protective, suggesting that it may be the glycemic control itself that leads to the mortality benefit demonstrated.[10]
- Thus, the use of insulin infusions may be impractical in settings where monitoring is limited. In settings where close monitoring for glucose levels is available, physicians should consider using insulin infusions for patients with insulin-dependent DM.
- Once patients are able to eat, outpatient diabetic medications can be resumed.
- Consider a step-up approach for those on high-dose sulfonylureas, administering doses at increasing increments until the patient's usual dose is reached.
- Minimize the length of time spent on insulin sliding scale if the patient is able to eat.
- If patients develop increased hyperglycemia, consider dextrose-containing intravenous solutions. Also consider infection or other types of physiologic stressors as a potential cause of poor glucose control.

MONITORING

- Patients using insulin infusions should have their glucose levels monitored every 1 to 2 h and have potassium levels monitored every 12 to 24 h.
- For patients who are eating and not on an insulin infusion, monitor glucose levels in the morning (fasting), before lunch and dinner, and at bedtime.
- All DM patients should be monitored clinically for signs of infection and cardiovascular ischemia.

INTRAVENOUS SOLUTIONS

- For patients not using insulin infusions, maintenance intravenous solutions that contain or do not contain dextrose can be prescribed, depending on whether such patients are receiving other forms of caloric nutrition.

GLUCOSE TARGETS

- For major cardiac surgical procedures or those procedures requiring postoperative ICU care, aim for normoglycemia: 80 to 110 mg/dL or 4.4 to 6.1 mmol/L.
  - A randomized controlled trial of hyperglycemic patients admitted to a surgical ICU postoperatively compared intensive insulin therapy to conventional insulin therapy. For 1548 patients who mostly underwent elective cardiac surgery, the intensive insulin group (glucose: 80 to 110 mg/dL or 4.4 to 6.1 mmol/L]) had a 4.6 percent mortality rate compared to the group on conventional insulin therapy (glucose: 180 to 200 mg/dL or 10 to 11 mmol/L), who had an 8.0 percent mortality rate (42 percent relative risk reduction). The rate of sepsis was also lower with the intensive controlled group compared the conventional group (25 versus 67 percent).[11]
- For all other surgical procedures, major surgery that is noncardiac or not requiring a postoperative ICU stay as well as minor surgical procedures, there are few studies evaluating glucose targets. There are indeed some published observational data by Finney and colleagues[10] suggesting the possibility of benefit for protection against adverse outcomes when a majority of glucose levels are less than 200 mg/dL (<11 mmol/L) among critical care patients as well as RCT evidence demonstrating benefit with even tighter glycemic control among surgical ICU patients. It is difficult to extrapolate these findings to patients undergoing major or minor surgery given the risks for developing hypoglycemia in less monitored patient settings. Therefore, based on expert opinion,[7] we recommend maintaining glucose levels below 200 mg/dL (<11 mmol/L).
- For patients with a higher risk of hypoglycemia, increase the lower boundaries of the glucose targets.

SUMMARY

- There are many approaches to managing the surgical patient with DM and little evidence to guide the clinician on the optimal management strategy. The recommendations provided here, while largely derived from the review of Jacober and Sowers,[7] represent one practical and rational approach to management. Ultimately, management of the diabetic patient will depend on the individual patient and the clinician's judgment.

REFERENCES

1. Lee TH, Marcantonio ER, Mangione CM, et al. Derivation and prospective validation of a simple index for prediction of cardiac risk of major noncardiac surgery. *Circulation* 100(10): 1043, 1999.
2. Eagle KA, Coley CM, Newell JB, et al. Combining clinical and thallium data optimizes preoperative assessment of cardiac risk before major vascular surgery. *Ann Intern Med* 110:859, 1989.
3. Clarke RS. The hyperglycaemic response to different types of surgery and anaesthesia. *Br J Anaesth* 42(1):45, 1970.
4. Trick WE, Scheckler WE, Tokars JI, et al. Modifiable risk factors associated with deep sternal site infection after coronary artery bypass grafting. *J Thorac Cardiovasc Surg* 119(1):108, 2000.
5. Lawrence VA, Gafni A, Gross M. The unproven utility of the preoperative urinalysis: Economic evaluation. *J Clin Epidemiol* 42(12):1185, 1989.
6. Latham R, Lancaster AD, Covington JF, et al. The association of diabetes and glucose control with surgical-site infections among cardiothoracic surgery patients. *Infect Control Hosp Epidemiol* 22(10):607, 2001.
7. Jacober SJ, Sowers JR. An update on perioperative management of diabetes. *Arch Intern Med* 159(20):2405, 1999.
8. Furnary AP, Zerr KJ, Grunkemeier GL, et al. A continuous intravenous insulin infusion reduces the incidence of deep sternal wound infection in diabetic patients after cardiac surgical procedures. *Ann Thorac Surg* 67(2):352, 1999.
9. Furnary AP, Gao G, Grunkemeier GL, et al. A continuous insulin infusion reduces mortality in patients with diabetes undergoing coronary artery bypass grafting. *J Thorac Cardiovasc Surg* 125(5):1007, 2003.
10. Finney SJ, Zekveld C, Elia A, et al. Glucose control and mortality in critically ill patients. *JAMA* 290(15):2041, 2003.
11. van den Berghe G, Wouters P, Weekers F, et al. Intensive insulin therapy in the critically ill patients. *N Engl J Med* 345(19):1359, 2001.

27 THYROID DISEASE

William Wertheim and Visala Muluk

INTRODUCTION

Thyroid disease is commonly encountered in patients undergoing surgery. Problems may include anatomic abnormalities, such as a goiter, or functional abnormalities with signs and symptoms of hypothyroidism or hyperthyroidism. Additionally, seriously ill hospitalized patients often have abnormalities in thyroid function tests, although many do not actually have thyroid disease.

This chapter focuses on various issues concerning thyroid disease primarily in patients undergoing nonthyroid surgery, but specific preparation for thyroid surgery is mentioned as well.

HYPOTHYROIDISM

- Hypothyroidism is classified as follows:
  - ***Primary.*** Disease of the thyroid gland itself, including surgical removal of gland due to other conditions.

- *Secondary.* Due to hypothalamic-pituitary disease.
- *Subclinical*. A clinical entity with mild elevation of TSH but no definite clinical symptoms of hypothyroidism. This may or may not progress to overt hypothyroidism.
- *Myxedema coma.* Severe hypothyroidism complicated by exposure to cold, trauma, infection, or administration of hypnotics and narcotics.

PATIENT-SPECIFIC RISKS (TABLE 27-1)

Hypothyroidism affects many organ systems, resulting in various clinical manifestations and potential effects on perioperative outcome.[1]

General Signs and Symptoms

- Related to slowing of metabolic process:
  - Fatigue, cold intolerance, weight gain, constipation, slow movement, bradycardia, delayed relaxation phase of deep tendon reflexes
- Related to accumulation of matrix substances in the interstitium:
  - Coarse, dry skin; hoarseness; macroglossia

Effects on Specific Organ Systems

- Cardiovascular
  - Clinical findings include decreased heart rate and contractility, leading to decreased cardiac output, dyspnea on exertion, and decreased exercise capability, hypertension due to increased peripheral vascular resistance, elevated diastolic pressure with narrow pulse pressure, and hyperlipidemia.
  - Electrocardiographic (ECG) abnormalities include bradycardia, decreased voltage, and flattening or inversion of T waves.
  - Reduced intravascular plasma volume, caused by increased capillary permeability and movement of albumin into interstitial space, can cause hemodynamic instability in the perioperative period.

TABLE 27-1 Risk Factors with Hypothyroidism

SYSTEM	PATIENT-SPECIFIC RISKS	SURGERY-SPECIFIC RISKS
Cardiac	Bradycardia CHF Pericardial effusion ECG low voltage	Intraoperative hypotension CHF exacerbation
Pulmonary	Dyspnea on exertion Hypoventilation Sleep apnea Pleural effusion	Depression of respiration drive Difficulty in weaning off ventilator
Gastrointestinal	Anorexia Constipation Paralytic ileus	Severe constipation GI bleed
Renal, fluid, and electrolyte	Hyponatremia	Depressed renal drug clearance leading to prolonged exposure to anesthetic agents Decreased renal perfusion and renal failure
Hematology	Normocytic anemia, Iron-deficiency anemia from menorrhagia Pernicious anemia	Bleeding complications due to reduced platelet adhesiveness Difficulty achieving therapeutic INR especially difficult in postoperative management of orthopedic and mechanical valve patients.
Neuromuscular	Excessive somnolence Delayed relaxation phase of deep tendon reflexes Proximal muscle weakness	May delay recovery from anesthesia Proximal muscle weakness may adversely affect rehabilitation potential in the postoperative period
Psychiatric	Depression Memory loss Personality change	Postoperative delirium Postoperative psychosis
Endocrine	Coexisting Addison's disease in primary hypothyroidism Decreased adrenal reserve in secondary hypothyroidism	Adrenal insufficiency leading to hemodynamic instability Stress-dose steroids to be considered
Infectious diseases	Viral thyroiditis, acute and subacute	Less likely to mount fever in response to infection and hence likely to be missed. Infection possibly triggering myxedema coma

CHF = congestive heart failure; ECG = electrocardiogram; INR = international normalized ratio.

- Pulmonary
  - Respiratory muscle weakness and diminished ventilatory drive in response to hypoxia and hypercapnea may lead to hypoventilation and somnolence.
  - Obesity and macroglossia may result in obstructive sleep apnea.
  - Patients may experience fatigue and dyspnea on exertion.
- Hematologic
  - Anemia may result from various mechanisms:
    - Decreased red cell mass, leading to normochromic normocytic anemia.
    - Menorrhagia, leading to iron-deficiency anemia in premenopausal women.
    - Autoimmune thyroiditis associated with pernicious anemia in some patients.
  - Bleeding complications may result from:
    - Decreased platelet adhesiveness.
    - Decreased concentration of plasma factor VIII.
  - Other changes include a prolonged half-life of some coagulation factors (II, VII, and X), requiring higher doses of warfarin to achieve a therapeutic international normalized ratio (INR).
- Gastrointestinal
  - These changes include constipation secondary to decreased motility, weight gain, and impaired hepatic drug metabolism.
- Renal, fluid, and electrolytes
  - Hyponatremia may result from impaired ability to excrete free water, probably related to the syndrome of inappropriate antidiuretic hormone (SIADH).
  - Renal perfusion, creatinine clearance, and renal drug clearance are decreased, which may lead to worsening renal insufficiency in the postoperative period.
- Neuromuscular
  - Proximal muscle weakness, myalgias, and paresthesias may occur.
- Psychiatric
  - Depression, memory loss, and dementia may increase risk of postoperative delirium and psychosis.

SURGERY-SPECIFIC RISKS (TABLE 27-1)

- Due to impaired hepatic metabolism and renal clearance of drugs, hypothyroidism increases sensitivity to anesthetic agents and other perioperative medications. As a result, these patients are more prone to prolonged unconsciousness, hypotension, and respiratory depression.
- In addition to hypotension, cardiac abnormalities caused by hypothyroidism are predictors of poor surgical outcome.
  - Ladenson et al. looked at perioperative complications in 40 hypothyroid patients compared to 80 matched controls. Hypothyroid patients had more intraoperative hypotension in noncardiac surgery and more heart failure in cardiac surgery.[2]
- Hypothyroid patients are less likely to develop fever, which may delay the diagnosis and treatment of infections.

PREOPERATIVE EVALUATION

Clinical Evaluation

- Clinically assess the patient's thyroid status on the basis of the signs and symptoms.

Thyroid-Stimulating Hormone (TSH) Measurement

- There is no indication for TSH as a routine screening test in preoperative evaluation.
- Obtain a TSH:
  - If significant hypothyroidism is suspected on the basis of signs and symptoms
  - To ascertain euthyroid state in a patient with hypothyroidism on thyroid hormone supplementation
- Severely ill patients and hospitalized patients may have abnormal thyroid function tests. This is referred to as the euthyroid sick syndrome or nonthyroidal illness. In these patients TSH and free T_3 will be low and reverse T_3 levels will be high. TSH testing in this group of patients is not useful unless there is a high clinical suspicion for hypothyroidism.

Whether to Postpone Surgery

- If a patient is severely hypothyroid—as indicated by myxedema coma, altered mental status, heart failure, or very low levels of thyroxine—postpone surgery until he or she has been adequately treated.
- Elective surgery is probably safe and generally need not be delayed in patients with mild to moderate hypothyroidism.
  - Weinberg et al. reviewed surgical outcome in 59 patients with untreated mild to moderate hypothyroidism. These patients were similar to the controls in all aspects including surgical outcome, perioperative complications, and length of hospital stay.[3]

Medications to Be Reviewed

- Medications like lithium, amiodarone, interferon, and interleukin-2 can cause hypothyroidism. Check TSH every 6 to 12 months in patients taking these medications chronically.
- In patients taking T_4, certain drugs like cholestyramine, iron, and carbamazepine can decrease the absorption of T_4, resulting in hypothyroidism.

- Iodine and iodine-containing agents like radiocontrast agents may worsen hypothyroidism.

PERIOPERATIVE MANAGEMENT

- Consider undiagnosed hypothyroidism in a patient in the postoperative period if there is difficulty weaning him or her from the ventilator, unexplained ileus, or heart failure.

Replacement of Thyroid Hormone in Noncardiac Surgery

- In patients with newly diagnosed or chronic mild to moderate hypothyroidism, start or continue thyroid supplementation as in an outpatient setting. However, most patients with mild to moderate hypothyroidism tolerate surgery well.
- Since levothyroxine has a long half-life, 5 to 9 days, the patient may, while being unable to eat, miss several doses without having any problems.
- When patients with severe hypothyroidism require urgent or emergent surgery, intravenous T_3, T_4, and glucocorticoids should be administered.[4]
    - Administer T_4 in a loading dose of 200 to 300 μg followed by 50 μg daily. Give T_3 simultaneously in a dose of 5 to 20 μg followed by 2.5 to 10 μg every 8 h, depending on the patient's age and coexistent cardiac risk factors.

Replacement of Thyroid Hormone in Cardiac Surgery

- The initiation of thyroid hormone supplementation in a hypothyroid patient undergoing cardiac surgery may precipitate acute cardiac events. However, an untreated hypothyroid patient undergoing cardiac surgery may be at risk for hypotension and cardiac failure.
- Although some studies favor supplementing after surgery, there is no clear conclusion; each case must be assessed individually.[5]

Myxedema Coma

- This is a rare complication seen in hypothyroid patients in the perioperative period.
- Precipitating factors include trauma, infection, and exposure to sedatives and narcotics.
- The hallmarks of myxedema coma are decreased mental status and hypothermia. Other findings include hypotension, bradycardia, hyponatremia, hypoglycemia, and hypoventilation.
- It is a medical emergency requiring immediate treatment with intravenous T_3 or T_4. Give stress-dose steroids until adrenal insufficiency is ruled out.
- Address the underlying cause and do not overlook infection, since a hypothyroid patient may not mount a fever response.
- Insert an oral airway to prevent obstruction by the tongue. Intubation may be necessary.
- Manage hypothermia by preventing heat loss and administering intravenous fluids warmed to body temperature. External warming may worsen hypotension.

HYPERTHYROIDISM

- Hyperthyroidism affects 1 to 2 percent of the population at large, making it a common problem encountered in the perioperative period. The main concern in a hyperthyroid patient is the risk of surgery precipitating thyroid storm.[6]
- Graves' disease accounts for the majority of patients with hyperthyroidism and has an 8:1 predilection for affecting women. It is followed in frequency of incidence by toxic multinodular goiter and functioning thyroid adenomas. Graves' disease has its peak incidence in the third and fourth decades, while multinodular goiter is more commonly diagnosed in older patients.
- Thyrotoxicosis, the spectrum of clinical and physiologic findings associated with excess thyroid hormone, occurs also in the destructive phase of subacute thyroiditis as well with amiodarone toxicity and metastatic rests of functioning thyroid tissue, such as follicular thyroid carcinoma and struma ovarii.[7]

PATIENT-SPECIFIC RISK FACTORS

- Surgical morbidity in hyperthyroid patients is related to the sympathetic excess and metabolic effects of thyroid hormone. Uncontrolled, untreated, or unrecognized hyperthyroidism increases the risk of perioperative complications.[7]
- The presenting features of thyrotoxicosis are varied and include the following:
    - ***Generalized symptoms:*** hyperactivity, irritability, insomnia, fatigue, weakness, weight loss, and increased appetite.
    - ***More specific symptoms:*** heat intolerance, diaphoresis, palpitations, diarrhea, polyuria, oligomenorrhea, and diminished libido.
    - ***Signs:*** tachycardia, moist skin, lid retraction, proptosis, enlarged thyroid (tender if thyroiditis is present), gynecomastia, tremor, hyperreflexia, and muscle weakness.
- Despite the myriad signs and symptoms of thyrotoxicosis, patients may be asymptomatic, particularly in the early phases of disease and in the elderly.

   - Older patients may present only with such nonspecific symptoms as weakness, weight loss, and fatigue; such patients are described as having "apathetic hyperthyroidism," since more clearly identifying symptoms may be absent. Consider subclinical hyperthyroidism in patients with related diseases, such as atrial fibrillation. Laboratory abnormalities such as elevated serum calcium, alkaline phosphatase, and serum transaminases; decreased creatine phosphokinase; and increased urinary calcium are all secondary to the effects of increased circulating thyroid hormone and may also provide a clue to thyrotoxicosis.[8]
- Cardiac risk factors include atrial ectopy and fibrillation, which may occur more commonly in the elderly. Tachycardia and increased oxygen requirements may precipitate myocardial ischemia and congestive heart failure.[9]
- Risk for pulmonary complications, including prolonged intubation, is increased related to dyspnea from increased oxygen consumption, respiratory muscle weakness, and decreased vital capacity.
- Thyrotoxic patients may also be malnourished from excess catabolism despite increased food intake.
   - Anemia, neutropenia, and thrombocytopenia may increase risk of infection and bleeding.

SURGERY-SPECIFIC RISK FACTORS

- The principal concern in surgical patients with thyrotoxicosis is precipitation of thyroid storm, a condition of exaggerated excess thyroid hormone symptomatology. Although urgent or emergent major surgery may be more likely to precipitate thyroid storm, it has been reported even in minor surgical procedures.
- Heavy sedation alone is not adequate prophylaxis. Avoid atropine, as it may result in adrenergic stimulation.
- The characteristic features of thyroid storm include abrupt onset of fever; tachycardia; gastrointestinal symptoms including nausea, vomiting, abdominal pain, and diarrhea; and central nervous system abnormalities including irritability, confusion, delirium, and coma. Hemodynamic complications may ensue, including heart failure, arrhythmia, and hypotension. The temperature typically exceeds 38°C (100.4°F).
- In addition to surgery, other conditions that may precipitate thyroid storm include trauma, stroke, infection, and diabetic ketoacidosis.
- Other than thyroid storm, surgical morbidity in hyperthyroid patients is related to the sympathetic excess and metabolic effects of thyroid hormone.
- Electrolyte abnormalities all increase surgical risk.
- Most surgical studies of hyperthyroid patients involved thyroidectomy. There are few data on nonthyroid surgery and hyperthyroidism.

PREOPERATIVE EVALUATION

- The history and physical examination should suggest the diagnosis.
- Laboratory testing confirms the diagnosis and assesses severity.
   - The elevated T_4 should suppress TSH. An undetectable TSH level indicates hyperthyroidism.
   - Free T_4 or calculated free thyroxine index (FTI) are elevated.
   - There are rare occurrences of pituitary tumors that produce TSH and T_3 toxicosis, in which the TSH level may be normal but total and free T_4 and T_3 are elevated (or in the case of T_3 toxicosis, total and free T_3 are elevated).[11]
- When elective surgery is planned for hyperthyroid patients, they should be treated to achieve a euthyroid state prior to the proposed procedure, either with antithyroid drugs or ablative therapy.[7,10] Treatment of Graves' disease consists of either blocking the synthesis of thyroid hormone by the gland or destroying the gland itself.
   - Both methimazole and propylthiouracil act by inhibiting thyroid peroxidase and reduce formation of thyroid hormone. Propylthiouracil also inhibits peripheral conversion of thyroxine to T_3.[11]
   - Iodide administration inhibits proteolysis of colloid and thus release of thyroid hormone.
      - Although iodide is more rapid in its effects on circulating thyroid hormone, the use of iodide should be concomitant with use of propylthiouracil or methimazole so as to prevent the accumulation of unreleased thyroid hormone.[11]
   - Either administration of radioactive iodine 131 (^{131}I) or subtotal thyroidectomy will result in destruction of the gland.
   - Not all of those receiving ^{131}I will become hypothyroid with the first dose. Some patients will be persistently hyperthyroid and will require a second dose, and some will be euthyroid. The effect of the ^{131}I may not be evident for up to 12 weeks. Nonetheless, over time the majority of patients will become hypothyroid, though it may take many years before that occurs. Because of the delay in action of ^{131}I and because of the possibility of a postradiation thyroiditis, pretreatment with antithyroid medication is required; often resumption of the medication is needed in those with large thyroid glands and significant thyrotoxicosis.[7]
   - Surgery is performed less frequently than prior to the advent of treatment with radioactive iodine, and it should be limited to those with large goiters, pregnant women, and those who either do not respond to or cannot tolerate antithyroid therapy. A surgeon with significant experience in thyroid surgery should perform the procedure.

TABLE 27-2 Hyperthyroid Patient: Risk-Reduction Strategies

	PREOPERATIVE	INTRAOPERATIVE	POSTOPERATIVE
Institution and maintenance of euthyroid state	Postpone nonemergent surgery Medical therapy to reduce thyroxine formation: PTU, methimazole Ablative therapy/surgical therapy	Administration of dexamethasone to delay peripheral thyroxine conversion Administration of iodine or propylthiouracil to reduce thyroxine release and peripheral conversion	Medical therapy to reduce thyroxine formation: PTU, methimazole Ablative therapy/surgical therapy
Management of sympathetic excess/arrhythmias	Long-acting (propranolol, atenolol) or short-acting (esmolol) beta blockers Other antiarrhythmic therapy as needed	Use of short-acting beta blockers (esmolol) Administration of fluids, glucose, and B-vitamin supplementation intravenously	Long-acting (propranolol, atenolol) or short-acting (esmolol) beta blockers Other antiarrhythmic therapy as needed
Management of thyroid storm			Intensive care unit monitoring Use of short-acting beta blockers (esmolol) Administration of fluids, glucose, and B-vitamin supplementation intravenously Administration of dexamethasone to delay peripheral thyroxine conversion Administration of iodine or propylthiouracil to reduce thyroxine release and peripheral conversion Fever reduction with acetaminophen and/or cooling blankets

PTU = propylthiouracil.

- Treat the adrenergic symptoms of thyrotoxicosis with beta-adrenergic blockade, usually propranolol or atenolol. Although these agents do not provide any meaningful reduction in circulating thyroid hormone, they are very helpful in giving symptomatic relief.[11]
- Patients with multinodular goiter also respond well to therapy. Control symptoms with beta-adrenergic blockade and treat with antithyroid drugs prior to ablative therapy with ^{131}I.

PERIOPERATIVE MANAGEMENT (TABLE 27-2)

- Patients on antithyroid medication should continue this medication throughout the perioperative period.
- If surgery is unavoidable despite the presence of thyrotoxicosis, control heart rate and other features of sympathetic stimulation with beta-adrenergic blockade to a target heart rate <80.
- Management of thyroid storm includes treatment of the effects of circulating thyroid hormone, attempts to reduce the release of thyroid hormone, and general supportive care.
- Use short-acting beta blockers like esmolol intraoperatively and longer-acting agents postoperatively.
  - If high-output heart failure is present, use of beta-adrenergic blockers may worsen this condition.
- Fluids, glucose, and B-complex vitamins should be administered to counter dehydration and the effects of diarrhea and electrolyte loss; high-dose glucocorticoids such as dexamethasone (2 mg every 6 h) should be given to delay the release of thyroid hormone as well as peripheral conversion of T_4 to T_3.
- To truly reduce the release of thyroid hormone from the gland, use iodide, because of its rapid effects on reduction of thyroid hormone, and high doses of an antithyroid agent such as propylthiouracil (300 to 400 mg every 4 h). If the patient is unable to take propylthiouracil by mouth, it may be crushed and administered via nasogastric tube or rectally.
- Other supportive measures include management of heart failure and arrhythmias, if they develop, and reduction of fever with acetaminophen and cooling blankets. Avoid salicylates, as they increase free thyroid hormone levels by competitively binding to thyroid-binding globulin; and in high doses, they further increase the metabolic rate.
- With this therapy, circulating T_3 levels generally return to normal within 36 to 48 h. Begin tapering dexamethasone at this time but continue antithyroid drugs and iodide until the metabolic state returns to normal.

REFERENCES

1. Davies TF, Larsen PR. The thyroid gland, in Larsen PR, Kronenbord HM, Melmed S, et al (eds), *Williams Textbook of Endocrinology*, 10th ed. Philadelphia: Saunders, 2003.
2. Ladenson PW, Levin AA, Ridgway EC, Daniels GH. Complications of surgery in hypothyroid patients. *Am J Med* 77:261, 1984.
3. Weinberg AD, Brennan MD, Gorman CA. Outcome of anesthesia and surgery in hypothyroid patients. *Arch Intern Med* 143:893, 1983.
4. Udelsman R, Ramp J, Gallucci WT, et al. Adaptation during surgical stress: A reevaluation of the role of glucocorticoids. *J Clin Invest* 77:1377, 1986.
5. Drucker DJ, Burrow GN. Cardiovascular surgery in the hypothyroid patient. *Arch Intern Med* 145:1585, 1985.
6. Davies TF, Larsen PR. Thyrotoxicosis, in Larsen PR, Kronenbord HM, Melmed S, et al (eds), *Williams Textbook of Endocrinology*, 10th ed. Philadelphia: Saunders, 2003:413–414.
7. Franklyn JA. The management of hyperthyroidism. *N Engl J Med* 330(24):1731–1738, 1994.
8. Surks MI, Ortiz E, Daniels GH, et al. Subclinical thyroid disease: Scientific review and guidelines for diagnosis and management. *JAMA* 291(2):228–238, 2004.
9. Osman F, Gammage MD, Franklyn JA. Hyperthyroidism and cardiovascular mortality. *Thyroid* 12(6):483–487, 2002.
10. Woeber KA. Update on the management of hyperthyroidism and hypothyroidism. *Arch Intern Med* 160:1067–1071, 2000.
11. Feek CM, Sawers JSA, et al. Combination of potassium iodide and propranolol in preparation of patients with Graves' disease for thyroid surgery. *N Engl J Med* 302:83, 1980.

28 ADRENAL INSUFFICIENCY

Gregory B. Seymann and David A. Halle

INTRODUCTION

ADRENAL PHYSIOLOGY

- The hypothalamic-pituitary-adrenal (HPA) axis plays an important role in the body's ability to cope with the stresses of surgery. In patients with an intact HPA axis who undergo surgery, the adrenal glands increase their baseline secretion of cortisol in response to increased levels of adrenocorticotropic hormone (ACTH), secreted by the anterior pituitary under the influence of corticotropin-releasing hormone (CRH) from the hypothalamus. This adaptation is essential to strengthening the action of the heart and inducing peripheral vasoconstriction to maintain cardiovascular tone. Gluconeogenesis, proteolysis, and lipolysis are also upregulated by cortisol to mobilize energy sources.
- The adrenal cortex secretes cortisol (the primary glucocorticoid), aldosterone (the primary mineralocorticoid), and androgens (predominantly dehydroeipandrosterone and androstenedione). The adrenal medulla secretes the catecholamines epinephrine and norepinephrine.
- ACTH stimulates the release of all adrenocortical hormones but primarily cortisol. By negative feedback inhibition, cortisol controls the secretion of CRH and ACTH as well as arginine vasopressin, which is a potent stimulant of ACTH release. Baseline daily cortisol production is about 15 to 20 mg.
- Aldosterone secretion is mainly regulated by the renin-angiotensin system. Aldosterone acts on the collecting duct to reabsorb sodium and excrete potassium. This results in the secondary retention of water and increased extracellular volume to maintain perfusion.

ETIOLOGY OF ADRENAL INSUFFICIENCY

- Inadequate adrenal function results from the destruction of the adrenal cortex (primary adrenal insufficiency of Addison's disease) or from adrenocortical atrophy caused by ACTH deficiency (secondary adrenal insufficiency).
    - **Primary adrenal insufficiency** is caused about 80 percent of the time by autoimmune destruction of the adrenal glands. Other causes include granulomatous diseases (histoplasmosis, sarcoidosis, tuberculosis) and infiltrative diseases (acquired immunodeficiency syndrome, adrenoleukodystrophy, amyloid, hemochromatosis, lymphoma, metastatic carcinoma). Clinical disease is associated with at least 90 percent destruction of the adrenal cortex.
    - **Secondary adrenal insufficiency** may be due to a wide variety of diseases that affect either the pituitary or hypothalamus, with a resultant decrease of ACTH production. These include pituitary tumors, infarction or ischemic necrosis, inflammatory disease (meningitis, abscess), infiltration (pituitary: hemochromatosis; hypothalamus: eosinophilic granuloma, sarcoidosis), destruction of pituitary stalk (surgery, trauma, mass), and empty sella syndrome. **Either current or recent administration of glucocorticoids in supraphysiologic doses is also capable of suppressing the HPA axis.**
- The serum ACTH level is increased in primary adrenal insufficiency as opposed to secondary adrenal insufficiency, where the levels are decreased. However, in both primary and secondary adrenal insufficiency, plasma cortisol and urinary metabolites are decreased.

  - Other laboratory findings in both disorders include variably decreased serum sodium, chloride, bicarbonate, and glucose, with elevated potassium levels.
  - Since aldosterone production is also decreased in primary adrenal insufficiency, the severity of hyponatremia and hyperkalemia is much greater.

PATIENT-RELATED RISKS

SYMPTOMS OF ADRENAL INSUFFICIENCY

- History and physical examination findings are helpful to increase clinical suspicion of patients who may have undiagnosed adrenal insufficiency.
  - Testing of the HPA axis should be performed if the clinical suspicions are high (see "Preoperative Evaluation and Testing," below).
- Clinically, patients with adrenal insufficiency may present with fatigue, mental depression, weight loss, anorexia, orthostatic hypotension, dizziness, nausea, vomiting, and diarrhea.[1]
  - Hyperpigmentation (from elevation of ACTH precursor peptides), and other autoimmune diseases (vitiligo, thyroid disease) are specific manifestations of primary adrenal insufficiency.
  - Associated manifestations of secondary adrenal insufficiency may include pale skin, amenorrhea, decreased libido, scant axillary and pubic hair, small testicles, delayed puberty, and diabetes insipidus.

POSTOPERATIVE COMPLICATIONS OF STEROIDS

- The goal is to treat patients with or at risk for adrenal insufficiency with a glucocorticoid replacement regimen that is of a physiologic dose.
- The use of perioperative steroids may contribute to perioperative morbidity, including but not limited to delayed wound healing, immunosuppression, myopathy, glucose intolerance, cardiac arrhythmias, myocardial infarction, pancreatitis, peptic ulcer disease, and neuropsychiatric disorders.[2]

SURGERY-RELATED RISKS

SURGERY IN PATIENTS WITH ADRENAL INSUFFICIENCY

- The theoretical dangers of adrenal insufficiency during surgery include hypotension, cardiovascular collapse, and death.
- The incidence of symptoms of acute adrenal insufficiency in surgical patients is low, ranging from 0.01 to 0.7 percent.[3]
- The standard for current perioperative glucocorticoid replacement has been based on two case reports from the early 1950s; these concerned young patients with rheumatoid arthritis who had their glucocorticoid therapy withdrawn prior to orthopedic surgery. The patients died unexpectedly and necropsy revealed diffuse atrophy and gross hemorrhage of the bilateral adrenal glands. Soon after, published recommendations for perioperative glucocorticoid coverage became the standard of care.
- Since the 1950s, there have been few clinical trials, and they have usually been of small sample size. In addition, limited longitudinal data and varying definitions of hypotensive crisis have limited definite conclusions on this topic.[4]
- The current guidelines for perioperative glucocorticoid treatment are based on the recommendations of Salem and colleagues from 1994.[5] They used their own clinical experience coupled with serum cortisol levels and correlated the recommended steroid therapy with the level of surgical stress.
- More recently, a few small studies have questioned the role of supplemental glucocorticoid therapy in the perioperative period. Most notable is a double-blind study in patients undergoing elective surgeries (mostly abdominal and orthopedic) who had been treated with glucocorticoids (at least 7.5 mg of prednisone daily for 2 months).[6] These patients also had secondary adrenal insufficiency as defined by ACTH stimulation testing (60-min cortisol level below 20 μg/dL). The intervention was treating one group of patients with the recommended glucocorticoid supplementation (one dose of hydrocortisone 100 mg IV given 1 h prior to the procedure, then 25 mg IV every 6 h for 48 hours, then 25 mg IV every 12 h for 24 h) and the other group with normal saline in the perioperative period. All patients continued to receive their usual daily dose of prednisone. The steroid-treated group (6 patients) and the saline-treated group (12 patients) each included 1 patient with hypotension, which resolved with volume replacement. The authors concluded that patients with secondary adrenal insufficiency "do not experience hypotension in the absence of supplemental steroids during the perioperative period."
- Despite this evidence and that of other small studies, more prospective randomized trials with larger patient samples and varying surgical procedures are needed to strengthen the evidence that there may be no benefit to treating patients on maintenance steroid therapy or those who recently received steroid therapy in the perioperative period. Until then, the standard of care will continue to be supplementation of this group of patients with "stress-dose" glucocorticoids in the perioperative period and to tailor the dose to the level of surgical stress.

ADRENAL CORTISOL RESPONSE TO SURGERY IN PATIENTS WITH A NORMAL HPA AXIS

- Serum cortisol and corticotropin levels begin to rise rapidly at the time of incision and return to baseline levels within 24 to 72 h.[3]
- The extent of the surgery directly correlates to the level of cortisol production in the perioperative period.
- Cortisol secretion in the first 24 h after the most extensive surgery rarely exceeds 300 mg/day.

ASSESSMENT OF GLUCOCORTICOID THERAPY AND SURGICAL STRESS

- To provide for the patient going for surgery who is or has been on glucocorticoids, ascertaining the dose (Table 28-1) and duration of glucocorticoid therapy is the first step in determining whether the HPA axis is intact or suppressed or whether this is unknown.
- The next step is to assess the level of surgical stress anticipated by the proposed procedure. There are three categories of surgical stress: minor, moderate, and major.
  - Minor surgical stress procedures (inguinal herniorrhaphy and those performed under local anesthesia) have a glucocorticoid target of **about 25 mg of hydrocortisone equivalent on the day of the procedure**.[5]
  - Moderate surgical stress procedures (open cholecystectomy, lower extremity revascularization, hemicolectomy, joint replacement, abdominal hysterectomy) have a glucocorticoid target of **about 50 to 75 mg/day hydrocortisone equivalent for 1 to 2 days**.
  - Major surgical stress procedures (Whipple, esophagogastrectomy, total proctocolectomy, coronary artery bypass grafting) have a higher glucocorticoid target of **about 100 to 150 mg of hydrocortisone equivalent/day for 2 to 3 days**.
- Table 28-2 makes specific recommendations on glucocorticoid supplementation for the three categories of surgical stress.

PREOPERATIVE EVALUATION AND TESTING

THE DECISION TO TEST

- **Routine perioperative testing of the HPA axis is not indicated in the majority of patients.** The history often reveals adequate information to guide decisions about perioperative steroid supplementation.
- It is appropriate to test when it is unclear if the patient has adequate adrenal reserve *and* there is sufficient time for preoperative testing. Examples of such patients include:
  - **Patients whose steroid dose or dosing schedule is in question.** Typically patients taking less than 5 mg of prednisone equivalent daily or those who take steroids less than once daily do not exhibit suppression of the HPA axis. Also, patients on steroids for less than 3 weeks do not need testing.
  - **Patients on intermediate doses of steroids.** Patients taking between 5 and 20 mg of prednisone equivalent daily are in the equivocal range; a percentage of these patients on low-dose steroids may retain adequate adrenal reserve. If time permits preoperatively, testing can be done and supplemental steroids avoided if the HPA axis is intact. Alternatively, short-term supplementation can be given with minimal risk and testing can be deferred.
  - **Patients who have recently discontinued steroids.** Studies report adrenal suppression for up to 1 year after stopping steroids; however the recovery period is variable.[7] Patients who have completed therapy within 1 year of surgery may warrant preoperative testing of the HPA axis.

TESTING THE HPA AXIS (FIG. 28-1)

- A number of tests are available to evaluate adrenal reserve; ideally the simplest tests will be used in the perioperative period so as to minimize delays in surgical care.

TABLE 28-1 Relative Comparative Steroid Potencies

GLUCOCORTICOID	GLUCOCORTICOID POTENCY	MINERALOCORTICOID POTENCY
Hydrocortisone (cortisol)	1	1
Cortisone	0.8	0.8
Prednisone	4	0.8
Prednisolone	4	0.8
Methylprednisolone	5	0.5
Betamethasone	30	0
Dexamethasone	40	0
Fludrocortisone	15	200

TABLE 28-2 Perioperative Supplemental Glucocorticoid Therapy

HPA AXIS	MINOR SURGICAL STRESS	MODERATE SURGICAL STRESS	MAJOR SURGICAL STRESS
Not suppressed 1. Less than prednisone 5 mg/day or equivalent for any duration 2. Any dose of glucocorticoid for less than 3 weeks	Give usual daily dose of glucocorticoid No supplementation	Give usual daily dose of glucocorticoid No supplementation	Give usual daily dose of glucocorticoid No supplementation
Suppression presumed or documented 1. More than prednisone 20 mg/day or equivalent for 3 weeks or more 2. Cushingoid appearance 3. HPA axis suppression by testing	Give usual daily dose of glucocorticoid No supplementation	Hydrocortisone 50 mg IV prior to induction of anesthesia, then 25 mg IV every 8 h for 24–48 h, then resume usual dose	Hydrocortisone 100 mg IV prior to induction of anesthesia, then 50 mg IV every 8 h, for 48–72 h, then resume usual dose
Suppression uncertain 1. Prednisone 5–20 mg/day or its equivalent for 3 weeks or more 2. Prednisone 5 mg/day or greater or its equivalent for 3 weeks or more in the year prior to surgery	Give usual daily dose of glucocorticoid No supplementation	Test HPA axis: if suppressed or clinical suspicion high, then hydrocortisone 50 mg IV prior to induction of anesthesia, then 25 mg IV every 8 h for 24–48 h, then resume usual dose	Test HPA axis: if suppressed or clinical suspicion high, then hydrocortisone 100 mg IV prior to induction of anesthesia, then 50 mg IV every 8 h for 48–72 h, then resume usual dose

SOURCE: Adapted from Schiff R, Welsh G. Perioperative evaluation and management of the patient with endocrine dysfunction. *Med Clin North Am* 87:175–192, 2003.

Pursuing testing must be considered carefully, because the short duration of steroid supplementation currently recommended perioperatively might make it more cost-effective to treat rather than test equivocal cases. Furthermore, there is poor correlation between results of the stimulation tests and outcomes.[4]

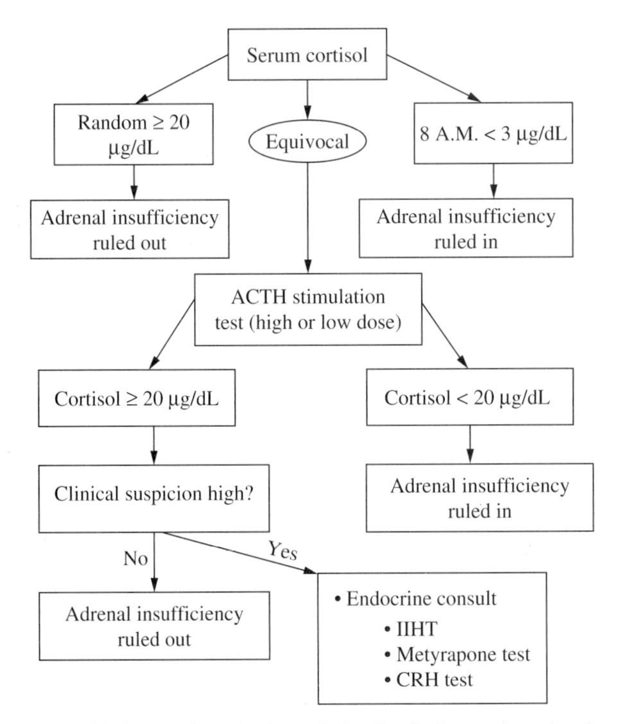

FIG. 28-1 Testing the hypothalamic-pituitary-adrenal axis. ACTH = adrenocorticotropic hormone; CRH = corticotropin-releasing hormone; IIHT = insulin-induced hypoglycemia. See text for details.

RANDOM SERUM CORTISOL

- A random serum cortisol level above 20 μg/dL rules out adrenal insufficiency. For an acutely ill patient, a random serum cortisol level below 20 μg/mL effectively rules it in.
- Cortisol levels peak in the morning, so an 8 A.M. cortisol level below 3 μg/dL suggests adrenal insufficiency.[7]

ACTH STIMULATION TEST

- Pituitary ACTH secretion is suppressed by administration of chronic glucocorticoids, and functional adrenal gland atrophy results from the loss of this trophic hormone. Administration of exogenous ACTH will not provoke a response from adrenal glands that have become atrophied.
- Patients who need HPA axis testing and cannot be diagnosed based on random cortisol testing should have ACTH stimulation testing done.
- The test involves administration of 250 μg of ACTH intramuscularly or intravenously after drawing a baseline serum cortisol level. Cortisol measurement is repeated 30 to 60 min later.
- Stimulation to cortisol levels above 19 μg/dL is considered normal. The incremental increase in serum cortisol is not felt to be as important by most authors. A relatively small percentage increase in pre- and poststimulation cortisol levels, suggesting relative adrenal insufficiency, may be more relevant in critically ill patients than in patients awaiting elective surgery.[3]
  - The standard ACTH stimulation test may miss patients with early adrenal insufficiency whose adrenal glands have not yet atrophied. A patient who is strongly suspected to be adrenally insufficient, especially of recent

onset, may need further workup if the standard ACTH stimulation test is negative or equivocal.

Low-Dose ACTH Stimulation Test

- The low-dose ACTH stimulation is performed similarly to the standard ACTH stimulation test, but a dose of 1 μg is injected. This test may be more sensitive to subtle or early adrenal insufficiency, although it is not clearly superior to the standard-dose test.[8,9]

Other Tests

- Other tests available include the insulin-induced hypoglycemia test, the overnight metyrapone test, and the CRH stimulation test. It is advisable to involve an endocrinologist at this stage unless the clinician has considerable clinical experience in this area.
  - Hypoglycemia is a potent stimulus to the adrenal axis and elevates ACTH secretion. The insulin-induced hypoglycemia test involves administering insulin to provoke hypoglycemia below 40 mg/dL, with an expected stimulated cortisol response to above 20 μg/dL. This test is considered the "gold standard" but obviously requires careful monitoring in an inpatient setting. A review of 6581 insulin-induced hypoglycemia tests noted 6 adverse events, all reversed successfully with glucose administration.[10]
  - Metyrapone interferes with cortisol synthesis; in normal subjects the drug produces a decrease in cortisol levels and a compensatory increase in ACTH. In patients with central adrenal insufficiency, no rise in ACTH is observed after overnight metyrapone administration. Acute adrenal crisis can occur, so this test should be done in the hospital.
  - CRH can be directly administered to test the HPA axis; normal subjects should respond with increases in both cortisol and ACTH within 2 h of injection. This test is comparable in accuracy to the insulin-induced hypoglycemia test and may be safely performed on an outpatient basis.[2,7]
- Testing in patients currently on steroids can be done 24 to 48 h after the last dose. If stopping the steroid is not an option, conversion to the equivalent dose of dexamethasone allows testing while therapy continues. Unlike all other steroid preparations, dexamethasone does not cross-react with the assay for cortisol.

PERIOPERATIVE MANAGEMENT (TABLE 28-3)

PREOPERATIVE

- Adequate hydration is essential. Hypotension is the main adverse perioperative outcome in patients with adrenal insufficiency. In studies of perioperative steroid supplementation, there were few documented episodes of hypotension; however, the majority of patients with hypotension in these studies were adequately resuscitated with fluids alone.[4]
- Given the increased likelihood of hyperkalemia and hyponatremia in patients with adrenal insufficiency, electrolytes should be checked and normalized preoperatively. Particular attention should be given to those patients with primary adrenal insufficiency, who are most likely to suffer electrolyte disturbances. Mineralocorticoid supplementation should be continued until the patient takes nothing by mouth, at which time isotonic saline should be administered.
- The level of surgical stress should be determined so steroid dosing matches physiologic requirements. Surgical stress levels of mild, moderate or severe warrant increasing amounts of steroid supplementation (see Table 28-2).

TABLE 28-3 Risk-Reduction Strategies

PREOPERATIVE	INTRAOPERATIVE	POSTOPERATIVE
Maintain adequate hydration	Maintain adequate hydration	Maintain adequate hydration
Normalize electrolytes	Avoid etomidate if possible	Taper steroids rapidly
Choose steroid dose to match surgical stress level	Be aware of effects of high-dose narcotics on HPA axis	Monitor for side effects of steroids
		Evaluate for other causes when hypotension is present; do not assume it is due to adrenal insufficiency if patient is receiving supplemental steroids

INTRAOPERATIVE

- Maintain adequate fluid balance to avoid hypotension.
- Etomidate, an anesthetic induction agent, has been shown to reduce cortisol levels for up to 8 h postoperatively.[2] It acts as an inhibitor of adrenal 11-B hydroxylase, the enzyme that converts deoxycortisol to cortisol. For patients undergoing low-risk surgeries, outcomes have not been affected, but critically ill patients who received etomidate had a doubling of their mortality rate.[3] Reliance on the discretion of the anesthesiologist is advised.
- High-dose opiates have been observed to attenuate the response of the HPA axis to surgical pain; cortisol and ACTH levels have been used as surrogate markers to measure successful anesthetic technique.[2] The implications for this in patients with adrenal insufficiency are unclear. It is unlikely to pose a problem unless

supplemental steroids are withheld perioperatively, as in a patient with clinically unrecognized disease of the HPA axis.

POSTOPERATIVE

- Hypotension in a patient receiving supplemental steroids is unlikely to be due to cortisol deficiency. Before increasing the steroid dose, make sure that other common causes—such as hypovolemia, anemia, sepsis, and cardiac dysfunction—have been ruled out (see Chap. 51).
- Hypotension in a patient with primary adrenal insufficiency is likely due to hypovolemia due to lack of aldosterone-mediated sodium retention. Administer isotonic saline at doses adequate to maintain hemodynamic stability and resume mineralocorticoid replacement once the patient is taking oral medications.
- Change steroid dosing from intravenous to oral once the patient resumes eating.
- Taper steroids rapidly to baseline dose.
- Monitor for side effects of high-dose steroids, such as hyperglycemia, fluid retention, and mental status changes. Monitor electrolytes and hemodynamics for signs of inadequate cortisol concentrations.
- Adrenal insufficiency is an important preoperative consideration in patients who require moderate or major surgery and have documented or presumed HPA axis suppression. The diagnostic evaluation of the patient's risk and the surgical procedure proposed determine whether perioperative prophylaxis with stress-dose steroids is recommended.

REFERENCES

1. Oelkers W. Adrenal insufficiency. *N Engl J Med* 335: 1206–1212, 1996.
2. Nicholson G, Burrin JM, Hall GM. Perioperative steroid supplementation. *Anaesthesia* 53:1091–1104, 1998.
3. Lamberts SWJ, Bruining HA, de Jong FH. Corticosteroid therapy in severe illness. *N Engl J Med* 337:1285–1292, 1997.
4. Brown CJ, Buie WD. Perioperative stress dose steroids: Do they make a difference? *J Am Coll Surg* 193:678–686, 2001.
5. Salem M, Tainsh RE, Bromberg J, et al. Perioperative glucocorticoid coverage: A reassessment 42 years after emergence of a problem. *Ann Surg* 219:416–425, 1994.
6. Glowniak JV, Loriaux DL. A double-blind study of perioperative steroid requirements in secondary adrenal insufficiency. *Surgery* 121:123–129, 1997.
7. Krasner AS. Glucocorticoid-induced adrenal insufficiency. *JAMA* 282:671–676, 1999.
8. Mayenknecht J, Diederich S, Bahr V, et al. Comparison of low and high dose corticotropin stimulation tests in patients with pituitary disease. *J Clin Endocrinol Metab* 83:1558–1562, 1998.
9. Weintrob N, Sprecher E, Josefsberg Z, et al. Standard and low-dose short adrenocorticotropin test compared with insulin-induced hypoglycemia for assessment of the hypothalamic-pituitary-adrenal axis in children with idiopathic multiple pituitary hormone deficiencies. *J Clin Endorinol Metab* 83:88–92, 1998.
10. Fish HR, Chernow B, O'Brian JT. Endocrine and neurophysiologic responses of the pituitary to insulin-induced hypoglycemia: A review. *Metabolism* 35:763–780, 1986.

29 PHEOCHROMOCYTOMA

Tariq Shafi and Gregory B. Seymann

INTRODUCTION

- Pheochromocytoma is a tumor of catecholamine-secreting chromaffin cells; it is most commonly found in the adrenal medulla.
- Symptoms typically include paroxysmal headaches, diaphoresis, palpitations, and hypertension. Sustained rather than paroxysmal hypertension is not unusual, particularly in norepinephrine-secreting tumors.
- Prevalence rates are not well known and are based on autopsy series or referral to tertiary care centers. Among the general population, approximately 5 individuals with pheochromocytomas are expected to be found per 100,000 hypertensive patients.[1] Incidence increases with advancing age and most tumors discovered at autopsy are in patients above age 60.
- The current availability of advanced diagnostic techniques allows accurate diagnosis and localization of most pheochromocytomas prior to presentation in the preoperative setting. The treatment of pheochromocytomas is surgical excision.
- Modern day perioperative management has resulted in a reduction of surgical mortality rates; these ranged from 13 to 45 percent and are now at 3 percent or less.[3] A number of varied and somewhat idiosyncratic perioperative approaches have been advocated. However, there is unanimous agreement that proper preoperative preparation of the patients, based on the understanding of the pathophysiology of the disease, along with an experienced team of physicians is the key to optimal outcomes.

PATIENT-RELATED RISKS

- There is paradoxical hyperactivity of the sympathetic nervous system in patients with pheochromocytoma despite high circulating levels of catecholamines.[1] This hyperactivity is due to loading of sympathetic nerve terminals with catecholamines, increased sympathetic nerve activity, and loss of inhibition of presynaptic $alpha_2$-receptor-mediated suppression of catecholamine release at the nerve endings.
- Noxious stimuli cause massive release of the stored catecholamines at the nerve terminals, leading to activation of the sympathetic nervous system and hypertensive crisis.
- Hypertensive crisis of pheochromocytoma, therefore, mimics the systemic administration of epinephrine and norepinephrine. There is an increase in cardiac output and systemic vascular resistance along with a decrease in vascular compliance, leading to a hyperdynamic and hypovolemic state. However, the hemodynamic profile of pheochromocytoma patients during steady state is similar to that of patients with essential hypertension.[1]

SURGERY-RELATED RISKS

SURGICAL TECHNIQUE

- Laparoscopic surgery is the preferred approach in pheochromocytoma resection. Small retrospective series confirm that laparoscopic surgery compared to the traditional abdominal approach is associated with fewer and less severe hypertensive episodes. In addition, there is less blood loss, less postoperative pain, and a 4- to 7-day decrease in length of hospital stay.[7,8] There is no difference in the duration of surgery.
- The safety of this procedure appears equivalent to that of laparoscopic adrenalectomy for other benign tumors, such as aldosteronoma and incidentaloma.[9]

ADRENERGIC HYPERACTIVITY

- The presence of sympathetic overactivity discussed above leads to hypertensive surges in response to painful stimuli and agents; this causes release of catecholamines from nerve endings. Intraoperatively, these stimuli include intubation, skin incision, and the creation of a pneumoperitoneum for laparoscopy.
- Manipulation of the tumor also releases catecholamines into the circulation. Palpation of the tumor or its manipulation during laparoscopy causes surges in systolic blood pressure (BP) to levels as high as 250 mmHg,[1] so careful handling is essential.
- High levels of catecholamines secreted by the tumor suppress catecholamine output from the contralateral adrenal gland. The patient's adrenergic receptors are also downgraded due to persistent stimulation. Removal of the tumor is often associated with a precipitous fall in BP and subsequently persistent hypotension.

PREOPERATIVE EVALUATION AND TESTING

DIAGNOSTIC TESTING

- Plasma free metanephrines offer the highest sensitivity (99 percent) in patients with pheochromocytoma, and a negative test excludes pheochromocytoma (Table 29-1).[1,10]
- In the biochemically confirmed patient, magnetic resonance imaging (MRI) provides the highest sensitivity (100 percent) for localizing the tumor.[1] However, MRI's specificity can be as low as 67 percent.
- ^{123}Iodinated metaiodobenzylguanidine (^{123}I-MIBG) scanning offers the best specificity (100 percent) and is used to aid in the diagnosis and localization of the tumor. Positron-emission tomography using 6-[^{18}F] fluorodopamine and octreotide receptor scintigraphy are useful in selective situations.[2]

CONTROL OF HYPERTENSION

- Adequate BP control is the cornerstone of successful perioperative management of pheochromocytoma. Although the principal focus is on alpha blockade, given the pathophysiology of the tumor, success with multiple regimens has been reported (Table 29-2).

TABLE 29-1 Sensitivity and Specificity of Diagnostic Tests for Pheochromocytoma

DIAGNOSTIC TEST	SENSITIVITY(%)	SPECIFICITY(%)
Plasma metanephrines	99	89
Plasma catecholamines	85	80
Urine catecholamines	83	88
Urine metanephrines	76	94
Urine vanillylmandelic acid	63	74
CT scan	98	70
MRI scan	100	67
^{123}I-MIBG scan	78	100

CT = computed tomography; ^{123}I-MIBG = ^{123}iodinated metaiodobenzylguanidine; MRI = magnetic resonance imaging.
SOURCE: Data from Bravo and Tagle[1] and Pacak et al.[10]

TABLE 29-2 Pharmacologic Agents Used in Perioperative Management of Pheochromocytoma

DRUG	DOSE	COMMENTS
α-ADRENERGIC ANTAGONISTS		
Phenoxybenzamine	Initial: 10 mg PO twice daily. Increase by 10-mg increments. Average dose required is 40 mg/day.	Longest experience among all therapies. Nonselective α-adrenergic blockade leads to many side effects. Long half-life can cause prolonged hypotension postoperatively.
Doxazosin	Initial: 1 mg daily. Increase as tolerated. Max 16 mg/day.	Selective α_1-adrenergic antagonist. Shorter half-life avoids postoperative hypotension. Less reflex tachycardia.
CALCIUM CHANNEL ANTAGONISTS		
Nifedipine gastrointestinal transport system (GITS)	30–90 mg daily	Avoids overshoot hypotension and coronary vasospasm. No orthostatic hypotension. Resistant hypertension may require addition of α-adrenergic antagonists.
Nicardipine	Intravenous infusion 5 mg/h. Increase 2.5 mg every 5 min. Max 15 mg/h.	For use intraoperatively.
OTHER AGENTS		
Atenolol	25–100 mg daily.	Cardioselective beta blocker. For control of tachycardia after adequate α-adrenergic blockade.
Labetalol	400–1600 mg daily.	Combined nonselective α and beta blocker. Can precipitate hypertensive crisis if used alone.
Esmolol	Initial: Bolus 500 μg/kg IV for 1 min, followed by 25–100 μg/kg/min for 4 min. Max of 300 μg/kg/min.	Short-acting parenteral cardioselective beta blocker. For control of tachycardia intraoperatively.
Sodium nitroprusside	Initial: 0.25 μg/kg/min Max: 10 μg/kg/min.	For control of hypertensive surges intraoperatively. Risk of cyanide toxicity with prolonged use.
Metyrosine	500–4000 mg daily.	Inhibits synthesis of catecholamines. Rarely used routinely.

ALPHA BLOCKADE

Phenoxybenzamine

- Many regard oral phenoxybenzamine as the drug of choice for alpha-adrenergic blockade. It is a nonselective alpha-adrenergic blocker with a half-life greater than 24 h.
- The initial dose is 10 mg once daily; this can be increased frequently until control of BP and symptoms is obtained. This therapy can be administered on an outpatient basis.
- Side effects of therapy include fatigue, nasal stuffiness, postural hypotension, somnolence, and tachycardia. The tachycardia is due to presynaptic alpha_2-adrenergic blockade, allowing uninhibited release of norepinephrine at the nerve endings. Administration of cardioselective beta blockers such as atenolol, after adequate alpha-adrenergic blockade has been achieved, abolishes this tachycardia.
- Intraoperative hypertension still occurs despite adequate alpha-adrenergic blockade.[1] The long half-life of the drug contributes to prolonged hypotension after removal of the tumor.[4] The alpha-adrenergic blockade also results in postoperative vasodilatation with interstitial fluid retention and peripheral edema.

Doxazosin

- Doxazosin is a selective alpha_1-adrenergic blocker with high bioavailability, once-daily dosing, and a shorter duration of action than phenoxybenzamine. The lack of presynaptic alpha_2-adrenergic blockade prevents tachycardia and reduces the need for beta blockers. Its shorter half-life prevents postoperative hypotension.[4]

- Doxazosin is started at 1 mg daily; the dose is gradually increased to a maximum of 16 mg daily.

OTHER ANTIHYPERTENSIVES

- Beta blockers, as mentioned above, are used in combination with phenoxybenzamine to reduce reflex tachycardia and perioperative ischemia.
- Calcium channel antagonists relax the arteriolar smooth muscle, thereby reducing catecholamine-mediated increased peripheral vascular resistance. They can effectively control BP while avoiding overshoot hypotension and orthostatic hypotension. The nifedipine gastrointestinal transport system (GITS) in doses of 30 to 90 mg/day has been used effectively without alpha-adrenergic blockers in patients undergoing surgery for pheochromocytoma.[5]
- Metyrosine inhibits tyrosine hydroxylase and decreases the synthesis of catecholamines. It is associated with a high incidence of undesirable side effects and is rarely used in practice.[6]

PREOPERATIVE MANAGEMENT

- The excess catecholamines from the pheochromocytoma can lead to hypertrophic cardiomyopathy or, rarely, dilated cardiomyopathy. Echocardiographic assessment of left ventricular function is helpful in managing hypotension, hypertension, and pulmonary edema in the perioperative period.
- Adequate hydration, along with alpha-adrenergic blockade, is essential to avoid excessive hypotension in the intraoperative period.
- Most authorities recommend control of hypertension and catecholamine-related spells for at least 1 week prior to surgery.
- Perioperative alpha-adrenergic blockade helps to control hypertension and may allow expansion of blood volume. Criteria for adequate alpha-adrenergic blockade are as follows[3]:
  1. BP well controlled below 160/90 mmHg for at least 24 h prior to surgery.
  2. Presence of orthostatic hypotension, with orthostatic readings greater than 80/45 mmHg before surgery.
  3. No electrocardiographic evidence of ST-T changes for 1 week before surgery.
  4. No more than one premature ventricular contraction every 5 min.

INTRAOPERATIVE MANAGEMENT

INTRAOPERATIVE MONITORING

- Placement of an intraarterial line is required for monitoring of BP. A central venous catheter is useful for monitoring of filling pressures and infusing medications including antihypertensive agents or vasopressors. Pulmonary artery catheterization may be necessary in selected patients with congestive heart failure.
- Pulse oximetry, continuous electrocardiography, and monitoring of urine output are essential.[3,6] Combined use of these approaches provides optimal management of these patients (Table 29-3).

ANESTHESIA

- Ketamine, ephedrine, morphine, meperidine, and droperidol can all cause hypertensive crises in patients with pheochromocytoma; they should be used cautiously.
- Halothane and desflurane have sympathetic stimulatory properties that make them less desirable anesthetic choices.[3,6]

HYPERTENSIVE SURGES

- Noxious stimuli (incision, intubation, tumor handling) can lead to hypertensive surges intraoperatively. A number of parenteral antihypertensive agents are available for treatment of these surges.
- Phentolamine is a parenteral alpha-adrenergic antagonist and is given in anticipation of the surge. Reflex

TABLE 29-3 Risk-Reduction Strategies

PREOPERATIVE	INTRAOPERATIVE	POSTOPERATIVE
Adequate hydration	Adequate hydration	Adequate hydration
Echocardiogram	Placement of arterial line	Monitor for hypotension
Blood pressure control	Placement of central venous catheter	Monitor for hypoglycemia
Assess level of alpha blockade	Parenteral antihypertensives for blood pressure surges	Follow up for recurrence
Control hyperglycemia	Attention to hypotension after tumor removal	

tachycardia is treated with labetalol or esmolol. Beta blockers are also useful in controlling sympathetically-mediated tachyarrhythmias.
- Sodium nitroprusside, nitroglycerin, nicardipine, and magnesium sulfate have all been used.[3,6] Use of drugs with short half-lives is preferable in anticipation of hypotension that occurs with the ligation of the venous supply of the tumor and its removal.

HYPOTENSION

- Tumor removal is often associated with hypotension due to sympathetic withdrawal. Hypotension may also persist due to lasting effects of preoperative phenoxybenzamine, a sudden increase in venous capacitance, or hemorrhage. Large-volume of fluid and colloid replacement, along with vasopressors, is often required.[3,6]

POSTOPERATIVE MANAGEMENT

HYPOGLYCEMIA

- Insulin secretion is antagonized by the stimulation of alpha$_2$-adrenergic receptors, and glycogenolysis is activated by sympathetic overactivity. Postoperatively, hypoglycemia results from rebound hyperinsulinism as the inhibitory effects of catecholamines are eliminated. Glucose concentrations should be monitored perioperatively.
- Beta blockers can impair the recovery from hypoglycemia and mask its clinical symptoms.[3]

HYPOTENSION

- Hypotension can persist in the postoperative period due to the factors discussed above. Aggressive intravascular volume resuscitation is indicated.
- Adrenal insufficiency may contribute to postoperative hypotension if the patient has undergone bilateral adrenalectomy; in such an instance, appropriate steroid replacement should be administered (Table 29-4).[3]

PERSISTENT HYPERTENSION

- BP remains elevated postoperatively in close to 50 percent of patients due to a number of factors:
  1. Residual effects of the circulating catecholamines and residual catecholamine stores in sympathetic nerve endings[3]
  2. Fluid overload during surgery
  3. Residual essential hypertension
  4. Residual tumor
  5. Inadvertent ligation of the renal artery

TABLE 29-4 Adrenal Steroid Supplementation in Bilateral Adrenalectomy

Day of surgery	Methylprednisolone 40 mg IV every 8 h for three doses
Postoperative Day 1	Methylprednisolone 20 mg IV every 8 h for three doses
Postoperative Day 2	Methylprednisolone 10 mg IV every 8 h for three doses
Maintenance	Prednisone 5 mg every morning and 2.5 mg every afternoon, with fludrocortisone 0.1 mg every morning

SOURCE: From Kinney et al.[3] Copyright 2002, with permission from Elsevier.

ADRENAL STEROID REPLACEMENT

- In patients undergoing bilateral adrenalectomy, give high-dose postoperative steroids briefly and then maintenance replacement doses indefinitely (Table 29-4).[3]
- Partial adrenalectomies are sometimes done in patients with hereditary pheochromocytoma to avoid the need for exogenous steroid replacement. Clinical outcomes are similar to those of total adrenalectomy, but recurrence can be as high as 33 percent. Close follow-up is essential.[10]

OUTCOMES

- Obtain a plasma metanephrine level at 6 months and 1 year after surgery to screen for recurrence.[10] Check levels sooner if hypertension persists more than 2 weeks postoperatively.
- Yearly follow-up for patients with familial pheochromocytoma is essential.
- Survival rates after surgical excision of pheochromocytoma are 97 to 100 percent in current series, with up to 38 percent of patients noted to have continued non-paroxysmal hypertension postoperatively.[10]

REFERENCES

1. Bravo EL, Tagle R. Pheochromocytoma: State-of-the-art and future prospects. *Endocr Rev* 24(4):539–553, 2003.
2. Ilias I, Pacak K. Current approaches and recommended algorithm for the diagnostic localization of pheochromocytoma. *J Clin Endocrinol Metab* 89(2):479–491, 2004.
3. Kinney MA, Narr BJ, Warner MA. Perioperative management of pheochromocytoma. *J Cardiothorac Vasc Anesth* 16(3):359–369, 2002.

4. Prys-Roberts C, Farndon JR. Efficacy and safety of doxazosin for perioperative management of patients with pheochromocytoma. *World J Surg* 26(8):1037–1042, 2002.
5. Ulchaker JC, Goldfarb DA, Bravo EL, Novick AC. Successful outcomes in pheochromocytoma surgery in the modern era. *J Urol* 161(3):764–767, 1999.
6. Prys-Roberts C. Phaeochromocytoma—Recent progress in its management. *Br J Anaesth* 85(1):44–57, 2000.
7. Sprung J, O'Hara JF Jr, Gill IS, et al. Anesthetic aspects of laparoscopic and open adrenalectomy for pheochromocytoma. *Urology* 55(3):339–343, 2000.
8. Kim HH, Kim GH, Sung GT. Laparoscopic adrenalectomy for pheochromocytoma: Comparison with conventional open adrenalectomy. *J Endourol* 18(3):251–255, 2004.
9. Kalady MF, McKinlay R, Olson JA Jr, et al. Laparoscopic adrenalectomy for pheochromocytoma. A comparison to aldosteronoma and incidentaloma. *Surg Endosc* 18(4):621–625, 2004.
10. Pacak K, Linehan WM, Eisenhofer G, et al. Recent advances in genetics, diagnosis, localization, and treatment of pheochromocytoma. *Ann Intern Med* 134(4):315–329, 2001.

30 ANEMIA AND TRANSFUSION MEDICINE

Gabriela S. Ferreira and Jeffrey L. Carson

INTRODUCTION

- Anemia is commonly present in patients prior to surgery.
- The causes of preoperative anemia are similar to those in the general population.
- Since blood loss commonly occurs during surgery, it is essential to identify and treat the anemia.
- Preoperative and postoperative anemia increase risk of mortality and morbidity. The risk associated with anemia may be greatest in patients with cardiovascular disease.
- Blood transfusion is the mainstay of therapy of anemia, although erythropoietin and methods to reduce blood loss are widely used techniques.

PREVALENCE

- The prevalence of anemia varies depending on the patient populations studied. Rates have been reported ranging from 5 to 58 percent.[1] Using hematocrit <36 percent as the definition of anemia, a study of 6301 veterans undergoing noncardiac surgery had a 33.9 percent prevalence of anemia. In a study of 27,370 hip fracture patients, the prevalence of anemia was 10 percent.

TABLE 30-1 Patient- and Surgery-Specific Risk Factors

PATIENT	SURGERY
Bleeding	Type
Hemolysis	Duration
Decreased bone marrow production	Hemodilution
Chronic disease—uremia, endocrine disease, malignancy, connective tissue disorders	Blood loss
Maturation abnormalities from vitamin B_{12} or folate deficiency	

PATIENT-RELATED RISK FACTORS (TABLE 30-1)

- Patient characteristics that increase the likelihood of anemia include increasing age and the presence of comorbid illness such as diabetes, hypertension, angina, congestive heart failure, cardiopulmonary disease, vascular disease, malignancy, and pregnancy.[1]
- The specific cause of anemia has not been demonstrated to be associated with risk of anemia during the perioperative time period.
- The specific causes of anemia may be categorized into four groups: red blood cell loss, increased destruction, reduced production, and iatrogenic (phlebotomy for blood tests) (see Chap. 59).
- Patients with chronic forms of anemia have more time to compensate for it by increasing 2-3 DPG than patients with acute causes of anemia. However, there is no evidence that patients tolerate chronic anemia better than the acute forms during the perioperative period or in any other clinical setting.
- The severity of anemia and patient's comorbidity influence the surgical risk.
- The preoperative hemoglobin concentration is associated with the odds of death in patients who decline blood transfusion for religious reasons[2] (Fig. 30-1).
- In patients with cardiovascular disease (defined as any history of coronary artery disease, congestive heart failure, cerebrovascular disease, or peripheral vascular disease), the risk of death or serious morbidity rises more rapidly as the hemoglobin concentration falls than it does in patients without cardiovascular disease.

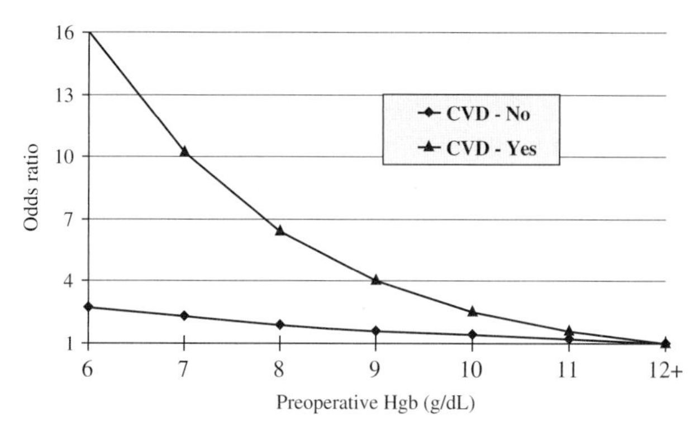

FIG. 30-1 Odds of death by preoperative hemoglobin concentration and presence of cardiovascular disease. (From Carson et al.,[2] with permission.)

TABLE 30-2 Techniques to Decrease Risk of Anemia

PREOPERATIVE	INTRAOPERATIVE	POSTOPERATIVE
Transfusion	Acute normovolemic hemodilution	See Chap. 59
Erythropoietin	Intraoperative recovery of blood	
Preoperative autologous donation	Synthetic oxygen carriers	
Iron therapy		

- The presence of acute or chronic pulmonary disease has not been established to increase the risk associated with anemia. However, in patients with hypoxemia, oxygen delivery to the peripheral tissues may be compromised by superimposed anemia.

SURGERY-RELATED RISK FACTORS

- Surgery-specific risk factors for anemia include the type of surgery, anticipated blood loss, and duration of surgery. These are discussed in detail in Chap. 59.
- These factors also independently contribute to increased perioperative mortality and morbidity.
- The risk of death associated with anemia rises with increasing operative blood loss and lower preoperative hemoglobin concentration.
- The postoperative hemoglobin concentration can be estimated based on the preoperative hemoglobin concentration and the estimated blood loss.

PREOPERATIVE EVALUATION AND TESTING TO STRATIFY RISK (TABLE 30-2)

- When there is time, the patient should undergo a thorough evaluation for anemia. Often patients must undergo surgery quickly. In those situations, it is advisable to obtain the diagnostic studies prior to transfusion or surgery.
- The evaluation of preoperative anemia should follow the approach used in the nonsurgical setting. A careful history and physical examination are essential to determine possible cause of anemia. In general the physical examination is not specific unless blood is detected in the stool or findings such as splenomegaly are identified.
- Laboratory evaluation should start with a reticulocyte count and complete blood count and peripheral smear to establish the degree of anemia and distinguish causes of acute blood loss and red cell destruction from hypoproliferative anemias.
- Examination of the peripheral smear for evidence of hemolysis and the morphology, size, and volume of red blood cells further refines the possible causes.
- Measurement of coagulation factors and a comprehensive chemistry panel, including, in some cases, total bilirubin and lactate dehydrogenase level can sometimes point to other causes of anemia such as uremia or liver disease.
- Additional laboratory testing should be guided by these initial findings, such as obtaining an iron level in microcytic anemia, B_{12} and folate levels in macrocytic anemias, and thyroid-stimulating hormone levels in normocytic anemias.
- Bone marrow biopsy should be reserved for those patients in whom etiology remains unclear after these initial steps.
- Perform an electrocardiogram to assess for ischemic changes. A cardiac evaluation should be performed, as outlined in Chap. 20.

PERIOPERATIVE RISK STRATIFICATION

- The perioperative risk of mortality and morbidity increases with increasing degree of preoperative and postoperative anemia, especially in patients with cardiovascular disease [2] (Fig. 30-1).
- In patients with cardiovascular disease, morbidity and mortality increases with a hemoglobin concentration below 10 g/dL.
- In patients without cardiovascular disease, the risk of anemia is lower. When the hemoglobin concentration falls below 5 to 6 g/dL, the risk of death is very high.

PERIOPERATIVE MANAGEMENT TO REDUCE RISK (TABLE 30-2)

- If there is time, identify the cause of anemia and delay surgery until anemia is corrected as much as possible. Many surgical procedures can and should be delayed.
- The management of preoperative anemia depends on the cause. Correct nutritional deficiencies as quickly as possible (iron, folic acid, and vitamin B_{12}). If oral iron cannot be used, administer sodium ferric gluconate complex (Ferrelicit) intravenously (125 mg for 8 doses). This iron preparation does not cause the anaphylaxis reactions seen with iron dextran.
- Bleeding should be stopped and coagulopathies reversed, if possible, depending on the acuity of surgery.
- If a cause for hemolysis is found, every effort should be made to either withdraw the offending trigger (such as medication), or treat with corticosteroids for immune-mediated causes.

BLOOD TRANSFUSION

- Blood transfusion is often required to treat anemia in the perioperative period. The indications remain controversial.
- The only adequately powered randomized clinical trial to evaluate the efficacy of blood transfusion on mortality and morbidity was performed in intensive care patients.[3] This trial found that a transfusion trigger of 7 g/dL was as safe as a transfusion trigger of 10 g/dL. In patients below 55 years of age and less ill (APACHE 2 score less than 20), mortality was lower in the group receiving 7 g/dL than in those given 10 g/dL. Whether these results can be applied to surgical patients is uncertain.
- An analysis of patients with ischemic heart disease from the trial in intensive care patients found a nonsignificant reduction in mortality in patients maintained above the threshold of 10 g/dL. This finding suggests (but certainly does not prove) that patients with underlying cardiovascular disease may benefit from a higher transfusion trigger.
- Several large observational studies evaluating the effect of a transfusion trigger in patients with underlying cardiovascular disease have come to different conclusions. One study in patients with myocardial infarction found that patients with hemoglobin concentrations below 11 g/dL who received a blood transfusion had a lower mortality than those who did not receive a blood transfusion.[4] A second study in patients with acute coronary syndrome found an increase in mortality and recurrent myocardial infarction in patients receiving transfusion.[5] A third study in hip fracture patients with or without cardiovascular disease undergoing surgical repair found no impact of transfusion on mortality.[6]
- A large clinical trial under way is comparing a threshold of 10 g/dL to a symptomatic threshold or 8 g/dL in patients with cardiovascular disease undergoing repair of hip fracture (Table 30-3).
- Therefore the optimal hemoglobin or hematocrit in surgical patients remains unclear. The authors recommend using a restrictive transfusion trigger of 7 to 8 g/dL in most patients. It may be prudent to use a higher transfusion trigger (9 to 10 g/dL) in patients with cardiovascular disease.[7]
- Transfusion decision should be modified by several other factors besides the hemoglobin concentration.
- If the patient has signs and/or symptoms of anemia, blood transfusion may be indicated. These symptoms include chest pain thought to be cardiac in origin, congestive heart failure, orthostatic hypotension, or tachycardia unresponsive to fluid resuscitation.
- Transfusion decision should take into account future blood loss. Prior to surgery, consideration should be given to the average blood loss associated with the surgical procedure. In patients undergoing a surgical procedure that frequently leads to a large blood loss, it is prudent to transfuse prior to surgery. In patients undergoing a surgical procedure associated with minimal blood loss, transfusion may be unnecessary.
- No set of guidelines should substitute for thoughtful individualized assessment of the patient's symptoms, signs, and underlying comorbidity.

TABLE 30-3 Techniques to Reduce Allogeneic Blood Transfusion

TECHNIQUE	COMMENTS
Restrictive transfusion threshold (7 g/dL)	Most effective approach to reduce allogeneic blood use. Clinical trial showed as safe and perhaps safer in younger or less ill patients. Has not been evaluated in surgical patients or those with underlying cardiovascular disease.
Predeposit autologous transfusion	Widely used in orthopedic surgery. Not recommended by authors since leads to greater risk of transfusion and blood is frequently wasted.
Acute normovolemic hemodilution	Requires removal of large amount of blood and blood loss to result in clinically significant reduction in transfusion.
Intraoperative blood collection	Cell savers widely effective in patients with large-volume blood loss.
Synthetic oxygen carriers	New class of drugs that hold great theoretical promise but none are close to FDA approval.

ERYTHROPOIETIN

- Erythropoietin is approved by the U.S. Food and Drug Administration (FDA) for the treatment of anemic patients with hemoglobin concentration >10 to ≤13 g/dL scheduled to undergo elective, noncardiac, nonvascular surgery to reduce the need for allogeneic blood transfusions. Most of the experience has been in patients undergoing joint replacement surgery.[8]
- The drug should be considered only in patients at high risk for perioperative transfusions with significant blood loss.
- Erythropoietin is administered either subcutaneously or intravenously. Since relative iron deficiency develops in many patients, supplemental iron should also be administered.
- The drug is contraindicated in patients with uncontrolled hypertension or known sensitivity to albumin. Rare side effects include pure red cell aplasia, seizures, and allergic reactions. The risk of thromboembolism may be increased and prophylaxis should be used.
- The recommended dose of erythropoietin alpha is 300 U/kg/day subcutaneously for 10 days before surgery, on the day of surgery, and for 4 days after surgery. An alternate dose schedule is 600 U/kg subcutaneously in once-weekly doses (21, 14, and 7 days before surgery) plus a fourth dose on day of surgery.
- The drug is expensive and reimbursement varies by insurer. The expense and need to administer by injection has been a barrier to widespread use in the perioperative setting.
- Darbepoietin alpha is new erythroid stimulator with a longer half-life. This drug is not FDA-approved for perioperative use, although it is likely to be as effective as erythropoietin alpha.

PREOPERATIVE AUTOLOGOUS DONATION

- Preoperative autologous donation is widely used in preparation for elective surgery (orthopedic) associated with significant blood loss. One to four units of blood are stored in the blood bank and administered during or after surgery.[8]
- The underlying premise of this treatment is that after a unit of blood is drawn and stored, the bone marrow will replete the stored blood. However, most studies demonstrate that the response to autologous donation is not adequate, and most patients go to surgery anemic.
- Another underlying premise of this treatment is that the risk of blood transfusion is reduced by eliminating the transmission of viral infections (i.e., HIV, hepatitis C), since the patient is receiving only his or her own blood. However, the risk of transmission of viral infections is very low (human immunodeficiency virus and hepatitis C, 1 per 2 million). The most common cause of life-threatening adverse effects of blood transfusion is from giving the wrong unit of blood to the wrong patient, a medical error. The use of autologous blood does not reduce this risk.
- Counterintuitively, clinical trials demonstrate that the overall rate of blood transfusion (autologous and allogeneic) is higher in patients undergoing preoperative autologous donation. Furthermore, approximately 50 percent of autologous units are wasted if the procedure is not limited to surgical procedures associated with high blood loss.
- It is likely that simultaneous administration of erythropoietin is required to reduce the use of blood. However, this strategy is expensive.
- The authors recommend against using this procedure.

SYNTHETIC OXYGEN CARRIERS

- None of these oxygen carriers have been approved for use and only one drug is currently in clinical trials.[8]

ACUTE NORMOVOLEMIC HEMODILUTION

- Acute normovolemic hemodilution involves removing blood from a patient in the operating room just prior to surgery and replacing it with crystalloid. Blood is collected in standard blood bags and stored in the operating room. After hemostasis is established, the blood is infused back into the patient.[8]
- Studies using mathematical models suggest that for hemodilution to save a clinically significant amount of blood, the hematocrit must be reduced to less than 20 percent and there must be substantial blood loss.
- Most patients cannot tolerate this degree of anemia. However, if blood substitutes become available, it may be possible to achieve significant reduction in allogeneic blood transfusion using this technique.
- The authors recommend against using this technique.

INTRAOPERATIVE RECOVERY OF BLOOD

- A cell-saver device is used to collect blood lost at the time of operation. The blood is washed and reinfused back into the patient.[8]
- This procedure is contraindicated in patients in whom there is the potential to reinfuse malignant cells, in the presence of infection, or when there is a significant risk of infusing other fluids such as amniotic fluid or ascites.

- This technique is cost-effective only in patients with heavy bleeding.

SPECIAL SITUATIONS

BLOODLESS SURGERY

- Bloodless surgery is surgery performed without the use of blood. These programs were developed to support patients who are Jehovah's Witnesses.[9]
- If possible, delay surgery in patients with anemia. Evaluate the cause of anemia and perform surgery only after the hemoglobin level is back to normal or as high as is achievable.
- In patients with the potential for significant blood loss or in those with potentially life-threatening hemoglobin concentrations, stimulate bone marrow with erythropoietin.
- Meticulous surgical technique to minimize blood loss is essential. Use a cell-saver device in patients with large-volume blood loss.
- There is a tendency to delay surgery in sick, complicated patients who decline blood transfusion in the hope that bleeding will stop. It is essential to stop the bleeding before it reaches the critical levels of 5 to 6 g/dL. Early surgery is recommended.

REFERENCES

1. Shander A, Knight K, Thurer R, et al. Prevalence and outcomes of anemia in surgery: A systematic review of the literature. *Am J Med* 116(7A):58S–69S, 2004.
2. Carson JL, Duff A, Poses RM, et al. Effect of anemia and cardiovascular disease on surgical mortality and morbidity. *Lancet* 348:1055–1060, 1996.
3. Hebert PC, Wells G, Blajchman MA, et al. A multicenter randomized controlled clinical trial of transfusion requirements in critical care. *N Engl J Med* 340:409–417, 1999.
4. Wu WC, Rathore SS, Wang Y, et al. Blood transfusion in elderly patients with acute myocardial infarction. *N Engl J Med* 345:1230–1236, 2001.
5. Rao SV, Jollis JG, Harrington RA, et al. Relationship of blood transfusion and clinical outcomes in patients with acute coronary syndromes. *JAMA* 292(13):1555–1562, 2004.
6. Carson JL, Duff A, Berlin JA, et al. Influence of perioperative blood transfusion on postoperative mortality. *JAMA* 279: 199–295, 1998.
7. Carson JL, Hebert P. Anemia and red cell transfusion, in Simon TL, Dzik WH, Snyder E, et al (eds), *Rossi's Principles of Transfusion Medicine*. Philadelphia: Lippincott, Williams & Wilkins, 2002.
8. Goodnough LT, Brecher ME, Kanter MH, AuBuchon JP. Transfusion medicine. *N Engl J Med* 340:438–447, 525–533, 1999.
9. Goodnough LT, Shander A, Spence R. Bloodless medicine: Clinical care without allogenic blood transfusion. *Transfusion* 43:668–676, 2003.

31 COAGULATION DISORDERS

Kurt Pfeifer and Majed Abu-Hajir

INTRODUCTION

Coagulation disorders can have a major impact on perioperative management and outcomes. Both hypercoagulable states and bleeding diatheses contribute to postoperative morbidity.

This chapter focuses on screening for coagulation disorders and perioperative management of those that have been identified prior to surgery. Coagulation disorders diagnosed in the postoperative setting are discussed in Chap. 59.

PATIENT-RELATED RISK FACTORS

- Patient-specific risk factors for coagulation abnormalities can be divided into two broad categories: inherited and acquired coagulopathies.
- Patients may have risk factors for both hypercoagulability and excessive bleeding, so the clinician must carefully assess patients' overall risk profiles in determining a preoperative hematologic risk-modification plan that will allow safe performance of surgery.

INHERITED COAGULOPATHIES

THROMBOPHILIAS

- Inherited thrombophilias pose a particular challenge in the perioperative setting because the postoperative state itself is a major risk factor for thrombosis.
- Many hereditary thrombophilias go undiagnosed, so their prevalence is likely higher than most clinicians perceive.
- Coinheritance of more than one hypercoagulable defect is common among those with inherited thrombophilia, and carriers of more than one defect have a much higher risk of venous thromboembolism (VTE).
  - ***Factor V Leiden (FVL):*** This is the most common form of inherited thrombophilia, found in up to 50 percent of cases of familial thrombosis. Mutation of the gene that encodes for coagulation factor V causes resistance to protein C–mediated degradation of activated factor V. Inhibition of this normal anticoagulation mechanism results in a hypercoagulable state. Homozygosity for FVL is rare, but heterozygosity also causes thrombophilia and is present in 5 percent of the U.S. population. The mutation is rare in African and Asian populations but even more common in patients

from Scandinavia, Greece, and the Middle East. Studies of the risk of VTE, recurrent deep venous thrombosis (DVT), and mortality in patients with FVL have generated conflicting results. In studies of patients with DVT, up to 30 percent are found to have FVL, with a 7-fold increase in relative risk in heterozygotes and 80-fold in homozygotes, based on retrospective assessment of risk. However, in prospective studies of FVL carriers, there was no significant increase in spontaneous VTE but a 3.5 percent risk of VTE per episode of surgery, trauma, or immobilization.[1] This level of perioperative VTE risk is much lower than that in other inherited thrombophilias and has not been found to be significant in other studies.[2] In summary, the published data suggest that FVL mutation confers less risk for VTE than most other known risk factors and appears to increase the risk of VTE events incurred by other coexisting risk factors.

- ***Prothrombin gene G20210A mutation (PTGM):*** This point mutation of the prothrombin gene results in elevated plasma levels of prothrombin, which leads to an increased risk of venous thrombosis. The original descriptive studies identified this thrombophilic defect in 18 percent of patients with a personal and family history of VTE; but like FVL, it is uncommon in African and Asian populations. In studies of patients with a history of VTE, up to 40 percent were found also to carry FVL. The relative risk of VTE in patients with PTGM alone is 2.8. Unlike other inherited thrombophilias, homozygosity for this mutation does not increase thrombosis risk markedly more than heterozygosity. Some studies also indicate an increased risk of arterial thrombosis, unlike most other disorders mentioned here.
- ***Deficiency of natural anticoagulants:*** Thrombosis risk is also increased by abnormalities of naturally occurring proteins that are important in controlling thrombin generation and preventing extension of clotting reactions beyond the necessary hemostasis field. Such natural anticoagulants include protein C (PC) and its cofactor protein S (PS) as well as antithrombin (AT), previously known as antithrombin III. Abnormalities of these proteins are inherited in an autosomal dominant manner, either as mutations that result in reduction of quantity, termed type I deficiency, or mutations resulting in normal quantities of dysfunctional molecules, termed type II deficiency. Both situations will result in reduced protein activity; thus this should be measured in screening suspected individuals.
  - AT deficiency is present in 1 per 2500 people in the general population. Relative risk of VTE in AT deficiency is increased by 20 times and the lifetime risk approaches 100 percent by the time the affected individual reaches 70 years of age. Unlike other disorders, this one is amenable to replacement therapy with an available concentrate approved in the United States.
  - PC deficiency is present in 1 per 200 to 500 individuals in the general population; VTE occurs in 75 percent of patients and is more likely to be spontaneous than in AT deficiency. PC and PS are vitamin K–dependent factors, and their deficiency is known for its association with warfarin-induced skin necrosis, although this has been described with other thrombophilias as well.
  - PS deficiency results in lifetime VTE risk of 75 percent in affected patients. Under normal circumstances, around half of the circulating protein S is bound by C4b-binding protein, so it can be measured as total and free plasma protein S antigen levels. The protein S activity measuring the functional component reflects the free form of the protein S antigen. This complicates interpretation of protein S assays, especially in women who are pregnant or receiving estrogen, since estrogen increases the levels of C4b-binding protein.
- ***Hyperhomocysteinemia:*** This thrombophilia was first described in patients with homocystinuria, a very rare condition caused by homozygous mutation of cystathionine-β-synthase and characterized by severely elevated serum levels of homocysteine. Unlike the previously described inherited defects, this condition was found to be associated with an approximately 50 percent prevalence of both arterial and venous thromboses. Subsequent studies also identified moderate elevations of homocysteine as an independent risk factor for arterial and venous thrombosis. In addition to various nongenetic causes, mutations of the methyltetrahydrofolate reductase (MTHFR) gene can increase the risk for developing some degree of hyperhomocysteinemia, especially when combined with certain nutritional deficiencies (i.e., pyridoxine, vitamin B_{12}, folate).
- ***Other inherited thrombophilias:*** There are several other rare inherited thrombophilias that are less well established, including plasminogen deficiency, heparin cofactor II deficiency, factor XIII mutations, dysfibrinogenemia, and excess plasminogen activator inhibitor 1 (PAI-1), whose complexity precludes discussion within the scope of this text. They require no specific evaluation or management prior to surgery but should be considered during DVT risk estimation and prophylaxis decision making. It is also important to note that there appear to be individuals with a clear history of familial thrombosis that have yet to be characterized. It is estimated that 30 percent of such individuals cannot be categorized by currently available testing; hence the importance of identifying a family history of thrombosis. Patients with such a history should be considered at high risk even in the absence of positive testing for the known thrombophilias.

Bleeding Diatheses

- Inherited bleeding diatheses are uncommon but can have a profound impact on postoperative care and morbidity. Unlike hereditary thrombophilia, genetic bleeding diatheses are usually diagnosed long before the preoperative evaluation. The exception to this is von Willebrand's disease (vWD), which may go undetected until a patient's first surgery.
    - ***Von Willebrand's disease:*** vWD is perhaps the most common hereditary bleeding disorder and is caused by deficiency (types 1 and 3) or dysfunction (type 2) of von Willebrand factor (vWF), which is responsible for platelet adherence to blood vessel walls. It has an estimated prevalence of 1 to 2 percent in the general population and can be inherited in both autosomal dominant (more common) and autosomal recessive patterns. The disease is manifest by failure of the primary phase of hemostasis, causing mucocutaneous bleeding, and also failure of the secondary phase of hemostasis, causing bleeding in soft tissue sites as well as postoperative bleeding.
    - ***Hemophilia A (factor VIII deficiency):*** Hemophilia A is an X-linked recessive disorder caused by mutation of the gene encoding factor VIII. It occurs in 1 per 5000 to 10,000 male births and has equal prevalence among all ethnicities. The disease is classified into three forms: severe (50 to 60 percent of patients), moderately severe (25 to 30 percent), and mild (15 to 20 percent). Severity of clinical manifestations is directly proportional to factor VIII level. Severe hemophilia A is seen with factor VIII activity <2 percent of normal and is characterized by spontaneous hemorrhage into joints and soft tissues. Patients with moderately severe hemophilia A have 2 to 5 percent of normal factor VIII activity and are prone to bleeding after minor trauma. In the mild form of hemophilia A, factor VIII activity ranges from 5 to 30 percent and bleeding typically occurs only with significant trauma or surgery.
    - ***Hemophilia B (factor IX deficiency):*** This is another X-linked recessive disorder caused by mutation of the factor IX gene. It is much less common than hemophilia A, accounting for 12 percent of total hemophilia cases, and is more frequently associated with de novo mutations. In approximately one-third of patients, factor IX antigen level will be normal, while antigen activity will be abnormal. However, bleeding complications correlate well with factor IX activity and are similar to those of hemophilia A.
    - ***Other inherited bleeding diatheses:*** Deficiencies of several other coagulation factors (II, V, VII, X, XI, and XIII) and congenital disorders of fibrinogen also predispose patients to bleeding, but they are very rare and beyond the scope of this text.

ACQUIRED COAGULOPATHIES

Hypercoagulable States

- The physiologic mechanisms of coagulation are complex, and a number of conditions increase the risk of thrombosis in poorly understood ways.
- Though thrombophilia is categorized as inherited or acquired, the clinician must understand that the two can interplay to create thrombotic risk. For instance, many patients with inherited thrombophilia do not sustain VTE unless they are exposed to one of the clinical conditions described below.
- Many clinical conditions (Table 31-1) are risk factors for thrombosis. Discussion of these conditions is limited to those of special interest and which fit within the scope of this textbook.
    - ***Pregnancy:*** Pregnancy causes a sixfold increase in relative risk for VTE. Pulmonary embolism (PE) is the most common cause of maternal death and accounts for 1 out of 8 deaths of pregnant patients. Mechanisms for this increased risk include venous stasis, increases in plasma coagulation proteins (i.e., coagulation factors, plasminogen-activator 2), and reduction in protein S activity. The risk of VTE is equally increased in each trimester throughout the pregnancy and during the postpartum period. A large percentage of pregnancy-related VTE is associated with coexistent inherited thrombophilias.
    - ***Exogenous estrogens/progestins:*** Observational studies have identified a two- to sixfold increased relative risk of VTE with use of either hormonal contraceptives or hormone replacement therapies (HRTs).[4] The thrombotic risk is higher with higher estrogen dose and products containing third-generation progestins, such as desogestrel and gestodene. However, VTE risk appears to be lower in progestin-only oral contraceptives and transdermal preparations. Furthermore, additional VTE risk factors, especially inherited thrombophilias, substantially increase the risk of thrombosis in patients using estrogens. The risk in postoperative patients receiving hormone replacement therapy (HRT) was also described in the Heart and Estrogen/Progestin Replacement Study (HERS). Patients in the HERS study had a severalfold increase in VTE risk for orthopedic and nonorthopedic surgery, which was present for 90 days after surgery.[5] A study of surgical patients using oral contraceptives (OCPs) demonstrated a non-statistically significant doubling of VTE risk compared to patients who discontinued OCP therapy the month prior to surgery.
    - ***Malignancy:*** All types of cancer cause hypercoagulability through a variety of mechanisms, including excessive elevation in coagulation factor levels, cytokines, and cancer procoagulant A.[3] VTE develops

TABLE 31-1 Patient-Related Risk Factors for Coagulation Disorders

THROMBOSIS	BLEEDING
Inherited	**Inherited**
Factor V Leiden	Von Willebrand's disease
Prothrombin gene mutation	Hemophilia A and B
Antithrombin III deficiency	
Protein C deficiency	
Protein S deficiency	
Hyperhomocysteinemia	
Acquired	**Acquired**
Advanced age	Bleeding with previous procedures
Obesity	Renal insufficiency
Pregnancy	Hepatic insufficiency
Trauma	Anticoagulants
Immobilization	Platelet-inhibiting medications
Postoperative state	Coagulation factor inhibitors
Nutritional deficiencies (B_6, B_{12}, folate-causing hyperhomocysteinemia)	Idiopathic thrombocytopenic purpura
Exogenous estrogens/progestins	Disseminated intravascular coagulation
Smoking	
Malignancy	
Prior VTE	
Nephrotic syndrome	
Congestive heart failure	
Diabetes mellitus	
Chronic obstructive pulmonary disease	
Polycythemia vera	
Paroxysmal nocturnal hematuria	
Heparin-induced thrombocytopenia	
Thrombotic thrombocytopenic purpura	
Antiphospholipid antibody syndrome	

in 10 to 20 percent of patients with cancer; the risk is especially high in those with adenocarcinoma (i.e., pancreatic, lung cancer) and other risk factors for thrombosis. Patients with cancer can also be at risk for thrombosis due to the adverse effects of some chemotherapeutic agents (i.e., asparaginase, mitomycin, selective estrogen receptor modulators). Catheter-related thrombosis is also a common problem in cancer patients with indwelling vascular access devices.

- ***Antiphospholipid antibody syndrome (APLAS):*** Like hyperhomocysteinemia, APLAS is characterized by a predisposition to both venous and arterial thromboses. It is estimated to be the cause of up to 15 percent of spontaneous DVT, one-third of strokes in patients under age 50, and 10 percent of cases of recurrent miscarriages. The exact pathophysiologic cause of APLAS is debated, but it may possibly be due to antibodies causing enhanced binding of beta$_2$-glycoprotein I to phospholipid cellular surfaces. APLAS is classically associated with systemic lupus erythematosus (SLE), thus its synonym lupus anticoagulant. An isolated elevated partial thromboplastin time (PTT) that does not correct with 1:1 mix study is a typical presentation on preoperative evaluation. However, the majority of cases of APLAS are encountered in other clinical conditions, including malignancy, infection, and other autoimmune diseases. The presence of persistent APLA more than 6 weeks later is an indication for long-term anticoagulation even in patients with triggered VTE. A subset of patients can develop the catastrophic antiphospholipid antibody syndrome (CAPS) if they undergo surgery without effective pharmacologic thromboprophylaxis. This is characterized by sequential thrombotic events, including bleeding resulting from organ infarction, and has a high mortality.

HEMOSTATIC DEFICIENCIES

- Normal hemostatic mechanisms may be disrupted by causes ranging from the consequences of thrombosis treatment to systemic disorders with complex effects on hemostasis (see Table 31-1).
  - ***Anticoagulant/thrombolytic medications:*** Patients undergoing treatment for acute or chronic thrombosis are at risk for bleeding caused by these therapies. Patients receiving thrombolytic therapy (i.e., tissue plasminogen activator, urokinase) are obviously at high risk for hemorrhage and cannot undergo surgery without discontinuation of treatment. Anticoagulants—including unfractionated heparin, low-molecular-weight heparin (LMWH), fondaparinux, lepirudin, and argatroban—also increase bleeding risk. However, some surgeries may be performed while patients have therapeutic levels of these medications (see Chap. 7A for details).
  - ***Platelet-inhibiting medications:*** Nonsteroidal anti-inflammatory drugs (NSAIDs) induce platelet dysfunction through inhibition of cyclooxygenase. Most NSAIDs cause reversible inhibition of this enzyme, but aspirin causes irreversible inhibition while cyclooxygenase 2 (COX-2)-specific agents (i.e., celecoxib) have little or no effect on platelets. Clopidogrel

and ticlopidine irreversibly block adenodiphosphate-mediated platelet aggregation, while cilostazol causes reversible platelet inhibition through its phosphodiesterase inhibition. Dipyridamole is rarely used alone and causes mild reversible platelet dysfunction.
- ◦ ***Renal insufficiency:*** Patients with renal disease have platelet dysfunction thought to be due to increased nitric oxide synthesis in platelets and endothelium. The degree of platelet dysfunction is directly related to the severity of renal insufficiency and generally becomes manifest with other signs or symptoms of uremia.
- ◦ ***Hepatic insufficiency:*** Liver disease disrupts normal hemostasis in several ways: it causes decreased hepatic synthesis of coagulation factors, thrombocytopenia (due to hypersplenism), and abnormal platelet function. The degree of hemostatic deficiency is proportional to the severity of hepatic insufficiency.
- ◦ ***Coagulation factor inhibitors:*** Approximately 5 percent of patients with hemophilia A and 3 percent with hemophilia B will develop inhibitors to coagulation factors VIII and IX, respectively, in response to exposure to various blood products. These inhibitors are antibodies that do not cause hemorrhage themselves but hamper attempts to treat bleeding in hemophiliacs. In addition to hemophilia-associated coagulation inhibitors, a number of reports have described spontaneous occurrence of factor VIII inhibitors.[6] These patients present with an unexplained elevation of PTT that does not correct with mixing studies; these patients may have autoimmune disease, pregnancy or malignancy.
- ◦ ***Immune thrombocytopenic purpura (ITP):*** This condition is characterized by variably decreased platelet counts due to autoantibody-mediated destruction of platelets. ITP affects 1 in 10,000 persons, is more common in women, and is most often diagnosed in the third decade of life. However, it can occur in either sex at any age. Platelet destruction leads to a greater number of larger, less mature platelets in plasma. These less mature platelets generally have more hemostatic potential than normal platelets, thus partially offsetting the bleeding potential in patients with ITP.
- ◦ ***Disseminated intravascular coagulation (DIC):*** DIC is a syndrome of diffuse, inappropriate thrombin generation followed by aggressive secondary fibrinolysis, which is seen in many different clinical settings including sepsis, obstetric complications, malignancy, and advanced liver disease. The initial thrombogenic phase causes diffuse microthrombi but can also cause large vessel thrombosis. However, bleeding complications can be observed in patients with fulminant decompensated DIC largely because of the depletion of coagulations secondary to increased consumption. Such patients usually have a significantly elevated prothrombin time (PT) and PTT and a low level of fibrinogen.
- ◦ ***Dilution coagulopathy:*** Also known as a massive transfusion syndrome, this can occur when a patient with severe bleeding receives large amounts of red cells but proportionately less amounts of plasma, thus diluting the amount of available clotting factors in the circulation. This is a more common issue in trauma patients undergoing emergency surgery than in those having elective surgery.

SURGERY-RELATED RISK FACTORS

SURGICAL SITE

- Intraoperative and postoperative bleeding is particularly important in surgeries involving critical body areas or where bleeding could seriously compromise the surgical result or go undetected until life-threatening blood loss has occurred. Examples of such surgical procedures include neurosurgery, ophthalmologic surgery, laparotomy, and laparoscopy.
- Cardiac surgery, hip and knee arthroplasty, lumbar spinal fusion, tonsillectomy, and prostatectomy also carry an increased risk of major hemorrhage, so preoperative hematologic evaluation must take these into account. A list of typical amounts of blood loss for common surgical procedures is given in Chap. 59. Further details on the bleeding risk of specific types of surgery can be found in Sec. II.
- Postoperative risk of VTE also varies depending on the type of surgery and is particularly high in intracranial surgery, hip fracture repair, hip arthroplasty, and knee arthroplasty. For further information on the VTE risk of various surgeries, see Chap. 46.

ANESTHESIA TYPE

- No definite association between thrombosis risk and type of anesthesia used has been documented.
- While anesthesia type does not influence the risk of surgical-site or systemic hemorrhage, neuraxial (spinal and epidural) anesthesia has been associated with spinal hematoma in patients with coagulopathies and/or those receiving anticoagulant therapy. This has led to several recommendations regarding the use of neuraxial anesthesia in patients at risk of bleeding: (1) avoid it in patients with known coagulopathies or who are currently receiving antithrombotic therapy (excluding aspirin); (2) do not insert spinal/epidural catheters within 12 h of the administation of a prophylactic dose of LMWH or unfractionated heparin or 24 h of a therapeutic dose; (3) when prophylactic anticoagulation is used

concomitantly with neuraxial analgesia, remove spinal/epidural catheters when the anticoagulant effect is at its lowest (i.e., just prior to a dose); (4) hold anticoagulant therapy for 2 h following removal of a spinal/epidural catheter; (5) limit the duration of neuraxial analgesia to 2 days in patients on warfarin therapy and do not remove the catheter unless the international normalized ratio (INR) is less than 1.5; and (6) defer administering pharmacologic thromboprophylaxis for 24 h if a bloody spinal tap has occurred.[7]

PREOPERATIVE EVALUATION AND TESTING

- Screen patients for bleeding or thrombotic disorders prior to surgery. The most effective method of screening is history and physical examination.
- Routine laboratory testing (platelet count, PT, or PTT) in patients without historical or physical examination evidence of bleeding or thrombosis is not cost-effective and is poorly predictive of perioperative complications.[8] Furthermore, even in patients suspected of having platelet dysfunction, bleeding time is an unreliable test that correlates poorly with postoperative bleeding.
- Preoperative evaluation begins with a thorough history and physical examination looking for evidence of a previously undiagnosed bleeding or thrombotic disorder. Table 31-2 lists history and physical examination findings and the hemostatic abnormalities they suggest.
- When this evaluation suggests evidence of a bleeding diathesis, initial laboratory evaluation should include a platelet count, PT, and PTT. Preoperative testing for thrombophilic conditions is rarely indicated, since it provides no additional prognostic information beyond the history.
- Further evaluation of a potential bleeding disorder proceeds based on the results of these assays (Fig. 31-1). Potential causes of thrombocytopenia are numerous and cannot be adequately covered in this chapter.
- In patients with ITP, hemophilia, and other coagulation deficiencies, measuring the levels of the deficient hemostasis component guides preoperative risk reduction measures.

TABLE 31-2 History and Physical Examination Findings Suggestive of Bleeding and Thrombotic Disorders

HISTORY/EXAMINATION FINDING	COAGULATION ABNORMALITY
Bleeding after surgery (including dental extractions)	
Immediate, mild	Platelet defect
Delayed, severe	Clotting factor deficiency
Gingival bleeding	Platelet defect
Prolonged or excessive menses	Platelet defect or clotting factor deficiency
Prolonged bleeding with minor trauma	Platelet defect
Prior history of venous or arterial thrombosis	Thrombophilia
Prior blood product transfusions	Platelet defect or clotting factor deficiency
History of iron-deficiency anemia	Any bleeding disorder
Recent antibiotic use	Clotting factor deficiency (from vitamin K deficiency)
Family history of excessive bleeding	Platelet defect or clotting factor deficiency
Family history of venous or arterial thrombosis	Thrombophilia
Hemarthroses	Clotting factor deficiency
Ecchymoses	
Small	Platelet defect
Large, palpable	Clotting factor deficiency
Telangiectasias	Liver disease–related coagulopathy

PERIOPERATIVE MANAGEMENT

PREOPERATIVE

Medication Management

(see Chap. 7 for details):

- NSAIDs, including aspirin-containing agents, are usually discontinued prior to any elective procedure. If urgent surgery is required, it can be safely performed without specific prophylactic measures. There is no evidence for providing empiric desmopressin or platelet transfusion to prevent bleeding from NSAID-induced platelet dysfunction.
- Optimal management of hormonal contraception and HRT in the perioperative setting remains controversial. The potential thrombotic risks associated with these therapies must be weighed against the potential risks of discontinuation and the relative risk of thrombosis from the planned procedure.
- Due to their noncritical importance and potential for causing perioperative complications, including bleeding and interference with DVT prophylaxis, all vitamins, herbal remedies, and nutritional supplements should be discontinued 1 to 2 weeks preoperatively and not resumed until the patient has finished any postoperative anticoagulation.
- Discontinue anticoagulant therapy prior to most elective procedures to prevent bleeding complications. However, there are exceptions to this rule, including

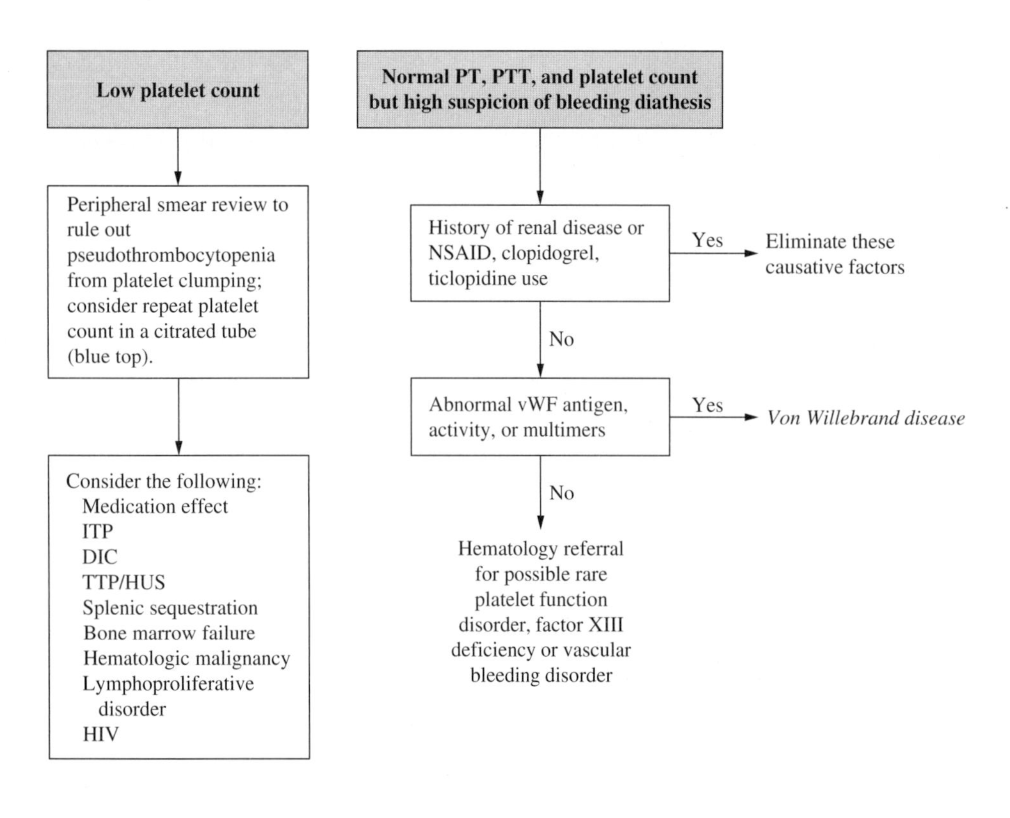

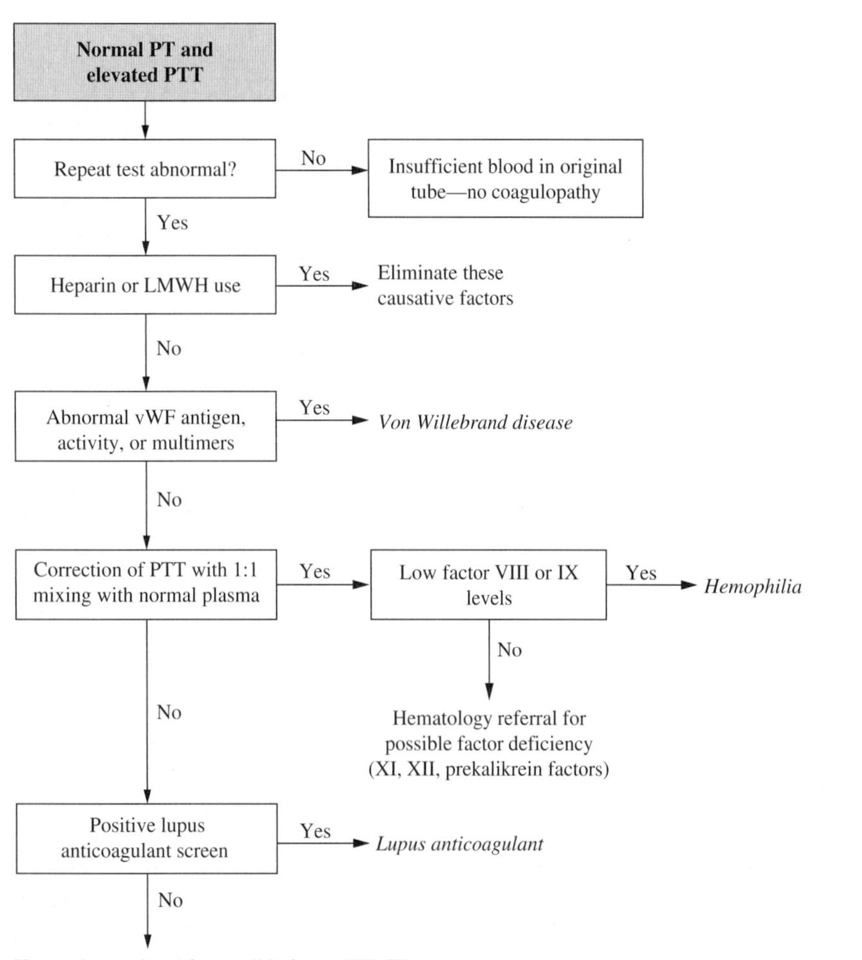

FIG. 31-1 Evaluation of abnormal screening hemostasis tests.

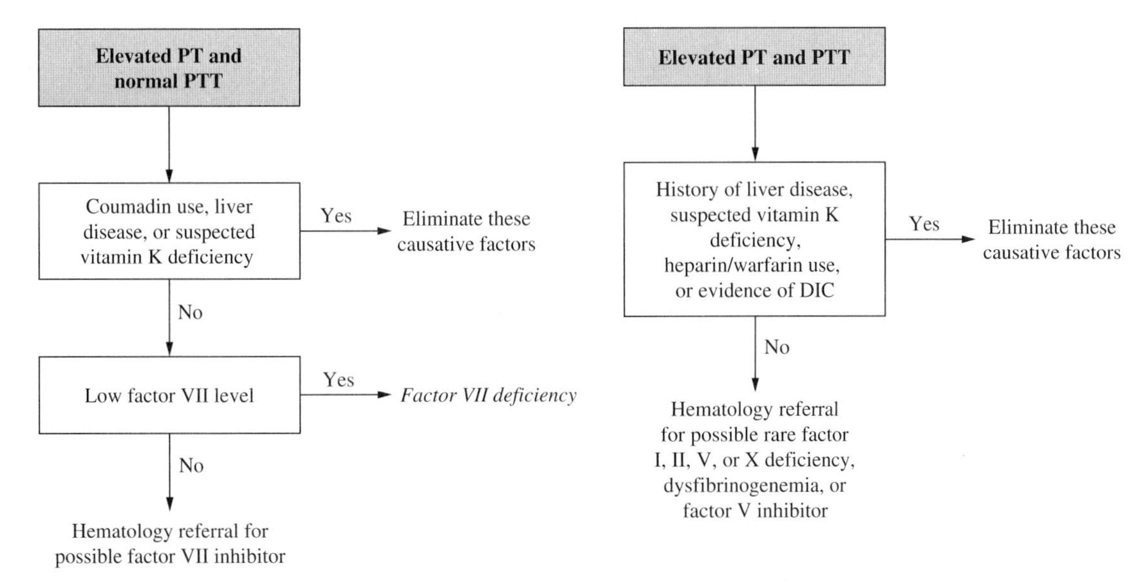

FIG. 31-1 (*Continued*)

cataract surgery. The patient's reason for chronic anticoagulation and risk of thrombosis must be factored into the clinician's plan for perioperative management. Management options include discontinuation with or without "bridging" short-acting anticoagulant therapy or rapid reversal of anticoagulation. This is discussed in detail in Chap. 7A.

Management of Specific Coagulation Abnormalities

- Previously documented or newly diagnosed coagulopathies require specialized preoperative management to reduce perioperative bleeding risk. These therapies and other perioperative risk-reduction methods are listed in Table 31-3.
- Cooperation with hematology and blood bank consultants in the management of coagulopathies is strongly advised.
- Regardless of the type of coagulation abnormality, blood product needs should be anticipated and an appropriate number of units made available.
  - ***Thrombocytopenia:*** Regardless of the cause of thrombocytopenia, maintain a perioperative platelet count greater than 50,000 for most surgeries except neurosurgery and ophthalmic surgery, where counts >100,000 are recommended.[9] Patients with ITP can be given prednisone, intravenous immunoglobulin (IVIG), or methylprednisolone to reduce autoimmune platelet destruction and raise platelet counts preoperatively. Further discussion of perioperative management of thrombocytopenia is provided in Chap. 59.
  - ***Platelet dysfunction:*** In addition to stopping culprit medications (i.e., NSAIDs, clopidogrel), patients with uremia-induced platelet dysfunction and vWD are candidates for further preoperative risk reduction strategies. Uremic patients should undergo dialysis.[10] Patients with a prior history of uremic bleeding should also be treated approximately 30 min preoperatively with desmopressin or cryoprecipitate. A factor VIII level should be determined in vWD patients and therapy instituted to maintain a level >50 percent of normal. Type I vWD patients undergoing minimally invasive procedures can be given desmopressin, but patients undergoing more invasive procedures or with type II or III vWD require intermediate-purity factor VIII concentrates infused at 30 to 50 IU/kg/day to maintain an adequate factor VIII level until healing is complete.[11] Antifibrinolytics [epsilon-aminocaproic acid (EACA) and tranexamic acid], estrogen, and recombinant factor VIIa have also been used successfully to prevent bleeding in vWD patients, especially those who have developed alloantibodies to factor VIII concentrates.
  - ***Coagulation factor deficiencies:*** Hemophilia A and B require 75 to 100 percent of normal factor VIII or IX (respectively) activity for safe performance of surgery, and these levels should be maintained for 72 h after the procedure. After that, trough levels should be maintained above 50 percent of normal until healing is complete, which typically takes 2 weeks. Recombinant or purified factor concentrates should be infused, and monitoring of peak and trough levels should be performed so as to modify doses as needed. Once the patient's responsiveness to the infused factor

TABLE 31-3 Perioperative Risk-Reduction Strategies

COAGULOPATHY	RISK-REDUCTION METHODS
Thrombocytopenia	Stop potential causative meds and agents causing platelet dysfunction. Transfuse platelets to maintain counts > 100,000 for neurosurgery and ophthalmic surgery and >50,000 for other surgeries.
ITP	Prednisone 1 mg/kg/day for 1 week prior to surgery Intravenous immunoglobulin 0.5–1.0 g/kg if urgent surgery or prednisone-unresponsive Platelet transfusion and methylprednisolone 1 g IV if major bleeding, emergency surgery, or above therapies have failed.
Platelet dysfunction	Stop potentially causative meds.
Uremia-induced	Adequate dialysis. Maintain hematocrit ≥ 30. Desmopressin 0.3 μg/kg IV or intranasally or cryoprecipitate if prior history of uremic bleeding. Platelet transfusions if bleeding despite above therapies.
Von Willebrand's disease	Desmopressin for minor procedures in type I vWD. Factor VIII concentrates to maintain factor VIII levels >50% until healing is complete. EACA, tranexamic acid, and recombinant factor VIIa for recalcitrant cases.
Coagulation factor deficiencies	Measure factor levels preoperatively.
Hemophilia A and B	Maintain 75–100% factor VIII or IX levels for 72 h after surgery and then 50% until healing is complete. Dose factor replacement and check factor levels every 8 h.
Coagulation factor inhibitors	Measure inhibitor levels preoperatively.
Factor VIII inhibitor	Recombinant factor VIIa.
Fibrinogen disorders	Cryoprecipitate at approximate dose of 12 units initially followed by 4 units daily until healing is complete.
Hepatic insufficiency	Vitamin K PO or IV. Transfuse FFP to maintain INR <1.5.
Hypercoagulable states	
Inherited	Most require prophylactic anticoagulation. For AT deficiency, AT concentrate to maintain AT activity at 100–120% for several days postoperatively, until INR is in target range in those receiving warfarin.
Acquired	Perform comprehensive VTE risk assessment and initiate prophylactic measures as appropriate.

AT = antithrombin; EACA = epsilon-aminocaproic acid; FFP = fresh frozen plasma; INR = international normalized ratio; ITP = immune thrombocytopenic purpura; VTE = venous thromboembolism; vWD = von Willebrand's disease.

concentrate is documented, daily trough levels must be measured to maintain the desired range. Each unit of factor concentrate increases factor levels by 2 percent per kilogram. An increasingly widespread practice has evolved recently, in the absence of clear data, of offering patients with bleeding disorders pharmacologic thromboprophylaxis once replacement therapy has been accomplished. The rationale is that VTE still occurs, albeit at perhaps reduced frequency, in this population, and anticoagulation in these patients is fraught with complications. By taking extra precautions to prevent VTE, one avoids these difficult scenarios. To adopt this practice is a difficult decision in the absence of clear data; each case should be assessed individually.

- ***Hepatic insufficiency:*** Patients with hepatic insufficiency should be given vitamin K orally to maximize the liver's limited production of coagulation factor. Fresh frozen plasma (FFP) can also be provided to temporarily reverse patients' coagulopathy and achieve an INR <1.5. Further information on perioperative hematologic risk management in liver disease is covered in Chap. 35.

INTRAOPERATIVE

- Communication between the anesthesiologist and surgeon is of prime importance in performing intraoperative monitoring and management of bleeding. If bleeding at the surgical site becomes difficult to manage, the surgeon can inform the anesthesiologist, who can then initiate appropriate laboratory evaluation and treatment.
- Meticulous local hemostasis is especially important in the patient at increased risk of bleeding. Extended observation of the surgical site before closure can help detect bleeding before severe postoperative hemorrhage occurs.
- For patients with disorders of primary hemostasis (i.e., platelet dysfunction, thrombocytopenia), topical use of thrombin preparations or fibrin sealant can help achieve improved local hemostasis.

POSTOPERATIVE

- Management of known bleeding diatheses is similar in the preoperative and postoperative settings and is described in previous sections of this chapter. In addition to monitoring of patients' coagulation profiles, hemoglobin levels and hemodynamics should be monitored closely for signs suggestive of hemorrhage.
- For patients with active bleeding, Chap. 59 provides further details on the evaluation and management of coagulation disorders.

- Recommendations for the duration and type of VTE prophylaxis (as described in Chap. 46) should take hypercoagulability disorders into account.
- Most patients with an inherited thrombophilia should receive anticoagulation for DVT prophylaxis in the postoperative setting. However, literature in this area is conflicting or nonexistent.
- Patients with acquired hypercoagulability should be assessed for overall VTE risk, as detailed in Chap. 46.

SUMMARY

In summary, although coagulation disorders may increase the risk of hemorrhagic and thrombotic complications, proper identification and management can allow surgery to be performed safely.

REFERENCES

1. Middeldorp S, Meinardi JR, Koopman MM, et al. A prospective study of asymptomatic carriers of the factor V Leiden mutation to determine the incidence of venous thromboembolism. *Ann Intern Med* 135(5):322–327, 2001.
2. Wahlander K, Larson G, Lindahl TL, et al. Factor V Leiden (G1691A) and prothrombin gene G20210A mutations as potential risk factors for venous thromboembolism after total hip or total knee replacement surgery. *Thromb Haemost* 87:580, 2002.
3. Gomes MP, Deitcher SR. Risk of venous thromboembolic disease associated with hormonal contraceptives and hormone replacement therapy: A clinical review. *Arch Inter Med* 164(18):1965–1976, 2004.
4. Manzullo EF, Weed HG. Perioperative issues in patients with cancer. *Med Clin North Am* 87(1):243–356, 2003.
5. Grady D, Wenger NK, Herrington D, et al. Postmenopausal hormone therapy increases risk for venous thromboembolic disease. *Ann Intern Med* 132:689–696, 2000.
6. Biss T, Crossman L, Neilly I, et al. An acquired factor VIII inhibitor in association with a myeloproliferative/myelodysplastic disorder presenting with severe subcutaneous haemorrhage. *Haemophilia* 9(5):638–641, 2003.
7. Geerts WH, Pineo GF, Heit JA, et al. Prevention of venous thromboembolism: The seventh ACCP conference on antithrombotic and thrombolytic therapy. *Chest* 126: 338S–400S, 2004.
8. Smetana GW, Macpherson DS. The case against routine preoperative laboratory testing. *Med Clin North Am* 87(1):7–40, 2003.
9. British Committee for Standards in Haematology, Blood Transfusion Task Force. Guidelines for the use of platelet transfusions. *Br J Haematol* 122(1):10–23, 2003.
10. Joseph AJ, Cohn SL. Perioperative care of the patient with renal failure. *Med Clin North Am* 87(1):193–210, 2003.
11. Mannucci PM. Treatment of von Willebrand's disease. *N Engl J Med* 351(7):683–694, 2004.

32 CANCER

Colleen G. Lance, Ellen Manzullo, and Harrison G. Weed

INTRODUCTION

- Cancer can make the perioperative period more challenging because of cancer-related concerns, including prognosis, comorbidities, and treatment side effects.

SURGERY-RELATED CONSIDERATIONS

- 75 percent of patients with solid tumors will have surgical resection for cure, and 90 percent will have surgery for either cure or palliation.[1]
    - The purpose of the surgery plays an important role in balancing the relative risks and benefits.
    - Surgeries in patients with cancer can be categorized as diagnostic, curative, palliative, or unrelated to the cancer.
        - Diagnostic (biopsy): Surgery to obtain tissue for prognosis and treatment planning.
        - Even if a patient chooses not to have additional treatment, prognostic information can be useful.
        - Curative: Patients and doctors are usually willing to incur greater risk of harm for the potential of a cure.
        - Palliative: The goals of palliative surgeries include relief of discomfort, improvement in quality of life, and prolongation of life.
            - They include procedures to excise or bypass tumors to relieve obstruction of the airway and of the gastrointestinal (GI) tract, to relieve pain, and to improve appearance.
        - Brachytherapy: The implantation of radioactive materials into or immediately adjacent to the tumor can be for cure or palliation.
            - Because brachytherapy does not involve resection of the tumor, the procedures are usually relatively minor and can often be performed with sedation and local anesthesia.
        - Surgery unrelated to cancer: Elective procedures are usually postponed if the recovery time will delay cancer treatment. Emergent procedures such as appendectomy may require special consideration of the cancer prognosis and of the impact of any cancer treatments on perioperative physiology.

PATIENT-RELATED CONSIDERATIONS BY ORGAN SYSTEM

CANCER AND TREATMENT-RELATED EFFECTS

CARDIOVASCULAR

- Chemotherapy and radiation can have cardiovascular effects that are important in perioperative management.
  - Table 32-1 lists some common cardiotoxicities of chemotherapy.

TABLE 32-1 Common Cardiotoxicities with Chemotherapy

DRUG	SIDE EFFECTS
Anthracyclines/anthraquinolones	CHF-all
Doxorubicin (Adriamycin)	
Daunorubicin (Cerubidine)	
Epirubicin (Ellence, Pharmorubicin)	
Idarubicin (Idamycin)	
Mitoxantrone (Novantrone)	
Aklylating agents	Endomyocardial fibrosis
Busulfan (Myleran)	Cardiac tamponade
Cisplatin (Platinol)	Ischemia, HTN, CHF
Cyclophosphamide (Cytoxan)	Pericarditis, myocarditis, CHF
Ifosamide (Ifex)	CHF, arrhythmias
Mitomycin (Mutamycin)	CHF
Antimetabolites	
Capecitabine (Xeloda)	Ischemia
Cytarabine, ARA-C (Cytosar)	Pericarditis, CHF
Fluorouracil (Adrucil)	Ischemia
Antimicrotubules	
Paclitaxel (Taxol)	Arrhythmias, CHF, hypotension
Vinca alkaloids	Ischemia
Biological agents	
Monoclonal antibodies	
Alemtuzumab (Campath)	Hypotension, CHF
Bevacizumab (Avastin)	HTN, CHF, DVT
Cetuximab (Erbitux)	Hypotension
Rituximab (Rituxan)	Hypotension, angioedema, arrhythmias
Trastuzumab (Herceptin)	CHF
Interleukins	
IL-2	Hypotension, arrhythmias
Denileukin (Ontak)	Hypotension
Interferon alpha	Hypotension, ischemia, CHF
Miscellaneous	
All-*trans* retinoic acid (Tretinoin)	CHF, hypotension, pericardial effusion
Arsenic trioxide (Trisenox)	QT prolongation
Imatinab (Gleevec)	Pericardial effusion, CHF, edema
Pentostatin (Nipent)	CHF
Thalidomide (Thalomid)	Edema, hypotension, DVT, bradycardia
Etoposide (Vepesid)	Hypotension

SOURCE: Adapted from Yeh et al.[3]

- Dexrazoxane is a cardioprotective agent used in patients receiving anthracyclines. It chelates iron, preventing formation of the anthracycline-iron complex that causes cardiotoxicity.[2]
  - Radiation therapy can damage all heart tissues.
    - The pericardium is most susceptible.
- Pericardial effusion is an early manifestation; fibrous thickening can occur after 18 months.[3]
- Radiation treatment also accelerates coronary atherosclerosis.

PULMONARY

- Table 32-2 lists chemotherapy agents and their associated pulmonary toxicities.
  - Bleomycin causes pulmonary fibrosis in 10 percent of patients receiving a cumulative dose above 450 U.
- Other chemotherapeutic agents are associated with bronchospasm. These agents include asparaginase, doxorubicin, epipodophyllotoxins, interferons, monoclonal antibodies, mitomycin, platinums, taxanes, and vinca alkaloids. Be prepared to support these patients

TABLE 32-2 Chemotherapeutic Agents and Pulmonary Toxicity

BRONCHOSPASM	PULMONARY FIBROSIS/ PNEUMONITIS
Asparaginase	Bleomycin
Doxorubicin	Chlorambucil
Epipodophyllotoxins	
Cyclophosphamide	
Etoposide	Melphalan
Tenoposide	
Methotrexate	
Interferons	Nitrosureas
6-Mercaptopurine	Carbomustine (BCNU)
Monoclonal antibodies	
Alemtuzamab	
Rituximab	
Mitomycin	
Procarbazine	
Platinums	
Carboplatin	
Cisplatin	
Taxanes	
Docitaxel	
Paclitaxel	
Vinca Alkaloids	
Vinblastine	
Vincristine	

with aggressive pulmonary toilet and bronchodilators in the postoperative setting.

Hepatic

- Cancer of the liver and metastasis to the liver have perioperative implications including coagulopathies, biliary dysfunction, and malnutrition.
- Chemotherapy may also have hepatotoxic effects. These are usually transient but may affect coagulation in the perioperative setting.
- Chemotherapy associated with hepatic toxicity includes methotrexate, L-asparaginase, cytosine arabinoside (ARA-C), plicamycin, streptozocin, and 6-mercaptopurine.

Gastrointestinal

- Patients with tumor primaries of the GI tract are at risk for malnutrition.
- Radiation therapy may also cause diarrhea, resulting in malabsorption, weight loss, and malnutrition. Vitamin deficiencies may also lead to coagulation abnormalities.

Urologic

- Renal insufficiency is a major comorbidity in the urologic cancer population. Cisplatin-based chemotherapy regimens are commonly used to treat these tumors, and the creatinine should be followed closely. Renal function may also be compromised due to the location of the tumor or renal vascular compromise due to tumor burden.
- Nitrosoureas such as carbomustine (BCNU) and semustine (methyl-CCNU) can also cause renal toxicity. Cyclophosphamide causes hemorrhagic cystitis.
- Patients with testicular cancer and retroperitoneal disease, particularly those who have had chemoradiation, are at high risk for postoperative complications. Those with germ cell tumors may have received bleomycin, which is associated with pulmonary toxicity and risk of postoperative pulmonary complications. Judicious intravenous fluid management helps minimize postoperative pulmonary complications.

Bone Marrow Transplant Patients

- The toxicities of chemotherapy and radiation therapy are more pronounced due to the increased dosing and prolonged periods of time for therapy.
- Immunodeficiency is the main complication. After high-dose chemotherapy, neutropenia persists much longer in these patients than in other cancer populations. B- and T-cell function is abnormal for up to 1 year posttransplant. Surgical interventions may have to occur in the face of concurrent infection. Cytomegalovirus (CMV), herpesvirus, fungi, and *Pneumocystis carinii* are common opportunistic infections.
- Use seronegative blood products for those patients who are seronegative for CMV. Also, irradiate and filter blood products for leukoreduction. Of note, irradiation may increase serum potassium levels.
- Graft-versus-host disease usually occurs in the first 100 days after transplantation. Involvement is with skin, the GI tract, and the liver. Treatment has traditionally been with corticosteroids, but other agents such as azathioprine, cyclosporine, tacrolimus, and pentostatin may be employed. In the perioperative setting, monitor nutritional status and coagulation.

Hematologic Considerations

- All cancer patients are hypercoagulable and at risk for postoperative deep venous thrombosis (DVT) due to higher levels of cytokines, clotting factors, and cancer procoagulant A. Postoperatively, there may be decreased levels of antithrombin III. Mucin-producing tumors such as adenocarcinomas of the pancreas, lung, and GI tract are particularly hypercoagulable. Perioperative DVT prophylaxis should be used in all patients.
- Disseminated intravascular coagulation (DIC) can occur after surgical manipulation of mucin-producing adenocarcinomas. It is also seen after induction chemotherapy for acute promyelocytic leukemia.
- Cancer patients can have pancytopenia (anemia, leukopenia, thrombocytopenia) either from the malignancy or as a result of treatment. They can also have thrombocytosis and polycythemia.
- Thrombocytosis can be caused by myeloproliferative disease, splenectomy, iron deficiency, or underlying inflammation.
- Polycythemia is associated with adrenal, hepatic, ovarian, renal, and uterine cancers. Perioperatively, there is risk of both bleeding and thrombosis.

Neurologic Considerations

- Brain metastasis occurs in up to 30 percent of cancer patients. The presentation usually includes headache, confusion, and focal neurologic deficits. Some cases of brain metastasis may be appropriate for surgical resection, although the most common modality of treatment is radiation. Suspect leptomeningeal disease in those with multifocal neurologic deficits.
- Spinal cord compression requires emergent attention. Treatment modalities include steroids, radiation, and surgical decompression.
- Neurologic paraneoplastic syndromes present with muscle weakness, peripheral neuropathies, radiculopathies, and degeneration of the central nervous system. Metastatic disease in the central or peripheral nervous system may present as multiple neurologic complaints. Obtain a metastatic workup prior to surgery.

- Eaton-Lambert syndrome is most commonly associated with small cell bronchogenic carcinoma. Myasthenia gravis occurs in 50 percent of patients with thymoma. In both conditions, calcium channel blockers are contraindicated. Anesthesia may exacerbate the underlying neuromuscular dysfunction and result in a prolonged intubation time.
- Radiation, cancer-related hypercoagulability, and direct tumor invasion can all contribute to an increased risk of perioperative stroke. Postoperatively, monitor neurologic status closely in patients with multiple risk factors for vascular disease.

Endocrine and Metabolic Considerations

- Ectopic production of adrenocorticotropic hormone (ACTH) is seen with small cell carcinoma of the lung, pancreatic carcinoma, carcinoid, and thymic tumors. Weight loss, muscle weakness, and hyperpigmentation are signs of this condition.
- The syndrome of inappropriate antidiuretic hormone (SIADH) is seen in small cell, large cell, and adenocarcinoma of the lung as well as pancreatic and duodenal carcinoma. Medications that reduce the excretion of free water may worsen hyponatremia. These medications include amitriptyline, chlorpropamide, clofibrinate, cyclophosphamide, morphine, selective serotonin reuptake inhibitors, thiazide diuretics, and vincristine. Asymptomatic hyponatremia is not a contraindication for surgery.
- Hypercalcemia is caused by ectopic production of a parathyroid hormone-like substance, prostaglandins, metastatic invasion of bone, and osteoclast-activating factor. Cancers most commonly associated with hypercalcemia include breast cancer, non-small cell lung cancer, and multiple myeloma.
- Hypoglycemia is seen in tumors like mesenchymal tumors, adrenocortical tumors, pancreatic non-islet cell tumors, and hepatocellular carcinoma. Check glucose frequently in the perioperative fasting period.
- Hyperglycemia is common with several chemotherapeutic agents. Occult diabetes is often unmasked during cancer therapy. Euglycemia in the perioperative period may improve wound healing and shorten hospital stays.
- Excessive renin production is seen in those with tumors of the kidney, Wilms' tumor, and hepatocellular carcinoma. Presentation is with hypertension, hypokalemia, and hyperaldosteronism. Continue angiotensin-converting enzyme inhibitors in the perioperative period.
- Adrenal insufficiency may occur in patients receiving chemotherapy regimens, including steroids. Courses of steroids lasting 2 weeks can have adrenal suppressive activity for up to 1 year. Treatment of breast, prostate, and adrenocortical tumors may include use of aminoglutethimide, metyrapone, or mitotane, all of which suppress adrenal function.
- Monitor patients who had surgery or radiation treatment of the head and neck for primary and central hypothyroidism.[4]

PREOPERATIVE EVALUATION AND PERIOPERATIVE MANAGEMENT

- Cancer patients often have multiple comorbidities and multisystem involvement related to their disease or to its treatment. Therefore perform a comprehensive preoperative history and physical examination.

GENERAL CONSIDERATIONS

- ***Performance status*** may decline because of the debilitating effects of cancer, its therapies, and the patient's underlying comorbidities. Validated tools to evaluate the status of a patient include the Karnofsky Performance Status, the Zubrod, and the ECOG Performance Status Scales. Disease-specific comorbidity scales include the Modified Kaplan-Feinstein Index (MKFI) and the Adult Comorbidity Evaluation (ACE-27).
- ***Nutritional status:*** Patients who have had cancer for a prolonged period of time or have completed chemoradiation prior to surgical intervention may have a poor nutritional status. Measurement of prealbumin is a helpful marker. Consider delaying surgery to provide enteral or parenteral nutritional supplementation in patients with severe malnutrition (<70 percent ideal body weight). There is evidence that in the severely malnourished, 7 to 10 days of preoperative parenteral nutrition can reduce morbidity. Postoperative nutritional support is also of benefit in those who are not able to eat within 7 days of surgery.[5]
- ***Pain:*** Patients and their physicians perceive cancer pain as a poorly treated condition. Reasons include lack of knowledge on the part of patients and the caregivers and lack of access or underutilization of analgesics.[6] A guideline for treating cancer pain is the Evidence-Based Program, associated with the Agency for Healthcare Research and Quality.[7] Assistance from a pain-management service may help prevent perioperative complications. Pain management is discussed in Chap. 63.
- ***Comorbid conditions:*** Evaluate the patient for the signs and symptoms of any comorbid condition that may occur with cancer, as previously noted.
- ***Substance abuse:*** Obtain a history of alcohol and tobacco use, particularly in patients with head and neck or lung cancer, and watch for evidence of alcohol or nicotine withdrawal postoperatively.

- ***Preoperative tests:*** More extensive preoperative testing is often warranted in cancer patients due to multisystem involvement. A complete blood count (CBC) with differential and platelet count, comprehensive metabolic panel (including electrolytes, glucose, BUN/creatinine, liver function tests, calcium, and albumin), prothrombin time (PT) and partial thromboplastin time (PTT), electrocardiogram, and chest x-ray are usually indicated for the reasons previously discussed.

SPECIFIC SYSTEMS

Cardiac

- Potential cardiac problems from cancer or its treatment include congestive heart failure (CHF), ischemic heart disease, hypertension, hypotension, pericarditis, and fibrosis.
- Consider delaying cancer therapy in patients with unstable coronary artery disease preoperatively. If treatment of the cancer cannot wait for the recovery time from cardiac catheterization or revascularization, proceed with surgery as a high-risk procedure, with a cardiologist involved in the perioperative care.
- Pericardial effusions occur due to metastatic disease, infection, and chemotherapy. Obtain an echocardiogram if there is any suspicion of a pericardial effusion. If there is global impairment or compromise of the diastolic filling pressure, take definitive measures prior to elective surgeries. Percutaneous drainage can be accomplished with local anesthesia. Sclerosis with bleomycin may provide longer-lasting relief. If these interventions fail, consider pericardectomy.

Pulmonary

- Consider preoperative spirometry and arterial blood gas in patients with significant cumulative doses of certain chemotherapeutic agents (Table 32-2), symptoms of pulmonary toxicity, or pleural effusions. Consider thoracentesis if the effusion is significant and surgery is elective.
- Airway management may be a potential problem in patients with head and neck cancer. There may be distortion of the anatomy from the tumor itself, radiation therapy, or previous surgery. Awake fiberoptic intubation or tracheostomy may be necessary.
- Airway problems may also be associated with the superior vena cava syndrome (SVCS), mediastinal masses, and obstructive sleep apnea.
  - The most common cause of SVCS is lung cancer, followed by lymphomas and tumors metastatic to the mediastinum. SVCS can cause airway edema, vocal cord paralysis, and compression of the airway. Treatment depends on the cause; if it is due to external compression by tumor and the tumor is radiosensitive, then x-ray therapy is the treatment of choice. If due to thrombosis, thrombolysis may be indicted. All intravascular access should occur from the lower extremities.
  - The most common mediastinal masses occur in the anterior and middle mediastinum and usually consist of lymphoma or metastatic bronchocarcinomas. If the purpose of surgery is biopsy, consider other possible biopsy sites, such as the axillary or supraclavicular nodes. Be aware of possible compression of mediastinal structures during surgery if postural wheezing, stridor, syncope, or cyanosis are present preoperatively. In this case, avoid general anesthesia if possible. Perform diagnostic computed tomography or magnetic resonance imaging of the chest in addition to upright and supine spirometry and echocardiography.
  - Observe for obstructive sleep apnea in the pre- and postoperative setting for patients particularly at risk. These include patients with head and neck tumors. The obstruction may be due to tumor, radiation, mandibulectomy, or flap reconstruction. Treat with continuous positive airway pressure (CPAP) or bilevel positive airway pressure (BiPAP).

Hepatic

- Obtain preoperative liver function tests, including PT and PTT, in patients with cancer of the liver or hepatic metastases. Thrombocytopenia may also be present in chronic liver disease. For those found to have coagulopathies, support with fresh frozen plasma and platelets.

Hematologic

- Cancer patients may have either thrombocytopenia or thrombocytosis. Platelet counts of ≥50,000 are usually considered adequate for most surgical interventions. For those with platelet counts greater than 2 million per cubic milliliter, use low-dose aspirin (81 mg/day) for prophylaxis against thrombotic events.[8]
- Use of erythropoietin can ameliorate anemia. Blood transfusion may increase the recurrence rate of certain tumors, including breast, cervical, colon, rectal, and soft-tissue sarcomas. Transfuse only when absolutely necessary (see Chap. 30). The use of cell-saver blood is currently controversial.
- Polycythemia is associated with both bleeding and thrombosis in the perioperative setting. The target hemoglobin preoperatively should be <15g/dL. Hydrate adequately and avoid hypotension and venous stasis. Start DVT prophylaxis immediately in the postoperative setting.
- Neutropenia (absolute neutrophil count <500/mm^3) occurs with most chemotherapy regimens. The nadir

is usually at days 7 to 14, with recovery from days 21 to 28. With high-dose chemotherapy, the nadir is markedly prolonged. Use of colony-stimulating factors like filgrastim and pegfilgrastim can shorten the length of neutropenia. Fever should immediately prompt obtaining cultures and initiating antibiotics.
- DIC can occur after surgical manipulation of mucin-producing adenocarcinomas or after induction chemotherapy for acute promyelocytic leukemia. Management of bleeding in the face of DIC includes replacement of clotting factors and platelets.

ENDOCRINE
- Ectopic production of ACTH is treated with the steroid inhibitors metyrapone and aminoglutethamide.
- Hyponatremia due to SIADH is treated with fluid restriction. Acute therapy consists of judicious use of saline and loop diuretics if needed. Intraoperative replacement of fluids with normal saline may be necessary.
- For hypercalcemia, the perioperative goal is to achieve a normal calcium level in addition to volume repletion; if this is not possible, however, calcium levels of less than 12 mg/dL are not associated with any increased risk in the asymptomatic patient. Acute treatment is with fluid hydration in combination with a loop diuretic. Long-term therapy includes bisphosphonates, mithramycin, calcitonin, and gallium.
- Stress-dose steroids for use in adrenal insufficiency are discussed in Chap. 28.

SUMMARY

Perioperative care of the cancer patient is challenging; however, by considering the multiple factors involved—including the diagnosis, extent of disease, prior treatment, prognosis, comorbidities, and planned surgical procedure—the consultant can play an integral role in the perioperative management team.

REFERENCES

1. Manzullo E, Weed HG. Perioperative issues in the patient with cancer. *Med Clin North Am* 87:243–256, 2003.
2. Poillart P. Evaluating the role of dexrazoxane as a cardioprotectant in cancer patients receiving anthracyclines. *Cancer Treat Rev* 30(7):643–650, 2004.
3. Yeh E, Tong A, Lenihan D, et al. Cardiovascular complications of cancer therapy. *Circulation* 109(25):3122–3131, 2004.
4. Manzullo E, Weber R. Pre-operative assessment, in Close LG, Larson DL, Shah JP (eds), *Essentials of Head and Neck Oncology*. New York: Thieme,1998:89–95.
5. Salvino R, Dechicco S, Seider L. Perioperative nutritional support: Who and how. *Cleve Clin J Med* 71(4):345–351, 2004.
6. Palos G, Mendoza T, Cantor S, et al. Perceptions of analgesic use and side effects: What the public values in pain management. *J Pain Sympt Mgt* 28(5):460–473, 2004.
7. Management of cancer pain: Summary of evidence report/technology assessment: Number 35. *J Pain Palliat Care Pharmacother* 16(2):91–102, 2002.
8. Schafer AI. Thrombocytosis. *N Engl J Med* 350(12):1211–1219, 2004.

33 HIV DISEASE

Howard Libman

INTRODUCTION

- Over the past decade, HIV disease has become a manageable chronic medical condition in many patients because of the availability of combination antiretroviral therapy.
- Patients are less likely to experience opportunistic infections and are living longer. However, because of this improvement in mortality, they may be at increased risk for other age-dependent chronic medical conditions.
- In addition, the long-term use of antiretroviral therapy may predispose to diabetes mellitus, hyperlipidemia, and premature atherosclerotic disease.
- All of the above considerations may be relevant to the preoperative care of this patient population.

EPIDEMIOLOGY

RISK OF TRANSMISSION FROM HEALTH CARE WORKER TO PATIENT

- This issue was first publicized in 1990 when a Florida dentist was conclusively identified as the source of HIV infection in six of his patients. The mechanism of this transmission remains an enigma to this day.
- Despite public concern regarding the possibility of HIV transmission during surgical procedures, only seven instances related to two cases have been reported in the literature.
- The Centers for Disease Control and Prevention (CDC) has initiated 66 "look back" investigations involving 22,759 patients with a history of invasive procedures by HIV-infected health care workers (HCWs).[1] Only

113 (0.5 percent) were noted to be HIV-infected, most of whom had been diagnosed in advance of surgery. In all other instances, the HIV strains of the patients differed from those of their HCWs.

- Modeling based on available data suggests that the risk of HIV transmission from HCW to patient during an invasive procedure is between 1 in 2.4 million to 1 in 24 million.
- The CDC has published recommendations for HIV-infected HCWs, but these are controversial. Most institutions do not have specific guidelines for this group of providers.

RISK OF TRANSMISSION FROM PATIENT TO HEALTH CARE WORKER

- Prospective studies show that occupational exposures to infectious agents occur in direct proportion to the frequency with which invasive procedures are performed. Surgeons average 12 percutaneous blood exposures per person-year.
- Based on prospective studies, the risk of HIV transmission from a percutaneous exposure has been estimated to be 0.3 percent. Of note, this risk is much lower than those of hepatitis B and hepatitis C transmission, which have been estimated as 6 to 30 percent and 2 percent, respectively.
- As of December 2002, a total of 57 cases of documented occupational HIV transmission had been reported to the CDC.[2] In addition, there were 139 cases of possible occupational transmission (no risk behaviors in patient and specific workplace exposure noted). Only 6 (11 percent) cases have involved physicians, none of whom were surgeons. Forty-eight (84 percent) of documented cases were related to "sharps."
- Significant risk factors for HIV seroconversion include the inoculum size and severity of the injury.[3] Deep injury is associated with a 15.0 adjusted odds ratio (AOR), visible blood on device with a 6.2 AOR, terminal illness in source patient with a 5.6 AOR, and procedure involving a needle in an artery or vein with a 4.3 AOR.
- Universal precautions are recommended to decrease the risk of HIV exposure among HCWs.[4] These include using gloves for any procedure involving contact with blood or any other potentially infected fluids, wearing masks and protective eyewear when fluid splatters are anticipated, and using gowns as appropriate based upon the clinical circumstances.
- Postexposure prophylaxis with antiretroviral drugs has been shown to decrease the risk of HIV seroconversion following a critical exposure by 80 percent. The CDC has published detailed recommendations on their use.[5]

PATIENT-RELATED RISK FACTORS

PREOPERATIVE TESTING FOR HIV INFECTION

- Routine preoperative screening for HIV infection is not recommended because of a lack of evidence that this information reduces the exposure risk to HCWs. Use universal precautions with all surgical patients regardless of their HIV serostatus.
- However, because knowledge of HIV serostatus may affect the patient's preoperative and perioperative care, a risk assessment should be performed. Indications and contraindications for HIV antibody testing are listed in Table 33-1. Pre- and posttest counseling is essential.
- Rapid tests that detect HIV antibody within 20 min have been developed. These enable clinicians to provide definitive negative and preliminary positive results immediately. A positive rapid HIV antibody immunoassay should be confirmed with the more specific Western blot test.

PATIENTS WITH ESTABLISHED HIV INFECTION

- The immunologic status of an HIV-infected patient is assessed by the CD4 cell count, which is a surrogate laboratory marker. The normal range is 350/mm^3 to

TABLE 33-1 Indications and Contraindications for HIV Antibody Testing

Historical indications
Men who have sex with men
People with multiple sexual partners
Current or past injection-drug users
Recipients of blood products between 1978 and 1985
People with current or past sexually transmitted diseases
Commercial sex workers and their sexual contacts
Pregnant women and women of childbearing age
Children born to HIV-infected mothers
Sexual partners of those at risk for HIV infection
Donors of blood products, semen, or organs
Persons who consider themselves at risk or request testing
Clinical indications
Tuberculosis
Syphilis
Recurrent shingles
Unexplained chronic constitutional symptoms
Unexplained generalized adenopathy
Unexplained chronic diarrhea or wasting
Unexplained encephalopathy
Unexplained thrombocytopenia
Thrush or chronic/recurrent vaginal candidiasis
HIV-associated opportunistic diseases
Contraindications
Inability of patient to understand implications of test result
Acute psychosis
Major depression or suicidality
Lack of adequate personal support system

1100/mm^3. Its clinical uses are to determine the need for antiretroviral therapy as well as the risk for opportunistic infections and need for antimicrobial prophylaxis.

- The HIV viral load predicts the likelihood of disease progression. It is performed by the measurement of RNA in plasma via the polymerase chain reaction (PCR) or branched DNA (bDNA) techniques. The range of this assay is generally from less than 50 copies to more than 100,000 copies per milliliter. Its clinical uses are to determine the need for antiretroviral therapy and to assess its effectiveness.
- Hematologic abnormalities are common in HIV-infected patients.
  - Anemia may be secondary to ineffective erythropoiesis, medications [e.g., zidovudine (ZDV), didanosine (ddI), stavudine (d4T)], nutritional deficiencies, or bone marrow infiltration. Perioperative transfusions may be necessary, preferably with leukocyte-depleted packed red blood cells if the patient is cytomegalovirus antibody-negative.
  - Leukopenia may be related to ineffective leukopoiesis, medications (e.g., ZDV, trimethoprim/sulfamethoxazole), or bone marrow infiltration. Marked neutropenia may predispose the patient to bacterial infections.
  - Thrombocytopenia may stem from immunologically mediated platelet destruction, medications, or bone marrow infiltration. Although HIV-related thrombocytopenia is generally mild, clinical bleeding is possible perioperatively.
- HIV-infected patients sometimes have underlying chronic renal or hepatic disease. Significant organ dysfunction may affect their surgical risk and/or necessitate modification of drug choice or dosage. Renal disease may be related to HIV infection itself or other comorbid conditions, such as diabetes mellitus. Hepatotoxicity may result from antiretroviral therapy, and coinfection with hepatitis C virus is common among injection drug users.
- Adrenal insufficiency has been reported with advanced HIV disease. It may be secondary to infection, malignancy, or medications. Affected patients, if unrecognized and untreated, are at risk of developing hypotension and electrolyte abnormalities.
- HIV-infected patients receiving long-term antiretroviral therapy may develop lipodystrophy syndrome, which is manifest by changes in body morphology (increased visceral and decreased peripheral fat), glucose intolerance (and less often diabetes mellitus), and/or hyperlipidemia. These factors may increase the risk of atherosclerotic disease.
- The nutritional status of HIV-infected patients varies and may also have an impact on surgical risk.

SURGERY-RELATED RISK FACTORS

EFFECT OF HIV DISEASE ON SURGICAL MORBIDITY AND MORTALITY

- Retrospective studies suggest that most surgical procedures can be safely performed in HIV-infected patients. There is no evidence of increased mortality. A higher risk of postoperative wound infections and delayed healing have been reported in some case series of anorectal and obstetric and gynecologic surgeries.[6,7]
- Postoperative bacterial complications may be more common in patients with lower CD4 cell counts.[8] The effect of the HIV viral load on perioperative risk is unknown.
- Case-control series suggest that undergoing surgery has no effect on HIV disease progression.[9]
- Elective cesarean section is recommended in HIV-infected women with viral loads of greater than 1000 copies per milliliter in order to decrease the risk of perinatal transmission.[10] Some reports suggest an increased risk of postoperative wound infection, endometritis, and pneumonia, especially in the context of low CD4 cell counts.[11]
- Organ transplantation has become more common in recent years in HIV-infected patients given the improved life expectancy of this population. Chronic renal failure can result from HIV disease, and chronic liver disease is often related to coinfection with hepatitis C virus. Experience to date suggests that patients with well-controlled HIV disease can tolerate the immunosuppressive therapies initiated following organ transplantation, although drug-drug interactions may be a concern in some instances.

PREOPERATIVE EVALUATION AND TESTING TO STRATIFY RISK

- A detailed medical history is an essential component of the preoperative evaluation of HIV-infected patients. Table 33-2 provides a preoperative preparation checklist.
- Assess the patient's HIV disease status, as evidenced by opportunistic diseases, lowest and most recent CD4 cell count, and highest and most recent HIV viral load. In addition, elicit any history of sexually transmitted diseases, viral hepatitis (A, B, and C), and tuberculosis exposure or infection.
- Obtain a careful history regarding depression, which is common in HIV-infected patients, as well as of any alcohol and substance abuse.
- Assess the patient's nutritional status by dietary history and augment it, if necessary, with appropriate supplements prior to elective procedures.

TABLE 33-2 Preoperative Preparation Checklist for HIV-Infected Patients

History
Opportunistic diseases
CD4 cell count
HIV viral load
Sexually transmitted diseases
Viral hepatitis
Tuberculosis
Nutritional status
Medications
Allergies
Depression
Alcohol and substance abuse
Medical directives
Health care proxy
Physical examination
Skin
Mouth
Lymph nodes
Lungs
Anogenital region
Laboratory tests
Complete blood and differential counts
Glucose
Electrolytes
Renal and hepatic function tests
CD4 cell count
HIV viral load

- Record a medication history, including prescribed, over-the-counter, and complementary therapies. Drug-drug interactions are common with protease inhibitors and non-nucleoside reverse transcriptase inhibitors. Some drugs may not be safely coadministered (Table 33-3) and others may require dosage adjustment.
- Obtain an allergy history. Adverse drug reactions occur frequently in HIV-infected patients. For example, the risk of toxicity to trimethoprim/sulfamethoxazole has been estimated to be as high as 25 to 50 percent.
- Discuss medical directives and health care proxy status with the patient prior to surgery.
- Perform a complete physical examination with attention to the skin and mucous membranes, lymph nodes, lungs, anogenital region, and any symptomatic areas.
- Preoperative laboratory studies should include a complete blood and differential counts, glucose, and renal and hepatic function tests to look for evidence of organ dysfunction. In addition, obtain a CD4 cell count and viral load to assess HIV disease status.
- Acute medical conditions may transiently decrease the CD4 cell count and increase the HIV viral load, so results should be interpreted cautiously in this setting.

TABLE 33-3 Drugs Contraindicated for Use with Antiretroviral Drugs

PROTEASE INHIBITORS	NONNUCLEOSIDE REVERSE TRANSCRIPTASE INHIBITORS
Antihistamine	Antihistamine
Astemizole (all)	Astemizole (DLV, EFV)
Terfenadine (all)	Terfenadine (DLV, EFV)
Antimycobacterial	Antimycobacterial
Rifabutin (SQV)	Rifabutin (DLV)
Rifampin (all except RTV)	Rifampin (NVP, DLV)
Rifapentine (all)	Rifapentine (all)
Calcium Channel Blockers	Ergot Alkaloids
Bepridil (RTV, FPV, ATV)	Ergotamine (DLV, EFV)
	Others in class (DLV, EFV)
Cardiac	
Amiodarone (RTV, IDV)	Gastrointestinal
Flecainide (RTV, LPV/rtv)	Cisapride (DLV, EFV)
Propafenone (RTV, LPV/rtv)	H2 blockers (DLV)
Quinine (RTV)	Proton pump inhibitors (DLV)
Ergot Alkaloids	Lipid-lowering
Ergotamine (all)	Lovastatin (DLV)
Others in class (all)	Simvastatin (DLV)
Gastrointestinal	Psychotropic
Cisapride (all)	Alprazolam (DLV)
Proton pump inhibitors (ATV)	Midazolam (DLV, EFV)
	Triazolam (DLV, EFV)
Lipid-lowering	
Lovastatin (all)	Other
Simvastatin (all)	Carbamazepine (DLV)
	Phenobarbital (DLV)
Psychotropic	Phenytoin (DLV)
Midazolam (all)	Voriconazole (EFV)
Pimozide (all)	
Triazolam (all)	
Other	
Fluticasone (RTV, LPV/rtv)	
Oral contraceptives (FPV)	
Voriconazole (RTV)	

ATV = atazanavir; DLV = delavirdine; EFV = efavirenz; FPV = fosamprenavir; IDV = indinavir; LPV/rtv = lopinavir/ritonavir; NFV = nevirapine; RTV = ritonavir; SQV = saquinavir.
SOURCE: From U.S. Public Health Service Guidelines. Guidelines for the use of antiretroviral agents in HIV-infected adults and adolescents (available as "living document" from AIDSinfo: Department of Health and Human Services. Web site at www.aidsinfo.nih.gov.)

- If not available on review of the medical record, consider additional tests to assess for common coinfections, including viral hepatitis (A, B, and C), syphilis and other sexually transmitted diseases, and tuberculosis.

PERIOPERATIVE MANAGEMENT TO REDUCE RISK

PREOPERATIVE

- Assess the patient for evidence of an opportunistic disease process and implement treatment for this condition prior to any elective procedure.

TABLE 33-4 Antimicrobial Prophylaxis for Opportunistic Infections

CD4 CELL COUNT	OPPORTUNISTIC INFECTION	DRUG OF CHOICE
<200/mm^3	*Pneumocystis* pneumonia	TMP/SMX
<100/mm^3	Toxoplasmosis*	TMP/SMX
<50/mm^3	*Mycobacterium avium* complex	Azithromycin
Any	Tuberculosis (latent)	Isoniazid

TMP/SMX = trimethoprim/sulfamethoxazole.
*In the context of positive IgG antibody.

- Confirm that the patient is on appropriate antimicrobial prophylaxis for opportunistic infections based upon the CD4 cell count (Table 33-4).
- In general, maintain antiretroviral drug therapy in the perioperative period. If necessary, a brief interruption of treatment does not generally undermine its long-term effectiveness. However, solicit advice from an HIV consultant if antiretroviral therapy must be stopped repeatedly or for more than 24 to 48 h.
- An HIV-infected woman who is carrying her pregnancy to term should be under the care of an experienced obstetrician in consultation with an HIV clinician familiar with such care. Interventions used to decrease the risk of vertical transmission include initiation of antiretroviral therapy in the mother during the second and third trimesters and its maintenance perioperatively, as well as consideration of elective cesarean section.[10]
- The indications for antibiotic prophylaxis in HIV-infected patients are the same as in seronegative persons. They are based on the type of surgical procedure and the presence of certain health conditions such as valvular heart disease.

POSTOPERATIVE

- HIV-infected patients generally have an uneventful postoperative course.
- The majority of postoperative complications—including delayed healing, wound infection, and sepsis—occur in patients with advanced HIV disease. Poor nutrition and neutropenia may also be contributing factors.
- Supplemental oral or intravenous nutrition may be necessary for some patients if oral intake is inadequate.
- Therapy with granulocyte colony-stimulating factor (G-CSF) is warranted if the absolute granulocyte count drops below 500/mm^3.
- If confusion, nausea/vomiting, or diarrhea interfere with the patient's ability to take oral medications on a short-term basis, hold all antiretroviral drugs until clinical circumstances improve. Liquid preparations are available for some of these agents.
- Subclinical adrenal insufficiency is common in patients with advanced HIV disease and may become manifest with the stress of surgery. It should be suspected in the postoperative period if there is unexplained hypotension, hyponatremia, or hypokalemia. Order a cosyntropin stimulation test in this setting (see Chap. 28).
- Medication side effects—including fever, rash, gastrointestinal symptoms, and liver function test (LFT) abnormalities—are common in HIV-infected patients and may occur postoperatively.
- Pneumonia, infected intravenous catheter, urinary tract infection, thrombophlebitis, and drug toxicity are responsible for most cases of postoperative fever. Opportunistic infections can occur postoperatively in patients with advanced HIV disease (CD4 count <200/mm^3) but should be prevented by the appropriate use of antimicrobial prophylaxis (see Table 33-4).
- Fever without localizing complaints may be caused by medications, some infections (e.g., cytomegalovirus, *Mycobacterium avium* complex, tuberculosis), lymphoma, or hypoadrenalism.
- Evaluate postoperative fever in the HIV-infected patient based on the clinical findings. Complete blood and differential counts, LFTs, blood cultures (including isolator culture if the CD4 count is <100/mm^3), urinalysis, and chest x-ray are often included. It is important to be aware that baseline leukopenia is common in HIV disease and that a "normal" white blood cell count may be tantamount to leukocytosis.
- Postoperative pneumonia is common in patients with advanced HIV disease.[12] *Staphylococcus aureus* and gram-negative bacilli are the most frequently isolated pathogens.
- Evaluation of postoperative pneumonia in the HIV-infected patient should include complete blood and differential counts, blood cultures, arterial blood gases or oximetry, and an induced sputum for Gram's, and acid-fast bacillus stains, and an immunofluorescent assay for *Pneumocystis carinii* if the CD4 cell count is <200/mm^3.

SUMMARY

- Surgical procedures can generally be performed safely in HIV-infected patients.

- However, preoperative risk factors should be assessed on an individual basis, and patient care may need to be tailored based on the nature of these and the type of surgical procedure being performed.

REFERENCES

1. Robert LM, Chamberland ME, Cleveland JL, et al. Investigations of patients of health care workers infected with HIV. The Centers for Disease Control and Prevention database. *Ann Intern Med* 122:653–657, 1995.
2. Centers for Disease Control and Prevention. HIV/AIDS Surveillance Data. (Web site at www.cdc.gov.)
3. Cardo DM, Culver DH, Ciesielski CA, et al. A case-control study of HIV seroconversion in health care workers after percutaneous exposure: CDC Needlestick Surveillance Group. *N Engl J Med* 337:1485–1490, 1997.
4. Centers for Disease Control. Universal precautions for prevention of transmission of human immunodeficiency virus, hepatitis B virus, and other bloodborne pathogens in health-care settings. *MMWR* 37:377–388, 1988.
5. U.S. Public Health Service guidelines for the management of occupational exposures to HBV, HCV, and HIV and recommendations for postexposure prophylaxis (available as "living document" from AIDSinfo: Department of Health and Human Services Web site at http://www.aidsinfo.nih.gov).
6. Morandi E, Merlini D, Salvaggio A, et al. Prospective study of healing time after hemorrhoidectomy: Influence of HIV infection, acquired immunodeficiency syndrome, and anal wound infection. *Dis Colon Rectum* 42: 1140–1144, 1999.
7. Grubert TA, Reindell D, Kastner R, et al. Rates of postoperative complications among human immunodeficiency virus-infected women who have undergone obstetric and gynecologic surgical procedures. *Clin Infect Dis* 34:822–830, 2002.
8. Albaran RG, Webber J, Steffes CP. CD4 cell counts as a prognostic factor of major abdominal surgery in patients infected with the human immunodeficiency virus. *Arch Surg* 133: 626–631, 1998.
9. Astermark J, Lofqvist T, Schulman S, et al. Major surgery seems not to influence HIV disease progression in haemophilia patients. *Br J Haematol* 103:10–14, 1998.
10. Centers for Disease Control and Prevention. Public Health Service Task Force recommendations for the use of antiretroviral drugs in pregnant women infected with HIV-1 for maternal health and for reducing perinatal HIV-1 transmission in the United States (available as "living document" from AIDSinfo: Department of Health and Human Services Web site at http://www.aidsinfo.nih.gov).
11. Semprini AE, Castagna C, Ravizza M, et al. The incidence of complications after caesarean section in 156 HIV-positive women. *AIDS* 9:913–917, 1995.
12. Tumbarello M, Tacconelli E, de Gaetano K, et al. Bacterial pneumonia in HIV-infected patients: Analysis of risk factors and prognostic indicators. *J AIDS Hum Retrovirol* 18:39–45, 1998.

34 CHRONIC KIDNEY DISEASE

Maninder Kohli

INTRODUCTION

- Patients with chronic kidney disease (CKD) and dialysis patients are at significant risk for morbidity and mortality from major surgery.
- Renal insufficiency is an important predictor of postoperative cardiac complications in patients undergoing a major operation.
  - Cardiac dysfunction and sepsis are significant causes of death after major surgery in patients with CKD.
  - Other complications include volume overload, hypertension, acidosis, electrolyte disturbances, bleeding, and hyperkalemia.
- Preoperative renal insufficiency is the most important risk factor for developing acute on chronic renal failure after a major surgical procedure. Postoperative renal failure is associated with a high mortality.[1]
- Patients on dialysis present unique management challenges in the perioperative period.
- As in other patients, the surgical risk in patients with CKD depends on the severity of the underlying kidney disease, presence of comorbid medical conditions, type of surgical procedure, and whether the surgery is emergent or elective. A careful preoperative assessment of patients with preexisting renal disease is imperative in predicting adverse postoperative events and implementing strategies to reduce operative morbidity and mortality.
- The incidence and management of postoperative renal complications (Chap. 58), fluid-electrolyte (Chap. 56) imbalances, and acid-base disorders (Chap. 57) are discussed separately.

PATIENT-RELATED RISK FACTORS (TABLE 34-1)

In general, few specific risk factors have been identified in controlled studies to predict postoperative complications in patients undergoing noncardiac surgery. Some potentially important factors are discussed below.

AGE

- Few studies have determined advanced age to be an independent predictor of developing postoperative renal failure.

TABLE 34-1 Factors That Predict Adverse Outcomes in Patients with Chronic Kidney Disease

PATIENT-RELATED	SURGERY-SPECIFIC
Advanced age	Aortic surgery
Mild to moderate kidney disease	Vascular surgery
Dialysis	Cardiac surgery
Cardiovascular disease	Surgery for obstructive jaundice
Anemia and bleeding diathesis	
Poor nutrition	
Volume overload	
Hypertension and hypotension	
Hyperkalemia	
Metabolic acidosis	

  - One study found age >65 years to be a multivariate predictor for developing postoperative acute renal failure after cardiac surgery; however, advanced age did not predict the need for dialysis.[2]
  - Advanced age was not predictive of postoperative renal failure requiring dialysis in a large prospective study of 4315 patients undergoing noncardiac surgery.[3]
- It is likely that age-related reductions in the glomerular filtration rate (GFR) and the presence of comorbid conditions can lead to renal dysfunction after surgery. Important variables that predict mortality in the elderly with postoperative renal failure are sustained perioperative hypotension, the need for mechanical ventilation, and multiorgan failure.

PREEXISTING RENAL INSUFFICIENCY

- Patients with a calculated GFR of >50 mL/min are unlikely to experience serious complications after major surgery. No specific precautions are necessary in these patients.
- In patients with mild to moderate renal insufficiency, the most serious complication is the development of acute postoperative renal failure. Diabetics with established nephropathy and patients with glomerular renal disease are particularly susceptible to postoperative renal dysfunction. This is more likely to occur in the presence of sustained perioperative hypotension.
- Patients with GFR <20 mL/min undergoing major noncardiac surgery are more likely to experience postoperative complications including volume overload, acidosis, hyperkalemia, and the need for initiating immediate dialysis after surgery.
- Patients with advanced CKD on dialysis are at increased risk for surgical morbidity and mortality.
  - A review of eight published trials of dialysis patients undergoing general surgery found the overall mortality to be 4 percent, ranging from 0 to a high of 47 percent in patients undergoing emergency surgery.[1]
  - There is also a risk of significant morbidity in the postoperative period. In a study of 312 dialysis patients, 64 percent experienced a major complication, the most frequent one being hyperkalemia.[4] Other important complications were hemodynamic instability, fluid overload, infections, arrhythmias, and bleeding.
  - Cardiovascular complications include postoperative myocardial infarction, congestive heart failure, and arrhythmias.
  - Hemodynamic derangements including hypertension and hypotension in the perioperative period are frequent in the dialysis patient.
  - Failure to metabolize and excrete anesthetics and analgesics can lead to toxic accumulation of these agents.[5]
  - Anemia, pericarditis, and clotting of vascular access ports can further complicate the day-to-day management of patients with CKD.
  - Patients on peritoneal dialysis undergoing abdominal surgery are at an increased risk for anastomotic leaks, poor wound healing, and incisional hernia formation.
  - Finally, dialysis patients frequently require intensive care support, including prolonged mechanical ventilation, vasopressor use, and a protracted length of stay.

SURGERY-RELATED RISK FACTORS

AORTIC AND VASCULAR SURGERY

- Patients undergoing major vascular surgery are at increased risk for mortality and major morbidity. Preoperative renal disease (in the elderly in particular) was a risk factor for postoperative renal failure and the need for dialysis in these patients. Other studies have also confirmed the presence of preexisting renal disease to predict postoperative renal failure.
  - In a study of 57 infrainguinal bypass procedures in 44 patients (33 diabetics) requiring maintenance dialysis, the perioperative mortality was 9 percent. The 30-day surgical morbidity rate was 39 percent, and the major complications were wound breakdown (19 percent), graft thrombosis (9 percent), and major limb amputation (4 percent). Patient survival was only 52 percent at 2 years.[6]
  - Other factors that increase the risk for postoperative renal failure include complicated aneurysms, such as those that have ruptured, suprarenal aneurysms, those that require renal artery bypass, intraoperative blood loss and hypotension, prolonged cardiopulmonary bypass, and cholesterol embolization.[1]

SURGERY FOR OBSTRUCTIVE JAUNDICE

- Patients undergoing surgery for obstructive jaundice have a high incidence of postoperative renal failure. Severity of preoperative jaundice, CKD, and perioperative hypotension predict postoperative renal impairment.
- Patients with obstructive jaundice appear to have significant postoperative reductions in the GFR. This effect may be explained by the fact that absorption of endotoxins is due to limited bile salt excretion in deeply jaundiced patients. The result of the endotoxinemia is enhanced renal vasoconstriction, which—in the presence of systemic hypotension or preexisting renal disease—can lead to worsening of renal function in the postoperative period.

ANESTHETIC CONSIDERATIONS

- The choice of anesthetic agents is best left to the anesthesiology team.
  - General anesthesia, and particularly spinal anesthesia, can cause hypotension and reduce effective renal blood flow. This effect may be proportional to the depth of the anesthesia achieved.
  - Propofol and isoflurane are well tolerated and widely used agents, although induction doses may need to be reduced. Ketamine can cause intraoperative hypertension.
  - The potential for hyperkalemia in patients with CKD who are given succinylcholine is well recognized. However, if the preoperative potassium level is <5.5 mEq/L, it may be safely administered.
  - Avoid long-acting muscle relaxants such as pancuronium. Vecuronium may be safe for induction, but the preferred agent is atracurium, since it does not accumulate in patients with preexisting renal disease.
  - Local and regional anesthetic agents are usually well tolerated.
- Exercise extreme caution with the use of perioperative sedatives and opiates.
  - Dialysis patients are particularly sensitive to the effects of benzodiazepines. The free fraction of these protein-bound drugs is increased in such patients. Midazolam is excreted as its active metabolite and can rapidly accumulate in renal failure.
  - Morphine may be used in patients with renal failure, but cautiously. Although the half-life of morphine is essentially unchanged, its metabolites can accumulate and are pharmacologically active.
  - Avoid meperidine in patients with advanced kidney disease, since its active metabolite normeperidine accumulates in toxic levels and can lead to seizures.

PREOPERATIVE EVALUATION

GENERAL ISSUES

- A basic evaluation of patients with CKD consists of a careful history and physical examination; a panel of laboratory tests including serum chemistry, calcium, phosphate, and magnesium levels; a complete blood count; a coagulation profile; and an electrocardiogram.
  - Specific risk factors requiring preoperative evaluation and possible intervention include creatinine >2 mg/dL, hyperkalemia, metabolic acidosis, severe anemia, and cardiac disease.
- Postpone elective surgery in patients with unexplained significantly abnormal renal function discovered during the preoperative evaluation so as to determine the etiology of the renal dysfunction.

CARDIOVASCULAR EVALUATION

- Cardiac disease is the most serious comorbidity in patients with CKD. It is estimated that 50 percent of all deaths in this patient population are from underlying cardiac disease.
  - Coronary artery disease (CAD) is the key factor in the development of significant cardiac disease in patients with CKD, with a prevalence of about 40 percent.[7]
  - In patients with advanced CKD on hemodialysis and peritoneal dialysis, the prevalence of cardiac failure is approximately 40 percent. Both CAD and left ventricular hypertrophy are risk factors for developing congestive heart failure.
  - Cardiovascular mortality approaches 9 percent per year in patients with CKD. In dialysis patients, the annual mortality is 10 to 20 times higher than in the general population.[7]
  - Preexisting renal disease (serum creatinine >2) has been shown to be an independent predictor of increased cardiac risk in patients undergoing major surgery.
- Given the high prevalence of cardiac disease, a careful cardiac risk assessment is mandated in CKD patients undergoing major surgery. Since many patients are asymptomatic and typical manifestations of coronary disease and cardiac failure are absent in patients with CKD, further preoperative evaluation is often necessary, particularly in dialysis recipients.
- Cardiac risk assessment for CAD in general is discussed in Chap. 20. However, some studies specifically related to the patient with CKD are discussed here.
- One study of cardiac risk stratification, particularly in patients with CKD undergoing renal transplantation, found that patients who had no risk factors (such as age >50, angina, congestive heart failure, type I diabetes, or an abnormal electrocardiogram) were at low risk for

cardiac events, with an overall cardiac mortality of 1 percent. Those with one or more risk factors had a 17 percent overall mortality.[8]

- A number of trials have studied the role of *noninvasive evaluation* in the preoperative assessment of cardiac risk in patients with CKD undergoing surgery. The majority of the patients were renal transplant candidates and thus represented a relatively healthy dialysis population. Many trials have noted limitations of exercise stress testing and dipyridamole thallium scanning in patients with CKD, reporting lower sensitivities and specificities for the detection of important coronary disease.[7]
- Recent reports of combined dipyridamole and exercise thallium scanning as well as the use of dobutamine echocardiography have shown favorable results in identifying significant coronary disease in patients undergoing renal transplantation:
  - Dipyridamole-exercise thallium imaging and coronary angiography were both performed prospectively in a study of 60 asymptomatic hemodialysis patients who were followed for major coronary events. After follow-up of almost 3 years, 47 percent of patients with abnormal thallium uptake experienced a coronary event, as compared with 9 percent of patients with a normal thallium uptake.[9]
  - In a study of 53 patients with insulin-dependent diabetes mellitus being considered for kidney and/or pancreas transplantation, cardiac event rates were 45 percent among those with an abnormal compared to 6 percent among those with a normal dobutamine stress echocardiogram.[10]
- Given the high prevalence of significant cardiac disease in dialysis patients, some authors have questioned the use of noninvasive testing before renal transplantation.
  - One study examined 126 renal transplant candidates who were classified as moderate (age ≥ 50 years) or high coronary risk (diabetes, extracardiac atherosclerosis, or clinical CAD) and underwent myocardial scintigraphy (SPECT), dobutamine stress echocardiography, and angiography. The prevalence of CAD was 42 percent, and the sensitivities and negative predictive values for the two noninvasive tests and risk stratification were <75 percent. The probability of event-free survival at 48 months was 94 percent in patients with <70 percent stenosis on coronary angiography and 54 percent in those with >70 percent stenosis. Multivariate analysis showed that the presence of critical coronary lesions was the sole predictor of cardiac events.[11]
- Consider preoperative echocardiography in renal patients with history or findings of congestive heart failure or valvular heart disease to evaluate left ventricular function.

PERIOPERATIVE MANAGEMENT

Perioperative management of CKD patients undergoing major surgery mandates aggressive metabolic, cardiovascular, hematologic, and pharmaceutical intervention.

FLUID MANAGEMENT

- Euvolemia is mandated in patients with CKD being prepared for surgery, as these patients have a limited ability to respond to volume expansion and depletion as well as other homeostatic changes.
  - Patients with mild-to-moderate reductions in the GFR may have impaired excretion of a large and rapid sodium load in the perioperative period. This may occur in circumstances where other comorbidities also inhibit sodium excretion, such as congestive heart failure, cirrhosis, and the nephrotic syndrome.
  - In patients with GFR <10 mL/min, administration of large quantities of intravenous fluids can quickly lead to volume overload.
- Manage *volume overload* preoperatively with aggressive sodium restriction and the use of diuretics.
  - Large doses of loop diuretics, such as furosemide or bumetanide, are often required in patients not already being dialyzed. At times, the judicious use of metolazone can enhance the effect of the loop diuretics. Maintenance infusions of furosemide are not recommended.
- The use of mannitol, low-dose dopamine, or calcium channel blockers has not been proven to prevent postoperative renal failure in patients with normal renal function or with preexisting renal disease. With careful preoperative resuscitation and control of fluid and electrolyte balance, the incidence of postoperative renal dysfunction can be minimized.
- In patients undergoing surgery for obstructive jaundice use only bile salts and/or lactulose after adequate preoperative hydration.

DIALYSIS (TABLE 34-2)

- Ideally, *dialysis patients* should be at or close to their "dry weight" by the time of surgery.
  - Preoperative consultation with the surgeon and anesthetist is useful to estimate the amount of fluids likely to be administered in the perioperative period.
  - Besides the type of fluid to be given, preferably isotonic saline and not lactated Ringer's, the timing and intensity of the preoperative dialysis can help to ensure a safe outcome.

Table 34-2 Management to Reduce Risk in Dialysis Patients

Basic laboratory evaluation
Manage fluids and electrolytes
Correct acidosis
Correct anemia and coagulation defect
Control blood pressure
Control dialysis dose, intensity, and timing
Evaluate cardiac risk
Address nutritional status
Achieve glycemic control

  - In general, dialyze the patient on the day before the procedure.
- Avoid *volume depletion* in patients with some preservation of renal function. Worsening renal function is likely in those with preoperative volume depletion who then experience sustained hypotension.
- Dialysis patients who undergo intensive preoperative dialysis are at risk for anesthesia-induced vasodilatation, which can lead to thrombosis of the vascular access graft.[4]
- The timing of *postoperative dialysis* depends on the amount of fluids administered perioperatively.
  - The critically ill and other patients who have received excessive fluids may need immediate postoperative dialysis.
  - Ultrafiltration provides a means to preferentially remove fluid in volume-overloaded patients. This must be balanced with the risk of hypotension, especially in patients with postoperative cardiac dysfunction or sepsis.
  - In stable patients, dialysis can be safely resumed 24 h after the surgery. The decision as to whether or not to use heparin with the dialysis should be made in consultation with the surgical and anesthetic team.
- Dialysis patients needing *emergency surgery* are at particular risk for serious morbidity and higher mortality.
  - If possible, perform a "no heparin" dialysis 2 to 3 h before surgery.
  - If necessary, dialysis can be continued throughout the surgical procedure.
  - Hypotension, hyperkalemia, and wound complications are common in the postoperative setting.
- *Peritoneal dialysis* patients present unique management challenges in the perioperative period.
  - Individualize dwells based on the preoperative assessment of fluid status, type of surgery, and expected fluid administration.
  - Exchange the dialysate before the start of surgery and maintain the dwell throughout the course of a short procedure.
  - For a longer procedure, an intraoperative exchange may be necessary. Adjust dialysate concentrations to manage excess fluid administration during surgery.
  - Postoperatively, resume dwells on a scheduled basis, with modifications to the dialysate based on volume status and serum electrolyte measurements.
  - For patients undergoing abdominal surgery, drain the peritoneal fluid completely just before the surgery. Alternative dialysis modes such as hemodialysis or continuous arteriovenous hemodialysis may be undertaken. Resume peritoneal dialysis after a few weeks, beginning with small volumes and short dwell times.

ELECTROLYTE MANAGEMENT

HYPERKALEMIA

- Hyperkalemia is the most important morbid complication in the perioperative period.
  - Obtain a preoperative electrocardiogram to assess the physiologic effect of hyperkalemia, although electrocardiographic changes may be seen only when the potassium concentration exceeds 6.0 to 6.5 meq/L.[5]
  - Patients with CKD usually tolerate a modest elevation in the serum level of potassium, but abrupt increases in potassium levels are poorly tolerated in dialysis patients.
  - In patients undergoing elective surgery, the preoperative potassium should be <5.0 meq/L.
  - Based on the preoperative serum potassium level, the dialysis flow rate, type of dialyzer, and potassium concentration of the bath, hemodialysis can adequately remove enough potassium.
- In cases of emergency surgery where time does not permit an adequate preoperative dialysis, other measures must be taken to stabilize the cardiac membrane.
  - In patients with electrocardiographic evidence of hyperkalemia, such as prolongation of the QRS or arrhythmias, give an infusion of one 10-mg ampule of calcium gluconate. This intervention can provide cardioprotection while attempts are under way to reduce the serum potassium.
- Medical management of severe hyperkalemia before surgery can reduce potassium by varying degrees and include the following[7]:
  - Insulin and glucose administered together cause a rapid shift of potassium to the intracellular space. The expected reduction in serum potassium is 0.9 meq/L.
  - Epinephrine and albuterol can be expected to reduce potassium by 0.3 meq/L; however, the $beta_2$ agonists can lead to arrhythmias.
  - Sodium bicarbonate has no effect on serum potassium in the absence of metabolic acidosis.

- Cation exchange resins are effective in removing excess potassium. The usual oral dose is 15 to 30 g, which can be repeated. If patients are unable to take anything by mouth, 50 to 100 g in 200 mL of water can be administered as a rectal enema. Of note, one complication of cation exchange resins is the risk of intestinal necrosis when administered within 1 week after abdominal surgery.[5]

Calcium and Phosphate

- Treat severe hypocalcemia (<6 mg/dL) beginning with control of the serum phosphate level.
  - Use phosphate binders early to aim for a level <5.5 mg/dL. In emergency situations, preoperative dialysis can also lower serum phosphate.
  - Replace calcium with 1.5 g of oral elemental calcium per day. Coadminister rapid-acting vitamin D derivative 1,25-dihydroxycholcalciferol in a dose of 0.25 to 0.75 μg/day.
  - Administer intravenous calcium in patients with signs and symptoms of severe hypocalcemia.

ACIDOSIS

- Patients with CKD are prone to metabolic acidosis. Although there is respiratory compensation, patients may be prone to severe acidemia due to perioperative ischemia. Impairment of renal function makes it difficult to buffer a large acid load.
  - The preoperative bicarbonate level should be >18 meq/L.
  - Bicarbonate administration with either oral replacement or intravenous infusion can raise the level without leading to significant volume expansion from the sodium load.

MANAGEMENT OF CARDIAC DISEASE

- Aggressive *perioperative management* of patients with CKD with cardiac disease is essential to reduce risk. Patients identified as being at increased cardiac risk by clinical risk stratification and noninvasive testing are potential candidates for various intervention strategies including preoperative coronary angiography, medical therapy, and perioperative hemodynamic monitoring.
  - There are no randomized trials of invasive intervention that have been shown to reduce perioperative risk in patients with CKD. Consider coronary revascularization in CKD patients if the coronary anatomy is severely compromised and amenable to either percutaneous coronary intervention or coronary artery bypass grafting.
  - Trials of medical therapy including beta blockers have shown a favorable immediate and long-term outcome in patients with established CAD or risk factors for CAD. Although the published trials were not specific to patients with CKD, the results indicate that, barring contraindications, almost all patients with CKD have enough CAD risk to justify the use of perioperative beta blockers. Ideally, these agents should be initiated several days or weeks before the surgery and titrated to a resting heart rate of 60 beats per minute.

MONITORING

- The use of a pulmonary artery catheter in the perioperative period is theoretically advantageous in patients with CKD. However, several studies have failed to demonstrate improved outcomes (although some excluded patients with renal failure).
- At present, the use of pulmonary artery catheters is probably justified only in CKD patients undergoing major operations who have preoperative volume or hemodynamic derangements or significant left ventricular dysfunction and in dialysis patients undergoing emergency surgery.

HYPERTENSION AND HYPOTENSION

- The incidence of *hypertension* is high in patients with CKD.
  - Excessive fluid retention and exaggerated catecholamine surges are primary mechanisms that can explain hypertension in dialysis patients.
  - Preoperative optimization can be accomplished by dialysis and ultrafiltration. Management of anxiety and continuation of usual antihypertensive agents throughout the operative day can help to control blood pressure.
  - For refractory hypertension that does not respond to preoperative dialysis and oral medications, intravenous labetalol, enalapril, or hydralazine can immediately lower the blood pressure. The use of intravenous nitroprusside should be limited to 1 to 2 days, since thiocyanate, a metabolite of nitroprusside, can accumulate in patients with advanced kidney disease, leading to anorexia, confusion, and psychosis.
- *Hypotension* in the dialysis patient is multifactorial and problematic, as the need for pre- and postoperative dialysis arises in the surgical patient.
  - Excessive preoperative fluid removal, congestive heart failure, autonomic dysfunction, hemorrhage, and the preoperative use of anesthetics and antihypertensive agents are important causes of hypotension.[5]

- Corrective measures to reduce and treat perioperative hypotension include adjusting the dry weight, increasing the dialysate sodium concentration, and the use of steady ultrafiltration. Use of erythropoietin to treat underlying anemia, higher calcium concentration in the dialysate, and cool-temperature dialysis can also favorably affect cardiovascular performance.

ANEMIA AND BLEEDING DIATHESIS

- Anemia is universally present in patients with significant CKD.
  - Since the anemia is chronic, it is usually well tolerated, and most patients with hematocrit levels of 20 to 24 percent tolerate even major procedures without the need for preoperative transfusions.
  - A preoperative transfusion is recommended for patients with a hematocrit of <20 percent.
- Patients with advanced CKD have defects in platelet aggregation and thus are at risk for postoperative bleeding.
  - The routine measurement of a preoperative bleeding time is not recommended; however, one may be obtained in patients with CKD who have a prior history of excessive bleeding.
  - Intensive preoperative dialysis is likely beneficial in patients with a prolonged bleeding time who require surgical procedures associated with excessive blood loss.
  - Intravenous desmopressin is recommended for urgent surgery. The duration of action is 8 h, although tachyphylaxis can develop after repeated doses.
  - Postoperative "no heparin" dialysis can be performed if the anticipated risk of postoperative bleeding is high.

NUTRITION

- Poor nutritional status is common in patients with advanced CKD. Poor wound healing and infections can complicate the postoperative course in malnourished patients. Diabetics with advanced CKD disease are also predisposed to hypoglycemic events.
- Earlier evidence suggests that patients with CKD who receive perioperative nutritional support have a lower mortality.[5]
- Patients with CKD undergoing major surgery should receive parenteral or enteral nutrition if oral intake cannot be resumed soon after major surgery.
- Since azotemia and fluid overload are issues in patients with advanced CKD, administration of essential amino acids and concentrated carbohydrates and lipids can minimize nitrogen and fluid excess.
- Frequent measurements of serum electrolytes are essential to avoid derangements in potassium, magnesium, phosphorus, and sodium.

SUMMARY

In conclusion, patients with CKD undergoing major surgery have a significant risk of postoperative morbidity and mortality. A careful assessment is mandated in such patients, with particular attention to those with cardiac disease or on dialysis. Preoperative optimization, perioperative monitoring, and specific interventions are frequently required to ensure a safe outcome.

REFERENCES

1. Kellerman PS. Perioperative care of the renal patient. *Arch Intern Med* 154:1674–1688, 1994.
2. Conlon PJ, Stafford-Smith M, White WD, et al. Acute renal failure following cardiac surgery. *Nephrol Dial Transplant* 14:1158, 1999.
3. Polanczyk CA, Marcantonio E, Goldman L, et al. Impact of age on perioperative complications and length of stay in patients undergoing noncardiac surgery. *Ann Intern Med* 134:637–643, 2001.
4. Pinson CW, Schuman ES, Gross EF, et al. Surgery in long-term dialysis patients. Experience with more than 300 cases. *Am J Surg* 151(5):567–571, 1986.
5. Soundararajan R, Golper TA. Medical management of the dialysis patient undergoing surgery. *UpToDate* (version 12.3), accessed January 5, 2005.
6. Baele HR, Piotrowski JJ, Yuhas J, et al. Infrainguinal bypass in patients with end-stage renal disease. *Surgery* 117(3):319–324, 1995.
7. Joseph AJ, Cohn SL. Perioperative care of the patient with renal failure. *Med Clin North Am* 87(1):193–210, 2003.
8. Le A, Wilson R, Douek K, Pulliam L, et al. Prospective risk stratification in renal transplant candidates for cardiac death. *Am J Kidney Dis* 24(1):65–71, 1994.
9. Dahan M, Viron BM, Faraggi M, et al. Diagnostic accuracy and prognostic value of combined dipyridamole-exercise thallium imaging in hemodialysis patients. *Kidney Int* 54(1):255–262, 1998.
10. Bates JR, Sawada SG, Segar DS, et al. Evaluation using dobutamine stress echocardiography in patients with insulin-dependent diabetes mellitus before kidney and/or pancreas transplantation. *Am J Cardiol* 15;77(2):175–179, 1995.
11. De Lima JJ, Sabbaga E, Vieira ML, et al. Coronary angiography is the best predictor of events in renal transplant candidates compared with noninvasive testing. *Hypertension* 42(3):263–268, 2003.

35 LIVER DISEASE

Calvin L. Chou and Kaleem M. Rizvon

INTRODUCTION

- Because the liver plays a crucial role during surgery, an otherwise routine surgical procedure in a patient with underlying liver disease may become risky.
- Patients with liver disease can develop (1) untoward and prolonged effects of anesthetics, opiates, benzodiazepines, and other hepatically metabolized medications; (2) bleeding due to inadequate coagulation factors and possible platelet sequestration in a large spleen; (3) wound dehiscence or poor wound healing due to poor protein synthesis or poor nutritional status; (4) infections, both locally at the wound site and systemically; and (5) ischemia due to peripheral shunting or intraoperative hypoxia.
- Because of the numerous possible perioperative risks, it is very difficult to anticipate and prevent many of these untoward effects. Most of the management of ill perioperative patients with liver disease is reactive rather than preventive.
- This chapter considers patient-related risk factors, procedure-related risk factors, laboratory testing, and interventions to assess the risk of surgery in patients with liver disease.
- Postoperative evaluation and management of the patient with jaundice (Chap. 60) is discussed separately.

PATIENT-RELATED RISK FACTORS (TABLE 35-1)

ACUTE HEPATITIS

- Acute viral or alcoholic hepatitis is a major risk factor for morbidity and mortality after general surgery.
  - Before 1974, it was common to perform exploratory laparotomy on all patients with jaundice to determine etiology. Patients who proved to have acute viral hepatitis had 10 percent mortality and 11 percent morbidity after laparotomy.[1]
  - Perioperative mortality rates among patients with acute alcoholic hepatitis range from 55 percent in open liver biopsy to 100 percent in exploratory laparotomy.[2]
- Few patients need to undergo laparotomy in the setting of acute viral or alcoholic hepatitis. In these patients, there is significant excess surgical mortality, likely due to the severe limitation in functional liver reserve necessary for the metabolic stress of surgery. Although the data are old and have not been recently corroborated, few advances in perioperative management of liver disease have appeared to decrease the risk of major surgery in these patients. No data exist on the risk of perioperative mortality for patients with acute liver disease due to toxic or ischemic causes.
- Active hepatitis B infection confers perioperative risk.
  - During the immune clearance phase of hepatitis B virus (HBV) infection, patients are at high risk of reactivation of viral replication, which can cause severe postoperative hepatitis and acute liver failure. Of patients with serologic evidence of active hepatitis B infection who underwent hepatoma resection, 24 percent developed severe postoperative hepatitis that could be monitored by DNA levels of hepatitis B virus.[3]

TABLE 35-1 Patient- and Surgery-Related Risk Factors for Perioperative Hepatic Complications

PATIENT-RELATED RISK FACTORS	PROCEDURE-RELATED RISK FACTORS*
Acute hepatitis (viral or alcoholic)	Emergent surgery
Cirrhosis with Child-Pugh score >7	Gastrointestinal luminal surgery
INR >1.6	Cardiac surgery (vascular or valvular)
Comorbid medical condition: Chronic obstructive pulmonary disease Pneumonia Congestive heart failure Ischemic heart disease Diabetes mellitus Renal insufficiency Hypoalbuminemia Malnutrition Preoperative infection	

*In patients with cirrhosis.

CIRRHOSIS

- The severity of a patient's underlying cirrhosis, which can be measured by Child-Pugh score or MELD ("model of end-stage liver disease") score (Table 35-2) (see "Risk Indices," below), is a significant predictor of perioperative risk.
- In a multivariate analysis, an international normalized ratio (INR) greater than 1.6 was separately associated with a greater than tenfold increased mortality risk.[4] A retrospective study of patients with cirrhosis and colorectal cancer showed that patients with prolonged prothrombin time were at significantly higher risk of postoperative mortality.[4]

TABLE 35-2 Calculation of Child-Pugh and MELD Scores*

CHILD-PUGH SCORE	1 POINT	2 POINTS	3 POINTS
Ascites	Absent	Slight to moderate	Tense
Serum bilirubin	≤2	2–3	≥ 3
Albumin	>3.5	2.8–3.5	<2.8
INR	≤1.7	1.8–2.3	≥2.4
Encephalopathy	None	Grade 1–2	Grade 3–4
Child-Pugh class	*Total number of points*		
A	5–6		
B	7–9		
C	10–15		

*MELD Score = 10 [0.957 Ln(Scr) + 0.378 Ln(Tbil) + 1.12 Ln(INR) + 0.643]
where Scr = serum creatinine in mg/dL; Tbil = total bilirubin in mg/dL; INR = international normalized ratio.
The calculation can be performed by logging onto the Mayo clinic website at www.mayoclinic.org/gi-rst/mayomodel5.html or The Drug Monitor at http://www.thedrugmonitor.com/meld.html.

OTHER COMORBID MEDICAL ILLNESSES THAT CONFER INCREASED RISK

- Patients with cirrhosis and a serious comorbid condition (see Table 35-1) had a significantly higher postoperative mortality rate.[5]

SURGERY-RELATED RISK FACTORS (TABLE 35-1)

- The type of surgical procedure appears to be the most important risk factor for the development of morbidity in patients with liver disease. Surgical procedures can be divided into relatively high risk versus low-risk operations.

HIGH-RISK SURGICAL PROCEDURES

- Emergent surgery in patients with chronic liver disease and cirrhosis is associated with a mortality risk of 47 to 86 percent, compared with 10 to 41 percent in patients undergoing elective surgery.

Gastrointestinal Luminal Surgery in Patients with Cirrhosis

- Gastric, small bowel, and colon surgery in patients with cirrhosis confers mortality rates of at least 35 percent. In a multivariate analysis, when compared with other forms of nonhepatic surgery, gastrointestinal surgery was the strongest predictor of postoperative mortality;[6] 39 percent of patients with GI operations died, with an odds ratio of 8.6; 81 percent of these died as a result of coagulopathy or sepsis.

Cardiac Surgery in Patients with Cirrhosis

- In two small series of patients with cirrhosis who required coronary artery bypass grafting, valve replacement, or both, there was a complication rate of greater than 50 percent; mortality ranged between 25 and 31 percent. All of the patients who died had Child-Pugh class B cirrhosis, and all who had class B cirrhosis experienced significant complications, including fluid overload and wound infection.[2]
- These studies may not have adequately controlled for the severity or type of surgery, so some of these comparisons may be of unclear significance.

LOW-RISK SURGICAL PROCEDURES

- Umbilical, ventral, and/or inguinal herniorrhaphy are relatively safe, commonly performed procedures in patients with large amounts of ascites.[2]
- Laparoscopic procedures, when compared with their open laparotomy counterparts, appear to confer lower operative morbidity and mortality in patients with cirrhosis.
- Small prospective studies have examined cirrhotic patients undergoing open or laparoscopic cholecystectomy. Intraoperative bleeding, wound infection, and wound dehiscence occurred more frequently in the groups undergoing open cholecystectomy; no mortality was reported in these studies.[2]
- Cirrhotic patients undergoing laparoscopic appendectomy have significantly decreased wound infections, bleeding, hospital stay, and ratings of postoperative pain.[2]
- The outcome of partial hepatectomy for patients with hepatocellular carcinoma depends on the underlying etiology and condition of the surrounding liver.
- Multiple retrospective studies have shown that over the last 15 years, morbidity and mortality after hepatectomy in all patients have declined, probably because of increased surgeon experience, more stringent patient-selection criteria excluding patients with known cirrhosis, and possibly earlier detection.
- In patients with hepatoma due solely to hepatitis B, surrounding liver parenchyma is typically not cirrhotic, and these patients have excellent long-term outcome after partial hepatectomy without subsequent transplantation/[7]
- Patients with hepatoma and Child class B or C cirrhosis had higher mortality rates and earlier recurrences.

Presence of portal hypertension, pathologic evidence of active hepatitis, and low expected remnant liver volume are correlated with increased surgical morbidity and mortality. Partial hepatectomy in these patients should be viewed more as a bridge to transplantation, since 5-year survival rates after hepatectomy remain at 25 to 40 percent, with disease-free 5-year survival at 10 to 30 percent.[2]

- Radiofrequency ablation, recently introduced as a method of treating patients with smaller tumors, appears promising; ongoing reproducible studies assessing long-term mortality benefit are needed.

PREOPERATIVE EVALUATION AND TESTING TO STRATIFY RISK

LIVER FUNCTION TESTING

- Assessment of baseline liver function tests in asymptomatic individuals is controversial.
- In patients with suspected acute liver disease, follow the progression of liver function tests (especially total bilirubin, transaminases, and prothrombin time/INR) daily before a proposed surgical procedure until the overall trend clearly delineates the severity of the disease.
- Transaminase levels and prothrombin time may rise rapidly in the setting of acute hepatitis and may precede other clinical signs of hepatic compromise (e.g., jaundice, encephalopathy). Among patients with jaundice, therefore, it is important to diagnose the etiology of acute liver disease (if unknown). However, no data establish that levels of bilirubin correlate with perioperative mortality.
- A history of recent alcohol use and high transaminases may aid in the diagnosis of alcoholic hepatitis; however, there are no data to suggest that transaminase levels or the slope of their rise predicts perioperative outcome.
- For patients with cleared hepatitis B infection or well-compensated hepatitis C infection, verify that liver function tests, prothrombin time, and platelet count are not substantially different from baseline values. No evidence suggests that patients with a past history of hepatitis A infection or with histologically stable hepatitis B or C infection are at increased risk for hepatic complications perioperatively.
- In patients with chronic hepatitis B infection, check alanine aminotransferase (ALT) levels preoperatively; if the ALT level is elevated, check hepatitis B viral DNA levels. During the immune-clearance phase of hepatitis B virus infection, patients are at high risk of reactivation of viral replication. This phase is characterized by immune-mediated lysis of infected hepatocytes followed by reactivation of viral replication, and can severely affect a patient's postoperative course. Preoperative measurement of HBV DNA levels does not appear to be extraordinarily valuable in predicting a postoperative flare of chronic hepatitis B, since these levels can reflect improved postoperative immune activity rather than greater HBV replication.

CREATININE, RENAL TRANSPLANTATION

- Renal insufficiency in patients with cirrhosis predicts high postoperative mortality, presumably due to recalcitrant fluid overload and a higher risk of developing hepatorenal syndrome. Also, measurements of serum creatinine overestimate renal function in patients with advanced liver disease because of reductions in overall creatinine synthesis by the liver.
- Up to half of all renal transplant recipients are infected with hepatitis C virus (HCV). Renal transplantation confers an overall survival benefit in HCV-positive patients on hemodialysis. In noncirrhotic patients, the efficacy of interferon alpha in clearing hepatitis C from patients with end-stage renal disease is up to 70 percent after 12 months of therapy. Pegylated interferon may confer similar treatment efficacy with fewer side effects.

LIVER BIOPSY

- Patients with bridging or multilobular necrosis on liver biopsy are at increased surgical risk. In patients undergoing partial resection for hepatocellular carcinoma, moderate to severe inflammation on liver biopsy correlated with increased postoperative complications, such as increased ascites and wound infection.
- Overall, however, the bulk of the literature does not support routine liver biopsy in preoperative patients. There is no causative evidence that the level of inflammation on biopsy is predictive of postoperative complications. Therefore obtain a liver biopsy only if an indication exists independent of the need for upcoming surgery.[2]

RISK INDICES

CHILD-PUGH CLASS (TABLE 35-2)

- In two retrospective case series of abdominal surgery in patients with cirrhosis, done at different institutions 13 years apart, Child-Pugh class correlated well with postoperative outcome. In both series, patients with Child class A cirrhosis had 10 percent mortality, patients with Child class B cirrhosis had 30 percent mortality, and patients with Child class C cirrhosis had approximately 80 percent mortality with general surgical procedures. Similarly, a retrospective case study of patients with cirrhosis and colorectal cancer showed that patients with Child-Pugh class A cirrhosis had a significantly lower postoperative mortality risk as compared with patients with class B or C cirrhosis.[1,2]

- With an odds ratio of 24.4, the Child-Pugh score independently predicts mortality in nonhepatic surgery.[8]
- Multivariate analysis showed that a Child-Pugh score of greater than 7 was associated with a statistically significant increase in mortality.[5]

THE MELD SCORE

- This score has been proposed as an additional method for estimating perioperative risk in patients with liver disease. Because calculation of the MELD score uses only objective laboratory values, it has a distinct advantage over the Child-Pugh score, which takes into account more subjective measures of the degree of ascites and encephalopathy. However, the MELD score has not yet been fully validated to estimate perioperative risk.

PERIOPERATIVE MANAGEMENT TO REDUCE RISK (TABLE 35-3)

PREOPERATIVE INTERVENTIONS

- Correct coagulation abnormalities, evidenced by an elevated INR, when possible with fresh frozen plasma and/or vitamin K treatment.
- In cirrhotic patients undergoing cholecystectomy, there was a nearly tenfold increase in mortality if prothrombin time was 2.5 s greater than control (83 percent) compared with a prothrombin time less than 2.5 s longer than control (9.3 percent).
- Although the standard of practice has been to give subcutaneous vitamin K or intravenous fresh frozen plasma for a prolonged prothrombin time,[5] there are no strong data to support it.
- Recent data suggest that administration of oral vitamin K, 1 mg, in asymptomatic patients with supratherapeutic INR due to warfarin overdose is more effective at lowering INR than subcutaneous vitamin K; however, this study did not include patients with liver disease.
- Platelet counts of greater than 100,000/mm^3 are thought to decrease the likelihood of intraoperative and perioperative bleeding.[5] Although some authors suggest that platelet counts of greater than 100,000/mm^3 are desirable, significant surgical bleeding may not occur in patients whose platelet counts are as low as 50,000/mm^3.
- Hepatic encephalopathy is exacerbated with hypokalemia, uremia, gastrointestinal bleeding, infection, overdiuresis, constipation, and medications (particularly sedatives and opiates). There is no experimental evidence, however, to indicate that prophylactic preoperative therapy can prevent postoperative encephalopathy.[5]
- Balance fluid intake and output to reduce the likelihood of fluid overload. More importantly, limiting sodium intake may be useful in decreasing fluid retention. No experimental evidence indicates that restricted intake of fluid in the absence of limited sodium intake decreases postoperative fluid overload. In fact, one study showed that fluid limitation does not prevent postoperative ascites.[9]
- Patients with long-standing chronic liver disease are typically malnourished and unable to complete adequate protein synthesis. Nutritional therapy is thought to reduce the catabolic response to surgery, improve protein synthesis, and promote liver regeneration.
- In one randomized controlled study in patients undergoing partial hepatectomy for liver cancer, patients were given oral and intravenous nutritional support for 2 weeks prior to surgery. There was a 33 percent reduction in overall postoperative morbidity in the

TABLE 35-3 Risk-Reduction Strategies

PREOPERATIVE	INTRAOPERATIVE	POSTOPERATIVE
Correct coagulation abnormalities.	Limit hepatically metabolized anesthetic agents.	Limit hepatically metabolized medications.
Replete platelets.		Treat encephalopathy with lactulose.
Limit factors associated with hepatic encephalopathy.		Administer thiamine in high-risk patients.
Balance fluid intake and output and limit sodium intake.		Balance fluid intake and output and limit sodium intake.
Optimize nutritional status.		Optimize nutritional status.
Give perioperative antibiotics if patients have active infections.		

group receiving nutritional supplementation and a 50 percent decrease in mortality.[10] There was no report of increased encephalopathy in these patients after nutritional intervention. This result has not yet been duplicated; further studies should be performed to corroborate these results before this support can be safely recommended.

- In patients with known severe portal hypertension, consider transjugular intrahepatic portosystemic shunt (TIPS) procedures. However, performing a TIPS procedure can subject a patient to a significant risk of postprocedure encephalopathy and thrombosis. Therefore TIPS for the sole purpose of improving the outcome of a single operation is not recommended.
- Use perioperative antibiotics if patients have active infections. No experimental evidence indicates that administration of prophylactic antibiotics (in addition to antimicrobial treatment already indicated for particular procedures) decreases the risk for perioperative infection. Because of the high risk for infection in cirrhotic patients with ascites, some review articles still recommend a 24-h perioperative course of prophylactic antibiotics (third-generation cephalosporin or fluoroquinolone).[5]

INTRAOPERATIVE INTERVENTIONS

- Strategies to reduce intraoperative risk are managed by anesthesiologists and surgeons. The internist can work with anesthesia colleagues to review the proposed operative anesthetic plan so as to reduce the potential effect of undermetabolized exogenous compounds.
- Use of anesthetic agents that are hepatically metabolized correlates with the likelihood of a toxic reaction. In terms of anesthetic agents, isoflurane, sevoflurane, and the newer volatile haloalkanes are favored because of their decreased hepatic toxicity. Atracurium is the favored neuromuscular blocking agent for similar reasons.[1]

POSTOPERATIVE INTERVENTIONS

- Review medication lists to reduce the potential effect of undermetabolized exogenous compounds. Patients with liver disease are at increased risk for untoward and prolonged effects of anesthetics, opiates, benzodiazepines, and other hepatically metabolized medications. Use of anesthetic agents that are hepatically metabolized correlates with the likelihood of a toxic reaction.[1]
- If the patient develops encephalopathy, begin lactulose by mouth (or via rectal enemas if necessary), approximately 30 mL every 4 h, titrated to two to three loose stools per day. Encephalopathy is a frequent postoperative complication in patients with cirrhosis.[5] Frequent monitoring in an intensive care unit setting may lead to earlier diagnosis.
- Postoperative administration of thiamine (vitamin B_1, 100 mg PO or IV daily) is a low-risk intervention to prevent postoperative Wernicke-Korsakoff syndrome in patients who are heavy users of alcohol or who have had bariatric surgery.

SUMMARY

In summary, patients with liver disease are potentially at increased risk of perioperative complications. Careful preoperative evaluation and anticipation of postoperative complications can reduce this risk. Patients with Child-Pugh class A cirrhosis can be classified as at relatively low risk for surgical complications.

REFERENCES

1. Friedman LS. The risk of surgery in patients with liver disease. *Hepatology* 29:1617, 1999.
2. Chou CL. Perioperative evaluation of patients with liver disease, in American College of Physicians (ed), *Physicians' Information and Education Resource,* 2005. Website: http://pier.acponline.org/index.html.
3. Kubo S, Nishiguchi S, Hamba H, et al. Reactivation of viral replication after liver resection in patients infected with hepatitis B virus. *Ann Surg* 233:139, 2001.
4. Gervaz P, Pak-art R, Nivatvongs S, et al. Colorectal adenocarcinoma in cirrhotic patients. *J Am Coll Surg* 196:874, 2003.
5. Ziser A, Plevak DJ, Wiesner RH, et al. Morbidity and mortality in cirrhotic patients undergoing anesthesia and surgery. *Anesthesiology* 90:42, 1999.
6. Mansour A, Watson W, Shayani V, et al. Abdominal operations in patients with cirrhosis: Still a major surgical challenge. *Surgery* 122:730, 1997.
7. Verhoef C, de Man RA, Zondervan PE, et al. Good outcomes after resection of large hepatocellular carcinoma in the noncirrhotic liver. *Dig Surg* 21:380, 2003.
8. del Olmo JA, Flor-Lorente B, Flor-Civera B, et al. Risk factors for nonhepatic surgery in patients with cirrhosis. *World J Surg* 27:647, 2003.
9. Lentschener C, Ozier Y. Anaesthesia for elective liver resection: Some points should be revisited. *Eur J Anaesthesiol* 19:780, 2002.
10. Fan ST, Lo CM, Lai EC, et al. Perioperative nutritional support in patients undergoing hepatectomy for hepatocellular carcinoma. *N Engl J Med* 331:1547, 1994.

36 ACID-PEPTIC DISORDERS

Vaishali M. Singh and Maninder Kohli

INTRODUCTION

- Common acid-peptic disorders that involve injury to gastroesophageal mucosa include gastroesophageal reflux disease (GERD), gastric and duodenal ulcers, and gastritis.
- This injury can occur in critically ill patients and/or in the setting of severe physiologic stress. In the operative /mechanical ventilation setting, "stress ulceration" has been associated with decreased splanchnic flow, which in turn leads to gastric hypoperfusion and ischemic damage.[1]
- The degree of ulceration depends on the patient's underlying illness. Left untreated, some deeper lesions can progress and erode into the submucosa, leading to perforation and/or hemorrhage.
- Acute upper gastrointestinal bleeding is a common problem in critical care medicine and accounts for some 300,000 hospital admissions annually.[2,3]
- Complications of GERD include esophagitis, esophageal stricture, and Barrett's metaplasia as well as extralaryngeal complications such as laryngitis, chronic cough, and reflex-induced asthma.
- This chapter addresses the patient and procedure related factors and their relation to perioperative management of acid-peptic disease.

PATIENT-RELATED RISK FACTORS (TABLE 36-1)

TABLE 36-1 Risk Factors and Risk-Reduction Strategies

RISK FACTORS	RISK-REDUCTION STRATEGIES
Age	Treat *H. pylori* and active PUD
Mechanical ventilation >48 h	PPIs or H_2 antagonist prophylaxis
Coagulopathy	Antireflux measures
H. pylori infection	Avoid ASA/NSAIDs in patients at risk for bleeding
Active PUD	
GERD	
Type of surgery: neurosurgery, trauma, burns, organ transplant	

ASA/NSAIDs = aspirin and other nonsteroidal anti-inflammatory drugs; GERD = gastroesophageal reflux disease; PPIs = proton pump inhibitors; PUD = peptic ulcer disease.

AGE

- Age-related changes to gastrointestinal physiology include decreased esophageal sphincter pressure and peristalsis, leading to increased risk of GERD, particularly in those 65 years of age and over.[4]
- In the U.S. population, the prevalence of *Helicobacter pylori* increases with age and is approximately 50 percent by age 60. Infection with *H. pylori* is an important cause of peptic ulcer disease (PUD) and gastritis.[5]
- Complications from PUD, specifically bleeding and perforation, are associated with a mortality rate of 30 percent in the elderly.[5]

MECHANICAL VENTILATION AND COAGULOPATHY

- A landmark study in 1994 reviewed risk factors in over 2000 patients for stress ulceration and the occurrence of clinically significant gastrointestinal bleeding.[6]
  - The study found that critically ill patients requiring mechanical ventilation greater than 48 h and patients with coagulopathy [defined as a platelet count <50,000/μL, international normalized ratio (INR) >1.5, or partial thromboplastin time (PTT) more than twice the control value] demonstrated an increased risk of stress-related mucosal disease (16-fold and 4-fold, respectively).
  - Of note, other factors noted *not* to be statistically significant by this study included shock (hypotension), sepsis, liver failure, enteral feeding, and glucocorticoids.
- Stress-related mucosal disease is widely believed to be the pathogenesis of severe postoperative erosive gastritis. Stress ulceration is seen in a majority of patients admitted to the surgical and trauma intensive care units. Once major bleeding has occurred, the mortality may approach 50 percent.

HELICOBACTER PYLORI INFECTION AND ACTIVE ULCER DISEASE

- Infection with *H. pylori* and its relationship to GERD, PUD, gastritis, and gastric malignancy has been well reported since its discovery by Marshall and Warren in 1984.
  - The majority of patients with chronic gastritis and duodenal ulcer (DU) are infected with *H. pylori.*
  - Smokers have a twofold greater risk of developing PUD than nonsmokers; however, after *H. pylori* infection is cured, smoking is no longer a risk factor for recurrent ulcers.
  - Family history of ulcer disease and the use of nonsteroidal anti-inflammatory drugs (NSAIDs) are other risk factors for the development of ulcer disease.

- The major concern in patients with active ulcer disease undergoing surgery is the risk of precipitating hemorrhage or perforation in the postoperative setting. Perioperative hypoperfusion and hypoxia may exacerbate mucosal changes in these patients.
- Patients undergoing nonulcer surgery with recent gastrointestinal bleeding are at significant risk for recurrent bleeding in the postoperative period. The risk is particularly high in the elderly patient.

GASTROESOPHAGEAL REFLUX DISEASE (GERD)

- Patients with GERD may experience exacerbations in the perioperative setting as a result of postoperative ileus, abdominal distention and insufflation, and prolonged nasogastric intubation.
- Patients with complicated reflux disease such as peptic stricture may be at risk for postoperative aspiration.[7]

SURGERY-RELATED RISK FACTORS

- Patients most at risk for postoperative bleeding from ulcers are:
  - Neurosurgical patients
  - Trauma patients
  - Patients with severe burns
  - Organ transplant patients

PREOPERATIVE EVALUATION

- Review basic coagulation panel (PT/INR, PTT, platelet count) and correct abnormalities as necessary with blood products and vitamin K.
- In general, avoid aspirin and other NSAIDs during the perioperative period not only for their antiplatelet function but also for their crucial role in the development of PUD as well as gastritis. However, a risk-benefit analysis should be done in deciding whether to continue these medications in the perioperative period (see Chap. 7).
- Provide counseling for smoking cessation.
- Assess patients with long-standing severe GERD symptoms for possible complications such as reflux asthma, otolaryngologic manifestations (laryngitis, laryngeal or tracheal stenosis), peptic stricture, or malignancy.
- As recommended by the American College of Gastroenterology, evaluate for and treat *H. pylori* in patients with known active peptic-acid disease or past history of documented peptic ulcers.[8]
  - Consider postponing elective surgery in patients with active ulcer disease to allow for preoperative evaluation and treatment.
  - Noninvasive evaluation for *H. pylori* includes urea breath testing and serologic testing using enzyme-linked immunosorbent assay (ELISA) technology. The stool antigen assay may be an alternative in patients who are not taking proton-pump inhibitors (PPIs) and who have not had recent acute gastrointestinal bleeding.
  - Upper endoscopy is the preferred test for preoperative detection of ulcer disease. Compared to barium contrast radiography, endoscopy has a higher sensitivity and specificity for the detection of peptic ulcers, gastritis, and gastric erosions. Biopsies of ulcers can be obtained to confirm the presence of *H. pylori*. The urease test on antral biopsy is the preferred first test when endoscopy is performed. If the urease test is negative, histology or serology is recommended to diagnose *H. pylori* infection.

PERIOPERATIVE MANAGEMENT TO REDUCE RISK

- Although acid-peptic diseases are common, there are few data to suggest that patients with simple GERD or *stable* PUD undergoing nonulcer surgery have adverse outcomes.
- Patients with symptoms suggestive of complicated reflux disease should be aggressively treated with PPIs and nonpharmacologic antireflux measures, including lifestyle and dietary modifications.
- Consider postponement of elective surgery in patients with recent *active* ulcer disease or recent gastrointestinal bleeding. Once ulcer disease is confirmed by noninvasive tests or endoscopy, patients should be treated intensively for at least 4 weeks before surgery.
- Eradicate *H. pylori* infection using one of the following regimens[8]:
  - The preferred regimen is triple therapy with a PPI, amoxicillin (1 g twice daily), and clarithromycin (500 mg twice daily) for 2 weeks. Metronidazole (500 mg twice daily for 2 weeks) may be substituted for amoxicillin in penicillin-allergic patients.
  - Combine a PPI with bismuth (525 mg four times daily) and two antibiotics (e.g., metronidazole 500 mg four times daily and tetracycline 500 mg four times daily) for 2 weeks.
  - Initial treatment with the above regimens can eradicate *H. pylori* in 85 percent of all patients.
- Although the incidence of postoperative ulceration is not known, the goal of active ulcer treatment must be ulcer healing. The presence of ulcer pain correlates poorly with the presence of an ulcer crater. Thus, symptom relief may occur early in the treatment of active ulcers and healing may lag, mandating treatment for an additional 2 to 4 weeks.

- If ASA/NSAIDs are necessary and cannot be stopped, the use of a PPI can protect against both duodenal and gastric ulcers. Alternatively, the use of a prostaglandin analogue such as misoprostol can mitigate the effects on the gastric and duodenal mucosa.

REFERENCES

1. Mutlu GM, Mutlu E, Factor P. GI complications in patients receiving mechanical ventilation. *Chest* 119:1222–1241, 2001.
2. Conrad CA. Acute upper gastrointestinal bleeding in critically ill patients: Causes and treatment modalities. *Crit Care Med* 30(6 suppl):S365–S368, 2002.
3. Terdiman JP, Ostroff JW. Gastrointestinal bleeding in the hospitalized patient: A case-control study to assess risk factors, causes, and outcome. *Am J Med* 104:329–335, 1998.
4. Greenwald DA. Aging and the gastrointestinal tract, and risk of acid-related disease. *Am J Med* 117:8s–13s, 2004.
5. Linder JD, Wilcox CM. Gastrointestinal disorders in the elderly. *Gastroenterol Clin North Am* 30(2):363–376, 2001.
6. Cook DJ, Fuller HD, Guyatt, GH, et al. Risk factors for gastrointestinal bleeding in critically ill patients. *N Engl J Med* 330: 377–381, 1994.
7. Ng A, Smith G. Gastroesophageal reflux and aspiration of gastric contents in anesthetic practice. *Anesth Analg* 93(2): 494–513, 2001.
8. Howden CW, Hunt RH. Guidelines for the management of *Helicobacter pylori* infection. Ad Hoc Committee on Practice Parameters of the American College of Gastroenterology. *Am J Gastroenterol* 93(12):2330–2338, 1998.

37 CEREBROVASCULAR DISEASE

Vinky Chadha and Frank Lefevre

INTRODUCTION

- A thorough assessment of the presence and severity of cerebrovascular disease is an important component of preoperative assessment for several reasons.
  - The general surgery population is expected to have a relatively high prevalence of cerebrovascular disease due to advanced age and other concomitant risk factors such hypertension, smoking, and hypercholesterolemia.
  - The incidence of postoperative stroke is higher in patients with preexisting cerebrovascular disease. While the overall rate of postoperative stroke is <1 percent, the rate for patients with a previous stroke or transient ischemic attack (TIA) is in the range of 2 to 5 percent range.[1-3] Risk-reduction strategies should be considered in this higher-risk population.
  - The presence of cerebrovascular disease is an important marker for atherosclerotic vascular disease and raises the possibility of widespread vascular disease. This may influence the pretest likelihood of ischemic cardiac disease and affect the decision to perform other diagnostic and/or therapeutic interventions preoperatively.
- Cerebrovascular disease may manifest itself as stroke, transient ischemic attack (TIA), or vascular dementia. A stroke is defined as a vascular central nervous system (CNS) insult that persists for more than 24 h, while a TIA resolves within 24 h. Vascular dementia is characterized by infarcts of small (lacunar) vessels in the CNS associated with stepwise decrements in cognition.

ASSESSING RISK

PATIENT-SPECIFIC RISK FACTORS

- There are numerous factors that increase the risk of stroke in general, although the precise contribution of these factors in the perioperative period is less certain. These factors are advanced age, hypertension, hypercholesterolemia, diabetes, smoking, and atrial fibrillation. The presence of structural heart disease, especially with systolic dysfunction, is also associated with an increased risk of stroke in general, and the same is likely to be true in the perioperative period.[4]
  - In one large series of patients undergoing general surgery (n = 2463), all patients with postoperative stroke or TIA had at least one clinical manifestation of atherosclerotic disease prior to surgery. Other significant predictors were age, hypertension, and heart disease.[1]
  - In a retrospective review from the Mayo Clinic between 1986 and 1996, a total of 61 patients were identified who suffered an ischemic event following a general surgical procedure. A history of prior cerebrovascular events was the variable most predictive of postsurgical ischemic stroke. Chronic obstructive pulmonary disease (COPD) and peripheral vascular disease (PVD) were also associated with an increased risk.[5]
  - In a large retrospective review of 19,475 vascular surgery patients from the Veterans Administration system,[6] the risk of postoperative stroke varied between 0.4 and 0.6 percent, depending on the specific type of operation. Independent risk factors for stroke were previous cerebrovascular accident

(CVA) (OR 4.2, 95 percent CI 2.7 to 6.4), postoperative myocardial infarction (MI) (OR 3.3, 95 percent CI 1.3 to 8.7), and need to return to the operating room (OR 2.2, 95 percent CI 1.4 to 3.5).

- When there is a history of prior stroke or TIA, the timing of the event in relation to elective surgery is important. The risk for recurrent CNS events is probably highest in the first 2 weeks, and increased risk may persist for up to 2 months. Elective surgery may be delayed appropriately during this time interval so as to minimize the risk of recurrent stroke perioperatively.
    - The underlying evidence supporting these general recommendations on timing of surgery following stroke is scant.[2] In 1968, DeWeese et al. reported on a series of patients who underwent general surgery following a stroke.[7] Mortality was 34 percent if the surgery was performed within 24 h of the stroke, 15 percent for surgery performed between 1 and 13 days following stroke, and 0 percent for surgery 2 weeks or longer following stroke. While other series have not confirmed this relationship, later studies are limited by the small numbers of patients who undergo surgery shortly after a stroke due to the high perceived risk.
    - Given the lack of empiric evidence, certain physiologic responses to stroke have been used to frame recommendations concerning the timing of surgery following stroke.[3] Cerebral autoregulation following stroke remains impaired for 1 to 2 weeks, and patients with impaired autoregulation may be less able to regulate cerebral blood flow in response to the hemodynamic stressors of surgery. In addition, inflammatory changes seen in cerebral tissue following stroke lead to softening of the tissue, which could make the surrounding areas vulnerable to hemorrhagic transformation and/or further ischemia. These alterations are likely to be resolved by 1 month following a moderately large stroke.
    - For patients with a prior stroke or TIA greater than 2 months before surgery, the risk of postoperative stroke is expected to return to baseline for patients with prior events (i.e., 2 to 5 percent).[1,2]
- Medications affecting the coagulation system may affect risk. Patients with preexisting cerebrovascular disease may be on aspirin or other antiplatelet agents, while patients with heart disease may be taking warfarin. The risk for stroke in the perioperative period may be increased or decreased by withdrawal of these medications. For example, withholding antiplatelet agents perioperatively may increase the risk of postoperative ischemic stroke while decreasing the risk for hemorrhagic stroke. While most medications that increase bleeding risk need to be held for at least some time perioperatively, the risks and benefits of withholding them need to be assessed individually.
- Asymptomatic carotid bruits are common on examination, present in approximately 10 percent of general surgery patients and 16 percent of vascular surgery patients.[2] The presence of a carotid bruit increases the likelihood of cerebrovascular disease and signifies a higher risk of postoperative stroke.
    - In a retrospective study, 224 general surgery patients were identified who, on ultrasound performed preoperatively, demonstrated a carotid stenosis ≥50 percent. In this group, there were 8 postoperative strokes, for an incidence of 3.6 percent. Increasingly severe carotid lesions did not result in significantly higher preoperative stroke risk, although there was a trend toward higher stroke rates as the degree of stenosis increased.[8]
    - However, the management of asymptomatic carotid stenosis remains controversial. While the benefit of carotid endarterectomy for high-grade symptomatic carotid stenosis is widely accepted, the risk/benefit ratio for interventions directed at asymptomatic lesions is not as clearly defined.
    - Despite the association of carotid bruits and the risk of stroke, revascularization of the carotid system is rarely if ever indicated to reduce the risk of postoperative stroke. In the best-case scenario, based on the Asymptomatic Carotid Atherosclerosis Study, the anticipated morbidity and mortality for carotid endarterectomy (CEA) at 30 days was 2.7 percent; complications in general practice are likely to be higher.[9] It is extremely unlikely that perioperative risk can be reduced enough to offset this complication rate.
    - One exception to this rule may be for coronary artery bypass graft (CABG) patients with high-grade carotid stenosis, in whom simultaneous CEA-CABG or a staged procedure may improve outcomes. For patients with indications for both CABG and CEA, the current controversy resolves around whether simultaneous procedures or staged procedures lead to better outcomes.
    - Some experts recommend the "symptomatic" approach to this situation, in which the area that is symptomatic is addressed first and the asymptomatic lesion(s) are operated on later.[3] When both lesions are equally symptomatic, especially in situations where both represent high risk, a combined approach may be recommended.

SURGERY-SPECIFIC RISK FACTORS

- The type of surgery is also important in determining the risk of postoperative stroke. The procedures with the highest rates of postoperative stroke are cardiac surgeries (including CABG), CEA, and aortoiliac procedures. For these types of procedures, the risk of postoperative stroke is in the range of 1 to 5 percent.[2,3]

PREOPERATIVE EVALUATION

- The main tools in assessing the presence of cerebrovascular disease are the history and physical examination. Prior stroke or TIA is usually evident on history, while a history of vascular dementia may be more difficult to elicit, since the typical stepwise decrements in cognition may be subtle and subclinical.
- Thoroughly question patients with TIA or stroke regarding symptoms of cardiac disease (exertional chest pressure, dyspnea, paroxysmal nocturnal dyspnea, orthopnea, edema), since 20 to 40 percent of patients with cerebrovascular disease may have unrecognized coronary artery disease (CAD).[10] Studies suggest that patients with asymptomatic CAD may benefit from further risk stratification. Based on a thorough clinical examination, estimate the probability of CAD and decide whether further preoperative testing is warranted.
- As previously noted, preoperatively address issues concerning any medications that affect clotting, such as warfarin and/or antiplatelet agents (see Chaps. 7 and 7A).
- For patients with prior stroke, carefully document the presence and severity of neurologic motor impairment preoperatively. This will enable a more accurate assessment of the risk for motor-related complications postoperatively, such as aspiration or deep venous thrombosis (DVT). Also, it will allow the clinician to establish a baseline, which may assist in evaluating new neurologic symptoms.
- It is likewise important to document the baseline level of alertness and cognitive function as part of the preoperative examination. This baseline may be crucial in assessing postoperative delirium and/or new cognitive deficits.
- Imaging of the CNS can confirm the presence of cerebrovascular disease, with magnetic resonance imaging (MRI) being the most sensitive modality in routine use. Imaging of the brain may be most helpful when there are unexplained or uncharacterized neurologic symptoms. In contrast, when there is a clear history of cerebrovascular disease and stable symptoms, neuroimaging is rarely useful preoperatively.
- Other diagnostic testing preoperatively should be directed toward the likelihood of widespread atherosclerotic vascular disease. Evaluate cardiac status according to the overall presence or absence of risk factors and symptoms. This may involve electrocardiography, echocardiography, or stress testing. Check renal function to assess for atherosclerotic renovascular disease.

REDUCING RISK

PERIOPERATIVE MANAGEMENT

- Risk factors for perioperative stroke are largely related to the risk of atherosclerotic vascular disease. However, even with the presence of multiple risk factors, the incidence of preoperative stroke in patients going for a general surgical procedure is low. Because of this low risk, the absolute benefit of reducing stroke risk is relatively limited.
- However, interventions prompted by the presence of cerebrovascular disease are likely to be useful in other ways. Risk-reduction strategies are likely to reduce other vascular complications, such as MI. In addition, the perioperative evaluation offers an opportunity to institute risk-factor modifications that are of long-term benefit in reducing vascular complications.
- Therefore, in the absence of specific data indicating the degree of risk reduction for stroke in this patient population, general recommendations can be made that will improve the patient's general medical condition while at the same time reducing the overall incidence of postoperative vascular complications. These are:
    - Consider an evaluation for the presence of CAD, based on the patient's overall likelihood for CAD. In some cases, preoperative evaluation is indicated, while in others, an evaluation following recovery from surgery is preferable. This decision will be determined by the pretest probability of CAD, the type of surgery planned, and the urgency of the surgery (see Chap. 20).
    - Strongly consider statin therapy pre- and postoperatively. Evidence for the long-term benefit of statins is indisputable, and there is accumulating evidence that these agents may have benefits for acute medical conditions such as MI and in the perioperative period.
    - Control blood pressure (BP) prior to surgery and postoperatively. Fluctuations of BP are of greater concern for patients with cerebrovascular disease, since they are more vulnerable to CNS damage as a result of underperfusion or overperfusion.
    - Initiate beta-blocker therapy for patients without contraindications. Beta-blocker therapy has been shown to be of benefit for patients at high risk for cardiac complications. While studies have not focused on populations with cerebrovascular disease, it is known that these patients are highly likely to have CAD.
    - For patients not already on antiplatelet agents, start them postoperatively as soon as the risk for bleeding is no longer elevated.

SUMMARY

- Cerebrovascular disease is common in patients presenting for general surgery. A thorough assessment of the presence and/or likelihood of cerebrovascular disease is an important component of preoperative assessment. Specific evidence on the benefit of risk-reduction strategies in this population is lacking. However, interventions that are likely to be of benefit in general for patients with atherosclerotic vascular disease should be considered in the perioperative period.

REFERENCES

1. Larsen SF, Zaric D, Boysen G. Postoperative cerebrovascular accidents in general surgery. *Acta Anaesthesiol* 32:698–701, 1988.
2. Lefevre F, Woolger JM. Surgery in the patient with neurologic disease. *Med Clin North Am* 87:257–271, 2003.
3. Blacker DJ, Flemming KD, Link MJ, et al. The preoperative cerebrovascular consultation: Common cerebrovascular questions before general or cardiac surgery. *Mayo Clin Proc* 79:223–229, 2004.
4. Blacker DJ. In-hospital stroke. *Lancet Neurol* 2:741–746, 2003.
5. Limburg M, Wijdicks E, Eelco F, et al. Ischemic stroke after surgical procedures: Clinical features, neuroimaging, and risk factors. *Neurology* 50:895–901, 1998.
6. Axelrod DA, Stanley JC, Upchurch GR, et al. Risk for stroke after elective non-carotid vascular surgery. *J Vasc Surg* 39:67–72, 2004.
7. DeWeese JA, Rob CG, Satran R, et al. Surgical treatment for occlusive disease of the carotid artery. *Ann Surg* 168:85–94; 1968.
8. Evans BA, Wijdicks FM. High-grade carotid stenosis detected before general surgery: Is endarterectomy indicated? *Neurology* 57:1328–1330, 2001.
9. Kelley RE. Stroke in the postoperative period. *Med Clin North Am* 85:1263-1276, 2001.
10. Adams RJ, Chimowitz MI, Alpert JS, et al. Coronary risk evaluation in patients with transient ischemic attack and ischemic stroke. *Circulation* 108:1278–1290, 2003.

38 SEIZURE DISORDER

Kevin J. O'Leary and Martin J. Arron

INTRODUCTION

- More than 10 percent of the population will experience a seizure at some point in their lives.[1] Common causes of secondary seizures include metabolic derangements, drug intoxication or withdrawal, central nervous system (CNS) infections, traumatic brain injury, cerebrovascular accidents, brain tumors, and vascular malformations.[2]
- Epilepsy is defined as recurrent seizures resulting from a congenital or acquired cause. The cumulative lifetime incidence of epilepsy is 0.5 to 3.0 percent.[3,4]
- Seizures are classified as partial or generalized.
  - Partial seizures are classified into two broad categories: simple and complex.
    - The symptoms of simple partial seizures depend on where the seizure originates in the brain. There is no loss of consciousness. Symptoms may be motor, sensory, autonomic, or psychic.
    - During a complex partial seizure, the patient appears awake but is not in contact with others in the environment. The patient may exhibit automatisms—repetitive behaviors such as grimacing, lip smacking, or repeating phrases. The seizure is often followed by a period of confusion.
    - Both simple and complex partial seizures may evolve into generalized tonic-clonic seizures.
  - The most common types of generalized seizures are absence seizures and generalized tonic-clonic seizures.
    - Absence seizures are characterized by a short period (10 s) of unresponsiveness. The onset and recovery are rapid. The patient may exhibit automatisms or mild clonic movements. Absence seizures usually begin in childhood but can begin at any age.
    - Generalized tonic-clonic seizures begin with an abrupt loss of consciousness, often in association with a scream or shriek. During the tonic phase, the muscles of the arms, legs, and back become stiff. The clonic phase follows, characterized by rhythmic jerking and twitching of muscles in the arms, neck, and face.
- For all seizure types, treatment is usually medical. Patients can be treated with one drug or a combination of antiepileptic drugs (AEDs). The treating physician must balance the efficacy of AEDs with their potential toxicity and interaction with other medications.
  - First-line AEDs for the treatment of partial seizures include carbamazepine, oxcarbazepine, phenytoin, valproate, topiramate, lamotrigine, and gabapentin.[5,6]
  - Absence seizures are usually treated with ethosuximide or valproate.
  - Generalized tonic-clonic seizures are most often treated with phenytoin, valproate, carbamazepine, or topiramate.
- Sedation, dizziness, and nausea are common side effects during the initiation of AED therapy. Most AEDs can also cause a rash during the initial weeks of therapy.
- The indications, pharmacokinetic issues, and side-effect profiles of various AEDs are illustrated in Table 38-1.
- Surgical treatment may be indicated for epilepsy that is refractory to medical treatment. These procedures

TABLE 38-1 Antiepileptic Drugs

ANTIEPILEPTIC DRUG	INDICATION	AVAILABLE IV	PHARMACOKINETIC ISSUES	METABOLISM	ADVERSE EFFECTS
Carbamazepine	Simple and partial complex, tonic-clonic	No	Enzyme induction, drug interactions	Hepatic	Rash, diplopia, hyponatremia, GI disturbances, hepatotoxicity, fever
Phenobarbital	Simple and partial complex, tonic-clonic	Yes	Enzyme induction	Hepatic	Sedation, GI disturbances, tolerance/dependence, behavior disorders
Phenytoin	Simple and partial complex, tonic-clonic	Yes*	Enzyme induction, drug interactions	Hepatic	Gingival hyperplasia, rash, hirsuitism, lymphadenopathy, confusion, hepatotoxicity, fever, neuropathy (with long-term use)
Valproate	Absence, simple and partial complex, tonic-clonic	Yes	Enzyme induction, blocks felbamate and lamotrigine metabolism	Hepatic	Weight gain, hair loss, tremor, GI disturbances, rare hepatotoxicity, rare pancreatitis
Ethosuximide	Absence	No	None		GI disturbances, sleep disturbances
Felbamate	Simple and partial complex, tonic-clonic	No	Enzyme inhibition	Hepatic	GI disturbances, anorexia, insomnia, diplopia, dizziness, ataxia, aplastic anemia, hepatotoxicity
Gabapentin	Simple and partial complex	No	None	Renal	Somnolence, dizziness, fatigue, weight gain
Lamotrigine	Simple and partial complex, tonic-clonic	No	None	Hepatic	Rash, fever, dizziness, red cell aplasia
Topiramate	Simple and partial complex	No	Minimal drug interactions	Hepatic/renal	Ataxia, decreased concentration, confusion, dizziness, fatigue, weight loss, kidney stones
Tiagabine	Simple and partial complex	No	Enzyme inducing AEDs can reduce half-life	Hepatic	Dizziness, tremor, impaired concentration
Levetiracetam	Simple and partial complex	No	None	Renal	Somnolence, asthenia, headache, behavioral disturbances, infection.
Oxcarbazepine	Simple and partial complex	No	None	Hepatic	Dizziness, diplopia, somnolence, nausea, ataxia, hyponatremia
Zonisamide	Simple and partial complex	No	None	Hepatic	Fatigue, dizziness, ataxia, anorexia

AED = antiepileptic drug; GI = gastrointestinal.
*Fosphenytoin is available only for intravenous administration.
SOURCES: Adapted from Refs. 3 to 6.

TABLE 38-2 Risk Factors and Adverse Outcomes in Patients with Seizure Disorder

PATIENT RISK FACTORS FOR SEIZURES	SURGERY-SPECIFIC RISK FACTORS	ADVERSE OUTCOMES OF PERIOPERATIVE SEIZURES
Noncompliance with AEDs	NPO: decreased AED level	Aspiration
Medications lowering seizure threshold	Anesthetic agents and certain narcotics	Delayed recovery from anesthesia
Metabolic derangements	Excess sedation	Disrupt surgical wound
Withdrawal syndromes	Resistance to muscle relaxants	
CNS tumors/infections	Intracranial surgery	

AED = antiepileptic drug; CNS = central nervous system; NPO = nil per os (nothing by mouth).

attempt either to resect the epileptogenic area or to interrupt seizure macrocircuits to prevent generalization.

- Status epilepticus is defined as more than 30 min of continuous seizure or a second seizure without recovery of consciousness between seizures. The treatment of status epilepticus is discussed in Chap. 61.

PATIENT-RELATED RISK FACTORS (TABLE 38-2)

- Breakthrough seizures in the perioperative period can result in aspiration, delayed recovery from anesthesia or surgery, and disruption of the surgical wound.
- AED noncompliance can raise the risk for perioperative seizure.
- A variety of medications used for other medical conditions can lower the seizure threshold (Table 38-3).
  - Antibiotics: beta lactams, quinolones, and isoniazid.
  - Antidepressants: tricyclic antidepressants, bupropion, and venlafaxine. Selective serotonin reuptake inhibitors appear safer.
  - Antipsychotic agents: phenothiazines and butyrophenones.
- Metabolic derangements—like hyponatremia, hypocalcemia, hypomagnesemia, and hypoglycemia—can precipitate seizures.
- Withdrawal syndromes from benzodiazepines, barbiturates, or alcohol may precipitate seizures.
- Patients with CNS tumors, infections, or prior stroke are at an increased risk for seizures.
- AEDs, particularly the older agents, can interfere with a variety of medications used for other medical conditions. For example, warfarin metabolism is increased by carbamazepine, phenytoin, and phenobarbital.[7] Digoxin levels may be lowered by phenytoin and topiramate.

TABLE 38-3 Drugs and Other Substances That Can Cause Seizures

Antimicrobials/antivirals	Psychotropics
β-lactams and related compounds	Antidepressants
Quinolones	Antipsychotics
Acyclovir	Lithium
Isoniazid	Theophylline
Ganciclovir	Sedative-hypnotic drug withdrawal
Anesthetics and analgesics	Alcohol
Meperidine	Barbiturates
Tramadol	Benzodiazepines
Local anesthetics	Drugs of abuse
Immunomodulatory drugs	Amphetamines
Cyclosporine	Cocaine
OKT3	Phencyclidine
Tacrolimus (FK-506)	Methylphenidate
Interferons	Flumazenil*
Radiographic contrast agents	

*In benzodiazepine-dependent patients.
SOURCE: Adapted from Lowenstein,[9] with permission.

SURGERY-RELATED RISK FACTORS (TABLE 38-2)

- Surgeries requiring a prolonged period of bowel rest present a challenge in administering maintenance AEDs to patients with epilepsy.
- Many AEDs can cause sedation, which may have an additive effect with anesthetic agents, narcotic analgesics, and sedative-hypnotics. AEDs that induce hepatic enzymes may cause some resistance to the effect of neuromuscular blocking agents and opiates.
- Many inhaled anesthetic agents have both proconvulsant and anticonvulsant properties. Isoflurane, desflurane, and halothane are generally considered to have stronger anticonvulsant properties. In fact, isoflurane and desflurane have been used to treat refractory status epilepticus.[8] Methohexital can activate epileptic foci and is often used during surgical therapy for epilepsy.
- Other medications used perioperatively can increase the likelihood of seizures. For example, large doses of meperidine, especially in patients on monoamine oxidase inhibitors, can cause seizures. Local anesthetic overdose can cause seizure (Table 38-3).

- Intracranial surgery carries a high risk for seizure. The risk is related to the location of surgery, the underlying pathologic condition, and the degree of brain manipulation.
  - Patients undergoing surgery for intracranial aneurysms are at risk for postoperative epilepsy, even if hemorrhage has not occurred.

PREOPERATIVE EVALUATION AND TESTING TO STRATIFY RISK

- Document the type and frequency of seizures.
- Note any associated medical and neurologic problems.
- Document current medications, including AEDs.
- Note use of benzodiazepine and barbiturates.
- Ask patients about illicit drug and alcohol use. Symptoms of prior withdrawal syndromes should raise concern of increased perioperative risk.
- Blood tests
  - Routine measurement of the plasma concentrations of AEDs is not likely to be helpful unless toxicity or noncompliance is suspected.
  - Consider checking liver enzymes in patients who are on phenytoin, carbamazepine, valproate, and felbamate.

PERIOPERATIVE MANAGEMENT TO REDUCE RISK

- The goal of perioperative management is to optimize seizure control in an effort to minimize breakthrough seizures.
- AEDs should be continued through the morning of surgery.
- Adjust diabetic medications in light of diet changes that will occur perioperatively.
- Monitor electrolytes and glucose closely and correct as needed.
- As noted above, isoflurane, desflurane, and halothane are potent anticonvulsants; however, the choice of a particular anesthetic agent is best left to the discretion of the anesthesiologist.
- AEDs that induce hepatic enzymes may cause some resistance to the effect of neuromuscular blocking agents and opiates.
- If prolonged bowel rest is needed or a patient experiences a seizure in the perioperative period, AEDs should be administered intravenously (Table 38-1).
  - Phenytoin can be given intravenously but must be infused slowly in order to avoid hypotension and asystole. It can also be given via feeding tube.
  - Phenobarbital can be given intravenously or intramuscularly.
  - Valproate can be given intravenously or via a feeding tube.
- If possible, avoid medications that may lower the seizure threshold or interact with AEDs.
- Monitor patients who consume excessive alcohol for signs and symptoms of withdrawal. If a patient has had a prior history of withdrawal or significant consumption, consider prophylactic benzodiazepine treatment.
- Resume prior AEDs as soon as the patient is able to take medications by mouth.

REFERENCES

1. Stoelting RK, Dierdorf SF. *Anesthesia and Co-Existing Disease.* Philadelphia: Churchill-Livingstone, 2002.
2. Delanty N, Vaughan CJ, French JA. Medical causes of seizures. *Lancet* 352:383–390, 1998.
3. LaRoche SM, Helmers SL. The new antiepileptic drugs: Scientific review. *JAMA* 291:605–614, 2004.
4. Kofke WA, Tempelhoff R, Dasheiff RM. Anesthetic implications of epilepsy, status epilepticus, and epilepsy surgery. *J Neurosurg Anesthesiol* 9:349–372, 1997.
5. Browne TR, Holmes GL. Epilepsy. *N Engl J Med* 344:1145–1151, 2001.
6. LaRoche SM, Helmers SL. The new antiepileptic drugs: Clinical applications. *JAMA* 291:615–620, 2004.
7. Patsalos PN, Froscher W, Pisani F, van Rijn CM. The importance of drug interactions in epilepsy therapy. *Epilepsia* 43: 365–385, 2002.
8. Mirsattari SM, Sharpe MD, Young BY. Treatment of refractory status epilepticus with inhalational anesthetic agents isoflurane and desflurane. *Arch Neurol* 61:1254–1259, 2004.
9. Lowenstein DH. Seizures and epilepsy, in Kasper DL, Braunwald E, Fauci AS, et al (eds), *Harrison's Principles of Internal Medicine,* 16th ed. New York: McGraw-Hill, 2005:2357–2372.

39 PARKINSON'S DISEASE, MYASTHENIA GRAVIS, AND MULTIPLE SCLEROSIS

Martin J. Arron and Kevin J. O'Leary

PARKINSON'S DISEASE

INTRODUCTION

- Parkinson's disease (PD) is present in 0.3 percent of the general population and in 1 percent of patients older than 60 years, with a mean age of onset between 55 to 65 years.

TABLE 39-1 Common Medications for Patients with Parkinson's Disease

MEDICATION CLASS	MEDICATION	ROUTE	ADVERSE EFFECTS
Dopaminergic drugs	Carbidopa/levodopa, levodopa/benserazide	PO	Nausea, vomiting, orthostatic hypotension, hypertension, confusion, hallucinations, cardiac dysrhythmias, dyskinesias
Dopamine agonists	Bromocriptine, pergolide, pramipexole, ropinirole	PO	Nausea, vomiting, somnolence, confusion, hallucinations, orthostatic hypotension, ankle edema, dyskinesias, pulmonary and/or retroperitoneal fibrosis (pergolide and bromocriptine), valvular heart disease
Monoamine oxidase type B inhibitors	Selegiline	PO	Dizziness, nausea, sleep disturbance, lightheadedness, hallucinations, orthostatic hypotension, cardiac dysrhythmias, drug interactions, meperidine induced serotonin syndrome
Indirect agonists	Amantadine	PO	Hallucinations, dry mouth, livido reticularis, ankle edema, orthostatic hypotension seizures,
Anticholinergic drugs	Trihexyphenidyl Biperiden Benztropine Diphenhydramine Orphenadrine Procyclidine	PO PO PO, IM, IV PO, IM, IV PO, IM, IV PO	Confusion, somnolence, sleepiness, dementia, confusion, hallucinations, blurred vision, constipation, dry mouth, urinary retention, glaucoma
Catechol *O*-methyltransferase inhibitors	Tolcapone Entacapone	PO	Dyskinesias, nausea, diarrhea, abdominal pain, vomiting, dizziness, insomnia, orthostatic hypotension, discolored urine, hallucinations, hepatotoxicity (with tolcapone)
Neuroleptics	Clozapine Quetiapine	PO	Somnolence, dizziness, weight gain, orthostatic hypotension, tachycardia, hyperlipidemia, hyperglycemia, fatal neutropenia (with clozapine)

SOURCES: From Samil et al.[1] and Jankovic,[13] with permission.

- The disorder is caused by injury to the dopaminergic neurons that originate in the substantia nigra and project into the striatum (caudate nucleus and putamen). This results in a deficiency of dopamine and a relative excess of cholinergic stimulation.
- Resting tremor, bradykinesia, rigidity, and postural instability are the cardinal symptoms.
- The diagnosis of PD depends on the history, physical examination, and response to dopaminergic therapy.
- Pharmacologic treatments include anticholinergic medications, levodopa, dopamine agonists, monoamine oxidase (MAO) inhibitors, and catechol *O*-methyltransferase (COMT) inhibitors (Table 39-1).[1] Levodopa is usually administered with a dopa-decarboxylase inhibitor (carbidopa or benserazide) to minimize side effects due to systemic conversion to dopamine.
- Some patients in the later stages of their disease develop an "on-off" phenomenon, with rapid and often unpredictable changes from mobility to immobility. The use of sustained-release levodopa preparations, COMT inhibitors, and dopamine agonists may alleviate wearing-off effects but are usually not effective in treating on-off phenomenon.
- Patients who are not optimally treated with medications because of intolerance or side effects are candidates for surgical intervention.

PATIENT-RELATED RISK FACTORS (TABLE 39-2)

- Respiratory disorders are frequently present. Obstructive lung disease is often seen, due to both upper and lower airway dysfunction. Reduced respiratory muscle strength, impaired cough, and sleep apnea are also common.[2]
- PD patients may have an increased risk of cardiac disease, which may be silent due to their limited mobility and dementia. Levodopa also increases heart rate and cardiac contractility and is associated with both hyper- and hypotension.

TABLE 39-2 Common Risk Factors and Management Strategies for Perioperative Complications in Patients with Parkinson's Disease, Myasthenia Gravis, and Multiple Sclerosis

RISK FACTORS	RISK-REDUCTION STRATEGIES
Respiratory disorders	Optimize medication therapy preoperatively
Cardiac disease	Continue medications perioperatively when possible
Swallowing abnormalities	Early mobilization
Psychiatric disorders	Bronchodilator therapy and lung-expansion maneuvers
Limited mobility	Prophylaxis against venous thromboembolism
Intraabdominal and intrathoracic surgery	
Adverse effects of medications	

- Oropharyngeal dysphagia and esophageal dysmotility may predispose to aspiration and thus impair postoperative nutrition.
- Dementia is seen in one-third of patients and is associated with an increased risk of perioperative complications, particularly delirium.
- Psychiatric disorders are more common in PD patients. Depression is found in 40 percent. Psychosis, including hallucinations, is common and is related to dopaminergic and anticholinergic therapies.
- Autonomic dysfunction is found in 15 to 20 percent of patients and may manifest as constipation, orthostatic hypotension, sialorrhea, or a neurogenic bladder.
- Voiding dysfunction is seen in up to 70 percent of patients; it usually consists of urinary frequency, nocturia, and urge incontinence from detrusor hyperreflexia. Some patients experience primarily obstructive symptoms.
- Patients may be at increased risk for venous thromboembolism due to advanced age and limited mobility.
- Patients with autonomic, motor, or cognitive impairment are at increased risk for postoperative falls.
- Limited mobility, dementia, delirium, and depression may increase the risk of decubitus ulcers.

SURGERY-RELATED RISK FACTORS

- Limited data are available regarding the impact of PD on the outcomes of specific surgeries.
- Aspiration pneumonia, urinary tract infections, and longer hospital stays are more common in PD patients undergoing gastrointestinal and prostate surgery than in those without this disease. Delirium may also be more frequent after these surgeries.[3]
- Intraabdominal and intrathoracic procedures are likely more risk-prone in PD patients due to their underlying pulmonary disease and reduced functional capacity (see Table 39-2).
- Surgeries associated with delayed enteral intake may also be more risky due to difficulty administering antiparkinsonian medications orally. Acute symptom exacerbation, including upper airway obstruction and respiratory failure, can occur with the short-term discontinuation of medication.[4]
- Surgeries requiring high doses of postoperative narcotic analgesic therapy may also be more risky. These medications can cause delirium, impair coughing, reduce mobility, and exacerbate constipation.

PREOPERATIVE EVALUATION AND RISK STRATIFICATION

- Identify and estimate the severity of any underlying lung or upper airway involvement. Formal pulmonary function testing may be useful in some patients.[2]
- Videofluoroscopy may be indicated for patients with dysphagia or symptoms suggesting aspiration.
- Carefully assess functional capacity and look for symptoms and signs of heart disease. A preoperative electrocardiogram is indicated for most patients.
- Look for evidence of autonomic dysfunction, including orthostatic hypotension, constipation, sialorrhea, and a neurogenic bladder.
- Perform an assessment of cognitive function, mood, and sleep patterns preoperatively.

PERIOPERATIVE MANAGEMENT TO REDUCE RISK

- Optimize antiparkinsonian therapy to maximize mobility and minimize side effects (see Table 39-2).
- Increased salt intake, fludrocortisone, and midodrine may be needed to treat orthostatic hypotension.
- Central cholinesterase inhibitors (rivastigmine, donepezil) may be effective for dementia and psychosis.
- Selective serotonin reuptake inhibitors are usually first-line treatments for depression. Venlafaxine may be useful, particularly in hypotensive patients, as it may increase blood pressure. Avoid tricyclic antidepressants.
- Clozapine or quetiapine may be useful treatments for hallucinations and delirium. Clozapine requires monitoring with complete blood counts to avert agranulocytosis. Avoid phenothiazines, butyrophenones, risperidone, and olanzapine.[5]
- Avoid postoperative withdrawal of antiparkinsonian medications if possible.[4,5] This can exacerbate rigidity and other symptoms of PD. It can also trigger the

parkinsonism-hyperpyrexia syndrome, which is similar to the neuroleptic malignant syndrome.
  - Most PD medications are administered on the morning of surgery. Reinstitute therapy as soon as possible postoperatively.
  - A levodopa/carbidopa solution can be continuously infused into the duodenum via a feeding tube if necessary.[6]
  - If the patient is taking nothing by mouth, use parenteral anticholinergic medications such as benztropine or diphenhydramine. In select cases, subcutaneous apomorphine may be cautiously administered to prevent or treat postoperative symptoms in patients unable to take oral medications. To minimize side effects, pretreat with trimethobenzamide hydrochloride for 3 days if possible.
  - Meperidine is contraindicated in patients also receiving selegiline.
- Incentive spirometry, bronchodilators, and chest physical therapy may be useful in preventing pulmonary complications in high-risk patients[2] (see Chaps. 24 and 25).
- Use prophylaxis against venous thromboembolism for patients with risk factors such as advanced age, limited mobility, and high-risk surgeries (see Chap. 46).
- Early mobilization will decrease the risk of deep venous thrombosis (DVT), minimize deconditioning, improve respiratory function, and reduce the risk of pressure ulcers.

MYASTHENIA GRAVIS

INTRODUCTION

- The prevalence of the disorder is 4 per 100,000 people, with a bimodal age distribution. One age peak is between 10 and 30 years and involves a predominance of women. The second peak, which is disproportionately male, occurs between 40 and 60 years.[7]
- Myasthenia gravis (MG) is an autoimmune disorder involving the destruction of acetylcholine receptors caused by antibodies, sensitized T cells, and complement.
- Muscle weakness and easy fatigability are hallmark symptoms. The extraocular muscles are often initially involved, resulting in diplopia and ptosis. Over time, the bulbar muscles, respiratory muscles, and somatic musculature may become affected.
- Patients experience frequent fluctuations in the severity of their symptoms. Acute exacerbations may be triggered by infections, surgery, pregnancy, other physiologic stress, and reductions in the doses of immunosuppressive medications. These exacerbations may be severe and can require mechanical ventilation.
- Certain medications can either cause or exacerbate the symptoms of MG.[8] These agents include aminoglycosides, ciprofloxacin, anticholinergics, phenytoin, beta blockers, quinidine, procainamide, and penicillamine.
- Diagnosis is based on the presence of typical symptoms, antiacetylcholine receptor antibodies, a positive edrophonium challenge test, and characteristic findings on electromyography. A chest computed tomography (CT) or magnetic resonance imaging (MRI) scan is usually performed to detect thymic abnormalities. Thymic hyperplasia and neoplasia (primarily thymomas) are present in 60 and 10 percent of patients, respectively.
- Acetylcholinesterase inhibitors (pyridostigmine, neostigmine), prednisone, cytotoxic medications (azathioprine, cyclophosphamide), and immunosuppressive drugs (cyclosporine, mycophenolate mofetil) are the main therapies. Plasmapheresis and intravenous immune globulin (IVIg) are used in severe cases (Table 39-3). Thymectomy is also pursued in select patients.[7]
- Cholinergic crisis may be precipitated by excessive anticholinesterase therapy. The presence of miosis, hypersalivation, excessive tearing, bradycardia, and increased weakness after edrophonium challenge are clues to the presence of this complication.
- A variety of other immune disorders are associated with MG, including hyperthyroidism, hypothyroidism, systemic lupus erythematosus, rheumatoid arthritis, pernicious anemia, and autoimmune hemolytic anemia.

PATIENT-RELATED RISK FACTORS (TABLE 39-2)

- Younger patients with MG tend to undergo a more limited range of surgeries, largely labor and delivery, thymectomy, and common gastrointestinal procedures such as appendectomy. Older patients are subject to a broader array of surgeries and have more comorbid conditions.[7]
- Respiratory muscle weakness can result in restrictive lung physiology, reduced ventilation, atelectasis, and impaired cough. Occasionally evidence of variable extrathoracic airway obstruction is present due to upper airway weakness. Sleep apnea is often present.
- Involvement of the bulbar musculature can predispose patients to aspiration.
- Muscle weakness limits mobility increasing the likelihood of pressure ulcers and the risk of venous thromboembolism.
- A myocarditis is seen in some patients, particularly those with thymoma; this may result in cardiac conduction disorders and dysrhythmias.
- Patients may experience exacerbations during pregnancy or the postpartum period and are more likely to experience complications during labor and delivery.

TABLE 39-3 Therapy for Myasthenia Gravis

TREATMENT CLASS	MEDICATION	ROUTE	ADVERSE EFFECTS
Cholinesterase inhibitors	Pyridostigmine Neostigmine Ambenonium	PO, IV, IM PO, IV, IM PO	Abdominal cramps, diarrhea, sialorrhea, bradycardia, hyperhidrosis, muscle fasciculations
Corticosteroids	Prednisone Methylprednisolone Dexamethasone	PO, IV, IM	Transient worsening of symptoms, hypertension, hypokalemia, diabetes, mood disorders, psychosis, avascular necrosis, myopathy, osteoporosis, infections
Cytotoxic agents	Azathioprine	PO	Vomiting, diarrhea, thrombocytopenia, leukopenia, liver dysfunction, flu-like symptoms
	Cyclophosphamide	PO	Nausea, vomiting, leukopenia, thrombocytopenia, hemorrhagic cystitis, infection, malignancy, infertility
Immunosuppressive agents	Cyclosporine		Hypertension, acute and chronic renal failure, opportunistic infections, tremor, headache, seizures, visual changes,
	Mycophenolate mofetil	PO, IV	Diarrhea, abdominal cramps, infections, bone marrow suppression
Immunoglobulin therapy	Immunoglobin-Ig Intravenous immune globulin (IVIG)	Intravenous	Headache, myalgias, rash, fluid retention, aseptic meningitis, hemolytic anemia, anaphylaxis (in IgA-deficient patients), acute renal failure, increased plasma viscosity, pseudohyponatremia, thromboembolism
Plasmapheresis		Intravenous	Hypokalemia, hypocalcemia, paresthesias, urticaria, myalgias, infections, catheter thrombosis, bleeding diathesis, drug clearance
Thymectomy		Transsternal or Transcervical	Infection (pneumonia, wound, empyema), phrenic and recurrent laryngeal nerve injury, venous thromboembolism, cardiac rhythm disturbances, transient worsening of symptoms

SOURCE: From Dillon,[7] with permission.

SURGERY-RELATED RISK FACTORS

SURGICAL SITE

- Thoracic and abdominal surgeries increase the risk of respiratory complications (see Table 39-2) (see Chaps. 24 and 25). Prolonged ventilation is often required postoperatively.

ANESTHESIA

- Patients may have resistance to succinylcholine and require higher doses. Anticholinesterase medications may also reduce the effectiveness of the plasma cholinesterases that degrade succinylcholine, resulting in a prolonged duration of action.[7]
- Patients may also have an increased sensitivity to nondepolarizing muscle relaxants.
- Epidural analgesia and anesthesia are preferred for labor and delivery.
- Local anesthetics from the amide group (lidocaine, bupivacaine) are preferred over members of the ester class (procaine, tetracaine) because they are not metabolized by serum cholinesterases.

PREOPERATIVE EVALUATION AND RISK STRATIFICATION

HISTORY

- Determine the patient's functional capacity, including exercise tolerance and ability to handle activities of daily living (see Chaps. 20 and 24).
- Identify any preexisting cardiac or pulmonary symptoms or disorders.
- Note the presence and severity of commonly associated comorbid disorders seen in patients with MG, particularly illnesses that may influence perioperative management. These include thyroiditis, systemic

lupus erythematosus, rheumatoid arthritis, diabetes mellitus, and inflammatory bowel disease.

Physical Examination

- Assess the patient for signs of respiratory compromise, including tachycardia, rapid shallow respirations, staccato speech, nasal voice tones, cough, the use of accessory muscles of respiration, weak neck flexion, and paradoxical breathing.[9]
- Identify any evidence of aspiration, such as dysphagia, coughing, and hoarseness.

Diagnostic Testing

- Clinicians should have a low threshold for diagnostic testing, given the limited functional capacity of these patients and the frequent occurrence of comorbid disorders, particularly those involving the respiratory system.
- Preoperative blood tests should include a complete blood count, renal and hepatic chemistry panels, and an electrocardiogram. Obtain an assay of thyroid-stimulating hormone (TSH) if this has not been checked recently.
- If there are signs or symptoms of pulmonary disease, obtain a chest radiograph, pulmonary function tests, and arterial blood gas analysis. Pulse oximetry is not an adequate screening test, as it does not detect mild or moderate degrees of hypoxemia or the presence of hypercapnea. Determine vital capacity, maximal inspiratory pressure (MIP or PI_{max}) and maximal expiratory pressure (MEP or PE_{max})[2,10] (Table 39-4).
- Consider videoflouroscopy if there are symptoms or signs of aspiration.
- Consider polysomnography preoperatively if there are symptoms suggesting sleep apnea.

PERIOPERATIVE MANAGEMENT TO REDUCE RISK

Medications

- Continue anticholinesterase medications until the time of surgery and restart them intravenously or orally immediately after surgery (see Table 39-2). Be aware that these agents can increase bronchial secretions, which can compromise respiratory status.
- Administer stress doses of corticosteroids for those patients on chronic or recurrent steroid therapy (see Chap. 28).
- Use appropriate prophylaxis against venous thromboembolism (see Chap. 46).
- Avoid narcotic analgesics if possible, as they can suppress respiration, impair coughing, and promote aspiration.
- If possible, avoid medications that can exacerbate MG.

TABLE 39-4 Measures of Respiratory Neuromuscular Performance

TEST	NORMAL VALUE	CRITICAL VALUE
Vital capacity	40–70 mL/kg	15 mL/kg
Maximal inspiratory pressure	Male ≥ 100 cmH_2O Female ≥ 70cmH_2O	−25 cmH_2O
Maximal expiratory pressure	Male > 200 cmH_2O Female > 140 cmH_2O	40 cmH_2O

SOURCE: From Wijdicks and Borel,[10] with permission.

Ventilation

- Controlled ventilation is often required for 24 to 48 h postoperatively. Extubated patients are generally monitored in a surgical intensive care unit (ICU) or step-down unit for 24 h prior to transfer to a general surgical floor.[7]
- Use biphasic positive airway pressure (BiPAP) or continuous positive airway pressure (CPAP) selectively for patients with postoperative respiratory failure.
- Monitor patients for evidence of respiratory dysfunction using serial measurement of oxygen saturation via pulse oximetry, mean inspiratory pressures (MIPs), and vital capacity.[10]
- Use incentive spirometry, early mobilization, frequent body repositioning, and, in select cases, chest physical therapy to prevent or treat pulmonary complications (see Chaps. 24 and 25).

MULTIPLE SCLEROSIS

INTRODUCTION

- Multiple sclerosis (MS) is an immune-mediated disorder of the central nervous system. Genetic and possibly environmental factors have an effect on susceptibility.[11]
- Pathologically, MS is characterized by inflammation and demyelination. Lesions are most often seen in the optic nerves, periventricular white matter, cerebellum, and spinal cord.
- Symptoms correlate with the site of lesions. Common initial symptoms include sensory loss, optic neuritis, weakness, paresthesias, diplopia, ataxia, vertigo, bladder symptoms, and Lhermitte's sign (trunk and limb paresthesias with neck flexion). Symptoms may worsen transiently with exercise and increases in body temperature (Uhtoff's phenomenon).
- The clinical course is variable and is divided into the relapsing-remitting type or the primary progressive type.
  - The relapsing-remitting type of MS accounts for 80 percent of patients. Symptoms usually develop over

the course of several days, stabilize, and then improve within weeks. The onset of the disorder is usually in the second or third decade of life. Females are affected twice as often as males. Many patients develop secondary progression, which is characterized by the gradual worsening of disability in between relapses.
  - Primary progressive MS accounts for 20 percent of patients and is characterized by a slowly progressive course without relapses and remissions. Males and females are affected equally.
- Diagnosis is usually made by clinical findings in conjunction with MRI features suggestive of MS. Cerebrospinal fluid often shows increased immunoglobulins of restricted specificity (oligoclonal bands) and a moderate lymphocytic pleocytosis.
- Treatment with corticosteroids can shorten the duration of acute relapses. Plasma exchange has also been used for acute relapses, but its efficacy is not yet proven. In patients with relapsing-remitting MS, interferon beta and glatiramer acetate reduce the frequency of clinical relapses and may decrease long-term disability. Common side effects of interferon beta include depression, flu-like symptoms, and injection-site reactions. Hepatotoxicity is an important albeit less common side effect. Glatiramer is generally well tolerated.

PATIENT-RELATED RISK FACTORS (TABLE 39-2)

- Patients may have significant neurologic deficits that predispose them to postoperative complications.
- Immobility may predispose to pressure ulcers and venous thromboembolism.
- Patients with bulbar or respiratory involvement may be at risk for postoperative pulmonary complications. Respiratory muscle weakness may cause restrictive lung physiology. Bulbar and respiratory muscle weakness may diminish the ability to cough and predispose patients to aspiration, atelectasis, and pneumonia.
- MS patients may be predisposed to urinary tract infection, urinary retention, and urinary incontinence.
- Depression and cognitive dysfunction may increase the risk for postoperative complications.
- Patients treated with corticosteroids may be at risk for secondary adrenal insufficiency (see Chap. 28).

SURGERY-RELATED RISK FACTORS

- Transient worsening of symptoms may occur postoperatively. Increases in body temperature are well known to exacerbate symptoms. Patients may have an increased risk of relapse in the postpartum period.
- Spinal anesthesia has been reported to exacerbate symptoms,[12] whereas epidural anesthesia seems to involve less risk. Significant hypotension can occur with either spinal or epidural anesthesia. General anesthesia is usually well tolerated.

PREOPERATIVE EVALUATION AND RISK STRATIFICATION

- Document any neurologic deficits preoperatively. This will help in the evaluation of new findings in the postoperative period. It may also clarify the risk for postoperative pulmonary complications (see Chap. 24) and pressure sores.[2]
- Note current medications and any recent adjustments.
- Consider a swallowing evaluation if aspiration is suspected.
- Obtain complete blood counts and liver functions tests in patients receiving interferon beta.

PERIOPERATIVE MANAGEMENT TO REDUCE RISK

- Monitor patients for the development of new neurologic deficits.
- Patients who have been on significant doses of corticosteroids may benefit from a stress dose of corticosteroids perioperatively.
- Treat fever aggressively with antipyretics and, if needed, cooling blankets.
- Avoidance of spinal anesthesia may be warranted.
- Use lung-expansion maneuvers for patients at increased risk for postoperative pulmonary complications (see Table 39-2) (see Chap. 24).
- Use appropriate prophylaxis for venous thromboembolism, especially in patients with limited mobility (see Chap. 46).

REFERENCES

1. Samil A, Nutt JG, Ranson BR. Parkinson's disease. *Lancet* 363:1783, 2004.
2. Oliveira E, Michel A, Smolley L. The pulmonary consultation in the perioperative management of patients with neurologic diseases. *Neurol Clin* 22:277, 2004.
3. Pepper PV, Goldstein MK. Postoperative complications in Parkinson's disease. *J Am Geriatric Soc* 47:967, 1999.
4. Galvez-Jimenez N, Lang AE. The perioperative management of Parkinson's disease revisited. *Neurol Clin* 22:367, 2004.
5. Frucht SJ. Movement disorder emergencies in the perioperative period. *Neurol Clin* 22:379, 2004.
6. Clinical Pharmacology. Levodopa:Carbidopa. Accessed 1/17/2005. URL:http://cp.gsm.com. Gold Standard 2005.

7. Dillon FX. Anesthetic issues in the preoperative management of myasthenia gravis. *Semin Neurol* 24:83, 2004.
8. Wittbrodt ET. Drugs and myasthenia gravis. *Arch Int Med* 157:399, 1997.
9. Rabinststein A, Wijdicks EFM. Warning signs of imminent respiratory failure in neurological patients. *Semin Neurol* 23:97, 2003.
10. Wijdicks EFM, Borel CO. Respiratory management in acute neurologic illness. *Neurology* 50:11, 1998.
11. Noseworthy JH, Lucchinetti C, Rodriguez M, et al. Multiple sclerosis. *N Engl J Med* 343:938, 2000.
12. Kytta J, Rosenberg PH. Anaesthesia for patients with multiple sclerosis. *Ann Chirug Gynaecol* 73:299, 1984.
13. Jankovic J. Movement disorders, in Goetz C (ed), *Textbook of Clinical Neurology,* 2d ed. Philadelphia: Elsevier, 2003: 655–679.

40 PSYCHIATRIC CONDITIONS

Donna L. Mercado and Jeffrey R. Allen

INTRODUCTION

- Psychiatric illness is increasingly prevalent in the general population, and medical consultants play an important role in preventing and treating perioperative psychiatric complications.
- Numerous studies have demonstrated that there are significant psychological effects related to surgery, regardless of the complexity of the procedure.
- Preexisting psychiatric vulnerability can have devastating effects on patient outcome, and psychiatric illnesses may be markedly exacerbated in spite of an excellent surgical cure. This can increase patient morbidity and is often associated with a longer length of hospital stay due to compromised postoperative rehabilitation.

RISK FACTORS FOR PERIOPERATIVE MORBIDITY (TABLE 40-1)

Although most patients with psychiatric illness do well in the postoperative setting, there are several predictors of increased morbidity.

TABLE 40-1 Risk Factors for Perioperative Morbidity

Risk Factors for Perioperative Morbidity
Panic/anxiety disorders
Major depression
Psychotic disorders
Dementia/cognitive impairment
Drug dependence
Somatization disorders
Personality disorders
Prior psychiatric complications in the perioperative setting
Postoperative pain
Altered functional status
Neuroleptic malignant syndrome
Medication interactions

PATIENT-SPECIFIC RISK FACTORS

PANIC/ANXIETY DISORDERS

- The literature suggests that inappropriately high levels of anxiety can adversely affect postoperative outcome. However, there are no randomized controlled trials to accurately assess the correlation of anxiety and specific postoperative complications [e.g., cardiac ischemia, deep venous thrombosis (DVT), pneumonia], length of hospital stay, or postoperative rehabilitation.
- Inappropriately low levels of anxiety have been seen in severely depressed patients. A higher postoperative mortality may be associated with surgery-related suicide in these patients.[1,2]

MAJOR DEPRESSION

- Severely depressed patients have more postoperative complications due to lack of motivation for rehabilitation; poor appetite, causing compromised healing; and difficult assessment of pain symptoms. These patients are also at higher risk for suicide.[1,2]

PSYCHOTIC DISORDERS

- Multiple studies have concluded that postoperative psychiatric morbidity is greatly increased in patients with preexisting psychotic disorders. However, postoperative medical complications are not necessarily increased in psychotic patients. Delusions and hallucinations may impair postoperative rehabilitation and assessment of pain, but several trials have not shown a rate of complications greater than that in nonpsychotic patients.[3]

DEMENTIA/COGNITIVE IMPAIRMENT

- Patients with dementia or impaired cognition have up to a three times higher incidence of postoperative delirium, depression, pneumonia, DVT, and cardiac complications than the general population.[3]

DRUG DEPENDENCE

- Withdrawal from medications (e.g., benzodiazepines, barbiturates), alcohol, or illegal substances can be associated with delirium, seizures, autonomic instability, and death. Additionally, substance abusers may have abnormal perceptions of pain symptoms or engage in drug-seeking behavior, which complicates postoperative treatment. An accurate drug and medication history is mandatory in the preoperative assessment.

SOMATIZATION DISORDERS

- Patients with somatization disorders present a cognitive challenge to physicians, since they are often dissatisfied with surgical results. An increased number of tests and surgical procedures can lead to a higher incidence of complications. Studies demonstrate that patients with these disorders have up to three times as many operations and hospitalizations than do patients with depressive disorders.[4]

PERSONALITY DISORDERS

- Poor compliance with postoperative care and rehabilitation are common. Interestingly, there is a higher incidence of litigation among these patients.

SURGERY-SPECIFIC RISK FACTORS

POSTOPERATIVE PAIN

- Uncontrolled pain may exacerbate psychiatric illnesses.

ALTERED FUNCTIONAL STATUS

- Postoperative physical function is often compromised; increased anxiety and depression can result.

NEUROLEPTIC MALIGNANT SYNDROME

- This is an inherited disorder that leads to an idiosyncratic reaction to neuroleptics. Clinical signs include fever, rigidity, mental status changes, rhabdomyolysis, and autonomic instability. Mortality rate can be as high as 20 percent. Neuroleptic malignant syndrome can mimic malignant hypothermia, which is a rare but serious adverse reaction to anesthetics.[5]

MEDICATION INTERACTIONS

- Psychotropic medications, narcotic analgesics, and anesthetic medications can have significant adverse interactions. A thorough preoperative history and discussion with the anesthesiologist can decrease perioperative morbidity.

PREOPERATIVE EVALUATION OF PSYCHIATRIC PATIENTS

HISTORY AND PHYSICAL

- Question the patient for stability of the psychiatric condition, compliance with medications, and ongoing psychological counseling.
- Obtain data relating to prior surgical procedures and outcomes. Certain procedures may exacerbate existing psychiatric illnesses (e.g., transplant surgery, bariatric surgery, trauma, reconstructive or disfiguring surgery).
- Anticipate perioperative pain and rehabilitation issues.
- Obtain a complete medication history (including nonprescription medications) and accurate drug and alcohol history, including history of withdrawal complications.
- Discuss use of "as needed" medications, history of untoward medication reactions, and any prior perioperative worsening of symptoms.

LABORATORY

- Measure serum levels of all psychiatric medications when appropriate (e.g., lithium, anticonvulsants) and evaluate for signs/symptoms of toxicity when drug levels are not available.
- Evaluate for abnormalities related to the use of psychotropic drugs and look for cardiac arrhythmias/conduction abnormalities as appropriate.

PERIOPERATIVE MANAGEMENT TO REDUCE RISK

PREOPERATIVE

- Discuss with the psychiatrist optimal dosing for difficult-to-use medications. For example, if doses of lamotrigine are missed, "makeup" doses should not be used, whereas a missed dose of lithium may result in subtherapeutic levels and requires extra dosing. If clozapine is held for more than 2 days, it must be restarted slowly (consult a psychiatrist regarding specific dosing); when it is started too quickly, hypotension may result.[6] In addition, because the risk of agranulocytosis is so

high with this medication, care must be taken that the white blood cell count remains in the normal preoperative range.
- If the patient is taking long-acting medications, a change to the short-acting formulation may be necessary postoperatively in those instances where the patient requires medications to be crushed.
- If the patient will be unable to take medications by mouth for a prolonged period, discuss with the psychiatrist which medications might require intravenous alternatives. In the case of such a patient, also consider which medications may be associated with significant withdrawal syndromes. In particular, both benzodiazepines and SSRIs are associated with withdrawal syndromes.

INTRAOPERATIVE

The use of psychoactive medications can cause a variety of hemodynamic and cardiac changes as well as prolongation of neuromuscular blockade and problems with oversedation. Some of the more commonly encountered medication side effects and interactions are as follows:

- ***Tricyclics:*** The most common side effects are anticholinergic and are likely to be additive with the effects of other anticholinergics. There have been rare reports of arrhythmias in patients on tricyclics who receive halothane.[7]
- ***Mood Stabilizers:*** Although lithium can prolong the action of depolarizing and nondepolarizing muscle relaxants, this has rarely been of clinical significance. Other mood stabilizers (valproic acid, gabapentin, lamotrigine) have no specific perioperative contraindications.
- ***Antipsychotics:*** The phenothiazines and butyrophenones (such as haloperidol, fluphenazine, chlorpromazine, and risperidone) usually do not cause significant perioperative problems but can enhance CNS depression induced by narcotics and barbiturates.[8] Abrupt stoppage of these agents can cause withdrawal dyskinesia and rebound agitation, so they should be continued perioperatively if possible.
- ***Selective serotonin reuptake inhibitors (SSRIs):*** Although there are no specific interactions between SSRIs and anesthetics, there is a recent report that SSRIs are associated with an increased risk of bleeding perioperatively. This may be related to serotonin-mediated platelet activation.[9] In addition, SSRIs can increase the international normalized ratio (INR) of patients on warfarin. Since stopping SSRIs can cause a withdrawal syndrome, however, consider continuing these agents perioperatively as long as the patient is not at significant bleeding risk, and, as appropriate, is having adequate INR monitoring if taking warfarin.
- ***Monoamine oxidase (MAO) inhibitors:*** These agents are occasionally used for depression that is resistant to other agents. They are associated with the development of hypertensive crises when used intraoperatively with sympathomimetics. Patients can also develop a neuroleptic malignant-type syndrome when combined with meperidine. When possible, hold these agents for 2 weeks preoperatively. However, when necessary, patients have undergone urgent surgery successfully while still on MAOIs. In this circumstance, minimize concurrent use of anticholinergics, sympathomimetics, and meperidine.[7]
- ***Benzodiazepines:*** Abrupt cessation of benzodiazepines preoperatively can result in a withdrawal syndrome. In addition, patients who take significant doses of benzodiazepines require less anesthetic medication and may require higher doses of postoperative narcotics.
- ***Herbal agents:*** Kava is used as a sleep agent and sedative, and it has been noted to occasionally cause severe hepatic injury. Also, it can enhance the sedative effects of anesthetic medications. Valerian is also used as a sedative and, like kava, can enhance anesthetic effects. There have been reports of significant withdrawal reactions when these agents stopped abruptly.[10] St John's wort induces the cytochrome P450 system and can affect the metabolism of multiple medications. It is unclear whether abrupt withdrawal can cause a withdrawal syndrome as do the structurally related SSRIs.

POSTOPERATIVE

- For optimal maintenance of psychiatric conditions, medication management includes maximization of pain control, "as needed" use of medications for anxiety and agitation, and continuation of the patient's usual psychiatric medications. Check drug levels of medications as appropriate.
- Nonpharmacologic measures to maintain psychiatric stability include reduction of environmental stimuli, maximization of postoperative education and support, use of bedside psychiatric liaison support, and use of family support.

SUMMARY

Psychiatric illness is an extremely important but often ignored aspect of perioperative care. It is critical to assess the stability of each patient's psychiatric condition, anticipate potential problems, and document a complete medication history. Recovery from surgery can be adversely affected if psychiatric issues are not addressed throughout the perioperative period. Most surgical patients with psychiatric conditions have a satisfactory outcome after a thorough preoperative evaluation has been done and a perioperative treatment plan developed.

REFERENCES

1. Goldmann DR, Brown FH, Guarnieri DM. *Perioperative Medicine: The Medical Care of the Surgical Patient,* 2d ed. New York:, McGraw-Hill, 1994.
2. Kammerer WS, Gross RJ. *Medical Consultation: Role of the Internist on the Surgical, Obstetric, and Psychiatric Services,* 2d ed. Baltimore: Williams & Wilkins, 1990.
3. Cutler BS, Fink MP. Postoperative complications in patients with disabling psychiatric illness or intellectual handicaps. A case controlled retrospective analysis. *Arch Surg* 125: 1436–1440, 1990.
4. Zoccolillo MS, Cloninger CR. Excess medical care of women with somatization disorder. *South Med J* 79:532–535, 1986.
5. Merli GJ, Weitz HH. *Medical Management of the Surgical Patient,* 2d ed. Philadelphia: Saunders, 1998.
6. Desan PH, Powsner S. Assessment and management of patients with psychiatric disorders. *Crit Care Med* 32(suppl): S166–S173, 2004.
7. Mercado DL, Petty BG. Perioperative medication management. *Med Clin North Am* 87:41–57, 2003.
8. Sarko J. Antidepressants, old and new. *Emerg Med Clin North Am* 18:637–654, 2000.
9. Movig KL, Janssen MW, de Waal Malefijt J, et al. Relationship of serotonergic antidepressants and the need for blood transfusion in orthopedic surgical patients. *Arch Intern Med* 163:2354–2358, 2003.
10. O'Hara MA, Kiefer D, Farrell K, et al. A review of 12 commonly used medicinal herbs. *Arch Fam Med* 7:523–536, 1998.

41 THE OBESE PATIENT

Judi Woolger-Kraft and Donna L. Mercado

INTRODUCTION

- Obesity is defined as a body mass index (BMI) of greater that 30, and overweight is defined as a BMI of greater than 25. Obesity has been deemed a worldwide epidemic, with the total number of overweight and obese individuals now numbering 1.7 billion.[1] Government statistics show that in the United States, two-thirds of all adults are overweight, and almost half of those are obese.[2] Obesity is the most common nutritional/metabolic disorder among patients going to surgery and is responsible for a variety of other comorbid conditions.
- Ideal body weight can be calculated as follows:
  Males: IBW (kg) = height (cm) − 100
  Females: IBW (kg) = height (cm) − 105
- Obesity is defined as a body weight of 20 percent or more above the ideal. The World Health Organization has established the following criteria:
  Grade I: Body mass index of 30.0 to 34.9 kg/m^2
  Grade II: Body mass index of 35.0 to 39.9 kg/m^2
  Grade III: Body mass index of ≥40.0 kg/m^2

PATIENT-RELATED RISK FACTORS (TABLE 41-1)

DEGREE OF OBESITY

- The degree of obesity often correlates with the number and severity of perioperative challenges and problems. Morbid obesity results in more pronounced physiologic and anatomic alterations.

COMORBID CONDITIONS

- Common comorbidities associated with obesity include hypertension, diabetes mellitus, hyperlipidemia, atherosclerotic vascular disease, and hypoventilation syndrome.

PULMONARY RISK FACTORS

Respiratory abnormalities can be found with almost any level of obesity and may represent the most difficult aspect of anesthetic care. These baseline abnormalities

TABLE 41-1 Patient- and Surgery-Related Risk Factors

PATIENT-RELATED RISK FACTORS	PROCEDURE-RELATED RISK FACTORS
Degree of obesity	Site and type of surgery probably do not affect risk
Presence and severity of pulmonary problems	
Presence and severity of cardiac problems	
Presence and severity of other comorbid conditions	

tend to worsen with exposure to anesthesia and sedatives, leading to a decline in pulmonary function intraoperatively and in the immediate postoperative period.[3]

Hypoventilation

- Because of the large volume of adipose tissue in the pharyngeal and thoracic structures, many obese patients have some level of upper airway obstruction, which will worsen in the recumbent position. As in any form of upper airway obstruction, airway patency is maintained by an activated state of inspiratory muscle tone assisted by gravity. When obese patients are sedated, that tone is either reduced or eradicated and airway obstruction worsens. This is dramatically demonstrated in the subgroup of obese patients who have obstructive sleep apnea (OSA, or pickwickian syndrome), who develop dangerous levels of hypoxemia and airway obstruction with sleep. The standard anesthetic combination of muscle relaxants and medications to depress consciousness may worsen airway obstruction severely and thus limit gas exchange even further.

Airway Management

- The above-mentioned airway obstruction is more difficult to overcome with usual means such as face masks. In addition, even endotracheal intubation may require special techniques, such as fiberoptic laryngoscopy.

Aspiration

- Although all patients are potentially at risk for perioperative aspiration and its complications, the obese patient's risk is increased because of altered gastrointestinal physiology. These changes can include delayed gastric emptying, hypersecretion of gastric acids, hiatal hernia, diminished esophageal sphincter tone, and increased potential for reflux.

Hypoxemia

- The combination of the recumbent position, muscle relaxants, anesthetic agents, and surgical maneuvers decreases the functional residual capacity (FRC) of any patient, but this worsens dramatically in the obese population. In addition, the changes persist into the postoperative period and often require additional monitoring and support equipment. Morbidly obese patients are also more likely to have reduced vital capacity, restrictive lung disease, and an increased work of breathing.

CARDIAC RISK FACTORS

Cardiovascular abnormalities are common in the obese population and can be associated with hemodynamic changes that may become significant in the surgical setting.

Atherosclerotic Disease

- Screen the obese patient for coronary artery disease, since the prevalence of hypertension and diabetes is so high in this population (see Chap. 20).

CARDIOMYOPATHY OF OBESITY

Chronic obesity may produce a series of hemodynamic changes termed the *cardiomyopathy of obesity*.[4] The syndrome includes a high-cardiac-output state with both systemic and pulmonary hypertension and possibly overt heart failure.

SURGERY-RELATED RISK FACTORS

SITE AND TYPE OF SURGERY

- Certain types of operations are associated with a longer duration of surgery and increased need for blood transfusion, whether the patient is obese or not.[5] There have not, however, been any consistent data to prove that the type or site of surgery puts the obese patient at greater risk for postoperative complications.

ANESTHESIA-RELATED CONCERNS

- There may be difficulties in maintaining an airway in the obese patient; therefore the anesthesiologist should carefully evaluate mouth opening, soft palate visualization, neck movement, and position of the larynx.
- Volume of distribution is altered in morbid obesity, requiring altered dosing of certain anesthetics.
- Because of the higher risk of aspiration in morbid obesity, rapid-sequence induction is often utilized.
- Regional anesthesia can be more difficult in the obese population. Anatomic landmarks are difficult to locate, longer-than-standard needles must be used, and the height of the regional block is less predictable.

PREOPERATIVE EVALUATION AND TESTING TO STRATIFY RISK (TABLE 41-2)

CARDIAC RISK

- Does obesity increase cardiac risk?
  - Despite the risk for atherosclerotic disease as well as the cardiomyopathy of obesity, it is not clear that

TABLE 41-2 Risk-Reduction Strategies

PREOPERATIVE	INTRAOPERATIVE	POSTOPERATIVE
Thorough evaluation for atherosclerotic disease and cardiomyopathy: Electrocardiogram Stress testing or echocardiography	Avoid premedication with opioids or benzodiazepines	Appropriate pulmonary toilet Incentive spirometry, Chest physiotherapy BiPAP CPAP
Pulmonary function testing only if symptomatic Lung-expansion maneuvers Arterial blood gas as needed Evaluate for sleep apnea	Monitoring: Telemetry Pulse oximetry Capnography Peak airway pressures	Monitor wounds: Infection Dehiscence Incisional hernias
Screening blood tests Glucose Thyroid	Pulmonary artery pressure monitor as needed	Control blood glucose
DVT prophylaxis	DVT prophylaxis	Early ambulation and DVT prophylaxis

BiPAP = biphasic positive airway pressure; CPAP = continuous positive airway pressure; DVT = deep venous thrombosis.

obesity per se increases the risk of perioperative cardiac events.

To determine the risk for atherosclerotic disease, an appropriate history and physical examination will elucidate which comorbid conditions are present, and guidelines [American College of Cardiology (ACC), American College of Physicians (ACP)] will help determine indications for further testing for reversible ischemia (see Chap. 20). How aggressively should cardiac testing be pursued?

- ◦ Make a decision to proceed with cardiac testing based on the type of surgery planned, the patient's cardiac reserve (as demonstrated by exercise tolerance), and the comorbid conditions. More liberal use of cardiac testing is expected in this patient population due to the high expected level of comorbid conditions and decreased exercise capacity.

- What methods are available to assess cardiac status in the morbidly obese patient?
  - ◦ Echocardiography and stress echocardiography are valuable tools for testing for the presence of atherosclerotic disease and cardiomyopathy. Pulmonary pressures can also be measured.
  - ◦ Obesity may preclude the ability to obtain a satisfactory cardiac window. In this situation, a dipyridamole (Persantine) or dobutamine test can look for the presence of reversible ischemia and assess ejection fraction. Another option is contrast echocardiography with an agent such as perflutren (Optison). If still unsuccessful in the case of an extremely morbidly obese patient, consider a dobutamine transesophageal echocardiogram.
- Should routine pulmonary testing be done?
  - ◦ Contrary to popular belief, obesity is not generally a risk factor for major postoperative pulmonary complications (see Chap. 24). Base the decision to proceed with pulmonary testing on other factors, such as abnormal pulmonary signs or symptoms.
  - ◦ There is a 10 percent incidence of OSA in the morbidly obese population. This subgroup suffers from severe hypoventilation at baseline and requires special attention to the risk for worsening hypoventilation, hypoxemia, and microaspiration.

PERIOPERATIVE MANAGEMENT TO REDUCE RISK

PREOPERATIVE

BLOOD TESTS

- ◦ ***Glucose testing:*** Because of the high degree of correlation between diabetes and obesity as well as the known issue of poor wound healing in hyperglycemic states, preoperative glucose testing is recommended.
- ◦ ***Thyroid testing:*** Thyroid function tests are usually performed on any patient being evaluated for obesity. If no recent test results are available and you suspect significant hypothyroidism, obtain thyroid function tests prior to elective surgery.
- ◦ ***Arterial blood gas (ABG):*** If there is suspicion of obesity-hypoventilation syndrome or resting dyspnea or hypoxia, obtain an ABG to help guide perioperative management.

CARDIAC TESTS

- ◦ ***Electrocardiograms*** should be considered in all obese patients anticipating surgery.
- ◦ ***Echocardiograms*** should be performed if there is a suspicion of heart failure or in the presence of

significant pulmonary disease. This will determine the ejection fraction, right-sided pressures, and wall motion abnormalities.
- ***Noninvasive stress testing*** follows the guidelines discussed in Chap. 20.

PROPHYLACTIC MEASURES
- ***DVT prophylaxis:*** Obesity is an independent risk factor for venous thromboembolism (VTE). Stratify the patient's risk and provide appropriate VTE prophylaxis as per the guidelines of the American College of Chest Physicians (ACCP) (see Chap. 46).
- ***Lung-expansion maneuvers:*** Start incentive spirometry or deep-breathing exercises preoperatively.
- ***Aspiration prophylaxis:*** Minimize the risk for aspiration pneumonitis by prophylaxis with an H_2 blocker or proton-pump inhibitor (see Chap. 36).

INTRAOPERATIVE

PREMEDICATION
- Avoid opiate premedication because of the risk of respiratory depression and delayed gastric emptying.
- Some practitioners also avoid benzodiazepines because of the risk of respiratory depression, particularly in patients with obesity-hypoventilation syndrome.

MONITORING
- Maintain the typical monitoring tools of electrocardiography (ECG), pulse oximetry, capnography, and peak airway pressure.
- With obese patients, intravenous access may be difficult, as may blood pressure monitoring (even with an appropriate-size cuff). If changes in pressure or very long procedures are expected, the anesthesiologist may consider an arterial line.
- Monitoring of pulmonary artery pressure or central venous pressure depends on individual situations.

POSTOPERATIVE

- Use of proper pulmonary toilet may decrease pulmonary risk.
- Early ambulation is imperative when it is safe from the surgical perspective. The supine position can further reduce the already decreased functional residual capacity. Additionally, the weight of the excess adipose tissue in the supine position can cause worsening of a restrictive pattern. Moving to a sitting position, or preferably walking, will help minimize these disturbances.
- Continue incentive spirometry and consider the use of chest physiotherapy (although that may be difficult in the morbidly obese), biphasic positive airway pressure (BiPAP), and continuous positive airway pressure (CPAP) to maximize alveolar inflation. Candidates for CPAP and BiPAP include those unable to perform deep-breathing exercises or those with OSA who use home CPAP.
- The obese population is at higher risk for wound dehiscence, infection, and incisional hernias. Carefully evaluate the wounds daily to minimize infectious complications.
- Evaluate the patient for postoperative hyperglycemia. Wound healing may be significantly delayed in the setting of hyperglycemia.
- Continue deep venous thrombosis (DVT) prophylaxis and encourage early ambulation as soon as it is safe from the surgical perspective.

SUMMARY

Overall, the obese patient undergoing surgery is at risk for the same types of complications found in the nonobese. Preoperative attention to comorbid conditions is imperative in providing the obese patient with a safe surgical experience. Attention should focus on potential cardiac and pulmonary abnormalities as well as aggressive DVT prophylaxis.

REFERENCES

1. Buchwald H, Avidor Y, Braunwald E, et al. Bariatric surgery: A systematic review and meta-analysis. *JAMA* 292:1724–1737, 2004.
2. National Center for Health Statistics, 2002 NHANES IV Report. Available at: http://www.cdc.gov/nchs/product/pubs/pubd/hestats/obes/obese99.htm2002.
3. Damia G, Masheroni D, Croci M, et al. Perioperative changes in functional residual capacity in morbidly obese patients. *Br J Anesth* 60:574–578, 1988.
4. Kasper EK, Hruban RH, Baughman KD. Cardiomyopathy of obesity: A clinicopathologic evaluation of 43 obese patients with heart failure. *Am J Cardiol* 70:921–924, 1992.
5. Dindo D, Muller M, Weber M, Clavien PA. Obesity in general elective surgery. *Lancet* 361:2032–2035, 2003.

42 ARTHRITIS OR SYSTEMIC AUTOIMMUNE DISEASE

Brian F. Mandell and Bruce E. Johnson

INTRODUCTION

- The systemic autoimmune diseases encompass a heterogeneous group of disorders that confront the patient, surgeon, and medical consultant with a number of unique concerns in the perioperative setting. With multisystem disease, the medical consultant should try to confirm the diagnosis by discussion with the patient's rheumatologist or review of prior records in order to predict the potential disease-specific risks of surgery. Then the consultant should assess disease activity and degree of any end-organ damage that may influence the patient's perioperative course.
- The consultant cannot assume that baseline laboratory tests will be normal, even in young, otherwise apparently healthy patients.
- Patients with these disorders are frequently utilizing many prescribed and "alternative" medications. These must be carefully reviewed.
- Before surgery, consider issues surrounding successful postoperative rehabilitation, since recommendations regarding pain control and the use of anti-inflammatory medication are likely to affect postoperative recovery. This is particularly important in patients with inflammatory arthritis undergoing arthroplasty.

INFLAMMATORY ARTHRITIS (RHEUMATOID ARTHRITIS, SPONDYLOARTHROPATHIES)

PATIENT-/DISEASE-SPECIFIC RISK FACTORS

- The duration, severity, and activity of the disease can affect surgical risk.
- Preoperatively assess involvement of the cervical spine, as this affects the ease and safety of endotracheal intubation.[1]
- Specific cardiovascular risks are associated with these disorders:
  - Patients with rheumatoid arthritis (RA) have an increased burden of cardiovascular disease compared to their age-/risk-matched counterparts without RA.
  - Patients with spondylitis or with the *HLAB27* gene, even without recognized spinal disease, are at risk for aortitis. This may be accompanied by aortic valve insufficiency, conduction disease, or atrial fibrillation.
- Patients with RA may have unrecognized interstitial lung disease or pleural effusions.
- Patients with RA have a greater risk of postoperative infected arthroplasties than patients with osteoarthritis.

PREOPERATIVE EVALUATION

Rheumatoid Arthritis

- Some 60 percent of patients with long-standing rheumatoid arthritis have radiographically demonstrable cervical instability. This predisposes the patient to cervical cord injury at the time of intubation or transfer.[2]
- More than 80 percent of patients with radiographic instability are asymptomatic. The neurologic examination in these patients may be complicated by peripheral joint destruction or peripheral compressive neuropathies. Hyperreflexia may indicate asymptomatic cervical myelopathy.
- RA does not generally involve the lumbar spine; thus epidural procedures may not be affected. However, the possibility of conversion from spinal to general anesthesia requires preoperative imaging of the cervical spine.
- Patients with recent-onset disease are unlikely to have significant cervical spinal instability, which occurs due to ligamentous laxity following years of inflammatory disease.
- C1-2 is the most common site of laxity and instability, followed by subaxial disease and then cranial settling. Pannus from synovial proliferation may also narrow the canal and put the cord at risk of injury.
- Preoperatively, obtain radiographs of the cervical spine in the neutral position as well as flexion and extension views to determine the presence of radiographic instability.
- If there are any symptoms or findings suggestive of cord compression, obtain a neurosurgical evaluation and magnetic resonance imaging (MRI) in flexion and extension to evaluate bone or soft tissue (pannus) compression of the cord prior to elective surgery.
- Communicate with the anesthesiologist and surgeon regarding potential problems.
- Cervical stabilization procedures have associated morbidity and mortality and are not routinely considered prior to other surgery.
- Temporomandibular joints are occasionally affected in RA, more commonly in patients with juvenile idiopathic arthritis. Assess joint motion in an effort to avoid problems at the time of attempted intubation.
- Hoarseness is a sign of cricoarytenoid joint dysfunction; its presence should prompt preoperative evaluation with an ear-nose-throat (ENT) specialist

in order to avoid a potential postextubation airway catastrophe due to vocal cord closure from joint dysfunction. If necessary, the inflamed joints can be injected with corticosteroids preoperatively.
- Patients may be unable to exert themselves sufficiently to provide an adequate history for the assessment of physiologically significant coronary artery disease. Patients with severe articular involvement are also likely to be deconditioned. Although not supported by data, it may be reasonable to consider the presence of long-standing RA as an intermediate-level factor in evaluating cardiovascular risk using the American Heart Association (AHA) guidelines.
- Sjögren's syndrome is common in patients with long-standing RA. Prior to long surgical procedures, a lubricating eye ointment (not drops) should be applied.

SPONDYLITIS

- Ankylosing spondylitis (AS) may involve all levels of the spine as well as peripheral joints. Unlike the case in RA, spinal involvement in AS is characterized more by fusion and reduced mobility than by instability. Hence the patient's ability to be intubated or positioned may be compromised.
- Patients with spondylitis are predisposed to develop heterotopic ossification around arthroplasties, adversely affecting outcomes. This is especially true in patients who had prior heterotopic ossification. This may be prevented (limited data) with the preoperative use of radiation, nonsteroidal anti-inflammatory drugs, or bisphosphonate therapy.[3]

PERIOPERATIVE MEDICATION MANAGEMENT (SEE TABLE 42-1 AND CHAP. 7)

NONSTEROIDAL ANTI-INFLAMMATORY DRUGS (NSAIDS)

- The traditional nonselective NSAIDs depress platelet function and are associated with surgical bleeding. They provide insufficient prophylaxis against perioperative thrombosis. They are generally discontinued 1 to 3 days prior to surgery; drugs with a longer half-life (e.g., piroxicam) should be stopped even earlier. Aspirin,

TABLE 42-1 Immunosuppressive and Rheumatic Disease Medications in the Perioperative Period

DRUG	PREOPERATIVE RECOMMENDATIONS	COMMENTS
NSAID (nonselective)	Stop 2-3 half-lives prior to surgery.	Reversibly inhibit platelet function, demonstrated increased postoperative bleeding. Can decrease renal function, decrease drug excretion.
Aspirin	Unless used as antithrombotic drug, stop ASA about 1 week preop.	Irreversible platelet inhibition. Increased postoperative bleeding.
COX-2-selective	Can continue through surgery unless renal concerns.	No antiplatelet effects. May be prothrombotic. Can decrease renal function. Effective as analgesic: narcotic-sparing.
Prednisone	Continue. Consider *short-term* hydrocortisone 50–100 mg IV q 8 h.	Concern with wound healing and infection with chronic use. Cause leukocytosis, hyperglycemia. *No need* for protracted tapering if "stress doses" are prescribed. Study shows baseline dosing is sufficient to avoid hypotension.
Hydroxychloroquine	Can continue.	Some antithrombotic effect (has been used as prophylactic antithrombotic in orthopedic surgery)
Methotrexate	Can continue.	Avoid administration within 24–48 h of possible acute renal insufficiency. Preop discontinuation associated with postoperative flares in RA. No evidence for increased infection if continued.
Azathioprine	Can continue.	
Leflunomide	Can continue.	Limited data.
Cyclophosphamide	Can continue.	Acute renal failure can cause buildup of metabolites.
Sulfasalazine	Can continue.	
Intravenous immunoglobulin	Can continue	Avoid within few days of potential acute renal injury (i.e., hypoperfusion), may cause intrarenal hypoperfusion.
Colchicine	Can continue in baseline chronic dose.	IV bioavailability is higher than oral; use IV route only with *extreme* care. Stop if renal insufficiency develops.
Allopurinol	Can continue.	Resume as soon as possible postop. Do not initiate therapy in the acute perioperative period.

unlike other NSAIDs, is an irreversible inhibitor of platelet cyclooxygenase. Platelet function returns to normal approximately 3 to 4 days following discontinuation of aspirin therapy. The nonacetylated salicylates do not affect platelet function.
- The cyclooxygenase 2 (COX-2)-selective NSAIDs do not affect platelet function. In small short-term trials, they have not adversely affected wound healing or bleeding. They may provide sufficient analgesia when given preoperatively to reduce the need for postoperative narcotics. There are concerns, however, regarding their association with increased cardiovascular morbidity. Rofecoxib and valdecoxib were recently withdrawn from the market.
- All NSAIDs are associated with (usually reversible) risk for renal insufficiency, particularly in the setting of decreased renal blood flow.
- Parenteral administration offers no gastric safety advantage over orally administered drugs.

METHOTREXATE (MTX)

- MTX is usually prescribed once weekly, along with daily folic acid (1 mg) to reduce side effects. Since the kidney excretes MTX, it should not be given immediately prior to any procedure likely to be associated with renal insufficiency. The drug is normally cleared rapidly from the circulation following each administration.
- There are no data strongly demonstrating that the use of MTX within the week prior to surgery adversely affects surgical outcome. Several small controlled studies have demonstrated the safety of providing the drug a week before surgery. Withdrawal of the drug can be associated with postoperative flare in the underlying disease, adversely affecting rehabilitation. Thus, there is no need to withhold the drug for a week or more prior to a procedure.[4]

LEFLUNOMIDE

- Leflunomide is a pyrimidine antagonist used in the treatment of RA and occasionally other inflammatory disorders. It has an extremely prolonged tissue half-life. Withdrawal preoperatively is thus not likely to affect tissue or plasma levels significantly. Results from a single small study suggest that continuation does not cause perioperative problems.

CORTICOSTEROIDS (SEE CHAP. 28)

- Patients with RA or spondyloarthropathy may be on daily low-dose or intermittent prednisone as therapy for their arthritis. Physiologic studies have repeatedly shown that patients taking supraphysiologic doses of prednisone for more than 2 weeks have submaximal cortisol release response to challenge with adrenocorticotropic hormone (ACTH). However, it has not been demonstrated that this blunting of the "stress response" has any clinically significant effect on the outcome of surgery.
- It has become routine practice to administer 50 to 100 mg of intravenous hydrocortisone prior to induction of anesthesia and every 8 h until the patient is stable. In many hospitals, all patients with documented or assumed blunted adrenal responses receive this regimen. Nonetheless, several small studies have shown that patients who receive their baseline corticosteroid dose or no supplementation do not suffer adverse effects.
- If perioperative corticosteroid supplementation is provided, baseline dosing (even if zero) should be utilized as soon as the patient is stable. There is no need for prolonged tapering regimens.
- Chronic corticosteroid therapy may adversely affect wound healing, although there are limited supportive data from controlled studies in humans.
- Administration of corticosteroids elicits neutrophilia and may also cause hyperglycemia and blunt a postoperative fever.

ANTI-TUMOR NECROSIS FACTOR (TNF) THERAPIES

- There are limited data on the perioperative effects of these drugs (adalimumab, etanercept, infliximab) on postoperative infection. In patients with inflammatory bowel disease, there is no suggestion from retrospective studies of an increased rate of wound infection.[5,6]
- In general, many rheumatologists suggest holding anti-TNF therapy for several half-lives of the drug prior to surgery, restarting it when the patient is stable postoperatively without evidence for infection.

POSTOPERATIVE COMPLICATIONS

- Flares in disease may occur due to the withholding of medications. Reinstitute anti-inflammatory medications as soon as possible. Low-dose corticosteroids (<7.5 mg prednisone daily) may be helpful, as may NSAIDs.
- Postoperative fever is not likely due to a flare in these diseases.
- A monoarticular "flare" should be assumed to be an infection until proven otherwise with arthrocentesis.
- Postoperative neurologic complications are commonly due to compressive neuropathies and rarely to myelopathy.

CRYSTALLINE ARTHRITIS

PREOPERATIVE EVALUATION AND MANAGEMENT

DISEASE-ASSOCIATED

- Try to document the validity of the prior diagnosis of gout or pseudogout. Frequently the finding of hyperuricemia alone has unreliably led to a diagnosis of gout.

- Ascertain the frequency of attacks and the need for aggressive prophylaxis from the patient and records.
- Note any prior episodes of postoperative attacks of arthritis.
- Obtain a careful cardiac history, as hyperuricemia is strongly associated with coronary artery disease and the metabolic syndrome.

MEDICATIONS

- Prophylaxis is important because postoperative flares are particularly common in patients with frequent attacks and may prolong their hospitalization.
- Continue allopurinol up to the time of surgery and restart it immediately thereafter.
- Continue low-dose colchicine prophylaxis (0.6 mg up to twice daily) up to the time of surgery and reinstitute it as soon as possible following surgery. Given orally, it can cause diarrhea or nausea, but it is not ulcerogenic. Drug interactions (i.e., with erythromycin) can increase colchicine levels and cause significant toxicity.
- NSAIDs can be used as prophylactic therapy, but owing to their many side effects in the postoperative setting, they are generally utilized only in the presence of an attack.

POSTOPERATIVE COMPLICATIONS

- Flares (attacks) are common and are frequently associated with fever.
- Acute arthritis in the postoperative setting warrants arthrocentesis to exclude infection. Indirect evaluation (presence or absence of fever, leukocytosis, hyperuricemia, elevation of the erythrocyte sedimentation rate) is inadequate to distinguish infection from crystalline arthritis.
- There is no diagnostic value in obtaining radiographs or nuclear imaging studies to distinguish between acute septic and crystalline arthritis.
- Treatment options include:
  - NSAIDs: selective versus nonselective based on the clinical concern for suppression of platelet function and induction of gastric injury. All NSAIDs can adversely affect renal function.
  - Corticosteroids in moderate to high doses (i.e., approximately 40 mg daily).
  - Colchicine oral or intravenous; the intravenous route is fraught with potentially life-threatening complications if an inappropriate dose is used. Hence many clinicians avoid this route of administration. High dose oral colchicine almost always causes diarrhea.
  - Do not initiate or significantly alter hypouricemic therapy in the setting of an acute flare of gout.
  - The measurement of serum urate is not a reliable diagnostic test, especially at the time of an attack.

MYOSITIS

PREOPERATIVE EVALUATION AND MANAGEMENT

- Patients with myositis are at increased risk for cardiomyopathy, cardiac conduction disease, interstitial lung disease, dysphagia, and respiratory muscle dysfunction. Assess these parameters preoperatively.
- Patients with active disease may be difficult to wean from a ventilator. Profound weakness in respiratory muscle function by objective testing or history may warrant the delay of major elective procedures.
- Consider obtaining baseline enzyme measurements. Transaminases, CPK MB, and (rarely) troponin may be elevated in patients with peripheral myositis (without cardiac involvement).
- Initiation of swallowing may be compromised. Inquire about the patient's ability to swallow pills.

MEDICATIONS

- Methotrexate, calcineurin antagonists, and azathioprine are frequently utilized in relatively high doses to maintain remission.
  - Myositis is not likely to flare with short-term holding of these medications, but there is no evidence that continuing them up until surgery compromises outcome.
  - Resume medications postoperatively as soon as the patient is stable and renal function is known.
- Hydroxychloroquine has some antithrombotic effect but seems to be an unlikely cause of bleeding. It can be continued in the perioperative period.
- Intravenous immunoglobulin (IVIg):
  - Some patients with myositis receive this in very high doses on a monthly basis to induce or preserve remission.
  - If possible, do not give IVIg in temporal proximity to any potential renal insult, since it rarely can cause intrarenal hypoperfusion and renal failure.

POSTOPERATIVE COMPLICATIONS

- Weaning from a ventilator may be difficult, and placing the patient in a seated position may help. Noninvasive ventilatory support may provide significant assistance.
- Diagnosis of myocardial infarction (MI) may be difficult due to the occasional baseline elevation of troponin or, more frequently, the baseline increase of the MB fraction of CPK (from regenerating skeletal muscle).

SYSTEMIC LUPUS ERYTHEMATOSUS

PATIENT-/DISEASE-SPECIFIC RISK

- SLE potentially affects multiple organ systems, which, in turn, can increase the risk of perioperative complications.
- Patients with SLE, like those with RA, are at an increased risk for coronary artery disease beyond that explained by traditional risk factors.[7]
- Pulmonary hypertension may be present and asymptomatic. Interstitial lung disease is less common.
- Patients with SLE may be at increased risk for bleeding (secondary to thrombocytopenia) or thrombosis (lupus anticoagulant, antiphospholipid antibodies).
- Renal function may be abnormal despite the young age of the patient and a normal creatinine.
- Patients with SLE may have myositis.
- Lupus affecting the central nervous system may be manifest by cognitive dysfunction and deficient memory.

PREOPERATIVE EVALUATION AND MANAGEMENT

- Cytopenias are common. Obtain a baseline complete blood count (CBC). Thrombocytopenia should prompt questioning regarding miscarriage or thrombosis (antiphospholipid antibody syndrome).
- While it is reasonable to obtain a partial thromboplastin time (PTT), do not assume, without a full coagulation laboratory evaluation, that a prolonged PTT reflects a lupus anticoagulant.
- Glomerulonephritis (GN) is usually asymptomatic. The urine in GN may have significant pyuria, although usually with red cells as well. Microscopic evaluation of a fresh urine sample is mandatory in the evaluation of possible GN. An abnormal preoperative urine dipstick (blood, leukocytes) should not be assumed to be due to urinary infection.

PERIOPERATIVE MANAGEMENT OF MEDICATIONS

- Drugs other than corticosteroids used to maintain remission may be held during the immediate perioperative period, as noted above and in Table 42-1, but they generally need not be discontinued in advance of surgery.
- Continue corticosteroids during the perioperative period. Some clinicians recommend a slight elevation in corticosteroid dose to prevent a flare in SLE induced by the stress of surgery. There are no data to strongly support or refute this practice.

POSTOPERATIVE COMPLICATIONS

- Flares in disease may occur in the perioperative setting and be difficult to distinguish from infection, corticosteroid withdrawal syndromes, drug reactions, or a surgical complication.
- Fever may be a manifestation of disease activity, thrombosis, infection,[8] or drug reaction.
- Antiphospholipid antibodies or lupus anticoagulant may be present in >30 percent of patients with SLE. This predisposes at least some of these patients to thrombosis. This subset of patients cannot be readily recognized other than by a history of prior thrombosis.
- In the absence of severe thrombocytopenia, it is prudent to provide aggressive prophylactic anticoagulation.

SCLERODERMA

PATIENT-/DISEASE-SPECIFIC RISK

- Severe disease may produce facial tightening, with decreased ability to open the mouth wide enough to permit easy intubation. Dental health may be poor.
- Central venous access may be necessary, as peripheral vascular access may be limited.

PREOPERATIVE EVALUATION

- Carefully evaluate the need for arterial lines. Ulnar occlusion is common, and digital circulation is often tenuous. Hence the placement of a radial artery line can produce severe tissue damage.
- Digital ischemia due to Raynaud's phenomenon may make digital oximetry unreliable.
- Pulmonary hypertension may be severe yet clinically unrecognized.[9] Modest hypovolemia can elicit severe hypotension.
- A baseline electrocardiogram (ECG) may reveal conduction disease or a pseudoinfarction pattern.

PERIOPERATIVE MEDICATION MANAGEMENT

- No specific drugs are effective in the treatment of scleroderma. Continue drugs given as symptomatic

therapy for Raynaud's phenomenon if they are tolerated. Low-dose beta blockade is generally tolerated.
- Continue aggressive antireflux therapies, including positioning in bed.

POSTOPERATIVE COMPLICATIONS

- Fever is not expected from the disease.
- Scleroderma involvement of the gut may make oral drug absorption slow and unreliable. Bacterial overgrowth is common. Postoperative ileus may be problematic.
- Reflux and esophageal dysmotility are often severe and place many patients at high risk for aspiration.
- Hypothermia may cause peripheral, renal, or central vasoconstriction. Severe vasospastic ischemia may warrant vasodilator therapy. Prostaglandin E infusion is well tolerated, effective, and easily titrated.
- Do *not* interrupt continuous epoprostenol (Flolan) infusion in patients being treated for pulmonary hypertension.

ANTIPHOSPHOLIPID ANTIBODY SYNDROME (APLAS)

- APLAS includes venous and arterial thrombosis.
- Patients with a history of thrombotic events and persistent antiphospholipid antibodies or the lupus anticoagulant are at extremely high risk for perioperative thrombosis.[10] They should receive aggressive prophylaxis with medication as well as intermittent compression whenever possible.
- Patients may be at particularly high risk for thrombosis at initiation of warfarin, especially if accompanied by the additional thrombotic risk of surgery.
- The presence of thrombocytopenia is not protective against thrombosis in the setting of APLAS. Corticosteroid or IVIg therapy may be used to increase the platelet count if necessary to permit anticoagulation.
- Immunosuppressive therapy is unlikely to be of benefit in preventing thrombosis.
- Women with a history of otherwise unexplained miscarriages and APLAS may also be at high risk for thrombosis.
- In the presence of a lupus anticoagulant, routine monitoring of the PTT may be unreliable. Dose low-molecular-weight heparin by weight. Alternatively, monitor factor Xa activity or thrombin time.
- Monitoring of the effect of heparin during bypass may be unreliable if the activated clotting time is used. Consider monitoring of heparin levels.

OSTEOARTHRITIS AND OSTEOPOROSIS

- Pain from osteoarthritis may limit activity; thus exertional symptoms of coronary artery disease or vascular disease may be absent.
- Severe kyphoscoliosis may decrease lung volumes.
- Attention should be devoted to the prescription and alternative medications that the patient is taking for pain relief (Table 42-1).
- Arthroplasty is discussed in Chap. 11.

REFERENCES

1. Grauer JN, Tingstad EM, Rand N, et al. Predictors of paralysis in the rheumatoid cervical spine in patients undergoing total joint arthroplasty. *J Bone Joint Surg Am* 86A:1420–1424, 2004.
2. Gurley JP, Bell GR. The surgical management of patients with rheumatoid cervical spine disease. *Rheum Dis Clin North Am* 23:317–332, 1997.
3. Pakos EE, Ioannidis JP. Radiotherapy vs. nonsteroidal anti-inflammatory drugs for the prevention of heterotopic ossification after major hip procedures: A meta-analysis of randomized trials. *Int J Radiat Oncol Biol Phys* 60:888–895, 2004.
4. Bridges SL Jr, Moreland LW. Perioperative use of methotrexate in patients with rheumatoid arthritis undergoing orthopedic surgery. *Rheum Dis Clin North Am* 23:981–993, 1997.
5. Marchal L, D'Haens G, Van Assche G, et al. The risk of post-operative complications associated with infliximab therapy for Crohn's disease: A controlled cohort study. *Aliment Pharmacol Ther* 19:749–754, 2004.
6. Aberra FN, Lewis JD, Hass D, et al. Corticosteroids and immunomodulators: Postoperative infection complication risk in inflammatory bowel disease patients. *Gastroenterology* 125:320–327, 2003.
7. Leung WH, Wong KL, Lau CP, et al. Association between antiphospholipid antibodies and cardiac abnormalities in patients with systemic lupus erythematosus. *Am J Med* 89: 411–419, 1990.
8. Bouza E, Moya JG, Muñoz P. Infections in systemic lupus erythematosus and rheumatoid arthritis. *Infect Dis Clin North Am* 15:335–361, 2001.
9. Blaise G, Langleben D, Hubert B. Pulmonary arterial hypertension: Pathophysiology and anesthetic approach. *Anesthesiology* 99:1415–1432, 2003.
10. Erkan D, Leibowitz E, Berman J, Lokshin MD. Perioperative medical management of antiphospholipid syndrome: Hospital for special surgery experience, review of literature, recommendations. *J Rheumatol* 29:843–849, 2002.

43 ALCOHOL DISORDERS

Adam J. Gordon

INTRODUCTION

- Alcohol problems are common among patients in the United States and are often overrepresented in surgical populations. As many as 43 percent of the patients admitted to a trauma service have detectable alcohol levels.[1]
- Alcohol use disorders (AUDs) constitute a range of problem drinking, from consumption of "at risk" amounts of alcohol to the diagnoses of alcohol abuse and dependence. AUDs contribute to significant preventable disability, disease, and mortality; it is estimated that more than one-third of adults in the United States consume enough alcohol to be at risk for alcohol-related harm.[2]
- Persons consuming "at-risk" levels of alcohol meet a quantity or frequency threshold that contributes to alcohol-related harm. The National Institute of Alcohol Abuse and Alcoholism (NIAAA) defines at-risk levels of alcohol drinking as the consumption of more than 14 standard drinks for men and more than 7 standard drinks for women (Table 43-1). In the United States, a standard drink is often defined as one 12-oz bottle of beer or cooler, a 5-oz glass of wine, or a 0.2-oz shot or jigger of spirits. These drinkers are at increased risk for all-cause mortality, certain cancers, other medical and psychiatric conditions, and progression to alcohol abuse and dependence.
- Alcohol abuse and alcohol dependence are defined by diagnostic criteria in the fourth edition of the American Psychiatric Association's *Diagnostic and Statistical Manual of Mental Disorders* (DSM-IV).

PATIENT-SPECIFIC RISKS

- Perioperative risk can be evaluated by considering the level of intoxication, toxic effects of alcohol, and likelihood or severity of withdrawal.
- The intoxicated patient may give an inadequate or misleading medical history or may be unable to provide any history. The patient may also be uncooperative with the physical examination.
- AUDs are often associated with tobacco use, other drugs of abuse, and psychiatric disorders, which complicate medical or surgical treatments and care.

MORBIDITY DUE TO ALCOHOL

- Physiologic effects of alcohol and alcohol intoxication can increase the risk of perioperative complications.
  - Increased gastric acid secretion, delayed gastric emptying, and depressed level of consciousness can increase the risk of aspiration.
  - Hypovolemia is poorly tolerated, increasing the risk of shock.
  - Cardiac contractility may be depressed, which, in conjunction with general anesthesia, increases the risk of developing congestive heart failure.
  - Intoxicated patients require less anesthesia.
- The end-organ damage from chronic alcoholism rather than the alcohol itself is the major risk factor for perioperative complications. AUDs are associated with metabolic, hematologic, gastrointestinal, cardiac, infectious, and neurologic comorbidity.
  - Electrolyte abnormalities—including hyponatremia, hypomagnesemia, and hypophosphatemia—are more frequent.
  - Anemia, thrombocytopenia, and coagulopathy increase the risk of bleeding.
  - Alcohol increases the risk of cirrhosis, gastritis, ulcer disease, and cancers of the upper digestive system.
  - Cardiomyopathy, congestive heart failure, hypertension, and arrhythmias may result.
  - Malnutrition, neutropenia, and impaired defense mechanisms may increase the risk of infection.
  - AUDs contribute to prolonged stays in the intensive care unit (ICU) and longer hospitalizations.

ALCOHOL WITHDRAWAL SYNDROME (AWS)

- Alcohol abuse and dependence increase the risk of AWS complications in the perioperative period and during hospitalization.
- Alcohol withdrawal syndrome (AWS)—that is, autonomic hyperactivity and impaired functioning—can occur when alcohol-dependent persons suddenly reduce their consumption of alcohol. This can occur in operative settings when the alcohol-dependent patient requires emergent surgery.
- Abstinence from drinking as imposed by a hospital admission places patients with abuse or dependence at risk for AWS.
- Patients with AWS experience tremulousness, increased blood pressure and pulse, and a variety of other nonspecific signs and symptoms. The signs and symptoms of AWS exist along a spectrum from mild to severe. Most patients who experience AWS have mild to moderate symptoms with no need for pharmacologic treatment. However, patients with severe AWS may have significant complications that require intervention.

TABLE 43-1 Definitions of Alcohol Use Disorders

CATEGORY	DEFINITION	PRIMARY DEFINING AUTHORITY
At-risk drinking	Quantity or pattern of use that places the person at risk for adverse consequences of alcohol consumption. This category includes harmful, hazardous, and heavy drinking.	WHO NIH
Harmful drinking	Clear evidence that the alcohol use is responsible for (or is substantially contributing to) physical or psychological harm. The nature of the alcohol-related harm is clearly identifiable and specified. The pattern of use has persisted for at least 1 month or has occurred repeatedly within the previous 12-month period. The subject does not fulfill criteria for alcohol dependence.	WHO ICD-10
Hazardous drinking	The quantity or pattern of use places person at risk for adverse consequences of alcohol consumption.	WHO NIH
Heavy drinking	The quantity or pattern of alcohol use exceeds a defined threshold.	WHO NIH
Alcohol abuse	A maladaptive pattern of alcohol use leads to clinically significant impairment or distress as manifest by one or more of the following over a 12-month period: Recurrent alcohol use resulting in a failure to fulfill major role obligations at work, school, or home Recurrent alcohol use in situations where it is physically hazardous Recurrent alcohol-related legal problems Continued alcohol use despite having persistent or recurrent social or interpersonal problems caused or exacerbated by the effects of the substance The symptoms have never met the criteria for alcohol dependence.	DSM-IV[11]
Alcohol dependence	Maladaptive pattern of alcohol use leading to clinically significant impairment or distress as manifest by three or more of the following, occurring at any time in the same 12-month period: 1. Tolerance, as defined by either of the following: a. Need for markedly increased amounts of alcohol to achieve intoxication or desired effect b. Markedly diminished effect with continued use of the same amount of the alcohol 2. Existence of a characteristic withdrawal syndrome for alcohol, alcohol being taken to relieve or avoid this 3. Alcohol often taken in larger amounts or over a longer period than was intended 4. A persistent desire or unsuccessful efforts to cut down or control use 5. A great deal of time spent in activities necessary to obtain alcohol, use alcohol, or recover from its effects 6. Loss or reduction of important social, occupational, or recreational activities due to alcohol use 7. Continued use of alcohol despite persistent or recurrent physical or psychological problems likely to have been caused or exacerbated the use of alcohol Physiologic dependence: Evidence of tolerance or withdrawal (i.e., either item 1 or item 2 is present)	DSM-IV[11]

DSM-IV = Diagnostic and Statistical Manual of Mental Disorders, 4th edition; ICD-10 = *International Classification of Diseases*, 10th edition; NIH = National Institutes of Health; WHO = World Health Organization.

- Although all patients with AUDs are at increased risk for perioperative complications, the development of AWS in alcohol-dependent patients constitutes an independent cause of increased morbidity.
- Identification of AWS may be delayed in the perioperative period, which may contribute to increased morbidity. In a study of 539 episodes of AWS, 21 percent of patients had adverse outcomes, such as increased

length of hospital stay, delirium, or seizures. Complications correlated with patient age over 70 years, history of seizures, or a delay in initial patient assessment. [3]
- Despite the increased incidence and related harm associated with AUDs and AWS in surgical populations, AUDs are often unrecognized; if recognized, they may not be treated.

SURGERY-SPECIFIC RISKS

- AUDs predispose patients to trauma, often necessitating emergent surgical interventions.
  - A large proportion of motor vehicle accidents and occupational, interpersonal, and intentional injuries of patients who are hospitalized are related to alcohol problems.
- The prevalence of AUDs in surgical settings is higher than in the general population; a study of inpatients found that 23 percent of general surgery admissions and 43 percent of otolaryngology admissions met the criteria for alcohol abuse. [4]
- The stress of surgery additionally predisposes patients to AWS or may exacerbate it if it already exists.
- The incidence of AWS is two to five times higher in surgical and trauma patients than in any other group of hospitalized patients.

PREOPERATIVE CONSIDERATIONS

IDENTIFICATION OF ALCOHOL USE DISORDERS

- Assess all patients who are undergoing elective or emergent surgical operations for alcohol consumption.
- The preoperative evaluation of patients with potential AUDs should include effective screening strategies to identify the presence of AUDs, detect end-organ damage secondary to alcohol consumption, and prompt intervention on the AUD prior to surgery. The identification and treatment of patients with AUDs in the perioperative period reduces surgical complications. Patients who may be at risk for alcohol abuse and dependence should be identified prior to surgery.
- The most effective means of screening for AUDs is through short, validated screening instruments. The identification of patient characteristics that are often associated with AUDs may assist in effective screening for AUDs. These include the presence of historical factors, comorbid medical or psychiatric conditions, physical examination findings, and laboratory characteristics. [2]
- Because perioperative patients are often unable to communicate or answer questions on AUD screening instruments, assessment may have to depend on physical and laboratory findings; the latter can also add to the sensitivity of detection when combined with history and screening instruments.
- Many instruments have been developed to screen for alcohol consumption, at-risk drinking, and alcohol abuse/dependence. Authorities recommend a screening strategy to identify the range of AUDs, from "at risk" to alcohol abuse and dependence disorders. The Alcohol Use Disorders Identification Test (AUDIT) is an excellent initial screening instrument for at-risk alcohol consumption. The AUDIT is a 10-item questionnaire that evaluates the quantity and frequency of alcohol consumption. Abbreviated AUDIT instruments (three- or one-item questionnaire) have been shown to be as effective as the 10-item questionnaire. The CAGE ("cut-down, annoyed, guilt, and eye-opener") questionnaire is an excellent initial screening instrument for alcohol abuse/dependence (Fig. 43-1).
- Screening for alcohol consumption can be incorporated into standardized preoperative questionnaires.

PREOPERATIVE INTERVENTIONS FOR ALCOHOL USE DISORDERS

- The preoperative diagnosis of AUDs allows the opportunity to anticipate operative and postoperative complications and offer preoperative interventions to reduce perioperative morbidity. Preoperative interventions for patients with AUDs but without alcohol dependence include assessment of complications secondary to alcohol, encouraged or controlled abstinence, referral for substance abuse counseling, and AWS prophylaxis.
- Patients who are suspected of having problems with alcohol consumption and who have AWS should have laboratory evaluations looking for complications secondary to alcohol consumption that may complicate surgical care.
  - These tests should include a complete blood count (CBC), liver enzymes, prothrombin time, electrolytes, glucose, and urinary drug screen.
  - An electrocardiogram should also be performed.
  - Obtain a blood alcohol level in an intoxicated or unconscious patient who requires urgent surgery. It will confirm the level of intoxication, provide a measure of the degree of tolerance, and serve medicolegal purposes. Also, alert the health care team to the patient's risk of developing withdrawal postoperatively.
  - Abnormal laboratory tests should prompt corrective interventions to reduce operative risk.
- Educate patients regarding safe alcohol consumption and advise them to reduce their consumption of alcohol prior to the surgical procedure. Encourage alcohol abstinence for at least 4 weeks prior to elective surgery. Abstinence has been associated with reduced surgical morbidity and improved perioperative outcomes.

THE ALCOHOL DISORDERS IDENTIFICATION TEST (AUDIT)

1. How often do you have a drink containing alcohol?
Never (0) | Monthly or less (1) | 2–4 times a month (2) | 2–3 times a week (3) | 4 or more times a week (4)

2. How many drinks containing alcohol do you have on a typical day when you are drinking?
1 or 2 (0) | 3 or 4 (1) | 5 or 6 (2) | 7 to 9 (3) | 10 or more (4)

3. How often do you have six or more drinks on one occasion?
Never (0) | Less than monthly (1) | Monthly (2) | Weekly (3) | Daily or almost daily (4)

4. How often during the last year have you found that you were not able to stop drinking once you had started?
Never (0) | Less than monthly (1) | Monthly (2) | Weekly (3) | Daily or almost daily (4)

5. How often during the last year have you failed to do what was normally expected from you because of drinking?
Never (0) | Less than monthly (1) | Monthly (2) | Weekly (3) | Daily or almost daily (4)

6. How often during the last year have you needed a first drink in the morning to get yourself going after a heavy drinking session?
Never (0) | Less than monthly (1) | Monthly (2) | Weekly (3) | Daily or almost daily (4)

7. How often during the last year have you had a feeling of guilt or remorse after drinking?
Never (0) | Less than monthly (1) | Monthly (2) | Weekly (3) | Daily or almost daily (4)

8. How often during the last year have you been unable to remember what happened the night before because you had been drinking?
Never (0) | Less than monthly (1) | Monthly (2) | Weekly (3) | Daily or almost daily (4)

9. Have you or someone else been injured as a result of your drinking?
No (0) | Yes, but not in the last year (2) | Yes, during the last year (4)

10. Has a relative or friend or a doctor or other health worker been concerned about your drinking or suggested you cut down?
No (0) | Yes, but not in the last year (2) | Yes, during the last year (4)

CAGE QUESTIONNAIRE

1. Have you ever felt you should CUT DOWN on your drinking?
2. Have people ANNOYED you by criticizing your drinking?
3. Have you ever felt bad or GUILTY about your drinking?
4. Have you ever had a drink first thing in the morning to steady your nerves or to get rid of a hangover (EYE OPENER)?

FIG. 43-1 The AUDIT and CAGE questionnaires. AUDIT questions are usually asked in context of consumption of alcohol in the prior 12 months.[8] Possible scores are from 0 to 40. A common cutoff score for hazardous drinking is a score of 8 or above. Abbreviated AUDIT questionnaires include the AUDIT-C (questions 1 to 3, positive score of 3 or greater) and the AUDIT-3 [positive score on question 3 (binge question) is any affirmative answer]. Any affirmative answer on the CAGE questionnaire should arouse suspicion of alcohol abuse/dependence; two affirmative answers are more likely to be clinically significant.[9]

- Alcohol-dependent patients at risk for AWS may undergo preoperative detoxification and rehabilitation, medical detoxification, and/or AWS prophylaxis prior to operative interventions (see "Postoperative Considerations," below).
- The decision to enter detoxification treatment requires a motivated patient, and the preoperative evaluation provides an excellent opportunity to educate patients about the consequences of at-risk alcohol use during the perioperative period. The urgency of surgery and the patient's attitudes about his or her alcohol use determine the feasibility of preoperative detoxification. While this approach may be promising as a preoperative treatment for patients with alcohol dependence, no studies have evaluated the effect of preoperative alcohol detoxification on surgical outcomes prior to elective or emergent surgical procedures.

- Consider AWS prophylaxis for patients who have AUDs and are at risk for AWS when abstinence prior to the operative procedure is not possible. These patients include those with a past history of AWS, alcohol-dependent patients who have refused preoperative detoxification or who require urgent surgery that does not permit time for detoxification, patients with ongoing hazardous drinking, and patients who present in an intoxicated state.
- Those patients who are given early and adequate prophylaxis for AWS appear to have fewer postoperative complications and a shorter length of hospitalization than alcohol-dependent patients who do not receive prophylaxis. AWS prophylaxis should begin on cessation of alcohol consumption or admission to the hospital and should not be delayed until the postoperative period.
- AWS prophylaxis is accomplished by using cross-tolerant medications during the immediate perioperative period. Evidence from a large metaanalysis and a review of AWS treatment strategies support the use of benzodiazepines as first-line treatment for AWS. Suggested regimens include diazepam 2.5 to 10 mg, lorazepam 0.5 to 2 mg, or chlordiazepoxide 5 to 25 mg every 6 h during the time of potential AWS.
- The use of AWS prophylaxis does not prohibit future detoxification and rehabilitation. Use the multiple contacts with providers that occur during the perioperative period to encourage patients to seek treatment for their AUDs. The need for surgery itself can be a powerful motivator for modifying the unhealthy behavior of these patients.
- An addiction specialist or psychiatrist experienced in the evaluation and treatment of AUDs may improve the ability of the referring surgeon to promote abstinence and perform preoperative detoxification, although there are no studies evaluating the impact of expert consultation on AUD treatment outcomes.

PERIOPERATIVE MANAGEMENT

OPERATIVE CONSIDERATIONS

- Provider awareness of a patient's AUD allows for anticipation of increased anesthetic and analgesic requirements and heightened responses to surgical stress. Due to the widespread and complex effects of alcohol on virtually all organ systems, it is important to recognize and modify dosages and intervals of administration of intraoperative medications in patients with AUDs.
- Acute alcohol consumption prior to surgery may prolong the duration of action of several medications used during surgery, including propranolol and phenobarbital. Chronic alcohol consumption induces the cytochrome P450 system, potentially shortening the duration of action of medications used during surgery.
- AUDs among surgical patients can complicate the administration and dosing of anesthesia and analgesia. Patients consuming greater than 40 g of alcohol per day for at least 2 years require more propofol to induce anesthesia than is needed for social drinkers (<40 g alcohol per day) or nondrinkers. Alcoholics require significantly larger doses of fentanyl than nondrinkers to achieve adequate analgesia.
- Acute physical stress, including surgery itself, activates the hypothalamic-pituitary-adrenal (HPA) axis, resulting in increased serum cortisol levels. The "surgical stress" response triggers multiple physiologic changes, including increased heart rate, elevated blood pressure, and increased levels of plasma catecholamine. The stress response begins at the time of incision, peaks on cessation of anesthesia and return of pain sensation, and continues throughout the postoperative period.
- Patients with AUDs exhibit increased responses to surgical stress compared with normal controls, as measured by increased levels of plasma catecholamines and cortisol. This exaggerated stress response may contribute to increased morbidity postoperatively through immunosuppression and increased cardiovascular demand. Due to similarities in pathophysiology, AWS and stress responses can have additive effects. Following surgery, patients with AWS have increased levels of norepinephrine compared with controls. The severity of withdrawal symptoms correlates with norepinephrine levels.
- Close attention to adequate hemostasis may prevent the development of complications. A study of patients with traumatic hemorrhage found that those with AUDs were less able to maintain adequate blood pressures during surgery.
- Intraoperative episodes of hypoxemia or hypotension increase the risk of postoperative delirium in patients with AUDs.

POSTOPERATIVE CONSIDERATIONS

- Patients with AUDs require close attention during the postoperative period to detect AWS and minimize complications, as the latter are likely to be greater in these patients as compared with normal controls or social drinkers. The most common complications encountered are infections, bleeding, and cardiopulmonary insufficiency, in addition to prolonged intensive care unit (ICU) and overall hospital stays.

- Perioperative arrhythmias can develop in patients with AUDs without preexisting cardiac disease. The "holiday heart syndrome" refers to arrhythmias classically occurring after episodes of binge drinking. Such behavior can be assessed through the third question of the AUDIT.
- Significantly higher bleeding times and an increased frequency of bleeding episodes, often requiring transfusion, have been observed postoperatively in patients with AUDs.
- Alcohol abuse is a significant independent risk factor for surgical-site infections.
- Possible mechanisms for increased complications in patients with AUDs include immune incompetence, cardiac disease, hemostatic imbalance, and decreased protein accumulation with impaired wound healing. Chronic alcohol use decreases T-cell activity and proliferation, and delayed type-hypersensitivity (DTH) reactions are decreased pre- and postoperatively in patients with AUDs. Chronic alcohol abuse is a known cause of cardiomyopathy, and patients with AUDs have decreased preoperative ejection fractions compared with controls. Depressed cardiac function may predispose patients to increased postoperative ischemia and arrhythmias.
- It is often difficult to diagnose AWS and establish the severity of symptoms in the postoperative period. Postoperative delirium is a common condition, and similarities in presentation between other causes of delirium and AWS may delay time to diagnosis.
- To adequately diagnose postoperative AWS, other common causes of postoperative delirium must be considered. Agitation, which is commonly seen in AWS, may be falsely attributed to postoperative pain, the use of restraints, medications, or continued pulmonary intubation. The use of a preoperative screening assessment of the level of alcohol consumption, the time from the last drink to delirium, and the use (or lack of use) of preoperative and operative AWS prophylaxis may also assist in determining whether a patient's agitation is due to AWS.

ALCOHOL WITHDRAWAL TREATMENT: ALCOHOL DETOXIFICATION

- Alcohol detoxification includes pharmacologic treatment to reduce the morbidity and mortality of AWS, specialized counseling to reduce future alcohol-related harm, and encouragement to attend to future alcohol treatments, alcohol rehabilitation, and aftercare.
- Treatment of AWS is guided by the severity of AWS signs and symptoms. An objective validated measure of AWS, the Clinical Institute Withdrawal Assessment Scale for Alcohol—Revised (CIWA-Ar), has been used to measure AWS severity (Fig. 43-2). Use of the CIWA-Ar along with symptom-triggered benzodiazepine dosing has been useful in reducing length of stay and the amount of benzodiazepines administered to patients undergoing medical detoxification.[5] However, administration of CIWA-Ar in the postoperative period may be complicated by endotracheal intubation, a decreased level of consciousness, or the patient's inability to communicate with the assessor.
- Pharmacologic treatment of AWS through detoxification includes long-acting benzodiazepines and barbiturates (Fig. 43-3). Use carbamazepine as an alternative to benzodiazepines. Treat alcoholic seizures with intravenous benzodiazepines.[6,7]
- The use of intravenous or oral ethanol-replacement therapies for AWS remains controversial; limited data are available to support this practice. It is not recommended for alcohol detoxification.
- Adjuvant therapies for AWS can include beta blockers and clonidine to reduce sympathetic overactivity and cardiovascular complications.
- Patients with AUDs, and especially patients with AWS, should receive daily multivitamins, high-dose thiamine (100 mg), and oral or parenteral thiamine (100 mg daily) during the preoperative and perioperative periods to prevent stress-induced Wernicke-Korsakoff syndrome.
- Educate patients with AUDs and/or AWS regarding the harm done by their alcohol consumption. Hospitalization after alcohol-related trauma may be an opportunity for alcohol interventions, as patients may then be more receptive to recognizing alcohol as a problem and therefore more likely to accept further treatment.

SUMMARY

Despite the great prevalence of AUDs and the harm to which these patients are vulnerable in undergoing operative procedures, this problem generally goes unrecognized by clinicians. In the perioperative period, consider risk-reduction strategies (Table 43-2). Medical consultants and surgeons should screen for AUDs in all surgical patients and consider alcohol detoxification or alcohol withdrawal prophylaxis and treatment in the perioperative period. Benzodiazepines are the mainstay therapy for AWS. Finally, the perioperative period can be a critical time to intervene with alcohol-dependent patients to reduce their consumption of alcohol and maintain abstinence postoperatively.

Patient: ____________ **Date:** (yy/mm/dd) ____/____/____ **Time:** (24 hr) ________

Pulse or heart rate: __________ **Blood pressure:** ____________

Nausea and vomiting- Ask"Do you feel sick to your stomach?" "Have you vomited?" Observation.

- ☐ 0 - no nausea and no vomiting
- ☐ 1 - mild nausea with no vomiting
- ☐ 2
- ☐ 3
- ☐ 4 - intermittent nausea with dry heaves
- ☐ 5
- ☐ 6
- ☐ 7 - constant nausea, frequent dry heaves and vomiting.

Tactile disturbances - Ask "Have you any itching, pins and needles sensations, any burning, any numbness, or do you feel bugs crawling on or under your skin? Observation.

- ☐ 0 - none
- ☐ 1 - very mild itching, pins and needles, burning or numbness
- ☐ 2 - mild itching, pins and needles, burning or numbness
- ☐ 3 - moderate itching, pins and needles, burning or numbness
- ☐ 4 - moderately severe hallucinations
- ☐ 5 - severe hallucinations
- ☐ 6- extremely severe hallucinations
- ☐ 7- continuous hallucinations

Tremor - Arms extended and fingers spread apart. Observation.

- ☐ 0 - no tremor
- ☐ 1 - not visible, but can be felt fingertip to fingertip
- ☐ 2
- ☐ 3
- ☐ 4 - moderate, with patient's arms extended
- ☐ 5
- ☐ 6
- ☐ 7 - severe, even with arms not extended

Auditory disturbances - Ask "Are you more aware of sounds around you? Are they harsh? Do they frighten you? Are you hearing anything that is disturbing to you? Are you hearing things that you know aren't there?" Observation.

- ☐ 0 - not present
- ☐ 1 - very mild harshness or ability to frighten
- ☐ 2 - mild harshness or ability to frighten
- ☐ 3 - moderate harshness or ability to frighten
- ☐ 4 - moderately severe hallucinations
- ☐ 5 - severe hallucinations
- ☐ 6 - extremely severe hallucinations
- ☐ 7 - continuous hallucinations

Paroxysmal sweats - Observation.

- ☐ 0 - no sweat visible
- ☐ 1 - barely perceptible sweating, palms moist
- ☐ 2
- ☐ 3
- ☐ 4 - beads of sweat obvious on forehead
- ☐ 5
- ☐ 6
- ☐ 7- drenching sweats

Visual disturbances - Ask " Does the light appear to be too bright? Is its color different? Does it hurt your eyes? Are you seeing anything that is disturbing you? Are you seeing things that you know aren't there?" Observation.

- ☐ 0 - not present
- ☐ 1 - very mild sensitivity
- ☐ 2 - mild sensitivity
- ☐ 3 - moderate sensitivity
- ☐ 4 - moderately severe hallucinations
- ☐ 5 - severe hallucinations
- ☐ 6 - extremely severe hallucinations
- ☐ 7 - continuous hallucinations

Anxiety - Ask "Do you feel nervous?" Observation.

- ☐ 0 - no anxiety, at ease
- ☐ 1 - mildly anxious
- ☐ 2
- ☐ 3
- ☐ 4 - moderately anxious, or guarded, so anxiety is inferred
- ☐ 5
- ☐ 6
- ☐ 7- equivalent to acute panic states as seen in severe delirium or acute schizophrenic reactions

Headache, fullness in head - Ask "Does your head feel different? Does it feel like there is a band around your head?" Do not rate dizziness or lightheadedness. Otherwise, rate severity.

- ☐ 0 - not present
- ☐ 1 - very mild
- ☐ 2 - mild
- ☐ 3 - moderate
- ☐ 4 - moderately severe
- ☐ 5 - severe
- ☐ 6 - very severe
- ☐ 7 - extremely severe

Agitation - Observation.

- ☐ 0 - normal activity
- ☐ 1 - somewhat more than normal activity
- ☐ 2
- ☐ 3
- ☐ 4 - moderately fidgety and restless
- ☐ 5
- ☐ 6
- ☐ 7 - paces back and forth during most of the interview, or constantly thrashes about.

Orientation and clouding of sensorium - Ask "What day is this? Where are you? Who am I?"

- ☐ oriented and can do serial additions
- ☐ cannot do serial additions or is uncertain about date
- ☐ disoriented for date by no more than two calendar days
- ☐ disoriented for date by more than two calendar days
- ☐ disoriented for place and/or person

This scale is not copyrighted and may be used freely

Total CIWA-Ar Score _____
Rater's initials _____
Maximum possible score - 67

FIG. 43-2 The Addiction Research Foundation Clinical Institute Withdrawal Assessment—Alcohol revised (CIWA-Ar) scale. A score above 8 is clinically significant and indicates a treatable level of alcohol withdrawal.[10]

Prevention of Alcohol-Related Harms

Correct any laboratory abnormalities
Administer:

- Thiamine 100 mg every day
- Folate 1 mg every day
- Multivitamin every day

Counsel to reduce alcohol consumption

Consider a consult to an addiction specialist

Monitoring
Monitor patients every 4 to 8 h by means of CIWA-Ar until score has been <8 to 10 for 24 h

Alcohol Withdrawal Prophylaxis: Fixed-Schedule Regimens

Chlordiazepoxide, 50 mg every 6 h for 4 doses, then 25 mg every 6 h for 8 doses
Diazepam, 10 mg every 6 h for 4 doses, then 5 mg every 6 h for 8 doses
Lorazepam, 2 mg every 6 h for 4 doses, then 1 mg every 6 h for 8 doses

Provide additional medication as needed when symptoms are not controlled (i.e., CIWA-Ar >=8 to 10) with above regimen.

Alcohol Detoxification: Symptom-triggered regimens

Administer one of the following medications every hour when CIWA-Ar is >= 8 to 10:

Chlordiazepoxide, 50 to 100 mg
Diazepam, 10 to 20 mg
Lorazepam, 2 to 4 mg

Repeat assessment with CIWA-Ar one hour after every dose to determine need for further medication

Provide additional medication as needed when symptoms are not controlled (i.e., CIWA-Ar >=8 to 10) with above regimen.

FIG. 43-3 Typical protocols for the treatment of alcohol abuse and dependence in the perioperative period.

TABLE 43-2 Risks and Perioperative Risk-Reduction Strategies for Alcohol Disorders in the Perioperative Period

PERIOPERATIVE RISKS OF ALCOHOL CONSUMPTION	PREOPERATIVE RISK REDUCTION	POSTOPERATIVE RISK REDUCTION
AUDs are not often recognized preoperatively. AUDs are strongly associated with use of other drugs of abuse and medical and psychiatric conditions. AUDs often contribute to trauma and need for emergent surgery. AUDs contribute to significant end-organ damage and poor health states. AWS may be deadly. Alcohol affects analgesic and anesthetic treatments.	Screen for AUDs with standard, evidenced-based screening instruments from "at-risk" consumption to alcohol abuse/dependence. Evaluate for laboratory abnormalities secondary to AUDs. Inform patients regarding risks of operative procedure due to AUDs. Consider delaying elective surgery until patient is abstinent from alcohol. Consider AWS prophylactic treatment with benzodiazepines. Inform surgeons and anesthesiologists regarding perioperative AUD treatments as well as anesthesia and analgesia management.	Treat AWS with alcohol detoxification using benzodiazepines. Encourage patients to maintain abstinence from alcohol. Encourage patients to continue with alcohol rehabilitation and aftercare. Support nutritional status and correct laboratory abnormalities secondary to AUDs. Consider consultation with an addiction specialist.

AUD = alcohol use disorder; AWS = alcohol withdrawal syndrome.

References

1. Craft PP, Foil MB, Cunningham PR, et al. Intravenous ethanol for alcohol detoxification in trauma patients. *South Med J* 87(1):47–54, 1994.
2. Gordon AJ, Saitz R. Identification and treatment of alcohol use disorders in primary care. *J Clin Outcome Mgt* 11(7): 444–462, 2004.
3. Foy A, Kay J, Taylor A. The course of alcohol withdrawal in a general hospital. *Q J Med* 90(4):253–261, 1997.
4. Moore RD, Bone LR, Geller G, et al. Prevalence, detection, and treatment of alcoholism in hospitalized patients. *JAMA* 261(3):403–407, 1989.
5. Saitz R, Mayo-Smith MF, Roberts MS, et al. Individualized treatment for alcohol withdrawal. A randomized double-blind controlled trial. *JAMA* 272(7):519–523, 1994.
6. Saitz R, O'Malley SS. Pharmacotherapies for alcohol abuse. Withdrawal and treatment. *Med Clin North Am* 81(4):881–907, 1997.
7. Mayo-Smith MF. Pharmacological management of alcohol withdrawal. A meta-analysis and evidence-based practice guideline. American Society of Addiction Medicine Working Group on Pharmacological Management of Alcohol Withdrawal. *JAMA* 278(2):144–151, 1997.
8. Babor TF, de la Fuente JR, Saunders J, Grant M. *The Alcohol Use Disorders Identification Test: Guidelines for use in primary health care.* Geneva: World Health Organization, 1989.
9. Mayfield D, McLeod G, Hall P. The CAGE questionnaire: Validation of a new alcoholism screening instrument. *Am J Psychiatry* 131(10):1121–1123, 1974.
10. Sullivan JT, Sykora K, Schneiderman J, et al. Assessment of alcohol withdrawal: The revised Clinical Institute Withdrawal Assessment for Alcohol scale (CIWA-Ar). *Br J Addiction* 84(11):1353–1357, 1989.
11. *Diagnostic and Statistical Manual of Mental Disorders,* 4th ed (DSM-IV). Washington, DC: American Psychiatric Association, 2005.

44 THE ELDERLY PATIENT

William Wertheim and
Margaret Beliveau-Ficalora

INTRODUCTION

- Surgical disease in the elderly is enormously common in the United States. Approximately one-third of all surgical procedures are performed on patients who are in the geriatric age group.
- As might be predicted, such patients are more likely to pose clinical challenges for the physicians caring for them during the perioperative period. Patients over the age of 65 are more than twice as likely as those under age 65 to require emergency surgery. Similarly, the burden of underlying illness is significant; up to 30% of patients over 65 have three or more concurrent chronic medical problems.

PATIENT-RELATED RISK FACTORS (TABLE 44-1)

- The hallmark of normal aging is declining physiologic functional reserve. While basal function may be adequately maintained, the ability to compensate for a variety of stresses, including surgery and anesthesia, is compromised. Age is a marker for subclinical disease or declining functional reserve, which is ubiquitous across organ systems and may contribute to many perioperative complications.[1]

TABLE 44-1 Components of Surgical Risk in the Elderly: Patient-Specific Risks and Common Conditions

Cardiac
Coronary artery disease
Hypertension
Valvular heart disease, especially aortic stenosis
Congestive heart failure
Peripheral vascular disease
Pulmonary
Chronic obstructive pulmonary disease
Respiratory muscle weakness
Obstructive sleep apnea
Aspiration risk
Renal
Diminished glomerular filtration rate and renal blood flow
Renal failure
Hepatic
Decreased hepatic function
Neurologic
Stroke
Dementia
Parkinson's disease
Gastrointestinal
Constipation
Gastroesophageal reflux disease
Musculoskeletal
Osteoarthritis
Osteoporosis
Endocrine
Diabetes
Malnutrition
Polypharmacy
Surgery-specific risk
Increased incidence of emergency surgery
Increased chance of "high-risk" surgery, e.g., cardiac, vascular

CARDIAC

- In the cardiovascular system, systemic vascular resistance increases with aging, resulting in systolic hypertension. This is due to a loss of arterial elasticity, a decrease in the cross-sectional area of the peripheral vascular bed, and declining responsiveness to beta-adrenergically mediated vasodilation. Ventricular hypertrophy results from these changes. The noncompliant, hypertrophied heart is more susceptible to ischemia and more reliant on atrial contraction to achieve adequate ventricular filling. Ventricular hypertrophy, coupled with decreased inotropic and chronotropic responses to catecholamines and age-related changes in autonomic control of cardiovascular homeostasis, render the elderly less capable of preserving their blood pressure and cardiac output. Therefore they are predisposed to congestive heart failure with even modest fluid overload.[2]
- Likewise, the elderly have difficulty compensating for even small decreases in absolute or relative intravascular volume and are prone to hypotension. An example is the increased likelihood of hypotension in the elderly due to the relative hypotension caused by the sympathectomy of spinal or epidural anesthesia.

PULMONARY

- Pulmonary changes with aging include a decrease in maximal minute ventilation because of diminished thoracic muscle mass and thoracic compliance. By age 65, declining elastic lung recoil results in a closing capacity that is greater than functional residual capacity.
- Anatomic and functional dead space increases. Ventilation/perfusion matching is altered. The effects of these changes include an increased alveolar-arterial oxygen gradient and lower resting Pao_2. At baseline, the central response to hypoxia is diminished. This is exacerbated by a variety of anesthetic and analgesic agents.
- Ciliary function and cough are reduced and limit the ability to clear secretions.
- Finally, the elderly are prone to aspiration because of limited pharyngeal sensation and motor function.[3]

RENAL

- The glomerular filtration rate (GFR) declines with age as a result of diminished renal blood flow, cortical atrophy, and glomerular sclerosis. However, because of diminished muscle mass, serum creatinine often does not reflect this. These changes limit the ability to excrete drugs and their metabolites, making dose adjustments necessary.
- Aging impairs sodium excretion and conservation and limits the ability of the kidney to excrete acid. Alterations in thirst mechanisms and release of antidiuretic hormone (ADH) combine with changes in renal function to restrict the ability of the kidney to fulfill its homeostatic role.[2,3]

PHARMACOKINETICS

Many factors contribute to the altered pharmacokinetics seen in elderly patients.

- Liver size decreases, and there is an associated decrease in hepatic blood flow. This results in a diminished clearance of drugs requiring biotransformation, such as opioids, barbiturates, and benzodiazepines.
- Aging steadily increases the relative ratio of lipid to aqueous tissue, especially in women. As a result, the volume of distribution of lipid-soluble drugs is increased.
- Absorption may be affected by decreased flow to the gastrointestinal tract as well as by changes in gastric acidity and altered motility (especially in patients with diabetes).[1,3]

IMMUNOLOGIC FUNCTION

- Elderly patients are more vulnerable to perioperative infection and poor wound healing. Response to foreign antigens is diminished, there may be an increased responsiveness to autologous antigens, and there is some evidence that the phagocytic response of polymorphonuclear leukocytes decreases with age.[2]

ALTERED PRESENTATION OF DISEASE

- The clinical presentation and natural history of some illnesses may be different in the elderly population. Most patients have multiple comorbidities and take multiple medications, both of which can alter disease presentation.
- Older patients may present with only nonspecific symptoms of illness.
- Older patients may have a higher pain threshold, and pain may be less of a localizing finding than it is in younger patients.
- Fever may not be as prominent a symptom in an elderly patient with sepsis. Hypothermia is more common in seriously ill patients.

COGNITIVE FUNCTION

- Preoperative identification of significant cognitive decline is essential in the preoperative assessment of the elderly surgical patient. Even mild to moderate dementia may significantly affect postoperative rehabilitation and return to full function. Patients with dementia may also have limited ability to understand the risks and benefits of a proposed surgical procedure and may be unwilling or unable to give full informed consent. These patients are at increased risk of postoperative delirium.

FUNCTIONAL STATUS

- Preoperative functional status is a key factor in identifying the risk of postoperative complications.[4] Studies have shown that an active lifestyle is associated with decreased surgical morbidity and mortality. There are many validated tools to assess functional status. Preoperative assessment of a patient's ability to perform activities of daily living (ADLs—dressing, ambulation, toileting, bathing, transfer, continence, grooming, and communication) and instrumental activities of daily living (IADLs—travel, employment, money management, reading, writing, cooking, shopping) may be better at predicting surgical risk than many technologies available for risk assessment. Unfortunately, many elderly patients may be limited in their abilities due to musculoskeletal complaints. This makes assessment of functional status more difficult. Careful and creative questioning may be needed to get a better "snapshot" of a patient's true functional abilities.

SURGERY-SPECIFIC RISK

- Operative mortality in the elderly is declining, most likely from a combination of improved surgical and anesthetic techniques as well as better preoperative evaluation and management. In general, the best-tolerated procedures are those involving less tissue injury and physiologic disruption.
- Emergency procedures carry a high risk of morbidity and mortality. This results from a combination of severity of surgical disease and a lack of time to optimize the patient medically prior to surgery.
- The elderly are more likely to undergo high-risk procedures: repair of an abdominal aortic aneurysm, peripheral vascular surgery, coronary artery bypass grafting or valve replacement, hip fracture repair or joint replacement, and cancer surgery.

GOALS OF SURGERY IN THE ELDERLY

- Many elderly patients are very concerned about maintaining their quality of life and functional status and less concerned about their overall lifespan. Surgical procedures that improve quality of life by relieving pain or maximizing function may be worthwhile despite some risk due to age or comorbidities.
    - For example, a total hip replacement rarely prolongs someone's life, but it serves to relieve pain associated with osteoarthritis and improve or preserve mobility and function. In some cases, a surgical procedure that accomplishes this goal may be preferred to a more radical procedure that offers a chance of "cure."
    - Do not overlook the goals of pain relief and symptom control. Preoperative assessment should include knowledge of the patient's goals for the procedure, and the patient should understand the likelihood of achieving those goals. Take into account treatment alternatives and the risks and benefits of each.
- Finally, the natural history of the disease and the patient's life expectancy should be part of the equation.

PREOPERATIVE EVALUATION

Preoperative risk assessment in the elderly is based on the same principles as in the younger patient; however, certain special areas warrant particular attention.

- Cardiac risk can be assessed utilizing the same criteria as with younger patients. Assessment of cardiac risk prior to noncardiac surgery is reviewed in Chap. 20; however, certain features merit discussion:
    - First, both the original articles discussing cardiac risk (Goldman,[5] Detsky[6]) and the clinical guidelines [American College of Physicians (APP), American College of Cardiology/American Heart Association (ACC/AHA)] largely employ clinical criteria to reach their conclusions about the individual risk, with a deemphasis on invasive or specialized testing.[4,7]
    - Second, each authority considers advanced age alone to be a small but consistent risk for cardiac complications. The physiologic changes outlined above most likely explain this persistent increase in risk.
    - Third, because of the frequency with which cardiac risk factors such as hypertension and hypercholesterolemia occur in the older population, serious consideration should be given to use of perioperative beta blockers and possibly statins in this setting.
- Assessment of pulmonary risk in the older patient is also similar to that in younger patients. Historically, pulmonary risk assessment had been plagued by variability and a paucity of useful studies. More recently, studies that looked at the risk of pulmonary complications demonstrated that age alone (above 80 years) is associated with an increased risk of both pulmonary morbidity and mortality.[8,9]
- Functional capacity, while not age-specific, is a very important measure in the elderly. Easy clinical assessments such as the Duke Activity Status Index are both

readily available and part of the ACC/AHA guidelines. Other studies have demonstrated the increased risk of specific surgeries such as vascular or cardiac surgeries in patients with impaired functional capacity as well as the increased risk associated with other simple assessments, such as the ability to walk stairs.
- In contrast to the straightforward role of functional capacity, assessment of cognitive function has an unclear role in assessing the risk of those undergoing surgery. At least two studies failed to show any link between preoperative cognitive function and postoperative complications; however, other studies demonstrated an association between preoperative cognitive impairment and postoperative delirium as well as between preoperative cognitive impairment and postoperative mortality. Assessment of preoperative cognitive status using simple bedside tools such as the Folstein Mini-Mental Status Examination may be helpful both in establishing a baseline and uncovering occult dementia.[10,11]

PERIOPERATIVE STRATEGIES TO REDUCE RISK (TABLE 44-2)

MEDICATION MANAGEMENT

- Polypharmacy is a significant problem for older patients, who are often taking multiple medications with complex dosing regimens. Drug regimens may include not only physician-prescribed drugs but also over-the-counter (OTC) drugs and supplements. Adverse drug reactions are more common. Noncompliance and nonadherence to complex drug regimens may further complicate the picture.
- A key component of preoperative assessment is a careful and complete review of all medications, including supplements and OTC medications. The preoperative setting may provide an opportunity to simplify drug regimens, identify adverse drug reactions, and eliminate potentially harmful combinations of drugs. A review of perioperative medication management can be found in Chap. 7.

PROPHYLAXIS FOR DEEP VENOUS THROMBOSIS (DVT)

- Perioperative DVT prophylaxis is discussed in detail in Chap. 46; however, certain features are relevant to the elderly and place them at increased risk for DVT.
  - First, advanced age itself is a risk factor for venous thrombosis.
  - Second, the elderly have a higher prevalence of comorbidities, such as heart failure and malignancy, that also increase risk for DVT.
  - Third, because of the decline in functional capacity related to medical comorbidities, the elderly may be more likely than younger patients to experience prolonged immobility in the perioperative period, again raising the risk of venous thrombosis.
  - Last, the types of surgeries that many elderly undergo include various high-risk procedures with specific recommendations for DVT prophylaxis, such as hip fracture repair and the replacement of hip or knee joints.[12]

TABLE 44-2 Perioperative Risk-Reduction Strategies for the Elderly

Medications
Medication review: reduce/eliminate unnecessary/toxic medications or medications with anticholinergic/CNS depressant effects
DVT prophylaxis
Consider age >60 as posing increased DVT risk even when procedure is not high risk
Cardiovascular
Beta-blocker therapy in those with CAD or at high risk for CAD
Attention to fluid shifts and intake/output intra- and postoperatively
Thermoregulation
Attention to core temperature; adjustment of ambient temperature and use of warming blankets intraoperatively
Skin
Careful attention to positioning intra- and postoperatively
Use of cushioning intraoperatively and while patient is bed-bound
Early mobilization
Attention to incontinence issues
Attention to nutrition status
Bowel/bladder function
Avoidance of anticholinergic drugs
Prompt elimination of indwelling bladder catheters: intermittent catheterization when necessary
Surveillance for urinary tract infection
Surveillance for, and treatment of constipation
Use of bedside commode
Systematic toileting (timed voids)
Cognitive function
Attention to preoperative risk factors: preexisting dementia, functional status, alcohol use
Avoidance of CNS-depressant drugs
Careful attention to hemoglobin and intraoperative blood loss

CAD = coronary artery disease; CNS = central nervous system; DVT = deep venous thrombosis.

INTRAOPERATIVE CONSIDERATIONS

- No special techniques or approaches are required for the optimal intraoperative care of geriatric surgical patients other than diligent application of the fundamental principles of anesthetic management: an anesthetic plan appropriate for the procedure and the physical status of the patient combined with proper monitoring and attention to detail.

- ***Positioning:*** The high incidence of arthritis and osteoporosis among the elderly mandates careful attention to proper positioning. Failure in this regard increases the likelihood of injuries such as neuropraxias. The preoperative interview should include questions about limitations in range of motion and position-associated discomfort. Also, ischemic pressure sores are more likely to occur among older patients due to the age-related loss of skin elasticity and subcutaneous tissue. Thus, proper intraoperative padding is essential to minimize these.
- ***Fluid therapy:*** As noted previously, the elderly have a limited ability to compensate for changes in intravascular volume. Many geriatric surgical patients present to the operating room with some degree of intravascular volume depletion from fasting, diuretics, preoperative bowel preparation, or disease processes. Intraoperative sympathectomy from anesthetic agents, blood loss, and fluid sequestration in the "third space" exacerbates this hypovolemia. Therefore careful intraoperative fluid management is essential. The goal should be to restore intravascular volume to a level that maintains adequate cardiac output and blood pressure while avoiding fluid overload. There are no compelling data to support routine administration of colloid versus crystalloid in elderly surgical patients.
- ***Thermoregulation:*** Perioperative hypothermia is associated with an increased risk of infection, myocardial infarction, coagulopathy; it also prolongs the effect of anesthetic agents. Since older patients have diminished thermoregulatory capacity that is exacerbated by the vasodilatory and central nervous system effects of many anesthetics, diligent monitoring and correction of core temperature may have a marked influence on perioperative outcome. Modalities include forced-air warming blankets, the use of warmed fluids, and increasing the ambient operating room temperature.
- ***Regional versus general anesthesia:*** The question often arises as to whether an operation should be performed under regional (neuraxial/spinal or epidural) or general anesthesia. Many of the operations commonly performed in elderly patients are amenable to regional anesthetic techniques. Since most general anesthetic agents depress cardiopulmonary function, use of regional techniques has been advocated in this population. Numerous studies have examined perioperative outcomes with regard to regional versus general anesthesia, particularly in orthopedic surgical patients. Early studies demonstrated decreased mortality, higher postoperative $Pa{O_2}$, and fewer mental status changes following hip surgery conducted under regional anesthesia. Other studies in this population found a decreased incidence of DVT and blood loss. There is, however, no conclusive evidence that any one technique is superior, and the decision is best left to the anesthesiologist.

POSTOPERATIVE CONSIDERATIONS

- ***Cognitive impairment:*** The development of postoperative delirium can have a significant negative impact on surgical outcomes, affecting both functional recovery and mortality. Risk factors include advanced age, preexisting cognitive dysfunction, preoperative frailty, alcohol abuse, and substantial medical comorbidities. The identification of high-risk patients remains problematic. A complete review of postoperative delirium can be found in Chap. 62.
- ***Mobility:*** One of the most devastating problems faced by elderly patients, especially those who were frail preoperatively, is immobility. The consequences of immobility and bed rest can be staggering, yet the elderly are more likely than younger patients to be put at bed rest postoperatively. Some common reasons for prolonged bed rest postoperatively include dementia, musculoskeletal problems such as arthritis and muscle weakness, and the increased caregiver time and expense required to encourage mobility. Bed rest can have effects on multiple organ systems, including the skin, cardiovascular system, lungs, musculoskeletal system, and gastrointestinal and genitourinary tracts. Early effects of deconditioning can be seen after only 24 to 48 h of bed rest. Bed rest will increase the risk of postoperative pulmonary complications including atelectasis, pneumonia, and pulmonary embolism. Immobility is also associated with a decreased cardiac output due to decreased stroke volume. The ensuing orthostatic hypotension may make mobilization increasingly difficult and perpetuate a vicious cycle, which will be difficult to overcome.
- ***Continence:*** Postoperative development of urinary incontinence may increase the risk of an elderly patient entering a nursing home. Take aggressive measures to restore normal voiding as soon as possible after surgery. Remove indwelling catheters as soon as possible postoperatively. Manage urinary retention, detected by postvoid residual or bladder scan, with intermittent catheterization. Seek and eliminate, if possible, factors that contribute to urinary retention and incontinence. Some contributing factors include immobility, anticholinergic medications, increased fluid intake secondary to intravenous fluids, and urinary tract infection. Postoperative delirium may increase the risk of incontinence. Systematic toileting and prompt responses to requests will help maintain continence. A bedside commode for patients with limited mobility will enhance their ability to maintain continence. Constipation may

also contribute to urinary incontinence. Elderly patients often need an aggressive bowel-management strategy postoperatively.

- ***Pressure ulcers:*** Pressure ulcers are a significant cause of morbidity and mortality among postoperative patients. Elderly patients are at particular risk because of age-related changes in the skin. These changes include an increase in dermal collagen, a decrease in elastic fibers, flattening of the dermoepidermal junction, decreased epidermal turnover, and a decreased number of dermal blood vessels. In patients with hip fracture, there is an increased incidence of pressure ulcers, which in turn increases the mortality associated with hip fracture. Intraoperative cushioning of pressure points is critical even during short surgical procedures. Postoperative mobilization and ambulation will further decrease risk. Adequate cushioning while a patient is in bed is also important. Pressure ulcers will increase length of stay and may increase the risk of transfer to a long-term-care facility postoperatively.
- ***Malnutrition:*** Malnutrition is common in elderly patients. Limited income and transportation problems may impede access to healthy, nutritionally valuable food. Appetite may be diminished due to altered taste sensation, medications, or coexisting medical illness. Patients with dementia may have little interest in food. Little is known about requirements for vitamins and trace minerals in the elderly.
  - Malnutrition may be identified preoperatively by measuring serum albumin levels, which were found to be excellent predictors of 30-day postoperative mortality. Elderly patients with a marginal nutritional status preoperatively are at high risk for the development of protein-calorie malnutrition from the stress of surgery and illness. Increased demands lead to depletion of visceral protein stores. This, in turn, will lead to loss of muscle mass, altered gastrointestinal function, impaired immune responses, and impaired wound healing.
  - Begin prevention of malnutrition preoperatively and carefully watch nutritional status postoperatively. Begin vitamin and mineral supplementation early in the postoperative course. Monitor voluntary food intake and implement nutritional supplementation promptly in patients with inadequate intake. Studies looking at overnight nasogastric tube feedings have shown a benefit in patients at risk; however, nasogastric feeding may be poorly tolerated, and oral nutritional supplementation may be adequate. Early recognition and intervention are key. It is easier to try to maintain good nutrition than to "catch up" once the patient has fallen behind. Use the enteral route whenever possible. Parenteral nutrition should be reserved only for those patients with altered gastrointestinal tract function, as elderly patients are particularly vulnerable to the complications of parenteral feeding.

SUMMARY

Overall, surgery in the elderly patient can be undertaken with appropriate preoperative evaluation and perioperative management. While the elderly often carry a greater burden of disease than a younger population and changes in physiology pose unique challenges to the physician managing these patients, with care and attention to specific areas, the elderly may tolerate surgery without incident.

REFERENCES

1. Beliveau M, Multach M. Perioperative care for the elderly patient. *Med Clin North Am* 87:273–289, 2003.
2. Dharmarajan TS, Ugalino JT. The physiology of aging, in Dharmarajan TS, Norman RA (eds, *Clinical Geriatrics*. New York: Parthenon, 2003:9–22.
3. Taffet GE. Age-related physiologic changes, in Cobbs EL, Duthie EH, Murphy JB (eds), *Geriatrics Review Syllabus*, 4th ed. Dubuque, IA: Kendall/Hunt, 1999:10–23.
4. American College of Cardiology/American Heart Association. ACC/AHA guideline update for perioperative cardiovascular evaluation for noncardiac surgery. *J Am Coll Cardiol* 39: 542–553, 2002.
5. Goldman L, Caldera DL, Nussbaum SR, et al. Multifactorial index of cardiac risk in noncardiac surgical procedures. *N Engl J Med* 297:845–850, 1977.
6. Detsky AS, Abrams HB, McLaughlin JR, et al. Predicting cardiac complications in patients undergoing non-cardiac surgery. *J Gen Intern Med* 1:211–219, 1986.
7. American College of Physicians. Guidelines for assessing and managing the perioperative risk from coronary artery disease associated with major noncardiac surgery. *Ann Intern Med* 127:309–312, 1997.
8. Arozullah AM, Khuri SF, Henderson WG, et al. Development and validation of a multifactorial risk index for predicting postoperative pneumonia after major noncardiac surgery. *Ann Intern Med* 135:847–857, 2001.
9. Polanczyk CA, Marcantonio E, Goldman L, et al. Impact of age on perioperative complications and length of stay in patients undergoing noncardiac surgery. *Ann Intern Med* 134:637–643, 2001.
10. Bernstein GM, Offenbartl SK. Adverse surgical outcomes among patients with cognitive impairments. *Am Surg* 57: 682–690, 1991.
11. Marcantonio ER, Goldman L, Orav EJ, et al. The association of intraoperative factors with the development of postoperative delirium. *Am J Med* 105:380–384, 1998.
12. Geerts WH, Pineo GF, Heit JA, et al. Prevention of venous thromboembolism: The Seventh ACCP conference on antithrombotic and thrombolytic therapy. *Chest* 126: 338S–400S, 2004.

45 THE PREGNANT SURGICAL PATIENT

Michael P. Carson and David A. Halle

INTRODUCTION

FETAL/MATERNAL OUTCOMES AND SURGERY

- The incidence of nonobstetric surgery in pregnant patients is 0.2 to 1.0 percent.[1]
- The most common nonobstetric surgical procedure is appendectomy (1 per 2000 pregnancies), followed by cholecystectomy (1 to 6 per 10,000 pregnancies).[2]
- The perioperative risks of nonobstetric surgery in the mother are similar to those of nonpregnant surgical patients. However, surgery any time in pregnancy poses a potential risk to the fetus—including preterm labor, spontaneous abortion, or stillbirth—with the risk being highest in the first trimester.[1] Studies have not conclusively found any increase in the rate of congenital abnormalities after nonobstetric surgery.
    - It is important to balance the maternal risks of the procedure against the fetal risks, so that the benefits of maternal health throughout the remainder of the pregnancy may have a positive effect on the health of the fetus.

COMMON PHYSIOLOGIC CHANGES

- Physical findings during pregnancy may mimic disease states.
- Laboratory changes are summarized in Table 45-1.

CARDIOVASCULAR PHYSIOLOGY

- Systemic and pulmonary vascular resistance falls during pregnancy.
- Systolic blood pressure decreases by about 10 to 20 mmHg and diastolic blood pressure decreases by about 10 mmHg, reaching a nadir at about 20 weeks of gestation. Then, by late pregnancy, the blood pressure rises to prepregnancy levels.
- Heart rate (HR) increases 10 percent and plateaus at about 32 weeks of gestation. The HR measured in the seated position is higher than in the left lateral decubitus position.
- Plasma volume increases throughout pregnancy, peaking at 28 to 32 weeks, when undiagnosed cardiac disorders may be unmasked.

TABLE 45-1 Laboratory Changes in Pregnancy

PARAMETER	EFFECT
Albumin and total protein	Decrease by 1 mg/dL. Dilutional.
Alkaline phosphatase	Increases due to output by the placenta.
Bicarbonate (serum)	Decreases to about 20 meq. Decreased ability to buffer acid loads. Other electrolyte levels should be normal.
Blood urea nitrogen	Should be ≤14 mg/dL.
Creatinine	Should be ≤0.8 mg/dL. Mean is 0.5 mg/dL.
Creatinine clearance	Increases by 50% to about 150 mL/min.
Creatinine kinase—myocardial	May be elevated after cesarean section. The MB fraction makes up 6% of the total enzyme from the uterus and placenta.
D-Dimer	May be elevated in normal pregnancy. Negative value may be useful, as in the nonpregnant population.
Erythrocyte sedimentation rate	Elevated. No clinical utility during pregnancy.
Fibrinogen	Elevated.
Glomerular filtration rate	50% increase can shorten the half-life of medications.
Hemoglobin	Decreases to 10–12 g/dL. Red cell mass increases less than plasma volume, leading to a normal dilutional anemia of pregnancy.
Leukocyte count	Slight increase. Mean 8–10 and up to 14×10^9/L after delivery.
P_{CO_2}	Decreases to 28–32 mmHg.
pH	Mildly alkalotic. Tends to run 7.44.
Plasma oncotic pressure	Decreases. Women are more susceptible to noncardiogenic pulmonary edema in the setting of infection, preeclampsia, surgery, tocolysis with beta-adrenergic agonists, or volume overload.
Platelets	No change.
P_{O_2}	Increases slightly due to hyperventilation and "blowing off" of P_{CO_2}.
Thyroid labs (TSH, free T_4, free T_3)	No change. Free hormones may be elevated during the first trimester in 40% of women with hyperemesis gravidarum.
Transaminases and bilirubin	No change.
Urine protein; 24-h collection	Up to 300 mg is normal.

- The plasma volume increases to a greater extent than the red blood cell mass, resulting in a physiologic (dilutional) anemia of pregnancy. The lowest

hemoglobins (10 to 11 g/dL) are seen between 30 and 34 weeks of gestation.
- ◦ Cardiac output and stroke volume increase by 50 percent and peak at about 16 weeks' gestation.

Cardiovascular Examination

- ◦ The arterial pulses are characterized by a rapid rise and a quick collapse.
- ◦ The jugular venous A and V waves are more prominent; however, the jugular venous pressure (JVP) remains normal.
- ◦ The point of maximal impulse (PMI) will shift leftward and cephalad. Because of the increased blood volume, the right ventricle may be palpated during the first half of pregnancy.
- ◦ Some 96 percent of women will develop a grade I to II early systolic murmur over the pulmonary and tricuspid areas. This pulmonary murmur will become softer with inspiration. A nonsustained S_3 gallop may be heard, but a sustained S_3 or fourth heart sound warrants further evaluation. A continuous venous hum may be appreciated over the sternum and a holosystolic murmur (mammary souffle) may be appreciated over the medial aspects of both breasts in late pregnancy or lactation.
- ◦ Preexisting cardiac murmurs will increase in intensity throughout pregnancy due to the increase in blood volume. Diastolic murmurs are uncommon and should be further evaluated.
- ◦ About one-third of women will develop lower extremity edema during pregnancy as a normal variant. If the onset of the edema is sudden and/or it is increasing, consider evaluation for preeclampsia and/or venous thromboembolism.

Pulmonary Physiology

- ◦ Throughout pregnancy, the diaphragm rises due to displacement of the abdominal contents by the uterus, and there is an increase in the anteroposterior dimensions of the thorax.
- ◦ There is a progesterone-mediated increase in minute ventilation due to the dramatic increase in tidal volume (about 40 to 50 percent).
- ◦ An important "clinical pearl" is recognizing that an increased respiratory rate is not a normal finding in pregnancy and warrants further evaluation.
- ◦ A respiratory alkalosis is normal in a pregnant patient. (See Table 45-1 for changes in arterial blood gas values.)
- ◦ The forced expiratory volume in 1 s (FEV_1) does not change significantly.
- ◦ Functional residual capacity may decrease up to 70 percent when a pregnant woman is supine. This leads to a lower oxygen reserve prior to the induction of anesthesia; therefore supplemental oxygen should be administered.

Renal Physiology

- ◦ The glomerular filtration rate (GFR) increases by 150 percent over the nonpregnant level and contributes to more rapid clearance of some medications.
- ◦ Normal 24-h urine protein excretion is up to 300 mg, whereas only 150 mg is acceptable for nonpregnant women.

Hepatic Physiology

- ◦ Hepatic blood flow and the metabolism of medications are not significantly altered.

APPROACH TO PRESCRIBING

- Changes in renal and hepatic physiology were noted above.
- The increase in plasma volume leads to an increase in the volume of distribution. Protein binding of medications decreases during pregnancy, with little effect on the unbound (free) levels of the drug.
  - ◦ Phenobarbital is an exception, where the unbound levels will significantly decrease during the pregnant state. Follow serum levels closely.
- Several principles should guide the selection of medications during pregnancy (Table 45-2).
  - ◦ Medications that have been used for long periods of time and proven safe to the fetus should be used in preference to newer medications.
  - ◦ To minimize fetal exposure, one may try to dose medications at the lower end of the therapeutic range, but it is important to remember that the increased renal clearance and/or volume of distribution may necessitate higher doses or more frequent administration.
  - ◦ Fetal well-being is dependent on maternal well-being. Consider what might happen if the medication were *not* administered. Overly cautious restriction of medications in pregnancy can lead to a decline in maternal health, thereby putting the fetus at risk.
  - ◦ With a few exceptions, the *absolute* risk to the fetus of prescribing medications to a pregnant woman is mostly unknown, but the maternal benefits of most medications are clear.
  - ◦ The U.S. Food and Drug Administration (FDA) categorization system is oversimplified. Utilize a reference text such as Briggs et al.[3] or information on medication teratogenicity available at http://orpheus.ucsd.edu/ctis/ (Table 45-3).

PATIENT-RELATED RISK FACTORS

- The most common anesthesia-related risk is loss of the maternal airway in nonobstetric surgery.[4] This has been attributed to edema of the vocal cords and

TABLE 45-2 Preferred Medications for Common Medical Diseases

CONDITION	DRUGS OF CHOICE
Acne	Topical: erythromycin, clindamycin, benzoyl peroxide
Allergic rhinitis	Topical: steroids, cromolyn, decongestants, xylometazoline, naphazoline, phenylephrine Systemic: diphenhydramine, dimenhydrinate, tripelennamine, astemizole
Constipation	Docusate sodium, glycerin, sorbitol, lactulose, mineral oil, magnesium hydroxide
Cough	Diphenhydramine, codeine, dextromethorphan
Depression	Tricyclics, fluoxetine
Diabetes	Insulin
Headache	Acetaminophen, codeine, dimenhydrinate
Hypertension	Labetalol, methyldopa
Hyperthyroidism	Propylthiouracil, methimazole
Bipolar disorder	Lithium, chlorpromazine, haloperidol
Nausea	Diclectin
Peptic ulcer disease	Antacids, magnesium hydroxide, aluminum hydroxide, calcium carbonate, ranitidine
Pruritus	Topical: moisturizing creams, aluminum acetate, zinc oxide, calamine lotion, steroids Systemic: hydroxyzine, diphenhydramine, astemizole, steroids
Thrombosis	Heparin (unfractionated), streptokinase, low-molecular-weight heparin [not mentioned in the original article]

SOURCE: Modified from Koren,[11] with permission.

TABLE 45-3 Drugs with Proven Teratogenic Effects in Humans

DRUG	TERATOGENIC EFFECT
ACE inhibitors	Renal failure and hypotension in the newborn, renal tubular dysgenesis, decreased skull ossification, hypocalvaria.
Carbamazepine	Neural tube defects. May be considered if other medications ineffective.
Cocaine	Growth retardation, uterine rupture.
Ethanol	Fetal alcohol syndrome: prenatal and postnatal growth deficiency, CNS anomalies, facial defects (short palebral fissures, hypoplastic philtrum, flattened maxilla), major organ-system malformations.
Isotretinoin	Retinoid embryopathy, CNS abnormalities, craniofacial defects, cardiovascular defects, thymic defects, decreased muscle tone, limb reduction, behavioral abnormalities.
Lithium	Ebstein's anomaly and other heart defects.
Phenytoin	Fetal hydantoin syndrome: prenatal and postnatal growth deficiency, motor or mental deficiency, short nose with broad nasal bridge, microcephaly, hypertelorism, strabismus, epicanthus, wide fontanelles, abnormally formed ears, positional deformities of limbs, hypoplasia of distal phalanges, hypospadias, hernia, webbed neck, low hairline, impaired neurodevelopment and low intelligence.
Thalidomide	Limb-shortening defects, loss of hearing, abducens paralysis, facial paralysis, anotia, microtia, renal malformations, congenital heart disease.
Valproic acid	Neural tube defects. May be considered if other medications ineffective for the disorder.
Warfarin	Fetal warfarin syndrome: skeletal defects, limb hypoplasia, low birth weight, hearing loss, ophthalmic abnormalities.

ACE = angiotensin-converting enzyme; CNS = central nervous system.

hypopharynx, leading to failed intubation and bleeding into the airways.

- Normal physiologic changes in pregnancy may increase the risk of certain perioperative complications:
  - Hypoxia: Due to decreased FRC when supine
  - Venous thromboembolism (VTE): Due to reduced venous flow and increased clotting factors
  - Aspiration: Due to decreased gastric motility (during labor) and reduced competence of the gastroesophageal sphincter
  - Urinary tract infection (UTI): Especially with catheterization, due to dilatation of the urinary collecting system
- Disease presentations may differ from the nonpregnant patient.
- Chronic stable disease may be exacerbated, improved, or unchanged in pregnancy. This pattern holds true for asthma in particular.
- Disease management and prescribing may need to be adjusted, even if a disease state was stable before pregnancy.

SURGERY-RELATED RISK FACTORS

SURGICAL TECHNIQUE: LAPAROSCOPY VERSUS LAPAROTOMY

- A laparoscopic approach is preferred so as to decrease both maternal (decreased blood loss, less analgesic use) and fetal risks (preterm labor) when compared to open laparotomy.[1]
- Some studies have found both surgical approaches to be associated with intrauterine growth restriction as well as preterm labor and delivery, but the cause of these outcomes is not always clear.

- Limit the intraabdominal insufflation pressure to 12 to 15 mmHg during the laparoscopic procedure in order to minimize a further decrease of the pulmonary functional residual capacity and cardiac preload.[5]

TIMING OF SURGERY

- The ideal time for semielective surgery, when possible, is the second trimester. First-trimester anesthesia has been associated with neural tube defects and hydrocephalus.[6,7] Third-trimester intraabdominal surgical procedures are more technically difficult due to the enlarged uterus and are associated with preterm labor.
- Avoid arbitrarily delaying nonobstetric surgery when possible. This is particularly true for symptomatic gallbladder disease, where delays contribute to maternal morbidity, including multiple return visits to the hospital, increased operative times, longer hospitalizations, and higher conversion to open cholecystectomy.

TYPE OF ANESTHESIA

- Consider regional anesthesia when possible, so as to avoid the morbidity associated with intubation and airway management in the pregnant surgical patient.

PREOPERATIVE EVALUATION AND TESTING TO STRATIFY RISK

CARDIAC TESTING

- The approach should be the same as in nonpregnant patients. Stress echocardiography is preferred for the evaluation of known ischemic heart disease that is not optimized or when ischemic heart disease is suspected.
- Perform nuclear stress testing and cardiac catheterization if stress echocardiography is not available (Table 45-4).
- Consider resting transthoracic echocardiography if the patient has a systolic murmur of grade III or higher, a diastolic murmur, or a sustained S_3 or S_4 (although an S_3 has been reported as normal in pregnant patients).

PULMONARY TESTING

- As in the approach in nonpregnant patients, consider pulmonary function tests if the patient has asthma with wheezing or increased symptoms despite appropriate medicines.

OTHER ORGAN SYSTEMS

- Test to see whether there are known or suspected abnormalities.

TABLE 45-4 Fetal Radiation Exposure of Various Radiologic Studies*

STUDY	FETAL EXPOSURE	PERMISSIBLE IN PREGNANCY	SOURCE
Single chest x-ray with abdominal shielding	0.001 rads	Up to 5000	[3513577]**
V/Q scan	0.02–0.05 rads	100	[3884214]**
ERCP	0.310 rad		[12591046]**
Head CT	≤0.013		
Helical chest CT, first trimester	0.002		[12147847]**
Helical chest CT, third trimester	0.013		[12147847]**
Arteriogram (pulmonary/coronary) via femoral vessels	0.2–0.4		Rosene-Montella et al.[12]
Arteriogram (pulmonary/coronary) via brachial vessels	0.05		Rosene-Montella et al.[12]
MRI	Apparently no adverse effect on the fetus		[8475280] [7489290]**

CT = computed tomography; ERCP = endoscopic retrograde cholangiopancreatography; MRI = magnetic resonance imaging; V/Q = ventilation/perfusion.

*Listed next to each test is the estimated fetal radiation dose out of the 5.0 rads (5000 mrad) of fetal exposure permissible during pregnancy. The third column lists the number of tests "permissible." We developed this information in order to allow patients to grasp the low relative risk of the various studies.

**PubMed 10.

- Inquire about a personal or family history of bleeding and anesthesia-related complications.

USE OF LOW-DOSE ASPIRIN

- Women with a past history of multiple pregnancy losses may be prescribed low-dose aspirin to decrease the risk of a recurrent loss.
- The CLASP trial randomized 9364 pregnant women to 81 mg of aspirin or placebo. Aspirin was not associated with an increase in bleeding during preparation for epidural anesthesia, but there was a slight increase in the use of blood transfusion after delivery.[8]

DIAGNOSTIC IMAGING

- Fetal radiation exposure in various radiologic studies is listed in Table 45-4.
- Obtain chest radiographs, ventilation/perfusion lung scans, magnetic resonance imaging studies, fluoroscopic procedures, and other tests as you would in a nonpregnant patient if the test result will clearly affect the treatment plan and benefit the patient.
- Most common radiographic investigations confer much less than the acceptable limit of 5.0 rads (5000 mrad) of fetal radiation exposure cumulatively over the course of the pregnancy.
- Exposures less that 2.0 rads do not carry any risk of fetal demise, nor do they increase the risk that the child exposed in utero will develop cancer later in life.
- Clinical diagnosis without appropriate radiologic confirmation may lead to inappropriate treatment. Therefore it is important to educate patients about the safety of radiographic studies and the importance of obtaining clinical information in making treatment decisions.
- Ventilation/perfusion scans do not increase the rate of congenital or developmental abnormalities.
- The intravenous iodinated contrast agents iobitridol and iohexol did not cross the placenta of pregnant rabbits in doses similar to those used for human angiography.

PERIOPERATIVE MANAGEMENT TO REDUCE RISK

COLLABORATION

- Enlist the aid of clinicians familiar with the specifics regarding medication and testing during pregnancy. Specialties include obstetric medicine, perinatology, and surgery.
- Obstetric anesthesiologists will be familiar with the physiologic changes, alterations in sensitivity to anesthetic agents, and high risk of airway complications.
- Perinatologists or the patient's general obstetrician will decide on the most appropriate way to monitor the fetus intra- and postoperatively.
- If possible, consider delaying surgery for medical diseases that are not optimized.

PREOPERATIVE

- Preoperatively, evaluate the pregnant patient in a similar fashion to a nonpregnant patient.
- Consider perioperative beta-adrenergic blockade as you would for a nonpregnant patient with appropriate cardiac risk factors. Beta blockers have yet to be studied in pregnant patients undergoing nonobstetric surgery (Chap. 20).

INTRAOPERATIVE

- To minimize hypotension, position the patient in the left lateral decubitus position, using a wedge under the right hip. Aortocaval compression by the uterus can affect venous return, cardiac output, and uteroplacental perfusion as early as 20 weeks. Similar compression of the vessels can occur if the mother is placed in a "fetal" position prior to a lumbar puncture or placement of an epidural catheter.
- When the fetal age is less than 24 weeks' gestation, fetal heart rate (FHR) monitoring is less reliable at assessing fetal well-being. Understand that FHR monitoring was designed for use during labor and can detect only severe alterations in fetal perfusion. While FHR changes suggestive of fetal stress can give the clinician an additional assessment of uterine perfusion, these changes are not likely to occur without other obvious signs of maternal distress, such as prolonged hypotension or hypoxia.
- Avoid overresponding to contractions. Tocolytic medications such as beta-adrenergic agonists are associated with maternal complications such as pulmonary edema, tachycardia, atrial fibrillation, chest pain, and electrocardiographic changes.
- Consider end-tidal CO_2 monitoring of the mother. Normal maternal $Paco_2$ is 28 to 32 mmHg. Animal studies are conflicting regarding whether or not intraperitoneal CO_2 insufflation can increase maternal Pco_2. Maternal hypo- or hypercarbia can lead to uterine artery contraction. Transcutaneous and end-tidal carbon dioxide monitoring correlates well with maternal $Paco_2$. Capnography can be used to adjust

ventilation and to help in the detection of accidental intravascular CO_2 insufflation and its related complications, such as pneumothorax and hemorrhage.[9]

- In critically ill patients, do not risk maternal well-being by withholding a medication that poses a theoretical risk to the fetus. If needed, ephedrine causes less uterine artery spasm than other pressor agents and is the vasopressor of choice, with phenylephrine as the second-line agent.[10] One should not equate a potential for uterine artery vasoconstriction with complete loss of blood flow to the uterus.

POSTOPERATIVE

- Minimize atelectasis by encouraging deep breathing, incentive spirometry, or early ambulation (walking).
- Prevent the gravid uterus from compressing the vena cava by keeping the patient in the left lateral decubitus position until she is ambulatory.

Continue fetal monitoring if there is maternal hemodynamic instability.

PROPHYLAXIS FOR DEEP VENOUS THROMBOSIS

- Administer DVT prophylaxis. Unfractionated heparin (UFH) and the low-molecular-weight heparins (LMWHs) do not cross the placenta. In spite of a lack of prospective trials, pregnancy is a hypercoagulable state, and it is reasonable to generalize data from the nonpregnant population.
- The dose of UFH shown to decrease the risk of perioperative DVT in nonpregnant patients is 5000 U given subcutaneously three times a day, not two. There are no prospective data in pregnancy to support one dose over another, but due to the increased rate of heparin clearance, some practitioners will use 7500 U twice daily in the second trimester and 10,000 U twice daily in the third trimester. Enoxaparin 40 mg daily or twice daily may be used.
- Nonpharmacologic methods can be used, such as compression stockings, pneumatic compression boots, early ambulation, and maintaining the patient's volume status, as dehydration can lead to venous stasis.
- In evaluating postoperative hypertension, pain should be the first item on the differential.

PREECLAMPSIA

- While this chapter focuses on the healthy pregnant patient, an internist may be called in to manage postoperative hypertension in a patient who has undergone a cesarean section. One should be able to differentiate postoperative hypertension from preeclampsia.
  - The classic syndrome involves new systolic blood pressure >140 or a diastolic blood pressure >90, proteinuria >300 mg per 24-h collection, *or* new proteinuria > "+1" on a urine dip.
  - In the history, ask about a new headache, visual changes, right-upper-quadrant pain, or new-onset edema of the hands or face.
  - Physical findings include retinal vasospasm, a sustained S_3 or S_4 gallop, pulmonary edema, tender liver, severe edema, and clonus.
  - Laboratory abnormalities may include elevated transaminases, thrombocytopenia, proteinuria, hemolysis, or elevated hemoglobin and serum creatinine (>0.8 mg/dL) from hemoconcentration.
  - These patients may have intravascular volume depletion from capillary leak.

PREFERRED MEDICATIONS

- Labetalol: Orally 200 mg two or three times daily to a maximum of 2400 mg/day, or intravenously for blood pressure >170/110 mmHg (not related to pain) 20-mg IV bolus; subsequent doses of 40 mg followed by 80 mg IV may be administered at 10- to 20-min intervals, or it may be infused at 1 mg/kg/h.
- Methyldopa (Aldomet): Widely considered the first-line agent for the treatment of hypertension during pregnancy, with no adverse effects on cognitive development among children with exposure in utero; limited to oral dosing: 250 mg two or three times daily, increasing every second day as needed but not to exceed 3 g/day.

OTHER MEDICATIONS

- Beta blockers: Metoprolol is preferred, because atenolol was associated with mild intrauterine growth restriction when used in randomized trials focusing on the treatment of chronic hypertension during pregnancy.
- Nifedipine: Appears safe in pregnancy. It is occasionally used to treat preterm contractions.
  - Suspect pulmonary embolism if the patient is newly dyspneic (Table 45-4).
  - Monitor for noncardiogenic pulmonary edema if tocolytics were administered.
    - The chest x-ray may show bilateral pulmonary infiltrates.
    - Pulmonary edema in this setting is due to the low oncotic pressure of normal pregnancy and increased capillary permeability from the medication, not to increased hydrostatic pressure from left heart failure. Therefore "cephalization" of pulmonary veins may be absent.

SUMMARY

If the physicians are aware of the anatomic and physiologic changes that occur during gestation, surgery in the pregnant patient can be performed safely, with morbidity and mortality approaching that in a nonpregnant woman. A team approach including physicians experienced in treating pregnant patients is recommended.

REFERENCES

1. Reedy MB, Kallen B, Kuehl TJ. Laparoscopy during pregnancy: A study of five fetal outcome parameters with use of the Swedish Health Registry. *Am J Obstet Gynecol* 177(3): 673–679, 1997.
2. Mazze RI, Källén B. Appendectomy during pregnancy: A Swedish registry study of 778 cases. *Obstet Gynecol* 77(6): 835–840, 1991.
3. Briggs GG, Freeman RK, Yaffe SJ, eds. *Drugs in Pregnancy and Lactation: A Reference Guide to Fetal and Neonatal Risk,* 6th ed. Baltimore: Lippincott, Williams & Wilkins, 2001.
4. Hawkins JL, Koonin LM, Palmer SK, Gibbs CP. Anesthesia-related deaths during obstetric delivery in the United States, 1979—1990. *Anesthesiology* 86(2):277–284, 1997.
5. Carson MP, Gibson PS. Perioperative management of the pregnant patient. PIER: Physicians Information and Education Resource. www.pier.acponline.org
6. Kort B, Katz VL, Watson WJ. The effect of nonobstetric operation during pregnancy. *Surg Gynecol Obstet* 177(4):371–376, 1993.
7. Kallen B, Mazze RI. Neural tube defects and first trimester operations. *Teratology* 41(6):717–720, 1990.
8. CLASP: A randomised trial of low-dose aspirin for the prevention and treatment of pre-eclampsia among 9364 pregnant women. CLASP (Collaborative Low-Dose Aspirin Study in Pregnancy) Collaborative Group. *Lancet* 343(8898):619–629, 1994.
9. Bhavani-Shankar K, Steinbrook RA, Brooks DC, Datta S. Arterial to end-tidal carbon dioxide pressure difference during laparoscopic surgery in pregnancy. *Anesthesiology* 93(2): 370–373, 2000.
10. Tong C, Eisenach JC. The vascular mechanism of ephedrine's beneficial effect on uterine perfusion during pregnancy. *Anesthesiology* 76(5):792–798, 1992.
11. Koren G, Pastuszak A, Ito S. Drug therapy: Drugs in pregnancy. *N Engl J Med* 338(16):1128–1137, 1998.
12. Rosene-Montella K, Larson L. Diagnostic imaging, in Lee RV (ed), *Medical Care of the Pregnant Patient*. Philadelphia: American College of Physicians, 2000:103–115.

Section IV
GENERAL PROPHYLACTIC MEASURES

Gerald W. Smetana, MD, Section Editor

46 VENOUS THROMBOEMBOLISM PROPHYLAXIS

Amir K. Jaffer, Scott Kaatz, and Peter Kaboli

INTRODUCTION

- Venous thromboembolism (VTE) is a common complication after surgery. Approximately 2 million cases of deep venous thrombosis (DVT) and approximately 200,000 deaths due to pulmonary embolism (PE) occur every year in the United States. It is estimated that about half of these cases of DVT are attributable to hospitalized patients, of which half are surgical and the other half medical.[1]
- The prevalence of postoperative VTE varies based on the patient's risk factors for VTE (Table 46-1), the type of surgery (Table 46-2), and finally the type and amount of prophylaxis.
- Postoperative VTE is often silent. This is suggested by multiple clinical trials that have used routine venography to study the prevalence of postoperative DVT in the absence of prophylaxis (see Table 46-2).
- Most symptomatic postoperative DVTs occur after hospital discharge. Reliance on signs and symptoms of early DVT is not useful, as the first manifestation of VTE may be a fatal PE. In addition, routine screening for postoperative DVT is unreliable and expensive; it is therefore not recommended.
- Therefore the best strategy to prevent both postoperative VTE and its chronic sequelae, such as postphlebitic syndrome and chronic pulmonary hypertension, is universal VTE prophylaxis for almost all surgical patients.
- One of the most important considerations in perioperative VTE prophylaxis is to develop a close working relationship with surgeons, anesthesiologists, nurses, and medical consultants.
- Evidence-based guidelines support several methods of prophylaxis in a variety of surgical settings; therefore one should respect individual practice preferences to avoid unwanted complications or conflicts in management.

PATIENT-RELATED RISK FACTORS

- Virchow's triad describes three underlying etiologic factors for venous thrombosis: stasis of blood flow, endothelial injury, and hypercoagulability. Important patient-related risk factors for VTE reflect these underlying pathophysiologic processes and include increasing age, prolonged immobility, malignancy, prior VTE, chronic heart failure, and other factors (see Table 46-1). However, the magnitude of risk conferred by these and other risk factors varies, as this table outlines.
- It is not known exactly how these factors interact to determine a patient's individual VTE risk, but fair evidence suggests that VTE risk increases in proportion to the number of predisposing factors.

SURGERY-RELATED RISK FACTORS

- Surgery is a state where all three elements of Virchow's triad are present. The supine position coupled with anesthesia leads to stasis. The surgery itself may lead to endothelial injury, and the extent of injury ultimately depends on the type of surgery. For example, trauma to blood vessels occurs more frequently with major joint replacement, such as total knee and total hip arthroplasty.

TABLE 46-1 Patient-Related Risk Factors for VTE

Strong risk factors (odds ratio >10)
Spinal cord injury
Moderate risk factors (odds ratio 2–9)
Central venous lines
Chemotherapy
Congestive heart failure
Respiratory failure
Hormone replacement therapy
Malignancy
Oral contraceptive therapy
Paralytic stroke
Pregnancy (postpartum state)
Previous venous thromboembolism
Thrombophilia
Weak risk factors (odds ratio <2)
Bed rest >3 days
Immobility due to sitting (e.g., prolonged car or air travel)
Increasing age
Obesity
Pregnancy (antepartum state)
Varicose veins

SOURCE: Modified from Anderson and Spencer,[9] with permission.

- Anesthesia also leads to the pooling of blood in the extremities; the subsequent decreased clearing of clotting factors leads to a hypercoagulable state (the final component of Virchow's triad).
- The risk conferred by the surgery itself may sometimes be so high that additional risk conferred by patient-related factors may not necessarily elevate the patient's risk sufficiently to require a change in planned prophylaxis. For example, patients undergoing major hip replacement are at one of the highest levels of risk regardless of advanced age or other risk factors, and this risk continues past hospital discharge.
- Table 46-2 lists the various types of surgeries, the associated odds ratio, and the prevalence of DVT in these patient groups in the absence of prophylaxis.

TABLE 46-2 Surgery-Related Risk Factors for VTE

	VENOGRAPHIC PREVALENCE OF DVT (%)
Strong risk factors (odds ratio >10)	
Fracture (hip or leg)	40–60%
Hip or knee replacement	40–60%
Major general surgery	20–40%
Major trauma	40–80%
Moderate risk factors (odds ratio 2–9)	
Arthroscopic knee surgery	10–20%
Weak risk factors (odds ratio <2)	
Laparoscopic surgery (e.g., cholecystectomy)	0–10%

PREOPERATIVE EVALUATION AND RISK STRATIFICATION

- During the routine preoperative evaluation, estimate VTE risk by carefully considering both patient- and surgery-specific factors. Both of these types of factors contribute to risk; the interaction between the two can increase the overall VTE risk.
- In addition, the various modalities for prophylaxis, both pharmacologic and nonpharmacologic, carry risk (e.g., bleeding, thrombocytopenia) and may be uncomfortable for patients (e.g., needle sticks, stockings, pneumatic devices).
- Use a standardized risk-factor assessment (RFA) at the time of preoperative evaluation and/or admission. Initiate appropriate VTE prophylaxis that incorporates patient- and procedure-related risk factors as well as patient and provider preferences. Standardized risk-assessment tools exist, but these tools have not been rigorously validated. One such RFA incorporates a scoring system with levels of thrombosis risk and makes specific evidence-based recommendations for prophylaxis based on the guidelines of the American College of Chest Physicians (ACCP).[2]
- The RFA identifies the well-established patient-related risks and risks associated with clinical situations. The authors established relative weights for these risks based on epidemiologic and clinical trial data, but no prospectively validated data exist. For example, the use of oral contraceptives receives a score of 1, age over 60 a score of 2, and the presence of antiphospholipid antibodies a score of 3.
- The most recent (i.e., seventh ACCP) guidelines stratify patients' risk based on the procedure (i.e., the surgical risk based on proximal DVT and PE rates among patients who do not receive prophylaxis) and also patient-specific risk factors.[3] The classification proposes four risk categories. Table 46-3 outlines the recommended VTE strategies for each of these:
  - ***Low Risk:*** Minor surgery in patients <40 years with no additional risk factors such as those outlined in Table 46-1 (rate of proximal DVT 0.4 percent, all PE 0.2 percent).
  - ***Moderate Risk:*** Minor surgery in patients with additional risk factors (see Table 46-1) or in patients 40 to 60 years of age with no additional risk factors (rate of proximal DVT 1 to 4 percent, all PE 1 to 2 percent).
  - ***High Risk:*** Surgery in patients >60 years, or 40 to 60 years of age with additional risk factors (see Table 46-1) (rate of proximal DVT 4 to 8 percent, all PE 2–4 percent).
  - ***Highest Risk:*** Surgery in patients with multiple risk factors (see Table 46-1), hip or knee arthroplasty, hip fracture surgery, major trauma, and spinal cord

TABLE 46-3 VTE Recommendations According to Type of Surgery and Patient-Related Risk Factors

LEVEL OF RISK*	EVIDENCE-BASED OPTIONS FOR VTE PROPHYLAXIS
Low	Early ambulation
Moderate	LDUH q 12 h or LMWH† daily or GCS or IPCs
High	LDUH q 8 h or LMWH† or IPC
Highest	LMWH or fondaparinux or warfarin or (IPC/GCS + LDUH q 8 h or LMWH†)

GCS = graded compression stockings; IPCs = intermittent pneumatic compression devices; LDUH = low-dose unfractionated heparin; LMWH = low-molecular weight heparin.
*See text ("Preoperative Evaluation and Risk Stratification") for definitions for low, moderate, high, and highest risk.
†Recommended LMWHs/dosing: Enoxaparin 40 mg SQ qd or dalteparin 5000 IU SQ qd.
For total knee procedures, consider enoxaparin 30 mg SQ q 12 h or fondaparinux 2.5 mg SQ qd.

injury (rate of proximal DVT 10 to 20 percent, all PE 4–10 percent).

- Some patient-specific risk factors confer more risk than others (see Table 46-1), but all risk factors are additive to varying degrees.
- If VTE prophylaxis is warranted, consider the risks associated with the recommended evidence-based modality.
  - Patients with a known history of immune-mediated heparin-induced thrombocytopenia (HIT) should not receive unfractionated heparin (UFH) or low-molecular-weight heparin (LMWH). If heparin is absolutely necessary, as in the case of open heart surgery, it should not be used postoperatively. In this case, consider alternatives such as direct thrombin inhibitors or off-pump surgery.
  - Another option for patients with a history of HIT is fondaparinux, which does not cross-react with heparin or cause HIT.
  - In consultation with surgical colleagues, consider the inherent surgery-specific bleeding risk and defer initiation of pharmacologic anticoagulation unless the benefit of VTE prophylaxis outweighs the bleeding risk. Specific high-risk groups for bleeding include neurosurgical patients and those with multiple trauma. In such patients, initiate VTE prophylaxis with nonpharmacologic methods (e.g., compression stockings, intermittent pneumatic compression devices) initially and add pharmacologic methods once the bleeding risk has been minimized.
  - Graded compression stockings have been shown to reduce the risk of DVT in many surgical settings, but they can increase the risk of DVT if they are not fitted properly.[4] Do not use stockings for VTE prophylaxis in patients with very large legs or for those in whom stockings cannot be fitted properly.
  - Finally, consider patient preference in situations where both pharmacologic and nonpharmacologic methods are safe and effective. Specifically, some patients do not like subcutaneous injections. In this case, daily use of a LMWH may be preferable to thrice-daily injections of UFH. Intermittent pneumatic compression (IPC) devices may be another option. Alternatively, some patients find IPC devices and compression stockings uncomfortable and may therefore limit their ambulation. Most of the time, these devices are not used properly in the hospital.

PERIOPERATIVE MANAGEMENT

PHARMACOLOGIC OPTIONS

- Aspirin is not very effective for prophylaxis against VTE, and the ACCP guidelines recommend *against* its use in any surgical group as a single prophylactic agent.
- UFH is inexpensive but has a shorter half-life than LMWH and therefore requires twice- or thrice-daily dosing for maximal benefit. The anticoagulant effect can, however, be easily reversed with protamine if necessary. However, UFH does carry a significant risk of heparin-induced thrombocytopenia (HIT). This number may be as high as 5 percent in orthopedic patients.
- Warfarin has the advantage of oral administration and is relatively inexpensive. However, it requires monitoring with an international normalized ratio (INR), has multiple drug and food interactions, and has a narrow therapeutic range. In addition, its onset of action takes several days and patients may be at increased risk for VTE while the INR is subtherapeutic. It is reasonable to use LMWH and/or IPC devices until the INR becomes therapeutic. Therefore we do not recommend primary prophylaxis with warfarin alone for the first few days postoperatively in orthopedic patients. Pooled analyses of randomized clinical trials that have compared LMWH to warfarin show less VTE but a trend toward increased bleeding with LMWH.
- LMWHs are well absorbed from subcutaneous tissue, have a rapid onset of action, can be dosed once or twice daily, and cause less HIT compared to UFH. Although these agents are more expensive, studies that have included costs due to complications suggest that they are more cost-effective than warfarin. LMWHs are cleared by the kidneys. In the case of enoxaparin, the recommendation for renal insufficiency is to decrease the prophylactic dose from 40 to 30 mg SC once daily.

- Fondaparinux is a synthetic pentasaccharide that inhibits factor X and has a long half-life, so the drug truly can be dosed once daily subcutaneously. It has a rapid onset of action, but the anticoagulant effect cannot be adequately and routinely reversed. Studies in healthy volunteers have used activated factor VII (Novo-seven) to reverse the anticoagulant effect of fondaparinux, but no studies exist for patients who are actively bleeding. These results suggest that activated factor VII may be useful to reverse the anticoagulant effect of fondaparinux in case of serious bleeding complications or need for acute surgery during treatment with fondaparinux. The drug is cleared renally and therefore contraindicated in patients with a creatinine clearance <30 mL/min. It may be more effective in preventing VTE compared to LMWHs after major joint replacement, but only if dosed within 6 to 8 h of surgery. This practice may, however, cause more bleeding. When initiated on postoperative day 1, as is the practice in the United States, fondaparinux and LMWHs are probably equal in efficacy.[5]

NONPHARMACOLOGIC OPTIONS

- Recommend early ambulation for all patients.
- Elastic stocking are effective alone and in combination with pharmacologic measures and are a strategy for lower-risk surgeries or as an adjunct in selected cases.[6]
- Clinical trials of pneumatic compression stockings confirm efficacy, but in practice patients may not wear them for the required 15 h daily to achieve the benefit suggested by these trials.[3]

NEURAXIAL BLOCKADE (SPINAL AND EPIDURAL) ANESTHESIA

- Spinal hematoma may complicate spinal or epidural anesthesia in patients receiving pharmacologic VTE prophylaxis if special precautions are not exercised. Detailed guidelines are available at www.asra.com. Some important recommendations include the following:
  - Delay the initiation of UFH for 1 h after needle placement and removal of epidural catheters until 2 to 4 hours after the last prophylactic dose.
  - LMWHs carry a boxed warning from the U.S. Food and Drug Administration (FDA) regarding the risk of spinal hematoma. Therefore exercise extreme caution when patients have received neuraxial blockade perioperatively and the use of LMWHs for VTE prophylaxis is planned.
  - Wait 24 h prior to insertion of a spinal needle or epidural catheter if patients received full-dose LMWH prior to surgery (e.g., patients receiving bridging therapy when off warfarin).
  - Wait 10 to 12 h after a prophylactic dose of LMWH to insert a spinal needle or epidural catheter.
  - Avoid concomitant dosing of LMWH in the presence of an epidural catheter.
  - Wait a minimum of 2 h after catheter removal prior to dosing LMWH.
- Withhold warfarin for 4 to 5 days prior to catheter insertion. Remove the catheter only after ensuring that the INR is <1.5.
- Few data are available regarding the optimal management of neuraxial anesthesia for patients who receive fondaparinux for VTE prophylaxis. The American Society of Regional Anesthesia and Pain Medicine currently makes no recommendation on how to manage catheters with this anticoagulant. Therefore it is best to avoid using fondaparinux in the setting of an epidural catheter and to wait at least a couple hours after an epidural catheter has been removed to start fondaparinux.

POSTDISCHARGE OR EXTENDED PROPHYLAXIS

- Certain patient-related risks and surgeries confer a high risk for VTE even after discharge from the hospital. Patients that benefit from extended prophylaxis include:
  - Abdominal and pelvic cancer surgery patients for up to 28 days after surgery.[3,5] A proven agent for this indication is the LMWH enoxaparin, with 40 mg being given subcutaneously once daily.
  - Patients who have undergone total hip replacement and hip fracture repair, who may receive prophylaxis for anywhere from 28 to 35 days postoperatively.[3,7]
- The timing of VTE complications in orthopedic patients is different between hip and knee surgery, with most such events occurring out-of-hospital with hip surgery and in-hospital with knee surgery.[8]
- In hip replacement and hip fracture patients, options for extended prophylaxis include LMWHs, fondaparinux, and warfarin.[3,7]

FINAL EVIDENCE-BASED RECOMMENDATIONS FOR VTE PROPHYLAXIS

- The American College of Chest Physicians 7th Conference on Antithrombotic and Thrombolytic Therapy provides comprehensive recommendations based on surgical level of risk for VTE (see Table 46-3)

TABLE 46-4 Recommendations for VTE Prevention for Patients According to Type of Surgery

TYPE OF SURGERY	TYPE OF PROPHYLAXIS*	DURATION
Low-risk general surgery	Early mobilization	Until ambulation or discharge.
Moderate-risk general surgery	UFH 5000 U SC bid or LMWH	Until ambulation or discharge.
High-risk general surgery	UFH 5000 U SC tid or LMWH plus IPC or GCS	Until ambulation or discharge; but up to 28 days in major abdominal or pelvic cancer surgery is preferred.
Vascular surgery	UFH 5000 U SC bid or tid or LMWH	Until ambulation or discharge.
Laparoscopic gynecologic surgery >30 min	UFH 5000 U SC tid or LMWH plus IPC or GCS	Until ambulation or discharge.
Major gynecologic surgery	UFH 5000 U SC tid or LMWH plus IPC or GCS	Until ambulation or discharge.
Urologic surgery other than low-risk	UFH 5000 U SC tid or LMWH plus IPC or GCS	Until ambulation or discharge.
Major joint replacement (e.g., total knee or hip replacement)	LMWH or VKA or fondaparinux†	At least 10 days and up to 28–35 days for THR is preferred.
Hip fracture surgery	Fondaparinux† or LMWH or VKA	At least 10 days and up to 28 days is preferred.
Neurosurgery		Until ambulation or discharge.
Extracranial	IPC ± GCS	
Intracranial	IPC ± GCS (LMWH or UFH can be added if risk of bleeding acceptable)	

GCS = graded compression stockings; IPC = intermittent pneumatic compression; LMWH = low-molecular-weight heparin; THR = total hip replacement; UFH = unfractionated heparin; VKA = vitamin-K antagonists (warfarin).
*LMWH dosing = enoxaparin 40 mg SC qd, dalteparin 5000 IU SC qd, or tinzaparin 75 IU/kg qd.
†Recommended dose of fondaparinux = 2.5 mg SC qd.
SOURCE: Adapted from Geerts et al.,[3] with permission.

and type of surgery[3] (Table 46-4). We strongly recommend that the medical consultant use one or a combination of these approaches to determine the optimal type and duration of VTE prophylaxis.

REFERENCES

1. Goldhaber SZ, Tapson VF, Committee DFS. A prospective registry of 5,451 patients with ultrasound-confirmed deep vein thrombosis. *Am J Cardiol* 93(2):259–262, 2004.
2. Motykie GD, Zebala LP, Caprini JA, et al. A guide to venous thromboembolism risk factor assessment. *J Thromb Thrombol* 9(3):253–262, 2000.
3. Geerts WH, Pineo GF, Heit JA, et al. Prevention of venous thromboembolism: The Seventh ACCP conference on antithrombotic and thrombolytic therapy. *Chest* 126(3 suppl): 338S–400S, 2004.
4. Best AJ, Williams S, Crozier A, et al. Graded compression stockings in elective orthopaedic surgery. An assessment of the in vivo performance of commercially available stockings in patients having hip and knee arthroplasty. *J Bone Joint Surg Br* 82(1):116–118, 2000.
5. Turpie AG, Eriksson BI, Lassen MR, Bauer KA. A meta-analysis of fondaparinux versus enoxaparin in the prevention of venous thromboembolism after major orthopaedic surgery. *J South Orthop Assoc* 11(4):182–188, 2002.
6. Amarigiri SV, Lees TA. Elastic compression stockings for prevention of deep vein thrombosis. *Cochrane Database Syst Rev* 3:CD001484, 2000.
7. Eikelboom JW, Quinlan DJ, Douketis JD. Extended-duration prophylaxis against venous thromboembolism after total hip or knee replacement: A meta-analysis of the randomised trials. *Lancet* 358(9275):9–15, 2001.
8. White RH, Romano PS, Zhou H, et al. Incidence and time course of thromboembolic outcomes following total hip or knee arthroplasty. *Arch Intern Med* 158(14):1525–1531, 1998.
9. Anderson FA Jr, Spencer FA. Risk factors for venous thromboembolism. *Circulation* 107(23 suppl 1):I9–I16, 2003.

47 ENDOCARDITIS PROPHYLAXIS

Harrison G. Weed

OVERVIEW

- Infective endocarditis is a devastating disease that was uniformly fatal in the preantibiotic era and continues to be associated with substantial mortality and morbidity.

- Bacteremia caused by surgical and dental procedures can sometimes cause endocarditis; prophylactic antimicrobials can reduce this risk.
- The most current guidelines for antimicrobial prophylaxis of procedure-associated endocarditis are those of the American Heart Association (1997) and the European Society of Cardiology (2004).[1,2]

WHAT IS INFECTIVE ENDOCARDITIS?

- Infective endocarditis is the growth of bacteria or fungi on the inner surface of the heart, including the heart valves.
- A model for the etiology has three steps:
  - An area of abnormal vascular endothelium leads to activation of the clotting system and deposition of a microscopic thrombus.
  - A bloodborne organism adheres to the thrombus or directly to the abnormal endothelium.
  - The organism proliferates and produces a complex colony (vegetation) that resists immune attack.
- Infective emboli can break off from the vegetation and distribute through the vascular tree. The vegetation also erodes into deeper layers of the heart, destroying the valve and sometimes producing an abscess.

DO PROCEDURES CAUSE INFECTIVE ENDOCARDITIS?

- The model of infective endocarditis given above predicts that bacteremia induced by invasive procedures could seed abnormal heart valves, causing endocarditis.
  - Evidence from animal experiments supports the model.
    - In animal experiments, endocarditis can be induced by denuding cardiac endothelium with an intravascular catheter and injecting pathogenic bacteria.[3]
  - Evidence in humans also supports the model; however, medical procedures are not a major cause of endocarditis.
    - Bacteremia has been demonstrated after invasive procedures, such as dental extractions, since the 1930s.[4]
    - In a population-based case-control study at 54 hospitals in the Philadelphia area, dental treatment in the previous 3 months was no more frequent among patients with infective endocarditis who were not users of injection drugs than among controls matched for age, sex, and neighborhood of residence.[5]

CAN ANTIMICROBIAL TREATMENT REDUCE THE RISK OF INFECTIVE ENDOCARDITIS?

- Evidence from animal experiments suggests that antimicrobial treatment can reduce the risk of infective endocarditis.
  - Prophylactic treatment with antimicrobials immediately before and up to 30 min after injection of bacteria can prevent experimental endocarditis in animals.[3]
- Evidence in humans suggests that antimicrobial treatment can reduce the risk of procedure-associated endocarditis; however, the magnitude of the risk reduction appears modest for most patients. Furthermore, the evidence is limited and unlikely to improve. Randomized controlled trials would be unethical, given our current understanding of the disease, and observational studies of adequate size would be prohibitively expensive, because of the rarity of procedure-associated infective endocarditis.
  - Oral amoxicillin prophylaxis reduces the incidence of positive blood cultures after dental extraction from 84 to 33 percent.[6]
  - In a retrospective review of 524 patients with prosthetic valves who underwent invasive procedures capable of causing bacteremia, 6 of 220 patients who did not receive antimicrobial prophylaxis immediately prior to the procedure developed endocarditis, whereas none of 304 who received an antimicrobial developed endocarditis.[7]
  - In 1983, Durack analyzed 52 cases of apparent failure of antimicrobial prophylaxis (mostly with penicillin) reported to a national registry.[8] In 27 (63 percent) of the 43 cases for which antimicrobial susceptibility data were available, the infecting microorganism was sensitive to the antibiotic(s) used for prophylaxis.
  - For patients with a low-risk condition for endocarditis, such as mitral valve prolapse without valve thickening or regurgitation, the risk of a fatal adverse reaction to penicillin is 10 to 100 times greater than the risk of developing fatal endocarditis after a dental procedure.[9]

WHAT ARE THE GUIDELINES FOR ENDOCARDITIS PROPHYLAXIS?

- Although procedure-associated endocarditis is rare, prevention is important because endocarditis is life-threatening. Therefore, interventions to minimize the risk of procedure-associated endocarditis should be a routine part of preoperative care.
  - Despite guidelines, antimicrobial prophylaxis is frequently both overused and underused.[10] Therefore it is important to use automatic reminders, preprinted

order sets, and other systems to ensure that at-risk patients receive appropriate treatment and that antimicrobial prophylaxis is not overused.
  - The American Heart Association (AHA) 1997 guidelines are available at http//www.americanheart.org.[1]
  - The European Society of Cardiology (ESC) guidelines are available at http://eurheartj.oxfordjournals.org.[2]

PATIENT-RELATED RISK FACTORS

- In a population-based case-control study at 54 hospitals, patient-related risk factors were the only significant risk factors for infective endocarditis.[5]
- Both the AHA and the ESC guidelines recommend antimicrobial prophylaxis for specific patient-related cardiac risk factors, as listed in Table 47-1.
  - Patients at highest risk for endocarditis include those with prosthetic valves, prior endocarditis, or complex cyanotic heart disease.
  - Patients at moderate risk include those with hypertrophic cardiomyopathy, congenital cardiac malformations other than complex cyanotic heart disease, or structurally abnormal valves, including thickened or regurgitant prolapsing mitral valves.
- Both the AHA and the ESC guidelines recommend against antimicrobial treatment for the specific heart-related patient conditions listed in Table 47-2.
  - Patients at no greater risk for endocarditis than the general population include those with isolated secundum atrial septal defects, surgically repaired atrial and ventricular defects (more than 6 months after successful repair), surgically repaired patent ductus arteriosus (more than 6 months after successful repair), prior coronary artery bypass, implanted cardiac pacemakers and defibrillators, and benign murmurs.

TABLE 47-1 Cardiac Conditions for which Endocarditis Prophylaxis Is Recommended

Prosthetic heart valves, including bioprosthetic and homograft valves*
Previous bacterial endocarditis*
Complex cyanotic congenital heart disease (e.g., single-ventricle states, transposition of the great arteries, tetralogy of Fallot)*
Noncyanotic congenital heart diseases (except for secundum-type atrial septal defect), including bicuspid aortic valves
Surgically constructed systemic pulmonary shunts or conduits
Acquired valve dysfunction (e.g., rheumatic heart disease)
Hypertrophic cardiomyopathy
Mitral valve prolapse with regurgitation and/or severe valve thickening

*High risk.
SOURCE: Adapted from Dajani et al.[1] and Horstkotte et al.,[2] with permission.

TABLE 47-2 Cardiac Conditions for which Endocarditis Prophylaxis Is Not Recommended*

Isolated secundum atrial septal defect
Surgically repaired atrial septal defect, ventricular septal defect, or patent ductus arteriosus (more than 6 months after successful repair)
Previous coronary artery bypass graft surgery
Mitral valve prolapse without valve regurgitation
Physiologic, functional, or innocent heart murmurs
Previous Kawasaki disease without valve dysfunction
Previous rheumatic fever without valve dysfunction
Cardiac pacemakers (intravascular and epicardial) and implanted defibrillators

*Risk of infective endocarditis is no greater than in the general population.
SOURCE: Adapted from Dajani et al.[1] and Horstkotte et al.,[2] with permission.

- In addition to heart-related conditions, other patient conditions that increase the risk for infective endocarditis are older age, conditions that promote the formation of thrombotic vegetations, and conditions that increase the risk for bacteremia, including disrupted skin and mucous membrane barriers and a compromised immune system.

PROCEDURE-RELATED RISK FACTORS

- Any procedure involving infected tissue at the surgical site is associated with a significant risk of bacteremia.
- Bacteremia can occur after upper aerodigestive tract procedures including dental extractions and implants, tonsillectomy, rigid bronchoscopy, esophageal sclerotherapy and dilation, biliary tract surgery, and other procedures that penetrate the oral or intestinal mucosa (Tables 47-3 and 47-4).

TABLE 47-3 Dental Procedures Likely to Produce Bacteremia: Endocarditis Prophylaxis Recommended

Dental extractions
Periodontal procedures including surgery, scaling and root planing, probing, and recall maintenance
Dental implant placement and reimplantation of avulsed teeth
Endodontic (root canal) instrumentation or surgery only beyond the apex
Subgingival placement of antibiotic fibers or strips
Initial placement of orthodontic bands but not brackets
Intraligamentary local anesthetic injections
Prophylactic cleaning of teeth or implants where bleeding is anticipated

SOURCE: Adapted from Dajani et al.[1] and Horstkotte et al.,[2] with permission.

TABLE 47-4 Procedures Likely to Produce Bacteremia: Endocarditis Prophylaxis Recommended

Respiratory tract
- Surgical operations that involve respiratory mucosa (e.g., tonsillectomy and/or adenoidectomy)
- Bronchoscopy with a rigid bronchoscope

Gastrointestinal tract
- Sclerotherapy for esophageal varices
- Esophageal stricture dilation
- Endoscopic retrograde cholangiography with biliary obstruction
- Biliary tract surgery
- Surgical operations that involve intestinal mucosa

Genitourinary tract
- Prostatic surgery
- Cystoscopy
- Urethral dilation

SOURCE: Adapted from Dajani et al.[1] and Horstkotte et al.,[2] with permission.

- Procedures with a negligible risk of bacteremia include restorative dentistry, local anesthetic injection, intracanal endodontistry (root canal), suture removal, adjustment of orthodontic appliances, endotracheal intubation, flexible bronchoscopy, tympanostomy, transesophageal echocardiography, and endoscopy without biopsy (Table 47-5).
- Procedures involving the lower gastrointestinal and genitourinary tracts that carry a risk of bacteremia include prostate surgery or biopsy, cystoscopy, and urethral dilation (see Table 47-4).
- Procedures with negligible risk include vaginal hysterectomy, normal vaginal delivery, cesarean section, uterine dilation and curettage, therapeutic abortion, tubal ligation, insertion and removal of intrauterine devices, and urethral catheterization (see Table 47-5).

TABLE 47-5 Procedures Unlikely to Produce Bacteremia: Endocarditis Prophylaxis Not Recommended

Respiratory tract
- Endotracheal intubation
- Bronchoscopy with a flexible bronchoscope, with or without biopsy
- Tympanostomy tube insertion

Gastrointestinal tract
- Transesophageal echocardiography*
- Endoscopy with or without gastrointestinal biopsy*

Genitourinary tract
- Vaginal hysterectomy*
- Vaginal delivery*
- Cesarean section
- In uninfected tissue:
  - Urethral catheterization
  - Uterine dilatation and curettage
  - Therapeutic abortion
  - Sterilization procedures
  - Insertion or removal of intrauterine devices

Other
- Cardiac catheterization, including balloon angioplasty
- Coronary stents
- Implanted cardiac pacemakers and defibrillators
- Incision or biopsy of surgically scrubbed skin
- Circumcision

*Prophylaxis is recommended for high-risk patients; it is optional for medium-risk patients.
SOURCE: Adapted from Dajani et al.[1] and Horstkotte et al.,[2] with permission.

TABLE 47-6 Prophylactic Regimens for Dental, Oral, Respiratory Tract, and Esophageal Procedures

SITUATION	AGENT	REGIMEN
Standard general prophylaxis	Amoxicillin	Adults: 2.0 g Children: 50 mg/kg* orally 1 h before the procedure
Unable to take oral medications	Ampicillin	Adults: 2.0 g Children: 50 mg/kg* IM or IV within 30 min before the procedure
Allergic to penicillin	Clindamycin	Adults: 600 mg Children: 20 mg/kg* orally 1 h before the procedure
	or	
	Cephalexin† or cefadroxil†	Adults: 2.0 g Children: 50 mg/kg* orally 1 h before the procedure
	or	
	Azithromycin or clarithromycin	Adults: 500 mg Children: 15 mg/kg* orally 1 h before the procedure
Allergic to penicillin and unable to take oral medications	Clindamycin or	Adults: 600 mg Children: 20 mg/kg* IV within 30 min before the procedure
	or	
	Cefazolin†	Adults: 1.0 g Children: 25 mg/kg* IM or IV within 30 min before the procedure

IM = intramuscular; IV = intravenous.
*Total children's dose should not exceed adult dose.
†Cephalosporins should not be used in people with immediate-type hypersensitivity reactions to penicillins, including urticaria, angioedema, and anaphylaxis.
SOURCE: Adapted from Dajani et al.[1] and Horstkotte et al.,[2] with permission.

ANTIMICROBIALS

- Focus antimicrobials for endocarditis prophylaxis on the most likely causative organisms.
  - *Viridans* (alpha-hemolytic) streptococci and staphylococci are the most common causative organisms in upper aerodigestive tract procedures.

TABLE 47-7 Prophylactic Regimens for Genitourinary/Gastrointestinal (Not Esophageal) Procedures

SITUATION	AGENTS	REGIMEN
High-risk patients	Ampicillin	Adults: 2.0 g Children: 50 mg/kg*
	plus	IM or IV within 30 min before the procedure
	gentamicin	Adults and Children: 1.5 mg/kg (not to exceed 120 mg) IM or IV within 30 min before the procedure
	6 h later: Ampicillin	Adults: 1 g Children: 25 mg/kg*
	or	IM or IV
	amoxicillin	Adults: 1 g Children: 25 mg/kg* orally
High-risk patients allergic to penicillin	Vancomycin†	Adults: vancomycin 1.0 g Children: 20 mg/kg*
	plus	IV over 1–2 h
	gentamicin†	Adults and Children: 1.5 mg/kg (not to exceed 120 mg) IM or IV within 30 min before the procedure
Moderate-risk patients	amoxicillin	Adults: 2.0 g Children: 50 mg/kg*
	or	orally 1 h before the procedure
	ampicillin	Adults: 2.0 g Children: 50 mg/kg* IM or IV within 30 min before the procedure
Moderate-risk patients allergic to penicillin	Vancomycin	Adults: vancomycin 1.0 g Children: 20 mg/kg* IV over 1–2 h

IM = intramuscular; IV = intravenous.
*Total children's dose should not exceed adult dose.
†No second dose of vancomycin or gentamicin is recommended.
SOURCE: Adapted from Dajani et al.[1] and Horstkotte et al.,[2] with permission.

  - Enterococci (*Enterococcus faecalis*) and facultative gram-negative bacilli are the most important causative organisms in procedures involving the lower gastrointestinal and genitourinary tracts.
- Oral amoxicillin or intravenous ampicillin is usually the antimicrobial of choice. In upper aerodigestive tract procedures, alternative antimicrobials for penicillin-allergic patients include clindamycin, cephalexin, cefadroxil, azithromycin, and clarithromycin. Erythromycin is no longer recommended because of the availability of better-tolerated alternatives (Tables 47-6 and 47-7).
- For procedures involving the lower gastrointestinal and genitourinary tracts, vancomycin is the primary alternative to ampicillin because of its activity against enterococci. In the highest-risk patients undergoing procedures of the lower gastrointestinal and genitourinary tracts, add gentamicin for more effective killing of enterococci and to kill gram-negative bacilli (see Table 47-7).
- Patients who chronically take antimicrobials, such as those who take penicillin for secondary prevention of rheumatic fever, are likely to be colonized with penicillin-resistant bacteria. For these patients, use an antimicrobial with a different mechanism of action than that of the agent taken chronically. For example, for the patient who is taking penicillin to prevent rheumatic fever, either clindamycin or azithromycin would be an appropriate alternative (see Table 47-6).

TIMING OF ANTIMICROBIAL ADMINISTRATION

- Animal experiments indicate that antimicrobials do not prevent endocarditis by interfering with bacterial adherence; they do so by killing bacteria after they have adhered. Antimicrobials active on the cell wall, including penicillins and vancomycin, can kill only actively growing bacteria. After adhering, bacteria may not begin to grow for a few hours.

- The short half-life (1 h) of penicillin may partly explain failures of penicillin endocarditis prophylaxis against penicillin-susceptible bacteria.[8] Therefore, to be effective, the prophylactic antimicrobial must be present in microbicidal concentrations for a few hours after the procedure.
- Administer antimicrobial prophylaxis no more than 2 h prior to the procedure, preferably within 30 min of the first incision.
- In high-risk patients, redose ampicillin about 6 h after the initial dose. Clindamycin, gentamicin, and vancomycin have substantially longer half-lives and do not require redosing.

REFERENCES

1. Dajani AS, Taubert KA, Wilson W, et al. Prevention of bacterial endocarditis. Recommendations by the American Heart Association. *JAMA* 277(15):1794–1801, 1997.
2. Horstkotte D, Follath F, Gutschik E, et al. Guidelines on prevention, diagnosis and treatment of infective endocarditis executive summary: The Task Force on Infective Endocarditis of the European Society of Cardiology. *Eur Heart J* 25(3): 267–276, 2004.
3. Glauser MP, Francioli P. Relevance of animal models to the prophylaxis of infective endocarditis. *J Antimicrob Chemother* 20(suppl A):87–98, 1987.
4. Okell CC, Elliott SD. Bacteremia and oral sepsis with special reference to the etiology of subacute endocarditis. *Lancet* 2:869–872, 1935.
5. Strom B, Abrutyn E, Berlin JA, et al. Dental and cardiac risk factors for infective endocarditis. A population-based, case-control study. *Ann Intern Med* 129(10)761–769, 1998.
6. Lockhart PB, Brennan MT, Kent ML, et al. Impact of amoxicillin prophylaxis on the incidence, nature, and duration of bacteremia in children after intubation and dental procedures. *Circulation* 109(23): 2878–2884, 2004.
7. Horstkotte D, Schulte HD, Bircks W, et al. Contribution for choosing the optimal prophylaxis of bacterial endocarditis. *Eur Heart J* 8(suppl J):379–386, 1987.
8. Durack DT, Kaplan EL, Bisno AL. Apparent failures of endocarditis prophylaxis. Analysis of 52 cases submitted to a national registry. *JAMA* 250(17):2318–2322, 1983.
9. Bor DH, Hummelstein DU. Endocarditis prophylaxis for patients with mitral valve prolapse. A quantitative analysis. *Am J Med* 7(4):711–717, 1984.
10. Seto TB, Kwiat D, Taira DA, et al. Physicians' recommendations to patients for use of antibiotic prophylaxis to prevent endocarditis. *JAMA* 284(1):68–71, 2000.

48 PREVENTION OF SURGICAL SITE INFECTION

Harrison G. Weed

SURGICAL SITE INFECTION IS COMMON AND DANGEROUS

- Surgical site infection (SSI) is second only to urinary tract infection as the most common type of hospital-acquired infection.[1]
  - SSI occurs in up to 5 percent of clean extraabdominal surgeries and in up to 20 percent of intraabdominal surgeries.[1]
- Patients who develop SSI are 60 percent more likely to spend time in an intensive care unit, five times more likely to be readmitted to the hospital, and twice as likely to die in the month after surgery.[1]

CAUSES OF SURGICAL SITE INFECTION

- The primary cause of SSI is the introduction of bacteria into a normally sterile body site.
  - Although some patient characteristics—such as extremes of age, extremes of body weight, diabetes mellitus, and cigarette smoking—are risk factors for SSI, the primary risk factor is the type of surgical wound (Tables 48-1 and 48-2).
  - Because the type of surgical wound is the primary risk factor for SSI, it is also the primary consideration in deciding which patients should receive prophylactic antibiotic treatment (Table 48-3).

TABLE 48-1 Patient Characteristics Associated with Surgical Site Infection

Extremes of age
Cachexia
Obesity
Diabetes mellitus
Cigarette smoking
Coexistent infection at another body site
Colonization with pathogenic microorganisms
Length of hospital stay prior to surgery

TABLE 48-2 Centers for Disease Control and Prevention: Surgical Wound Classification

Class I. Clean: An uninfected operative wound in which no inflammation is encountered and the respiratory, alimentary, genital, and urinary tracts are not entered. The wound is closed primarily and, if necessary, is drained with closed drainage. An operative incisional wound for nonpenetrating (blunt) trauma that meets other criteria. **Examples:** craniotomy, adrenalectomy, cardiac surgery, open reduction and internal fixation (ORIF) of a closed fracture, splenectomy, cataract surgery, inguinal hernia repair, orchiectomy, mastectomy

Class II. Clean contaminated: An operative wound in which the respiratory, alimentary, genital, or urinary tract is entered under controlled conditions and without unusual contamination. Specifically, operations involving the biliary tract, appendix, vagina, and oropharynx are included in this category provided that there is no evidence of infection or any major break in sterile technique. **Examples:** cholecystectomy or appendectomy in the absence of acute inflammation, vaginal or abdominal hysterectomy, prostatectomy, rhinoplasty, oral surgery, thoracotomy, colon resection, low anterior resection of the rectum, abdominoperineal resection of the rectum.

Class III. Contaminated: An open, fresh, accidental wound or operation with a major break in sterile technique (e.g., open cardiac massage) or gross spillage from the gastrointestinal tract, or in which acute, nonpurulent inflammation is encountered. **Examples:** any major break in sterile technique, appendectomy (inflamed or ruptured but not gangrenous), acute cholecystitis, ORIF of a compound fracture more than 8 h old, penetrating abdominal trauma without perforated viscera.

Class IV. Dirty or infected: An old traumatic wound with retained devitalized tissue or involving preexisting clinical infection or perforated viscera. Organisms causing infection are present in the operative field before the operation. **Examples:** gunshot wounds, traumatic wounds with retained devitalized tissue or embedded with foreign materials (e.g., grass or soil).

REDUCING THE RISK OF SSI

BEFORE SURGERY

- Some patient-related risk factors for SSI can be improved prior to surgery. If the surgery is elective or semielective, consider postponing it to allow time to improve patient-related risk factors. Although smoking cessation or weight loss is usually difficult, a desired surgery can sometimes provide the impetus to enable a patient to succeed.
  - Abstaining from smoking for at least 1 month before surgery reduces the risk of SSI.
  - In an obese patient, modest weight loss may reduce the risk of both SSI and deep venous thrombosis.
  - Some studies show a reduction in SSIs in cachectic patients treated with a week or more of intensive preoperative nutrition.
    - In general, do not postpone surgery for cachectic patients but do initiate intensive nutritional support as soon as feasible, either before or after surgery.
    - Use enteral nutrition whenever possible; reserve parenteral nutrition for severely cachectic patients (serum albumin below 2.5 g/dL) who have no enteral access. (See Chap. 49 for more information on perioperative nutrition.)
  - Because uncontrolled diabetes mellitus is a risk factor for SSI and other postoperative complications, adjust medications and diet as needed to control diabetes before surgery.
  - Colonization with pathogenic microorganisms increases the risk of SSI.
    - Because shaving creates microabrasions that increase pathologic skin colonization, advise patients not to shave near the surgical field for 2 days prior to surgery.
    - For selected surgeries, consider having the patient bathe with a chlorhexidine-based soap prior to the procedure.
  - Because coexistent infection at another body site increases the risk of SSI, detect and treat any coexistent infections before surgery.

IN THE SURGICAL SUITE AND AFTER SURGERY

- In addition to standard sterile technique for minimizing introduction of microorganisms into normally sterile body sites, the maintenance of good blood perfusion and oxygenation of the surgical site reduces the risk of SSI.
  - Maintain optimal blood pressure, body temperature, and blood oxygen concentration during surgery to minimize SSI.
- Tight blood sugar control may reduce the risk of SSI.
  - Consider intensive insulin treatment for selected patients. For example, continuous infusion of insulin for patients in the surgical intensive care unit can reduce the risk of sepsis. (See Chap. 26 for more information on diabetes mellitus.)
- In general, blood transfusion beyond that required for severe anemia (hemoglobin 7 g/dL, depending on the patient's condition) does not reduce SSI and may actually increase the risk of sepsis and other complications.[2]

PROPHYLACTIC ANTIBIOTICS

RISKS VERSUS BENEFITS

- Prophylactic antibiotics can dramatically reduce SSI.[3]
  - Prophylactic antibiotics continue to be underused and improperly used.[4]
  - In choosing which patients to treat with prophylactic antibiotics, which antibiotics to administer, and when to administer them, weigh the benefits of reducing risk for SSI and possibly other infections against the risks and costs of antibiotic treatment.
    - Risks of antibiotic treatment include allergic reactions, direct toxic effects, adverse interactions with other medications, selection pressure for the

TABLE 48-3 Suggestions for Choosing a Preoperative Prophylactic Antibiotic*

PROCEDURE	ANTIBIOTICS
Colorectal†	Prep is administered orally the day before surgery: neomycin and erythromycin Antibiotics are administered IV at the time of surgery: cefotetan or cefoxitin, or cefazolin and metronidazole
Appendectomy: Nonperforated	Cefotetan, or cefoxitin, or cefazolin and metronidazole
Ruptured viscus: Contaminated	Cefotetan, or cefoxitin, or ampicillin-sulbactam, or cefazolin and metronidazole plus or minus gentamicin
Gastric and biliary: Laparoscopic and open cholecystectomy	Cefazolin (only if high-risk)‡
Inguinal herniorrhaphy	Cefazolin
Mastectomy and other breast procedures	Cefazolin
Head and neck surgery: No incision through oral or pharyngeal mucosa, e.g., thyroidectomy, parotidectomy	Cefazolin
Head and neck surgery: Incision through oral or pharyngeal mucosa	Ampicillin-sulbactam, or clindamycin and gentamicin, or clindamycin and ciprofloxacin
Solid-organ transplant: Liver, pancreas, kidney, kidney/pancreas	Cefotetan, or cefoxitin, or cefazolin and metronidazole
Vascular surgery: Abdominal aorta, groin incision, lower extremity amputation	Cefazolin
Carotid endarterectomy with prosthetic	Cefazolin
Neurosurgery: Craniotomy, cervical fusion, lumbar, laminectomy, VP shunt placement	Cefazolin plus topical bacitracin for shunts and ventriculostomies
Abdominal/vaginal hysterectomy	Cefotetan, or cefoxitin, or cefazolin and metronidazole
Orthopedic surgery: Joint replacement, internal fixation of fracture, spinal fusion, arthroscopic procedure	Cefazolin
Cesarean section	Cefotetan, or cefoxitin, or cefazolin and metronidazole post–cord clamping (only if high risk)§
Thoracic surgery (noncardiac)	Cefazolin
Cardiothoracic surgery: CABG, valve replacement, device implant, heart transplant	Cefazolin
Lung transplant	Piperacillin-tazobactam
Genitourinary: Open and transurethral	Cefazolin

*Also consider local experience and resistance patterns (see Table 48-6 for suggested dosages and dosing intervals).
†Oral bowel preparation combined with intravenous antibiotic reduces SSI more than either alone. Use neomycin sulfate 1 g plus erythromycin base 1 g orally at 19, 18, and 9 h before surgery.
‡"High-risk" is a patient above 65 years of age or one with pancreatitis, jaundice, or acute cholecystitis.
§"High-risk" is emergent labor, active labor, or prolonged rupture of membranes.
SOURCE: Adapted from Bratzler et al,[3] with permission.

emergence of resistant organisms, and antibiotic-associated diarrhea.
- Costs of antibiotic treatment include purchase cost, administration cost, and costs to treat antibiotic-associated complications.

Which Antibiotic to Use

- Direct prophylactic antibiotic treatment against the most likely infecting organisms; it is not necessary to cover every possible pathogen (see Table 48-3).
  - If skin is the only bacteria-colonized tissue at the surgical site, the most likely infecting organisms are streptococci and staphylococci. Cefazolin is effective against these organisms and is the most appropriate prophylactic antibiotic for most clean surgeries.
  - Prophylactic antibiotics for surgeries involving the oral cavity should also cover oral anaerobic bacteria.
  - Prophylactic antibiotics for surgeries of the lower gastrointestinal tract should cover gram-negative enteric bacteria and bowel anaerobes, including *Bacteroides fragilis*.
  - Third- and fourth-generation cephalosporins and carbapenems are contraindicated as antibiotic prophylaxis for at least three reasons:
    - Most are less active than cefazolin against the organisms most likely to cause SSI, such as staphylococci.
    - They are active against organisms unlikely to cause SSI and therefore will cause unnecessary disruption of the normal flora, thus promoting the emergence of resistant organisms such as enterococci.
    - They are more expensive than the more effective alternatives.

Methicillin-Resistant *Staphylococcus aureus*

- It may be appropriate to use vancomycin as a prophylactic antibiotic for patients at "high-risk" of methicillin-resistant *Staphylococcus aureus* (MRSA) SSI.
  - However, there is no consensus on what constitutes a high-risk patient.
  - Furthermore, in a randomized trial of 855 patients undergoing cardiac surgery at an institution with a high rate of MRSA SSI, cefazolin and vancomycin were equivalent except that there were significantly fewer infections with methicillin-sensitive *S. aureus* in patients treated with cefazolin.[5]
  - In a retrospective multivariate analysis, the two most important risk factors for the development of MRSA SSI were (1) continuation of antibiotics longer than 24 h after surgery and (2) discharge to a long-term care facility.[6]

Beta-Lactam Allergy

- About 85 percent of patients who report an "allergy" to "penicillin" will not have any apparent allergic reaction when they are skin tested and can safely receive a beta-lactam antibiotic for surgical prophylaxis.
  - The medical history is sufficient to rule out an allergic reaction or other serious adverse drug reaction in a substantial proportion of these patients (Table 48-4).
  - Some medical centers have arranged for patients reporting penicillin allergy to be routinely evaluated by an allergist and to receive skin testing if indicated before surgery. These institutions have markedly reduced their use of vancomycin.[7]
    - For most preoperative settings, this is not feasible; a careful drug-reaction history to rule out serious adverse drug reaction to beta-lactams is the only available diagnostic tool.
- Use clindamycin or vancomycin for patients with a confirmed or suspected serious adverse reaction to beta-lactams (Table 48-5).
  - Because clindamycin and vancomycin do not have activity against gram-negative bacilli, add gentamicin or another agent that has activity against gram-negative bacilli when the risk of gram-negative infection is significant.

TABLE 48-4 Allergic and Other Serious Drug Reactions

Urticaria, hives
Diffuse pruritus
Angioedema
Bronchospasm
Hypotension
Cardiac dysrhythmia
Drug fever
Drug-induced hypersensitivity syndrome (fever, rash, adenopathy, hepatitis)
Toxic epidermal necrolysis

When to Start a Prophylactic Antibiotic

- A prophylactic antibiotic is most effective if it is started within 1 h of the first incision (within 2 h for antibiotics that require longer infusion times, such as fluoroquinolones or vancomycin).

TABLE 48-5 Alternate Antibiotics for Patients with Confirmed or Suspected Beta-Lactam Allergy*

EXPECTED BACTERIA	ANTIBIOTICS
Gram-positive†	Clindamycin or vancomycin
Gram-positive and gram-negative	Clindamycin or vancomycin plus gentamicin
Anaerobic	Clindamycin or metronidazole

*See Table 48-6 for suggested dosages and dosing intervals.
†Clindamycin does not cover enterococci; vancomycin and gentamicin do.

TABLE 48-6 Suggested Dosages and Dosing Intervals

ANTIBIOTIC	HALF-LIFE IN PATIENTS WITH NORMAL RENAL FUNCTION (hours)	HALF-LIFE IN PATIENTS WITH END-STAGE RENAL DISEASE (hours)	INFUSION DURATION (minutes)	STANDARD DOSE (grams)	WEIGHT-BASED DOSE (grams)	REDOSING INTERVAL (hours) (2–4 × half-life)
Ampicillin-sulbactam	1	6–24	15–60	1.5–3.0	Below 80 kg: 1.5 Above 80 kg: 3.0	2–4
Aztreonam	1.5–2.0	6	15–60	1–2	Below 80 kg: 1 Above 80 kg: 2	3–6
Cefazolin	1.2–2.5	40–70	15–60	1–2	Below 80 kg: 1 Above 80 kg: 2	2–4
Cefotetan	2.8–4.6	13–25	15–60	1–2	Below 80 kg: 1 Above 80 kg: 2	5–11
Cefoxitin	0.5–1.1	6.5–23	15–60	1–2	Below 80 kg: 1 Above 80 kg: 2	2–4
Cefuroxime	1–2	15–22	15–60	1.5–3.0	Below 80 kg: 1.5 Above 80 kg: 3.0	2–4
Ciprofloxacin	3.5–5.0	5–9	60	0.4	0.4	7–12
Clindamycin	2.0–5.1	3.5–5.0	15–60	0.6–0.9	Below 80 kg: 0.6 Above 80 kg: 0.9	4–8
Gentamicin	2–3	50–70	30–60	2 mg/kg	See footnote.* Redose:1.5 mg/kg	4–8
Metronidazole	6–14	7–21	30–60	0.5–1.0	Below 80 kg: 0.5 Above 80 kg: 1.0	6–12
Piperacillin-tazobactam	0.5–1.5	6–24	15–60	3.375–4.5	Below 80 kg: 3.375 Above 80 kg: 4.5	2–4
Vancomycin	4–6	44–400	120	10–15 mg/kg	See footnote.*	8–12

*Ideal body weight (IBW meant:) in pounds: For men: 106 + 6 for each inch above 5 ft. For Women: 100 + 5 for each inch above 5 ft. 2.2 lb = 1 kg. If patient's weight is more than 30 percent greater than IBW, then dosing weight (DW) = IBW + [0.4 × (weight – IBW meant)].

SOURCE: Adapted from Bratzler, Houck, and SIPGW Workgroup,[3] with permission.

- ◦ Starting an antibiotic more than 2 h before surgery provides substantially less protection.
- ◦ Starting an antibiotic after surgery provides no protection.
- ◦ To make sure that the antibiotic reaches the surgical site in adequate concentrations, complete the infusion of prophylactic antibiotic before inflation of any surgical site tourniquet.
- ◦ Starting prophylactic antibiotic soon after the start of surgery might be effective.
  - ▪ In an experimental SSI animal model, starting prophylactic antibiotic up to 3 h after inoculating the wound with *S. aureus* produced the same low infection rate as starting the antibiotic before inoculation.[8]

How to Dose a Prophylactic Antibiotic

- Very few studies of SSI prophylaxis have compared doses or dose intervals.
  - ◦ Studies have demonstrated insufficient blood and tissue concentrations of antibiotics in obese patients given usual doses of antibiotics.
    - ▪ In general, give larger patients a double dose of prophylactic antibiotic (Table 48-6).
- Antibiotics for treatment are often administered at dosing intervals that are four times the antibiotic's half-life.
  - ◦ Nonetheless, the most recent consensus guidelines recommend repeat administration of prophylactic antibiotic after two half-lives if the surgery is still in progress.[3]
  - ◦ Therefore antibiotics with half-lives less than 1 h, such as ampicillin and cefoxitin, are inconvenient to use for operations lasting more than 2 h because they must be readministered frequently (see Table 48-6).

How Long to Continue Antibiotic Treatment

- Most studies show no benefit of continuing antibiotic treatment after wound closure, and most published guidelines recommend that antibiotic prophylaxis be discontinued within 24 h after surgery.
  - ◦ Some surgeons prefer to continue antibiotics for 2 or 3 days after surgery with the rationale that surgical site drains and intravenous catheters provide conduits for bacterial seeding of the surgical site; however, the evidence does not support this practice.[9]
  - ◦ Therefore discontinue prophylactic antibiotics at the time of wound closure or no more than 24 h after surgery.
  - ◦ Continue treatment antibiotics, such as those administered for a class IV dirty or infected surgical wound, as guided by clinical evaluation of the wound and the patient.

DISCHARGE CARE

- Most patients are discharged soon after surgery, before their surgical wounds are fully healed. Appropriate education of the patient, family, and/or provider about postdischarge care of the surgical site can reduce surgical SSIs.
  - ◦ Ensure that patients are adequately educated and have supplies for postoperative wound care. For example, educate patients about handwashing and the use of protective gloves.
  - ◦ Make sure patients understand that they should avoid intimate contact between pets and the surgical site. Bacteria from the mouths of pets that slept with their owners or licked their owners' surgical wounds have caused *Pasteurella multocida* infection.[10]

References

1. Mangram A, Horan TC, Pearson ML, et al. Guideline for prevention of surgical site infection, 1999. Centers for Disease Control and Prevention (CDC) Hospital Infection Control Practices Advisory Committee. *Am J Infect Control* 27(2):97–132, 1999.
2. Carson J, Duff A, Berlin JA, et al. Perioperative blood transfusion and postoperative mortality. *JAMA* 279(3):199–205, 1998.
3. Bratzler DW, Houck PM, and the SIPGW Workgroup. Antimicrobial prophylaxis for surgery: An advisory statement from the National Surgical Infection Prevention Project. *Clin Infect Dis* 38(12):1706–1715, 2004.
4. Bratzler DW, Houck PM, Richards C, et al. Use of antimicrobial prophylaxis for major surgery: Baseline results from the national surgical infection prevention project. *Arch Surg* 140(2):174–182, 2005.
5. Finkelstein R, Rabino G, Mashiah T, et al. Vancomycin versus cefazolin prophylaxis for cardiac surgery in the setting of a high prevalence of methicillin-resistant staphylococcal infections. *J Thorac Cardiovasc Surg* 123(2):326–332, 2002.
6. Manian FA, Meyer PL, Setzer J, et al. Surgical site infections associated with methicillin-resistant *Staphylococcus aureus*: Do postoperative factors play a role? *Clin Infect Dis* 36(7): 863–868, 2003.
7. Park MA, Li JTC. Diagnosis and management of penicillin allergy. *Mayo Clin Proc* 80(3):405–410, 2005.
8. Burke J. The effective period of preventative antibiotic action in experimental incisions and dermal lesions. *Surgery* 50:161–168, 1961.
9. Coskun H, Erisen L, Basut O. Factors affecting wound infection rates in head and neck surgery. *Otolaryngol Head Neck Surg* 123(3):328–333, 2000.
10. Octavio J, Rosenberg W, Conte JE Jr. Surgical wound infection with *Pasteurella multocida* from pet dogs. *N Engl J Med* 345(7):549, 2001.

49 NUTRITIONAL EVALUATION

Anjala V. Tess

INTRODUCTION

- Malnutrition is common among hospitalized patients, though it is often underrecognized by caregivers. One study demonstrated that 40 percent of inpatients were malnourished, yet only half of these patients had any nutritional information documented in the record.[1]
- Nutritional status affects the immune system, regulation of blood chemistry, utilization of fat and muscle stores, and metabolic response to physiologic stress. Malnutrition contributes to an increased risk of poor wound healing, increased susceptibility to infection, overgrowth of bacteria, and increased frequency of decubitus ulcers. Malnourished patients are more likely to require longer stays in the hospital as well.
- In a large prospective study of hospitalized veterans undergoing surgery, those with severe nutritional deficiency had an increased infection rate (42 percent) versus the control group (16 percent), and a higher rate of noninfectious complications as well (21 percent versus 9 percent, respectively).[2]
- Given the risks associated with malnutrition, the preoperative evaluation should include attention to the patient's nutritional state and identification of patient risk factors for preexisting malnutrition.
- This chapter reviews patient-related risk factors, surgery-related risk factors, and potential interventions.

PATIENT-RELATED RISK FACTORS

- Both patient- and procedure-related factors contribute to the risk of perioperative complications of malnutrition (Table 49-1).

TABLE 49-1 Patient- and Surgery-Related Risk Factors for Complications from Malnutrition

PATIENT-RELATED RISK FACTORS	PROCEDURE-RELATED RISK FACTORS
Recent weight loss	Esophageal surgery
Recent hospitalization or surgery	Pancreatic surgery
Alcohol or drug use	Extensive bowel resection
Increased age	General anesthesia
Malignancy	
Chronic renal or liver disease	
Diabetes	
Chronic lung disease	
Inflammatory bowel disease	

RECENT WEIGHT LOSS

- Recent weight loss or being underweight is a risk factor for malnutrition because weight loss itself can lead to loss of fat, muscle, and skin. This may occur due to inadequate intake, increased metabolic demand due to physiologic stresses, or both.
- Since studies confirm that surgery further depletes these stores, identification of patients with recent weight loss is important in assessing perioperative nutritional requirements. In general, more than 10 percent of weight loss over a 3-month period confers increased risk.

RECENT HOSPITALIZATION

- Patients who have been recently hospitalized or have had recent surgery are at higher risk for malnutrition.
  - In a study in England, 48 percent of patients were malnourished on admission to the hospital. After 20 weeks in the hospital, two-thirds of these patients showed further deterioration in clinical parameters, including vitamin levels, weight, anthropometric measures, and laboratory values including albumin or hematocrit. Impressively, these values were also lower after 2 weeks in 75 percent of those patients admitted with normal nutritional parameters. Other studies have shown that patients lose an average of 5.4 percent of their admission weight after even a 1-week hospitalization.

ALCOHOL OR DRUG USE

- Malnutrition is common among patients with alcohol or intravenous drug use. These patients are at risk for complications of malnutrition at the time of surgery.
  - In alcoholics, the majority of calories consumed may come from alcohol alone. For example, in one recent study from the United Kingdom of patients who consumed more than 100 g of ethanol per day (>10 drinks per day), one-third of patients were below normal body weight and all had at least one or more deficiency in macronutrients. Some 60 percent of calories came from alcohol. Other work showed that 25 percent of alcoholic men had albumin levels of less than 2.8 mg/dL. Other anthropometric markers of malnutrition, such as triceps skinfold thickness, are also abnormal in alcoholics, though this may represent myopathy associated with alcohol use.
  - In a study of intravenous drug users admitted to the hospital, almost 20 percent had evidence of severe

protein-calorie malnutrition and 30 percent met other criteria for malnutrition.

ADVANCED AGE

- The prevalence of malnutrition in the elderly has been well documented; rates range from 40 to 71 percent, depending on the study and living situation.
- As part of the normal aging process, muscle stores may decrease and fat stores increase. This is known as sarcopenia.
- Older patients have higher rates of malnutrition and are more likely to have a longer length of stay when hospitalized.
- Factors that predict a likelihood of malnutrition in the elderly include dysphagia, slow eating, low protein intake, poor appetite, presence of a feeding tube, and advanced age. Other mechanisms include anorexia, change in metabolism, concomitant psychiatric disease, and medications that may cause gastrointestinal symptoms or anorexia.

CHRONIC MEDICAL CONDITIONS

- Chronic medical conditions can increase the risk of preoperative malnutrition by four mechanisms: decreased intake, increased metabolic demands, poor absorption of nutrients, or frank nutrient loss. All of these place the patient at higher risk at surgery.
    - Decreased intake from psychiatric illness, such as depression or anxiety, can profoundly affect nutritional stores. Eating disorders such as anorexia nervosa or bulimia can lead to extreme weight loss and volume and electrolyte disorders.
    - Reduced intake due to mechanical difficulties with eating, as in patients with dysphagia or neurologic compromise, can also lead to reduced nutritional stores.
    - Burns, infections, fever, hyperthyroidism, and HIV can increase risk of malnutrition due to increased metabolic needs.
    - Malabsorption or nutrient loss occurs with many illnesses. Chronic diarrhea can decrease absorption through inflammatory changes in the mucosal wall of the gut. Short-gut syndrome resulting from extensive bowel resection can lead to chronic nutrient and protein deficiency from inability to absorb foods.
    - Chronic diarrhea can lead to water, electrolyte, and protein loss. Protein loss can occur in patients with draining wounds.

MALIGNANCY

- Hospitalized patients with malignancy have at least a twofold higher rate of malnutrition than those without malignancy. This is due to increased metabolic demand, impaired intake from either mechanical problems or anorexia, and possibly decreased absorption.

CHRONIC RENAL DISEASE

- Depending on the definition of malnutrition, up to 70 percent of patients with end-stage renal disease are malnourished. Malnutrition in this population confers a poor prognosis; one study reported a 50 percent increase in rate of progression to end-stage renal disease or death over 12 months. Similarly, this group had a 79 percent likelihood of acute hospitalization over 1 year.
- Malnutrition in this population results from anorexia and subsequent inadequate protein intake as well as increased protein loss during dialysis itself.

CIRRHOSIS

- The prevalence of malnutrition in patients with cirrhosis approaches 50 percent; up to 30 percent of patients have reduced protein and/or fat stores.
- Surgical mortality is almost three times higher for abdominal surgery in cirrhotic patients who are malnourished compared with those who are adequately nourished.[3]

DIABETES

- Although diabetic patients are commonly obese, specific factors may lead to malnutrition in this population. Mechanical difficulty due to gastroparesis, reflux disease, and diarrhea from the autonomic complications of diabetes can limit intake and absorption.

CHRONIC OBSTRUCTIVE PULMONARY DISEASE

- Chronic obstructive pulmonary disease can predispose to malnutrition; rates are as high as 30 to 70 percent. Pulmonary cachexia is a progressive reduction in lean body mass due to several factors, including increased metabolism from work of breathing, decreased exercise capacity from loss of protein stores, inflammation, and medications (e.g., corticosteroids) that increase wasting. This loss of protein stores decreases diaphragmatic muscle bulk and correlates with increased mortality.

INFLAMMATORY BOWEL DISEASE

- The prevalence of malnutrition in patients with Crohn's disease or inflammatory bowel disease is 50 to 70 percent.
- The etiology of malnutrition is multifactorial; decreased intake, malabsorption, and increased nutrient loss all play a role.
- Malnourished patients with inflammatory bowel disease are at high risk for perioperative wound infections and sepsis.

SURGERY-RELATED RISK FACTORS

- Surgical stress causes a hypermetabolic state (increasing protein and energy requirements) due to increased skeletal muscle breakdown. Patients can develop protein-calorie malnutrition in as little as a few days after surgery.
- Surgery of the gastrointestinal tract poses a particular risk because oral intake and absorption of nutrients are limited owing to intestinal resection or postoperative ileus.
- Anesthesia may delay initiation of feeding due to ileus.
- One study stratified specific complication rates by surgical site and found that esophageal and pancreatic surgeries conferred a high risk regardless of the preoperative albumin level. Patients undergoing colon surgery had the fewest complications across all levels of albumin.[4]
- Surgical patients who are malnourished have impaired wound healing; this can contribute to further nutrient loss.

PREOPERATIVE EVALUATION AND TESTING TO STRATIFY RISK

HISTORY

- Obtain a careful history to determine baseline nutritional status and elicit risk factors for malnutrition, including recent hospitalization, prior surgery, and those chronic medical conditions that increase risk.
- The social history may identify substance abuse or socioeconomic factors that affect nutrition, such as whether the patient can do his or her own shopping and cooking.
- Determine the highest nonpregnant weight (in women), usual weight, and current weight. Specifically question whether any weight loss was intentional. In general, more than 10 percent of weight loss over 3 months increases the risk of malnutrition.
- In the review of systems, specific questions regarding dysphagia, dental problems, nausea, vomiting, abdominal pain, or diarrhea may reveal a patient at risk as well.

PHYSICAL EXAMINATION

- In addition to vital signs and a complete examination, measure the patient's height and weight in order to calculate his or her body mass index (BMI). In general, a BMI <18 kg/m^2 indicates an underweight individual.
- Other physical signs of malnutrition include hair loss, glossitis, stomatitis, poor dentition, edema, muscle wasting, evidence of peripheral neuropathies, and pressure ulcers or poorly healing wounds.
- Anthropometric measures, including triceps skinfold thickness and the circumference of the upper arm may be more detailed than necessary in the preoperative setting.

LABORATORY EVALUATION

- A targeted history and physical examination are the most important parts of the preoperative evaluation and are usually adequate to assess the risk for malnutrition.
- Reserve evaluation of protein stores for cases where the physical examination does not indicate malnutrition but the history suggests that the patient is malnourished. Laboratory evaluation is also helpful in those patients for whom a diet or weight history cannot be obtained.
- Serum albumin is the most commonly measured laboratory parameter. It has a half-life of 18 to 20 days and provides a measure of stores over the preceding 2 to 3 months. A level of less than 2.2 g/dL indicates severe malnutrition. Albumin is a strong predictor of mortality in surgical patients.
  - One large study of over 50,000 patients showed the serum albumin level to be the single strongest measure of postoperative 30-day morbidity and mortality, even stronger than weight loss itself.[5]
- Serum transferrin has a half-life of 8 to 9 days and reflects stores over the preceding 2 to 4 weeks. Serum prealbumin has a half-life of only 2 to 3 days and reflects levels in the preceding week.
- Clinicians may also measure serum electrolytes and BUN/creatinine to assess volume status. Low calcium, magnesium, and potassium levels may suggest inadequate intake of nutrients or electrolyte losses.

TOOLS AND DEFINITIONS FOR CLINICIANS

- There is no universally accepted clinical indicator, measurement, or laboratory test that strictly defines a patient's nutritional status. The Subjective Global Assessment (SGA) is a tool that uses the history and physical examination to help clinicians assess a patient's nutritional status. Using this tool, one classifies patients into the following three categories: well-nourished, mildly malnourished or suspected of malnutrition, or severely malnourished[6] (Table 49-2).
- The Nutrition Risk Index (NRI) was derived by the authors of the VA Cooperative Trial and utilizes serum albumin levels and the amount of weight loss to classify patients as borderline, mildly malnourished, or severely malnourished[2]:

$$\text{NRI} = 1.519 \times \text{serum albumin (g/L)} + [41.7 \times (\text{current body weight/usual body weight})]$$

  An NRI of 97.5 to 100 = borderline malnourished; 83.5 to 97.5 = mildly malnourished, and <83.5 = severely malnourished.
- Both the SGA and NRI correlate with outcomes in surgical patients.
- If screening for risk factors for malnutrition reveals that a patient may be malnourished, consider using these tools to further stratify the patient's risk.
- Documentation of the degree of malnutrition may help guide the choice of nutritional support.

PERIOPERATIVE MANAGEMENT TO REDUCE RISK

Strategies to reduce the risk of complications of malnutrition span the perioperative period (Table 49-3).

PREOPERATIVE INTERVENTIONS

- In patients who are malnourished or at risk for malnutrition after surgery, consult a nutritionist to assess caloric requirements and determine the potential need for supplementation.
- For patients who are malnourished, use preoperative enteral nutrition (EN) whenever possible. Because of the risk of infectious complications, consider total parenteral nutrition (TPN) only in severely malnourished patients.
  - Several small randomized trials have demonstrated a benefit of preoperative EN with two- to fourfold reductions in mortality compared with no supplemental support.
  - The benefit of preoperative TPN is less clear. Early prospective studies of patients with gastrointestinal cancer showed up to a twofold mortality benefit. However, in a subsequent large randomized controlled study, patients receiving a week of preoperative TPN and a few days of postoperative TPN had increased infection rates (14 versus 6 percent) and a nonsignificant decrease in mortality compared with controls (4.9 versus 7.3 percent). In the subgroup analysis, only severely malnourished patients had a lower rate of infectious complications, suggesting that only this group may benefit from preoperative TPN.[2]
  - A meta-analysis of studies of the perioperative use of TPN found no decrease in mortality rate but did suggest a decrease in the overall complication rate. The issue remains unclear, however, due to study heterogeneity in this analysis.
- Consider delaying elective surgery in patients for whom preoperative supplementation may be possible.

INTRAOPERATIVE INTERVENTIONS

- Consider placement of a gastrostomy or jejunostomy tube to prepare for postoperative feeding in patients who are at risk for not maintaining adequate nutrition after surgery. Discuss this possibility with the surgeon.
- Recommend careful attention to electrolyte and volume resuscitation during the procedure.

POSTOPERATIVE INTERVENTIONS

- Start postoperative supplementation with EN in malnourished patients. Restrict the use of TPN to patients who cannot receive EN, but recognize that postoperative TPN appears to confer some increased risks.
  - Multiple small studies have evaluated postoperative enteral feeding. Results include decreased infections, a reduced need for antibiotics, and less weight loss.
  - For example, in a study of elderly women undergoing orthopedic surgery, patients who received enteral feeding via nasogastric tube had shorter rehabilitation stays and a trend toward an improvement in mortality (8 versus 21 percent).[7] This benefit can also be achieved by using oral supplements.
  - Studies of postoperative TPN have been disappointing, but TPN may be the only option in patients who cannot tolerate oral or enteral feeding. As an example, in one report, investigators randomly assigned patients undergoing resection for pancreatic cancer to TPN or standard therapy. The rate of infection was higher in the intervention group than in the control group. All complications were more common in the TPN

TABLE 49-2 The Subjective Global Assessment Tool

History	Weight change	Overall loss in past 6 months	_______kg ________% weight loss
		Any change in past 2 weeks	☐ Increased ☐ No change ☐ Decreased
	Dietary intake	Ask about change relative to normal	☐ No change
			☐ Change If so: Duration: _______ weeks Type: ☐ Suboptimal solid diet ☐ Full liquid ☐ Hypocaloric liquid ☐ Starvation diet
	GI symptoms	Ask about any new symptoms in last 2 weeks	☐ No change
			☐ Change If so: ☐ Nausea ☐ Vomiting ☐ Diarrhea ☐ Anorexia
	Functional capacity	Ask about change relative to normal	☐ No change
			☐ Change If so: Duration: _______ weeks Type: ☐ Working but suboptimally ☐ Ambulatory ☐ Bedridden
	Disease effects	Diagnosis:	
		Assess metabolic stress	☐ None ☐ Low ☐ Moderate ☐ High
Physical Exam	(Specify 0 = normal, 1+ = mild, 2+ = moderate, 3+ = severe)		
	Loss of subcutaneous fat (triceps, chest)		
	Muscle wasting (quadriceps, deltoids)		
	Ankle edema		
	Sacral edema		
	Ascites		

Step II: Determine Subjective Rating

- Looking at the overall data, assessment of rank is meant to be subjective:
  A = Well-nourished
  B = Moderate or suspected of being malnourished
  C = Severely malnourished
- Weight loss, poor dietary intake, loss of subcutaneous fat, and muscle wasting should carry the most influence. Other historical questions are meant more to support the rater's overall assessment and guide intervention.
- For example:
  - If a patient has recently gained weight and has no physical evidence of malnutrition, he or she should receive an A rank.
  - If a patient has had a weight loss of at least 5 percent, reduction in intake, and mild or few physical exam findings, he or she should receive a B rank. Even with a less significant weight loss, if there are exam findings of malnutrition, a B rank is likely appropriate.
  - If a patient has had at least a 10 percent weight loss and clear evidence of physical exam findings, he or she should receive a C rank. Most patients with severe physical findings often have the weight loss history and dietary change noted as well.

SOURCE: Adapted from Detsky AS, McLaughlin JR, Baker JP, et al. What is subjective global assessment of nutritional status? *J Parenter Enteral Nutr* 1987; 11:8–13, with permission from the American Society for Parenteral and Enteral Nutrition (A.S.P.E.N.). A.S.P.E.N. does not endorse the use of this material in any form other than its entirety.

TABLE 49-3 Risk-Reduction Strategies

PREOPERATIVE	INTRAOPERATIVE	POSTOPERATIVE
Recognize patient-related risk factors and assess the degree of malnutrition.	If the patient will need postoperative feeding, discuss placement of a gastrostomy or jejunostomy tube with surgeon.	Use tube feedings or oral nutrition when possible.
Consult with nutritionist to help with assessment and calorie modification.	Pay close attention to volume and electrolyte replacement in the operating room.	
When possible, use preoperative EN support rather than TPN.		

EN = enteral nutrition; TPN = total parenteral nutrition.

group, including intraabdominal abscesses, fistulas, and peritonitis. Other studies have reproduced these findings.

IMMUNONUTRITION

- The newest addition to perioperative nutritional support is the use of immunonutrition or additives including the essential amino acids glutamine and arginine and/or ribonucleic acid (RNA).
- Randomized trials have demonstrated that perioperative use of glutamine decreases the risk of infection and shortens length of stay. However, there was no difference in mortality rates.
- Three meta-analyses of immunonutrition with multiple additives in critically ill and surgical patients have confirmed decreased rates of infection and shortened length of stay. In these trials, the subgroups who had received formula with high levels of arginine appeared to benefit the most.
- Trials that have examined the optimal timing of perioperative immunonutrition suggest that its use for at least 5 days after surgery may improve outcome.

REFERENCES

1. Pirlich M, Schutz T, Kemps M, et al. Prevalence of malnutrition in hospitalized medical patients: Impact of underlying disease. *Dig Dis* 21:245, 2003.
2. The Veterans Affairs Total Parenteral Nutrition Cooperative Study Group. Perioperative total parenteral nutrition in surgical patients. *N Engl J Med* 325:525, 1991.
3. Garrison RN, Cryer HM, Howard DA, et al. Clarification of risk factors for abdominal operations in patients with hepatic cirrhosis. *Ann Surg* 199:648, 1984.
4. Kudsk K, Tolley E, DeWitt C, et al. Preoperative albumin and surgical site identify surgical risk for major postoperative complications. *JPEN* 27:1, 2003.
5. Gibbs J, Cull W, Henderson W, et al. Preoperative serum albumin level as a predictor of operative mortality and morbidity: Results from the National VA Surgical Risk Study. *Arch Surg* 134:36–42, 1999.
6. Detsky AS, McLaughlin JR, Baker JP, et al. What is subjective global assessment of nutritional status? *JPEN* 11:8, 1987.
7. Bastow MD, Rawlings J, Allison SP. Benefits of supplementary tube feeding after fractured neck of femur: A randomised controlled trial. *Br Med J* 287:1589, 1983.

Section V
POSTOPERATIVE COMPLICATIONS

Gerald W. Smetana, MD, Section Editor

50 FEVER

James C. Pile and Harrison G. Weed

INTRODUCTION

DEFINITION OF FEVER

- Fever is a regulated elevation of the body's normal temperature.
- Although Wunderlich's 1868 definition of "normal" body temperature as 37.0°C (98.6°F) has persisted, more recent work has demonstrated that normal body temperature is usually in the range of 36.6 to 36.8°C (97.9 to 98.2°F). Furthermore, there is significant circadian variation: a person's temperature is generally lowest in the early morning and highest in the late afternoon or early evening.
- In the 1990s Mackowiak precisely defined fever as an oral temperature of more than 37.1°C (98.8°F) in the early morning or more than 37.7°C (99.8°F) at any time of the day[1]; however, Wunderlich's 1868 definition of fever as a body temperature of 38.0°C (100.4°F) or more is robust and time-honored.

PATHOPHYSIOLOGY OF FEVER

- Fever is one manifestation of an inflammatory response that includes elevated acute-phase reactants, leukocytosis, thrombocytosis, anemia, cachexia, increased lipolysis, and a negative nitrogen balance.
- Our current understanding of the pathophysiology of fever is incomplete. A simple model is that a variety of stimuli, ranging from endotoxin to tissue trauma, provoke the release of endogenous pyrogens from mononuclear phagocytes. These pyrogens—particularly the cytokines interleukin-1 (IL-1), interleukin-6 (IL-6), tumor necrosis factor-alpha (TNF-α), and interferon gamma (IFN-γ)—act on the preoptic area in and adjacent to the hypothalamus. The preoptic area then releases fever-inducing prostaglandins, particularly prostaglandin E_2, by activating cyclooxygenase. Body temperature rises through some combination of shivering, peripheral vasoconstriction, and endogenous thermogenesis by brown adipose tissue.
- Fever is probably adaptive. It occurs in a wide variety of vertebrate and invertebrate species. Nonetheless, it is not clear when a fever is beneficial and when it should be suppressed. Although supporting data are scant, suppression of fever is appropriate to relieve patient discomfort or when the metabolic costs of the fever seem unacceptably high—for example, in a patient with limited cardiac reserves.

INCIDENCE AND TIMING

- The frequency of postoperative fever varies from 14 to 91 percent, depending on the definition of fever and on the type of surgery.[2] Most postoperative fevers occur shortly after surgery, are self-limited, and are apparently benign.[3–6]
- Most fevers in the first 2 days after surgery are caused by the trauma-induced release of cytokines (IL-1, TNF-α) that stimulate the production of IL-6. Nonetheless, do not automatically dismiss fevers occurring soon after surgery as inconsequential, because medication reactions and fulminant infections can present within hours after surgery and even during the procedure.
- Fevers of 40°C (104°F) or greater may be less likely to be benign even in the immediate postoperative period. Additional evaluation should be considered for such patients.

DIAGNOSIS

DIFFERENTIAL DIAGNOSIS OF POSTOPERATIVE FEVER

- There are many infectious and noninfectious causes of postoperative fever (Table 50-1).
- Although surgical site infection, urinary tract infection, and pneumonia are the most frequently identified causes of postoperative fever, the frequency of different causes varies widely depending on procedure- and patient-specific factors.
- The timing of fever onset after surgery is a useful clue to the cause (Table 50-2). Fevers occurring after postoperative day 3 are more likely to have an identifiable cause (Fig. 50-1).

"CAN'T MISS" CAUSES

- Several relatively rare causes of postoperative fever must remain high in the differential diagnosis, because early diagnosis and treatment can be lifesaving.
  - Acute bacterial peritonitis can result from peritoneal soilage after any surgery involving the abdominal cavity, due either to inadvertent bowel perforation or to leakage from a bowel anastomosis. Rarely, perioperative hypotension or emboli can cause ischemic bowel, leading to peritoneal soilage. Abdominal pain and tenderness are often present, but recent surgery and sedating and analgesic medications can mask these findings. Abdominal computed tomography (CT) scanning can be helpful in making the diagnosis. Prompt surgical treatment is essential.
  - Necrotizing fasciitis or fulminant myonecrosis of the surgical site causes fever and surgical site necrosis. Emergent surgical debridement is mandatory; antibiotic treatment is important but adjunctive. Myonecrosis usually occurs in the first few hours to days after surgery and generally results from either *Clostridium* or beta-hemolytic streptococcal infection. Surgical site inspection can establish the diagnosis but requires removal of the bandages.
  - Toxic shock syndrome causes fever, hypotension, and flushing and can occasionally result from colonization of wound dressings with either *Staphylococcus aureus* or group A *Streptococcus*.
  - Adrenal insufficiency causes hypotension unresponsive to fluid resuscitation and can cause a low-grade fever. It occurs in patients whose high-dose corticosteroids (e.g., more than 20 mg/day of prednisone) are inadvertently discontinued and in those with hypophyseal or bilateral adrenal hemorrhage. Glucocorticoid replacement is lifesaving.

TABLE 50-1 Causes of Fever after Surgery

Infectious	
Bacterial infections	**Viral infections**
Urinary tract infection	Transfusion-associated (especially cytomegalovirus)
Surgical site	Reactivation (after transplant)
Superficial wound infection	**Noninfectious**
Wound myonecrosis	*Not* atelectasis
Intraabdominal infection (i.e., abscess, peritonitis after abdominal or pelvic surgery)	Direct surgical trauma (most common cause of postoperative fever)
Pneumonia	Aspiration pneumonitis (without infection)
Endovascular	Medications (especially beta-lactams, sulfonamides, and phenytoin)
Catheter-related	Hematoma
Cardiac device– or prosthetic valve–related	Venous thromboembolism
Grafts, stents	Fat embolism
Orthopedic devices (especially prosthetic joints)	Transplant rejection (lung > kidney, liver > heart)
Clostridium difficile infection	Adrenal insufficiency
Endocarditis	Hyperthyroidism
Sinusitis	Myocardial infarction
Osteomyelitis	Gout/pseudogout
Otitis media	Pancreatitis
Parotitis	Hepatitis/cirrhosis
Acalculous cholecystitis	Bowel infarction
Toxic shock syndrome	Drug/alcohol withdrawal
Staphylococcal	Transfusion reactions
Streptococcal	Stroke
Fungal infections	Cancer/neoplastic
Candida albicans, Candida glabrata	
Aspergillus	

SOURCE: Adapted from Weed and Baddour,[8] with permission.

TABLE 50-2 Differential Diagnosis and the Timing of Fever

Immediate (during surgery or within 1 h afterward):
- Medication reaction (often accompanied by hypotension)
  - Malignant hyperthermia
  - Antibiotic-related (sometimes with rash)
- Transfusion reaction (blood products)
- Infection present prior to surgery
  - Pneumonia (e.g., prior to fall and hip fracture)
- Fulminant surgical site infection
  - Group A *Streptococcus*
  - *Clostridium perfringens* myonecrosis
- Trauma suffered prior to or during surgery
- Adrenal insufficiency (hypotension unresponsive to volume, fever)

Acute (in the first week after surgery):
- Nosocomial infections
  - Pneumonia (especially if ventilated, poor gag reflex, or recent emesis)
  - Urinary tract (especially if urethral catheter is present)
  - Surgical site
  - Catheter-associated (especially if catheter was inserted emergently or under nonsterile conditions)
- Noninfectious
  - Pancreatitis (abdominal pain, vomiting)
  - Myocardial infarction
  - Pulmonary embolism
  - Thrombophlebitis
  - Alcohol withdrawal (delirium, low-grade fever)
  - Acute gout/pseudogout

Subacute (from one to four weeks following surgery):
- Surgical site infection
- Catheter-associated infection
  - Catheter entry site
  - Endovascular
- Thrombophlebitis
- Antibiotic-associated diarrhea
  - *Clostridium difficile* and others
- Drug fever
  - Antimicrobials (especially penicillins and sulfonamides)
  - H_2 blockers
  - Procainamide
  - Phenytoin
  - Carbamazepine

Delayed (more than 1 month after surgery):
- Surgical site infection (indolent organisms, more common with implanted device or prosthesis)
  - Coagulase-negative staphylococci
  - Nontuberculous mycobacteria
- Cellulitis due to impaired lymphatic drainage (e.g., lower leg after saphenous venectomy, arm after axillary node dissection)
- Infective endocarditis (after valve replacement or from perioperative bacteremia and preexisting abnormal heart valve)
- Postpericardiotomy syndrome
- Infection from blood-product transfusion (rare)
  - Viral
    - Cytomegalovirus (CMV)
    - Hepatitis B (HBV)
    - Hepatitis C (HCV)
    - Human immunodeficiency virus (HIV)
  - Parasitic
    - *Toxoplasma gondii*
    - *Trypanosoma cruzi*
    - *Babesia microti*
    - *Plasmodium* species

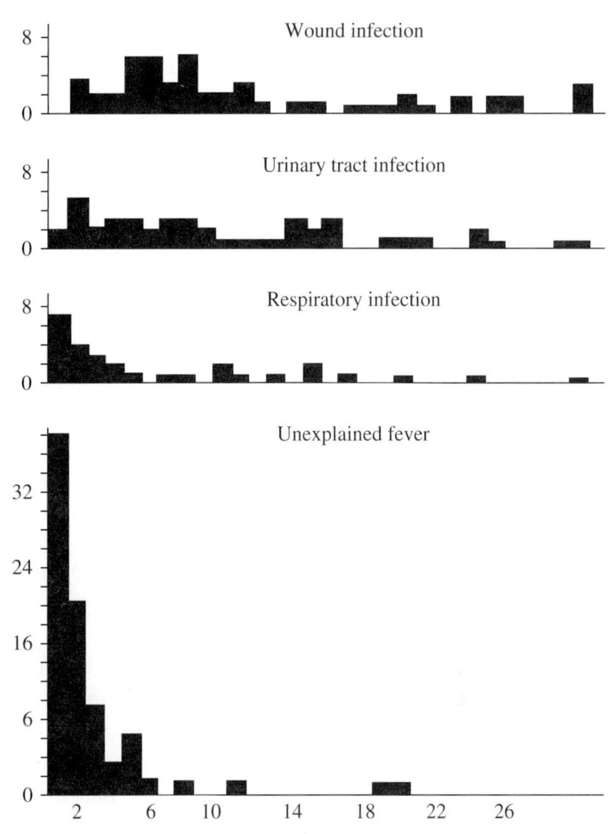

FIG. 50-1 Days of onset for postoperative infections and unexplained fever. The timing of fever after surgery is one of the most important characteristics in ordering the differential diagnosis of fever in postoperative patients. (Data from Garibaldi et al.,[11] with permission.)

- Pulmonary embolism is common and often unrecognized, even in the most technically advanced settings. In patients at risk, any combination of chest pain, dyspnea, tachypnea, hypoxemia, and low-grade fever should prompt consideration of the diagnosis. Although appropriate prophylactic measures substantially decrease the risk of pulmonary embolism, it must remain in the differential diagnosis of high-risk patients.
- Patients undergoing withdrawal from alcohol or other sedatives develop low-grade fever, hypertension, tachycardia, tremor, diaphoresis, and delirium. Recognition of alcohol withdrawal is important, as treatment with benzodiazepines improves symptoms and reduces the risk of delirium, seizures, and death. In febrile patients undergoing alcohol withdrawal, also consider other causes of fever, such as aspiration pneumonia.

INFECTIOUS CAUSES

- Surgical site infection (SSI) is either the most or the second most common cause of postoperative infection in most series. SSIs usually arise more than 3 days after surgery. Most SSIs are superficial and apparent on examination; however, fever and/or pain may be the only manifestations of deep infections, such as intraabdominal abscesses and prosthetic joint infections.

- In some series, urinary tract infection (UTI) is the most common infection after surgery. The frequency of UTI is proportional to the frequency and the duration of urinary catheterization.
- Pneumonia is also common after surgery and is more frequent in patients with compromised lung function and/or risk factors for aspiration. Underlying lung disease, mechanical ventilation, thoracic surgery, and upper abdominal surgery confer an increased risk of postoperative pneumonia. The microbiology of postoperative pneumonia differs markedly from that of community-acquired pneumonia. Empiric treatment should be directed at hospital-acquired gram-negative bacteria and should be based on local resistance patterns (see Chap. 54 for details).
- Antibiotic-associated diarrhea with colitis, usually caused by *Clostridium difficile*, can cause fever. Sometimes diarrhea is absent and the only clues to a significant colitis are fever and leukocytosis. Any systemic antimicrobial treatment can predispose patients to colitis, and illness may not occur until a week or more after the discontinuation of antimicrobial treatment. Recognition of *C. difficile*–associated colitis, discontinuation of antibiotic treatment when feasible, and treatment with metronidazole or vancomycin can be lifesaving.
- Intravenous catheter–associated infections are common. Peripheral intravenous catheters usually cause no more than superficial cellulitis or thrombophlebitis; however, central intravenous catheters can cause bloodstream infections. There is usually no inflammation at the entry site of an infected central intravenous catheter. Infection is more common if the catheter is placed emergently or without sterile technique including chlorhexidine skin preparation. In considering catheter-associated bloodstream infection, draw blood cultures from both the catheter and a peripheral site. In addition to removing the catheter, empiric treatment should usually include vancomycin to cover methicillin-resistant staphylococci while awaiting the results of blood cultures.

NONINFECTIOUS CAUSES

- In addition to adrenal insufficiency, pulmonary embolism, and alcohol withdrawal, a variety of other noninfectious processes can cause fever after surgery.
  - Deep venous thrombosis (DVT) with thrombophlebitis can cause low-grade fevers, even without pulmonary embolism. Always maintain a high index of suspicion in at-risk patients, because physical findings may be absent.
  - Gout and pseudogout are common after surgery. A history of the disease is not invariably present. Patients may not complain of joint pain, but the inflamed joint is usually evident on examination.
  - Hematomas, especially if large, can cause both fever and leukocytosis.
  - Myocardial infarction occurs in 2 to 3 percent of patients undergoing major surgery. A low-grade fever can be one manifestation.
  - Drug fever is an important and frequent noninfectious cause of postoperative fever. Rash and eosinophilia can be clues but are usually absent. Common offending medications include penicillins, sulfonamides, phenytoin, and H_2 blockers.
- Atelectasis, though traditionally touted as the cause of transient postoperative fevers, is probably usually only coincidental. That is, both transient fevers and atelectasis occur after surgery, but atelectasis does not cause fever. For example, Engoren found no correlation in individual postthoracotomy patients between atelectasis and fever.[7] In the entire cohort, atelectasis became more prevalent as the fevers resolved. Tissue trauma–related cytokine release explains the majority of fevers traditionally attributed to atelectasis.

APPROACH TO THE PATIENT WITH POSTOPERATIVE FEVER

INITIAL EVALUATION

- Most fevers in the first 2 days after surgery are self-limited and benign. However, until additional history and physical findings are reviewed, presume the fever to have a serious cause. Fevers that develop for the first time on postoperative day 4 or later are likely to have an identifiable and treatable cause (Table 50-3).
- Review the operative note and, if feasible, ask the surgeon and anesthesiologist about details of the procedure.
- Determine all recent and current treatments and medications, including preoperative antibiotics, venous thromboembolism prophylaxis, and blood product transfusions.
- Determine past medical history, including gout and atherosclerotic vascular disease.
- Nursing staff can provide valuable details, including the patient's sputum quantity and quality, stool volume and characteristics, skin breakdown at dependent sites, and fluctuations in arousal or orientation.

PHYSICAL FINDINGS

- Review all vital signs. Consider charting a temperature curve.

TABLE 50-3 Evaluation of the Patient with Postoperative Fever*

History—review:
1. Details of hospital course, both pre- and postoperative
2. Specifics of surgical procedure, including any complications or unanticipated difficulties
3. Past medical history, particularly presence of diabetes, atherosclerotic disease, valvular heart disease, gout, alcohol abuse
4. Allergies
5. Medications, especially antimicrobials
6. Administration of blood products
7. Location and duration of catheters
8. Nursing information regarding sputum production, diarrhea, skin breakdown, and evidence of delirium
9. Additional information from the patient

Physical examination:
1. Review vital signs—temperature, heart rate, blood pressure, respiratory rate, pulse oximetry readings
2. Paranasal sinuses/ears
3. Lungs for dullness and adventitious sounds
4. Heart
5. Abdomen for distention, bowel sounds, and tenderness
6. Surgical site
7. Skin for rash and hematoma
8. Catheter sites for inflammation or adjacent thrombophlebitis
9. Legs for evidence of deep venous thrombosis
10. Joints for acute arthritis

Laboratory/imaging (should be obtained in appropriate setting only):
1. Urine analysis and culture
2. Sputum Gram's stain and culture
3. Blood cultures, drawn both from catheters and peripherally
4. Swab from draining wounds for Gram's stain and culture
5. Complete blood count (CBC) with differential
6. Chest radiograph
7. Additional laboratory or imaging testing as dictated by clinical scenario (e.g., hepatic enzymes and hepatic ultrasound in a patient with right-upper-quadrant pain and tenderness at risk for acalculous cholecystitis.)

*A general caveat: Most early postoperative fevers will prove benign and self-limited, but none should be ignored.
SOURCE: Adapted from Weed and Baddour,[8] with permission.

- Tailor the physical examination to the patient's clinical situation. Generally the examination should include at least inspection of the skin, surgical site, catheter entry sites, and limbs; auscultation of the lungs, heart, and abdomen; palpation of the abdomen and any inflamed sites; and a screening neurologic examination for gross cognitive or focal motor deficits.

LABORATORY TESTING

- Laboratory tests are generally useful only when guided by the history and physical examination.
- Studies have shown that at least half of all "fever workups" in postoperative patients are unnecessary and do not benefit the patient.
- If a patient with fever in the first 48 h after surgery appears generally well and the history and physical examination do not identify a specific concern, it is reasonable to follow the patient with periodic reevaluation and not to obtain laboratory tests.
- Many studies have shown that blood cultures are grossly overutilized in this situation. Restrict their use to patients with suspected bacteremia; for example, those with additional evidence of infection or with sepsis syndrome including hypotension, tachycardia, unexplained hypoxemia, or delirium.
- Imaging studies should also be ordered judiciously. Chest radiography has a low yield if the findings on chest auscultation and the sputum quantity and quality are normal. Conversely, CT of the abdomen and pelvis can detect occult intraabdominal infection, hematoma, and thrombosis, so the threshold for obtaining CT should be relatively low in patients who develop fevers more than 3 days after pelvic or abdominal surgery.

TREATMENT

EMPIRIC TREATMENT

- In general, reserve empiric antibiotic treatment for patients who are likely to have a serious infection and direct treatment at the most likely pathogens (for example at gram-negative and anaerobic bacteria for suspected intraabdominal abscess). Broadly treat any patient with possible septic shock with antimicrobial therapy, but carefully consider, with surgical consultation, the need for reoperation.

SURGERY-SPECIFIC APPROACH

- In addition to the general considerations above, consider specific causes of fever based on the type of surgery.

CARDIOTHORACIC

- ◦ Careful assessment of the sternal wound is mandatory. Risk factors for sternal wound infection include emergent surgery, longer surgery, internal mammary artery grafting, diabetes, renal failure, and smoking.[8] Evidence of inflammation or instability should prompt imaging or reexploration to assess for mediastinitis and sternal osteomyelitis.
- ◦ Maintain a high index of suspicion for infective endocarditis with *Staphylococcus aureus* and coagulase-negative staphylococci after heart valve surgery.

NEUROSURGERY

- ◦ Bacterial meningitis can be difficult to differentiate from chemical meningitis caused by meningeal irritation from surgery and hemolyzed blood. Both can produce headache, photophobia, and nuchal rigidity. In a series of 70 patients, chemical meningitis was

infrequent after spinal or sinus surgery and was rarely associated with cerebrospinal fluid (CSF) rhinorrhea or otorrhea or a temperature above 39.4°C (102.9°F).[9] Furthermore, chemical meningitis was not associated with an inflamed or purulent surgical site, delirium, seizure, coma, a CSF white blood cell count (WBC) above 7500/µL, or with a CSF glucose below 10 mg/dL. Of the 70 patients studied, 30 were diagnosed with chemical meningitis and did not receive antibiotic. Patients who do require empiric antibiotic treatment for suspected bacterial meningitis after neurosurgery should receive agents directed against *S. aureus* (e.g., vancomycin) and hospital-acquired gram-negative bacilli, including *Pseudomonas aeruginosa* (e.g., ceftazidime plus or minus an aminoglycoside).
- Venous thromboembolism is common after neurosurgery due to limited patient mobility and less aggressive anticoagulation to avoid surgical site hemorrhage.

VASCULAR

- Vascular graft infections can be difficult to diagnose. They are more common after inguinal and upper leg surgeries. Scanning with CT, magnetic resonance imaging (MRI), or radiolabeled white blood cells can be helpful, but unrevealing images do not rule out infection. CT can identify fluid collections for aspiration and is usually the best initial test.
- Low-grade fevers can also be caused by peripheral ischemia due to sterile arterial emboli from atherosclerotic plaque broken off during the procedure.

ABDOMINAL

- Consider peritonitis (early) and intraabdominal abscess (later) when fever occurs after abdominal surgery. CT is useful in making the diagnosis, but keep in mind the possibility of an early false-negative result.
- Investigators have proposed three indicators of postoperative abdominal infection.[10]
  - A WBC below 5000 or above 10,000/µL
  - Blood urea nitrogen above 15 mg/dL
  - Fever onset after postoperative day 2
- Pancreatitis can cause fever, is more likely after upper abdominal surgeries, and is usually manifest by vomiting in association with epigastric or back pain.

OBSTETRIC AND GYNECOLOGIC

- Endometritis, cellulitis, and UTI are usually manifest by purulent vaginal discharge, skin inflammation, and dysuria, respectively.
- If no localizing physical findings are present, fever in the first 2 days after surgery does not require further testing or empiric antibiotic treatment as long as the patient is periodically reevaluated.
- For persistent fevers, consider pelvic suppurative thrombophlebitis in addition to abdominal and pelvic abscesses, especially after cesarean delivery. Diagnosis is often difficult and imaging with either CT or MRI can be helpful. Treatment is with broad-spectrum antibiotics and heparin, although the latter remains controversial.

ORTHOPEDIC

- Early prosthetic joint infections are usually caused by virulent organisms, most often *S. aureus*. Joint aspiration is necessary to confirm the diagnosis.

Venous thromboembolic disease is relatively common, even with optimal DVT prophylaxis.

SOLID-ORGAN TRANSPLANTATION

- The timing of the fever after solid-organ transplantation largely dictates the most common infectious causes.
  - In the initial weeks after transplantation, usual bacterial infections such as surgical site infections, UTIs, and pneumonia predominate, along with reactivation of herpes simplex virus.
  - From 1 month until 6 months posttransplant is a period of high risk for opportunistic pathogens, including cytomegalovirus, fungi (e.g., *Aspergillus* and *Candida*), *Toxoplasma, Pneumocystis,* and *Nocardia*.
- Noninfectious causes of fever are also common. These include drug reactions, organ rejection (particularly after lung transplantation), and lymphoproliferative disease.

REFERENCES

1. Mackowiak PA. Temperature regulation and the pathogenesis of fever, in Mandell GL, Bennett JE, Dolin R (eds). *Principles and Practice of Infectious Diseases,* 6th ed. Philadelphia: Elsevier, 2005:707.
2. Dellinger EP. Approach to the patient with postoperative fever, in Gorbach SL, Bartlett JG, Blacklow NR (eds). *Infectious Diseases,* 3rd ed. Philadelphia: Lippincott Williams & Wilkins, 2004:817.
3. Freischlag J, Busuttil RW. The value of postoperative fever evaluation. *Surgery* 94:358, 1983.
4. Lim E, Motalleb-Zadeh R, Wallard M, et al. Pyrexia after cardiac surgery: Natural history and association with infection. *J Thorac Cardiovasc Surg* 126:1013, 2003.
5. De la Torre SH, Mandel L, Goff BA. Evaluation of postoperative fever: Usefulness and cost-effectiveness of routine workup. *Am J Obstet Gynecol* 188:1642, 2003.
6. Shaw JA, Chung R. Febrile response after knee and hip arthroplasty. *Clin Orthop Rel Res* 367:181, 1999.

7. Engoren M. Lack of association between atelectasis and fever. *Chest* 107:81, 1995.
8. Weed HG, Baddour LM. Postoperative fever, in Rose BD (ed). *UpToDate.* Wellesley, MA: UpToDate, 2005.
9. Forgacs P, Geyer CA, Freidberg SR. Characterization of chemical meningitis after neurological surgery. *Clin Infect Dis* 32:179, 2001.
10. Mellors JW, Kelly JJ, Gusberg RJ, et al. A simple index to estimate the likelihood of bacterial infection in patients developing fever after abdominal surgery. *Am Surg* 54:558, 1988.
11. Garibaldi RA, Brodine S, Masumiya S, Colman M. Evidence for the non-infections etiology of early postoperative fever. *Infect Control* 6:273, 1985.

51 HYPERTENSION/ HYPOTENSION

Tariq Shafi and Steven L. Cohn

INTRODUCTION

- Hypertension affects almost one in three U.S. adults.
- As blood pressure control in the ambulatory setting is often suboptimal, a common request to clinicians caring for hospitalized patients is to assist in the management of patients with uncontrolled postoperative hypertension.
- This chapter reviews the causes of postoperative hypertension, contributing factors, and guidelines for management.

INCIDENCE

- The reported frequency of postoperative hypertension varies due to a lack of standard definition and criteria. The incidence ranges from 3 to 91 percent, depending on the definition of hypertension and the type of surgery (Table 51-1).

TABLE 51-1 Frequency of Postoperative Hypertension by Surgical Procedure

PROCEDURE	FREQUENCY OF POSTOPERATIVE HYPERTENSION (%)
Intracranial neurosurgery	57–91
Abdominal aortic surgery	33–75
Carotid endarterectomy	9–64
Cardiac surgery	22–54
Release of flexion contractures	46
Radical neck dissection	10–20
Elective general surgery	3–20

SOURCE: Modified from Kaplan,[4] with permission.

RISK FACTORS

- A history of severe uncontrolled hypertension predicts postoperative hypertension more reliably than the blood pressure (BP) just before surgery ("admit BP").[1] Elevated admit BP can be due to anxiety, rebound from discontinued medications, or the "white coat" effect.
- Patients with a prior history of diastolic BP >110 mmHg are prone to have elevated BP in the postoperative period.
  - Patients with uncontrolled hypertension in general tend to experience more perioperative BP lability than nonhypertensive patients or those with controlled hypertension. The presence of antihypertensive medication "on board" may decrease this lability to some degree.
- The risk of postoperative hypertension is greatest after vascular procedures, including peripheral vascular surgeries and aortic aneurysm resections.[1]
  - Patients more frequently receive intravenous fluid challenges during vascular procedures than during other surgeries.
  - Renal blood flow is decreased during vascular procedures.
  - It is likely that this combination of salt and water overload combined with decreased renal perfusion may contribute to the elevation of the BP after vascular surgeries.

TIMING AND CAUSES

- Perioperative hypertension can occur at various times:
  - Preoperative: upon admission to the hospital or upon entry to the operating room.
  - Intraoperative: during induction and intubation, after surgical manipulation, or with extubation.
  - Postoperative: early, in the recovery room, or later, (24 to 48 h) in the postoperative period.
- The causes of postoperative hypertension differ based on timing after surgery[2,3] (Fig. 51-1).

IMMEDIATE POSTOPERATIVE PERIOD

- Reversal of anesthesia reduces the vasodilatory effect of the anesthetic agents. The resulting increase in peripheral vascular resistance combined with volume overload from intraoperative intravenous fluids leads to elevation of the BP.
- Postoperative pain, hypothermia, shivering, and hypoxia induce sympathetic stimulation, which contributes to an increase in BP.

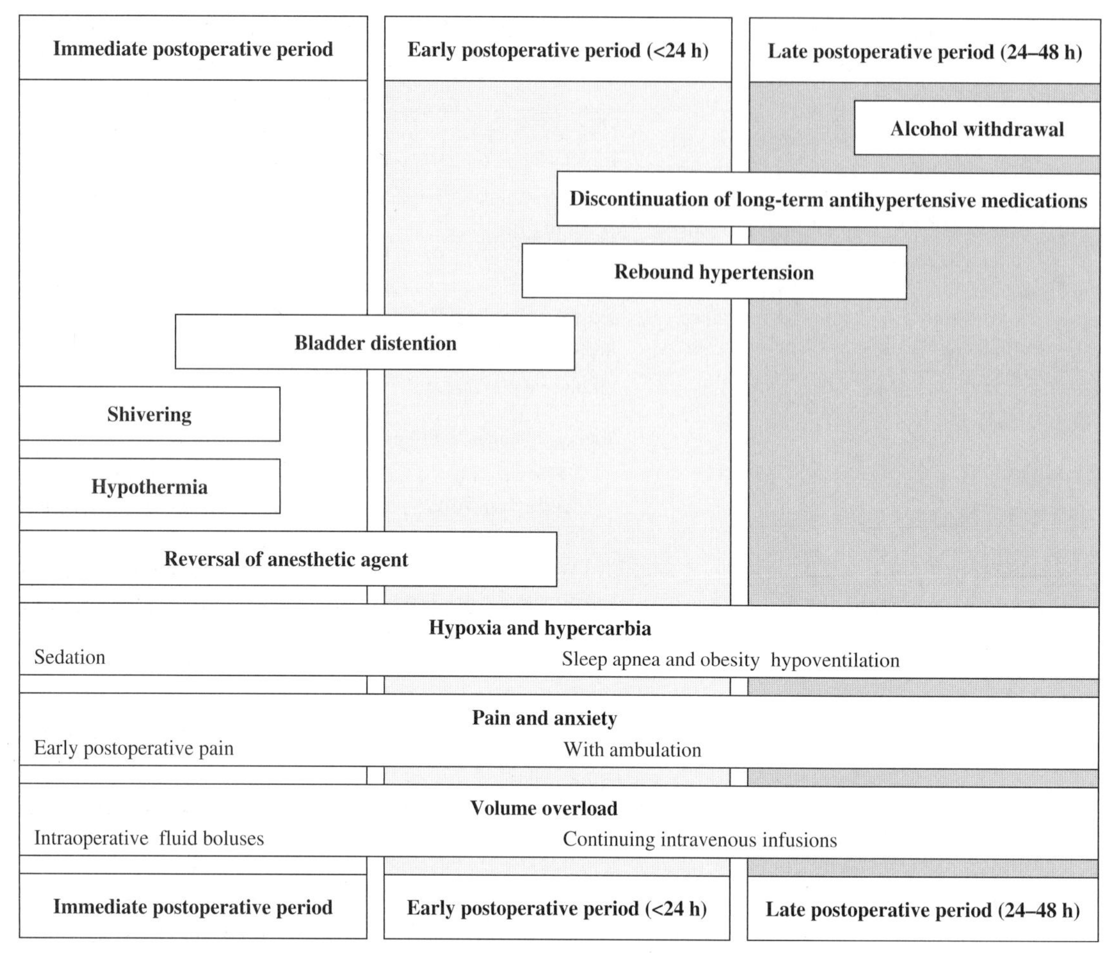

FIG. 51-1 Causes of postoperative hypertension based on time of occurrence.

EARLY POSTOPERATIVE PERIOD (<24 H)

- During this time, discontinuation of epidural anesthesia reduces peripheral vasodilation. This leads to a return of fluid into the central circulation and an elevation of BP.
- Rebound hypertension due to abrupt withdrawal of beta blockers and centrally acting sympatholytic agents (e.g., clonidine) contributes to uncontrolled hypertension. Patients on chronic therapy with both these classes of drugs are especially susceptible if the sympatholytic agent is withdrawn and the beta blocker is continued. The ensuing hyperadrenergic withdrawal state is similar to the pheochromocytoma crisis. Selective beta blockade with unopposed alpha-receptor stimulation by the circulating catecholamines can cause severe elevation of the BP.[4]
- Pain, hypercarbia, hypoxia, and bladder distention can all continue to contribute to the elevated BP.

LATE POSTOPERATIVE PERIOD (24 TO 48 H)

- Discontinuation of or failure to restart the patient's usual long-term antihypertensive medications may increase BP in the late postoperative period. This is especially important for patients who are unable to take medications orally.
- The effect of rebound hypertension can continue into the postoperative period. Hypoxia and poorly controlled pain are other contributing factors.
- Alcohol withdrawal and resulting sympathetic hyperactivity can complicate the recovery during this period, and worsen the hypertension.
- Narcotics for pain control may worsen sleep apnea, resulting in hypoxia, hypercarbia, and increased sympathetic activity, which can raise the BP.
- Continuing saline infusions lead to plasma volume expansion and the potential for worsening hypertension.

- Fluid shifts, particularly the volume that is "third spaced" during intraabdominal operations and now returns to the vascular space, can cause fluid overload and hypertension.

PRINCIPLES OF MANAGEMENT

- Continue most antihypertensive medications through the morning of surgery. This strategy decreases the risk of postoperative hypertension.
- Patients should take essentially all of their antihypertensive medications, with the possible exception of diuretics, with a sip of water on the morning of surgery (see Chap. 7).

ADAPTATION TO LONG-STANDING UNCONTROLLED HYPERTENSION

- Patients with long-standing uncontrolled hypertension adapt to chronic elevations of arterial pressure by the development of arteriolar hypertrophy. As a result, they are able to tolerate arterial pressures that would cause complications in a normotensive individual. This phenomenon, initially described for the cerebral circulation, occurs in other vascular beds as well.
- As a result, a patient with previously well-controlled hypertension in the range of 120/80 mmHg may be markedly symptomatic with an acute elevation of the BP to 180/110 mmHg. In this case, one should lower the BP relatively quickly to prevent acute target-organ injury and encephalopathy.
- On the other hand, a hypertensive individual with poor BP control prior to surgery may be completely asymptomatic at much higher pressures. In this circumstance, sudden lowering of the BP with short-acting agents can precipitate acute cerebral, renal, and myocardial ischemia.

BLOOD PRESSURE TREATMENT THRESHOLDS

- A threshold for treatment is difficult to define. The use of any absolute BP criterion (such as BP >180/110 mmHg) is fraught with the risk of overtreating certain individuals and undertreating others who may be at high risk for complications.
- In treating acute BP elevations, take into account the overall condition of the patient and baseline BP, rather than the level of the mercury column.
- Drug trials that have evaluated the efficacy of individual agents in the treatment of postoperative hypertension have either used a fixed threshold (e.g., systolic BP >160 mmHg, diastolic BP >90 mmHg, or mean BP >110 mmHg) or a relative change from baseline (e.g., an increase in systolic BP or diastolic BP >20%).[3]
- However, investigators designed most of these trials to compare the BP-lowering efficacy of a newer agent compared to an older established drug rather than to determine an optimal treatment threshold.
- Studies of intraoperative changes in the BP demonstrate an increase in the postoperative cardiac and renal complications, with a 20 percent change in the mean BP compared to the preoperative level.[5]
- In the absence of level-one evidence, the goal of treatment should be to maintain the BP within 20 percent of the preoperative BP level. Initiate treatment if the postoperative BP is >20 percent above the preoperative BP level.
- When acute BP lowering is necessary, do not acutely lower the mean arterial pressure by more than 20 percent or to less than 160/100 mmHg.

PATIENT EVALUATION AND DECISION MAKING

- All patients with elevated postoperative BP must undergo a careful evaluation to determine whether an urgent or emergent situation is present.
- The key to initiating or intensifying treatment is the presence and severity of target-organ damage, such as encephalopathy, retinal hemorrhages or exudates, papilledema, worsening renal failure, pulmonary edema, and chest pain.
- Progressive target-organ damage indicates a hypertensive emergency. Patients at excessive risk of hemorrhage from suture lines and vascular anastomoses also have hypertensive emergencies. These patients will need treatment in an intensive care unit with parenteral antihypertensive agents. A number of short-acting antihypertensive agents are available for this purpose (Table 51-2).
- If a hypertensive emergency is not present, evaluate the likely etiology of the hypertension and reverse any precipitating factors before resorting to antihypertensive medications.
  - Treat pain, hypervolemia, hypercarbia, and hypothermia.
  - In elderly men, make sure that bladder distention is not present.
  - Restart the patient's usual antihypertensive medications. If this is not possible because the patient is taking nothing by mouth, consider parenteral alternatives.
- Figure 51-2 provides a suggested algorithm for the management of postoperative hypertension.

TABLE 51-2 Short-Acting Antihypertensive Agents

DRUG	DOSE	EFFECT	COMMENTS
Sodium nitroprusside	Initial: 0.25 μg/kg/min Titrate: Double dose every 5 min Max: 10 μg/kg/min	Onset: 30 s –2 min Duration: 1–3 min.	Coronary steal Cyanide/thiocyanide toxicity with prolonged infusion, renal insufficiency, high infusion rate Reflex tachycardia ↑ Intracranial pressure
Nitroglycerin	Initial: 5–10 μg/min Titrate: 5–10 μg/min every 3–5 min. If no response at 20 μg/min, titrate by 10–20 μg/min Max: 100 μg/min	Onset: 2–5 min Duration: 3–5 min	Coronary vasodilatation Tolerance with prolonged use Can ↑ intracranial pressure
Hydralazine	Initial: 10 mg IV bolus over 3–5 min, increase 5–10 mg every 20–30 min Usual dose: 10–20 mg IV every 4–6 h Max: 50 mg IV per dose	Onset: 10–20 min Duration: Unpredictable, 3–8 h	Reflex tachycardia Safe in pregnancy
Nicardipine	Initial: 5 mg/h Titrate: 1–2.5 mg/h every 5–15 min Max: 15 mg/h	Onset: 5–10 min Duration: 1–4 h	Long elimination half-life Phlebitis at IV site Reduced cerebral vasospasm in subarachnoid hemorrhage
Enalaprilat	Initial: 0.625–1.25 mg IV every 6 h Titrate: Double dose every 6 h Max: 5 mg every 6 h	Onset: 15–30 min Duration: 6 h	Long residual effect First-dose hypotension with volume depletion May reset cerebral blood flow autoregulation
Fenoldopam	Initial: 0.1 μg/kg/min (or 0.03–0.1 μg/kg/min) Titrate: 0.05–0.1 μg/kg/min every 15–20 min Max: 1.6 μg/kg/min	Onset: 5–15 min Duration: 10–15 min	↑ Renal blood flow and natriuresis No coronary steal Can transiently ↑ intracranial pressure Can be used safely in renal failure Infusion can be abruptly discontinued
Esmolol	Initial: Bolus 500 μg/kg IV for 1 min, followed by 25–100 μg/kg/min for 4 min Titrate: Repeat bolus if inadequate response after 5 min, ↑ rate in increment of 50 μg/kg/min to max of 300 μg/kg/min	Onset: 1–2 min Duration: 10–20 min	Rapid, controllable onset Short duration Easily titratable
Labetalol (IV)	Initial: Bolus 20 mg IV over 2 min Titrate: Repeat bolus dose of 40–80 mg every 10–15 min up to max of 300 mg Infusion: 0.5–2.0 mg/min	Onset: 5–10 min Duration: 3–6 h	Does not ↑ intracranial pressure Prolonged action Not easily titratable
Clonidine (Oral)	Initial: 0.1–0.2 mg PO every 1 h (max 0.6 mg) Usual dose: 0.2–1.2 mg/day PO in 2–4 divided doses Max: 2.4 mg/day	Onset: 30–60 minutes Duration: 6–10 h	• Prolonged unpredictable effect • Rebound hypertension with abrupt cessation • Sedation, dry mouth, and bradycardia
Captopril (Oral)	Initial: 6.25 mg–12.5 mg Usual dose: 12.5–50 mg every 8 h Max: 450 mg/day	Onset: 10–15 min Duration: 4–6 h	• Long residual effect • First dose hypotension with volume depletion • May reset cerebral blood flow autoregulation
Labetalol (Oral)	Initial: 200–400 mg, repeat every 2–3 h Instructions post IV: 200 mg, followed in 6-12 h by 200 mg–400 mg; titrate at 1-day interval Max: Total dose 2.4 g/day divided BID or TID	Onset: 30 min–2 h Duration: 8–12 h	• Does not ↑ intracranial pressure • Prolonged action

SOURCE: Modified from Shafi,[8] with permission.

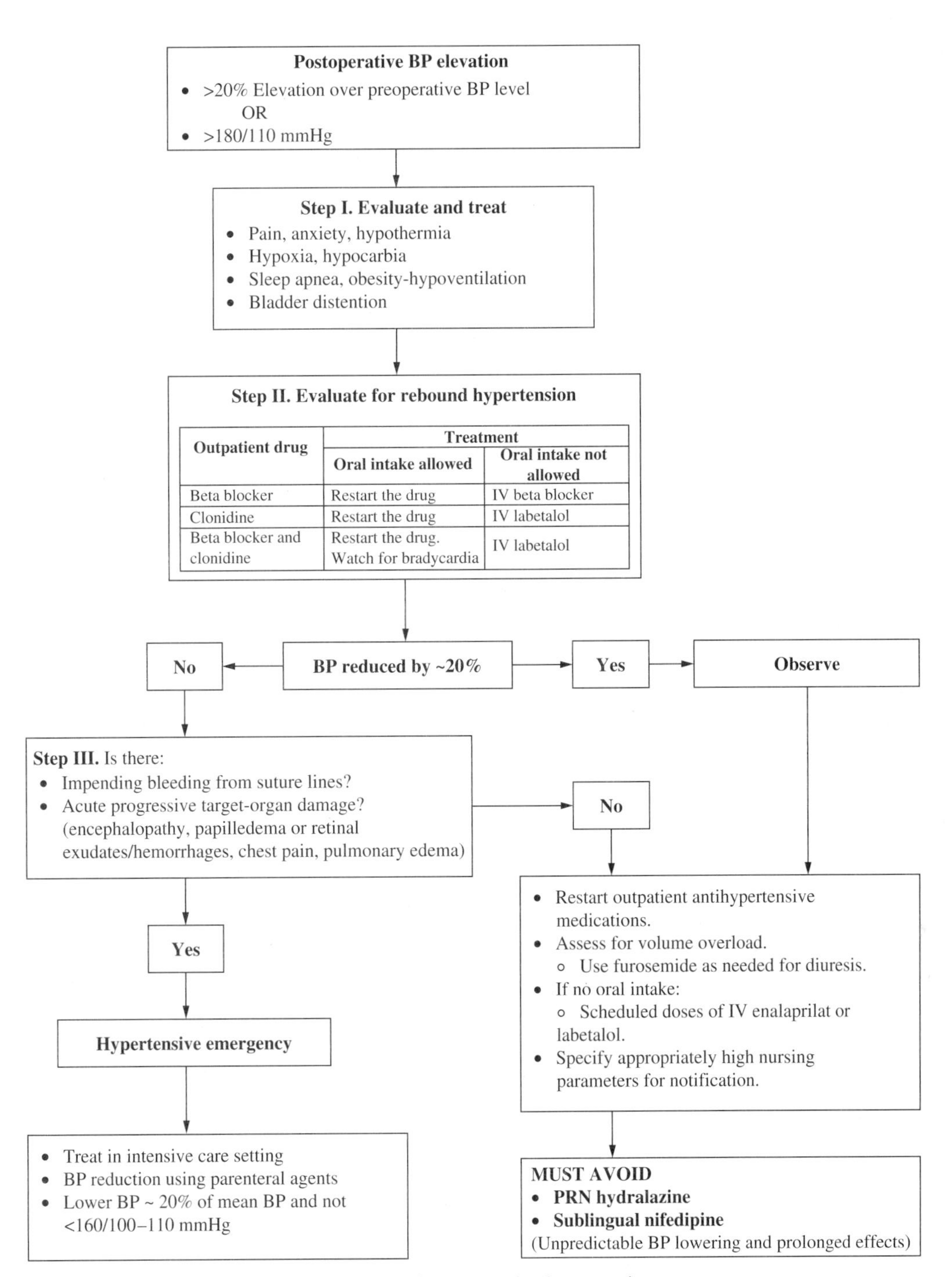

FIG. 51-2 Algorithm for the management of postoperative hypertension.

POSTOPERATIVE HYPOTENSION

- Postoperative hypotension is a predictor of postoperative cardiac complications in hypertensive patients.[6]
- The differential diagnosis for postoperative hypotension is extensive; a careful clinical evaluation is necessary to determine the underlying mechanism and specific etiology.

INTRAVASCULAR VOLUME DEPLETION

- Preoperative volume depletion may result from inadequate fluid intake, diuresis, or catecholamine excess in the patients with pheochromocytoma.
- Intraoperative hemorrhage can contribute to the volume depletion.
- Postoperatively, inadequate volume replacement, surgical site bleeding, and fever contribute to the fluid loss.

PERIPHERAL VASODILATION

- A decrease in peripheral resistance occurs with the administration of inhalational agents for induction of anesthesia.[1,7] This may occur with halothane, isoflurane, desflurane, and sevoflurane.[2] Anesthesiologists use the vasodilatory action of these agents to control BP surges intraoperatively.
- Spinal anesthesia causes peripheral vasodilatation, leading to peripheral pooling of the blood.

MYOCARDIAL DEPRESSION

- Myocardial ischemia reduces myocardial contractility.
- Inhalational anesthetic agents also reduce myocardial contractility by about 25 percent.[7]

OTHER CAUSES

- A variety of other conditions can cause postoperative hypotension. These include sepsis, pulmonary embolism, gastrointestinal hemorrhage, anaphylactoid reactions to medications, and acute myocardial infarction.
- The stress of surgery may unmask preexisting adrenal insufficiency.

TREATMENT

- The underlying pathophysiology and etiology guide the treatment of postoperative hypotension.
- Fluid replacement will correct hypotension caused by volume depletion or vasodilation. Blood transfusions may be required in some patients with anemia and hypotension.
- If hypotension secondary to significantly reduced peripheral resistance does not respond to volume expansion, use vasopressors. If possible, adjust the level of anesthesia to reduce the peripheral vasodilation.
- Use inotropic agents (dopamine, dobutamine) to treat hypotension resulting from a decrease in myocardial contractility.

REFERENCES

1. Goldman L, Caldera DL. Risks of general anesthesia and elective operation in the hypertensive patient. *Anesthesiology* 50(4):285–292, 1979.
2. Weitz HH. Perioperative cardiac complications. *Med Clin North Am* 85(5):1151–1169, 2001.
3. Haas CE, LeBlanc JM. Acute postoperative hypertension: A review of therapeutic options. *Am J Health Syst Pharm* 61(16): 1661–1673, 2004; quiz 1674–1665.
4. Kaplan N. *Kaplan's Clinical Hypertension,* 8th ed. Philadelphia: Lippincott, Williams & Wilkins, 2002.
5. Charlson ME, MacKenzie CR, Gold JP, et al. Intraoperative blood pressure. What patterns identify patients at risk for postoperative complications? *Ann Surg* 212(5):567–580, 1990.
6. Charlson ME, MacKenzie CR, Gold JP, et al. Preoperative characteristics predicting intraoperative hypotension and hypertension among hypertensives and diabetics undergoing noncardiac surgery. *Ann Surg* 212(1):66–81, 1990.
7. Prys-Roberts C, Meloche R, Foex P. Studies of anaesthesia in relation to hypertension: I. Cardiovascular responses of treated and untreated patients. *Br J Anaesth* 43(2):122–137, 1971.
8. Shafi T. Hypertensive urgencies and emergencies. *Ethn Dis* 14(suppl 2):S32–S37, 2004.

52 CHEST PAIN AND DYSPNEA

*Shaun Frost and Ahsan M. Arozullah**

INTRODUCTION—THE PROBLEM

INCIDENCE

- Postoperative chest pain and dyspnea are common.
- Perioperative myocardial ischemia and postoperative myocardial infarction (PMI) generally occur among patients with known coronary artery disease or who are at risk for coronary artery disease.
- PMI is rare among patients who do not have known heart disease or risk factors for heart disease.
- Consider perioperative myocardial ischemia and infarction as ends of a continuum of myocardial injury. What distinguishes ischemia from infarction depends on variable criteria used for their definitions. Because of this variability, the precise incidence of perioperative myocardial ischemia and PMI is not known.

TIMING

- Perioperative myocardial ischemia and PMI occur most frequently during anesthesia recovery or shortly thereafter.[1] This time period is characterized by ischemia-provoking stimuli such as tachycardia, hypertension, sympathetic discharge, and hypercoagulability.

*Dr. Arozullah is supported as a Research Associate in the Advanced Career Development Award Program of the VA Health Services Research and Development Service.

- Perioperative myocardial injury increases the risk of early and late postoperative adverse cardiac outcomes and death.

CAUSES

- The etiology of chest pain and dyspnea that occurs following surgery is similar to that of chest pain and dyspnea occurring in other settings.
- The exact etiology of perioperative myocardial ischemia and PMI is controversial.
- Autopsy studies of patients suffering fatal PMI have found evidence of plaque disruption and thrombosis involving the coronary artery supplying the infarct area. These findings are similar to those of autopsies after myocardial infarction in nonsurgical settings, suggesting that PMI and nonoperative myocardial infarction occur by similar mechanisms.[2]
- Angiographic studies of survivors of PMI suggest that infarction is due to inadequate collateralization around total occlusions rather than abrupt closure of high-grade stenoses. Angiography conducted within days following PMI has often failed to find evidence of vessel thrombosis or plaque rupture.[2] Most PMIs are non-ST-segment elevation and non-Q-wave events. These observations suggest that PMI results from prolonged myocardial ischemia due to a mismatch of oxygen supply and demand rather than acute plaque rupture and coronary artery thrombosis.
- The perioperative stresses underlying the mismatch of coronary artery oxygen supply and demand may also produce a physiologic milieu capable of destabilizing atherosclerotic plaque, leading to coronary artery thrombosis. Identifying the exact mechanism of PMI therefore may be less important than identifying and managing the perioperative stresses that lead to myocardial injury (Table 52-1).

TABLE 52-1 Perioperative Stresses That Precipitate Myocardial Ischemia and Infarction

Adrenocorticotropic hormone release
Catecholamine release
Alterations in arachidonic acid metabolism
Tachycardia
Blood loss
Fluid shifts
Hypertension
Hypotension
Hypothermia
Hyperthermia
Platelet activation
Coagulation abnormalities
Alterations in pulmonary function
Alterations in sleep patterns
Alterations in pain perception

DIAGNOSIS

DIFFERENTIAL DIAGNOSIS

- The causes of chest pain and dyspnea following surgery (Table 52-2) are similar to those in nonsurgical settings.
- Clinical findings among patients with perioperative pulmonary embolism include sudden hypoxemia, sinus tachycardia, and lower extremity edema (see Chap. 55). Lung fields are usually clear on auscultation; however, rales associated with perioperative atelectasis may create diagnostic confusion.
- Dyspnea, fever, and occasional pleuritic chest pain are symptoms of perioperative pneumonia (see Chap. 54). Lung auscultation frequently reveals rales or signs of consolidation.
- Postoperative cardiac arrhythmia may be associated with chest pain, palpitations, pulmonary edema, or syncope (see Chap. 53).
- Consider nonthoracic sources of chest pain. Gastroesophageal reflux occurs frequently following surgery. Pancreatitis and biliary pathology may occur from trauma sustained during intraabdominal procedures. Peptic ulcer disease may develop among patients subjected to significant postoperative stresses, such as prolonged mechanical ventilation and coagulopathy. Orthopedic procedures on the spine and shoulders may result in chest pain referred from these sites.

TABLE 52-2 Differential Diagnosis of Postoperative Chest Pain and Dyspnea

Myocardial infarction
Myocardial ischemia
Pulmonary embolism
Tachyarrhythmia
Pneumonia
Bronchospasm
Pneumothorax
Pericarditis
Chest wound infection
Gastroesophageal reflux
Peptic ulcer disease
Pancreatitis
Biliary pathology
Musculoskeletal disorders

- Myocardial ischemia and infarction can cause chest pain and dyspnea following noncardiac surgery and can lead to significant morbidity and mortality. A number of investigations have evaluated testing and monitoring strategies to assist in diagnosing perioperative myocardial ischemia and infarction.

MYOCARDIAL ISCHEMIA AND INFARCTION

- The diagnostic criteria for postoperative myocardial ischemia and infarction vary among research studies. Accordingly, reported rates of PMI among patients at elevated risk undergoing major noncardiac surgery range between 1 and 26 percent, while rates of myocardial ischemia range between 15 and 41 percent.
- Most PMIs occur within the first 48 h after surgery.[1]
- PMI is rare among patients who do not have known heart disease or risk factors for heart disease.

SYMPTOMS AND SIGNS

- Symptoms and signs of perioperative myocardial ischemia and infarction are identical to those resulting from myocardial ischemia and infarction in nonsurgical settings. However, anesthesia, analgesia, and competing somatic stimuli likely alter the normal perception of symptoms and the physiologic manifestations of myocardial injury. For example, postsurgical patients have a higher incidence of painless myocardial infarction than do nonsurgical patients.
- Some 55 to 85 percent of patients with PMI experience at least one sign or symptom, while 15 to 60 percent complain of chest pain.
- Some 84 to 97 percent of perioperative ischemic episodes diagnosed by continuous electrocardiogram (ECG) monitoring occur without symptoms.[3–5]
- Of postoperative ischemic episodes diagnosed by continuous ECG monitoring, 80 percent occur without acute changes in heart rate.[4]
- Of intraoperative ischemic episodes diagnosed by continuous ECG monitoring, 77 percent occur without acute changes in blood pressure.[4]
- Patients experiencing postoperative myocardial ischemia or infarction have significantly higher baseline heart rates than patients without these complications. Tachycardia is most common on postoperative days 1 and 2[5] and is an independent predictor of elevated postoperative levels of troponin T.[6]

LABORATORY TESTING

- ***Electrocardiographic features*** of perioperative myocardial ischemia and PMI:
  - Most PMIs are non-ST-segment elevation and non-Q-wave events.
  - Postoperative episodes of ischemia detected by ECG are more frequent, more severe, and longer in duration than intraoperative episodes. This suggests that the stresses of anesthesia and surgery are less severe than stress experienced in the postoperative recovery period.[3–5]
  - Postoperative ECG evidence of ischemia is most common during the first 3 days after surgery. ECG evidence of ischemia occurring after postoperative day 3 ("late" ischemia) is rare among patients who do not exhibit ischemia prior to postoperative day 3 ("early" ischemia). The relative risk of late ischemia after early ischemia is 8.5.[5] This suggests that monitoring for ischemia beyond postoperative day 3 may be necessary only among patients who demonstrate ischemia earlier in their postoperative recoveries.
  - Obtaining ECGs preoperatively, immediately postoperatively, and on the first 2 postoperative days appears to be cost-effective for high-risk patients.[7]
  - Postoperative ST-segment changes suggestive of ischemia are harbingers of future myocardial infarction and adverse cardiac outcomes. Some 85 to 100 percent of patients who develop either PMI or unstable angina have ECG evidence of transient ischemia preceding these events.[3,5] Furthermore, patients with postoperative myocardial ischemia have a 2.2-fold increase in the rate of subsequent cardiac complications over the 2 years following surgery.[8] Patients with ECG-detected postoperative ischemia warrant aggressive follow-up, including postoperative cardiac risk stratification and/or treatments to modify cardiac risk.
  - Recognize that ST-segment changes do not always indicate ischemia. Nonspecific perioperative ECG changes may result from a variety of factors such as alterations in blood pressure and temperature, fluid shifts, position changes, fluctuating serum electrolyte concentrations, and drug administration.
- ***Biochemical evidence*** of myocardial injury is common:
  - Concentrations of troponin T (TnT) and troponin I (TnI) are sensitive and specific markers of perioperative myocardial injury. Creatine kinase is a nonspecific marker of myocardial injury among postoperative patients and is less diagnostically useful than troponin measurement.
  - Troponin elevation is most likely to occur prior to postoperative day 3.
  - Postoperative elevation of troponin is associated with early and late adverse outcomes. Compared to patients without elevated TnT concentrations, elderly patients with postoperative TnT levels >0.02 ng/mL are 10 times more likely to die within 30 days of surgery and 15 times more likely to die within 1 year of surgery.[6]
  - There is a "dose-response" effect between increasing troponin levels and adverse outcomes, including

risk for future death. For example, in one investigation, the odds ratio for death 6 months following surgery was 1.3 [95 percent confidence interval (CI) 0.4 to 4.4] for TnI between 0.4 and 1.5 ng/mL, 4.3 (95 percent CI 0.8 to 24.3) for TnI between 1.6 and 3.0 ng/mL, and 4.9 (95 percent CI 1.9 to 19) for TnI greater than 3.0 ng/mL.[9]
  - In the absence of clinical, ECG, or hemodynamic evidence of acute myocardial ischemia or infarction, reserve the use of biochemical markers to screen for postoperative cardiac complications in patients at high risk who undergo major noncardiac procedures.[7]
- ***Transesophageal echocardiography*** (TEE) can demonstrate regional myocardial wall motion abnormalities indicative of intraoperative ischemia. Few studies have evaluated this strategy, but experience suggests that TEE adds little incremental value beyond routine operating room monitoring techniques for predicting significant cardiac complications.[7]
- ***Hemodynamic data*** collected by right heart catheterization (RHC) may not assist in diagnosing perioperative myocardial ischemia and infarction.
  - Observational studies indicate that the use of perioperative RHC is not associated with improved outcomes among patients undergoing major noncardiac surgery. To the contrary, RHC may be associated with prolonged hospitalization and significant postoperative complications, including pulmonary edema.[10]
  - Recent investigations suggest that maneuvers designed to intentionally increase cardiac index and oxygen delivery beyond normal parameters are not useful and may be harmful. In one randomized controlled investigation among high-risk surgery patients, RHC afforded no short- or long-term mortality benefit and was associated with a significantly higher incidence of pulmonary embolism.[11]
  - Patients who might benefit from monitoring by RHC include those with recent myocardial infarction and associated heart failure, those with known significant coronary artery disease undergoing surgery associated with significant hemodynamic stress, and those with significant valvular disease, cardiomyopathy, or left ventricular dysfunction undergoing high-risk surgery.[7]

TREATMENT

MYOCARDIAL ISCHEMIA AND INFARCTION

- After diagnosing myocardial ischemia or PMI, employ therapies that maximize oxygen delivery and the stabilization of coronary artery atherosclerotic plaque (Table 52-3).
- ***Pain control:*** Diligent postoperative pain control is necessary to minimize tachycardia and hypertension.

TABLE 52-3 Therapies for Perioperative Myocardial Ischemia and Infarction

Pain control
Oxygen
Aspirin
Beta-adrenergic blockade
Nitroglycerin
Heparin
Angiotensin-converting enzyme inhibitors
Statins
$Alpha_2$ adrenoreceptor agonists
Maintenance of normothermia
Urgent revascularization

Some studies suggest that pain control can reduce catecholamine surges and hypercoagulability. Opioids may also reduce the adhesion and migration of neutrophils and may be directly cardioprotective in patients susceptible to ischemia.
- Use *beta-adrenergic blockers* to treat PMI and ischemia in the same fashion as in the nonoperative setting. Beta blockers are also the cornerstone therapy for the prevention of perioperative myocardial ischemia and infarction among high-risk patients (see Chap. 20). If beta blockade is discontinued following hospital discharge, taper the dose gradually, as abrupt discontinuation increases the incidence of adverse cardiac events.
- ***$Alpha_2$-adrenoreceptor agonists*** such as clonidine also have cardioprotective effects among patients at risk for perioperative myocardial ischemia. This is likely related to sympatholytic effects. Consider $alpha_2$-adrenoreceptor agonists to treat perioperative myocardial ischemia and infarction when beta-adrenergic blockade is contraindicated.
- ***"Statins"*** (HMG-CoA reductase inhibitors commonly used to treat hyperlipidemia) may be cardioprotective among high-risk patients. Although further investigation is needed, strongly consider the use of these drugs among patients with perioperative myocardial ischemia and infarction.
- There is insufficient evidence to support the use of intraoperative nitroglycerin for the prevention of perioperative myocardial ischemia and infarction.[7] Consider nitroglycerin, however, in the treatment of PMI in the same fashion as in the treatment of nonoperative myocardial infarction.
- Maintenance of normothermia may reduce the incidence of adverse perioperative cardiovascular events.
- Unless strongly contraindicated, employ other routine therapies for myocardial ischemia and infarction (i.e., aspirin, heparin, angiotensin-converting enzyme inhibition, etc.).

- Consider angioplasty and emergent percutaneous therapy for patients suffering symptomatic ST-segment-elevation PMI due to acute thrombotic coronary artery occlusion.[7]
- Survivors of PMI or unstable angina have a 14-fold increase in the incidence of adverse cardiac events within 2 years.[8] Hospital discharge planning should therefore include strategies to modify future risk, such as the initiation of preventive therapies, and plans for additional cardiac testing and/or cardiology consultation. Furthermore, the physician assuming primary care of the patient must be fully informed.

CONCLUSIONS

- The differential diagnosis for postoperative chest pain and dyspnea is large.
- Consider perioperative myocardial ischemia and infarction as ends of a continuum of myocardial injury. Even subtle signs of minimal injury (i.e., transient ST-segment depression on ECG or slight elevation of cardiac enzymes) predict higher rates of immediate and long-term cardiac morbidity.
- Closely survey high-risk patients who undergo major noncardiac surgery for cardiac injury. Consider surveillance strategies such as ECG monitoring, biochemical blood work analysis for troponin levels, or combinations of these tests.
- Promptly and thoroughly evaluate patients for cardiac disease who exhibit evidence of perioperative myocardial injury.

REFERENCES

1. Landesberg G. The pathophysiology of perioperative myocardial infarction: Facts and perspectives. *J Cardiothorac Vasc Anesth* 17:90–100, 2003.
2. Priebe H. Triggers of perioperative myocardial ischemia and infarction. *Br J Anesthesiol* 93:9–20, 2004.
3. Mangano D, Browner W, Hollenberg M, et al. Association of perioperative myocardial ischemia with cardiac morbidity and mortality in men undergoing noncardiac surgery. *N Engl J Med* 323:1781–1788, 1990.
4. Mangano D, Hollenberg M, Fegert G, et al. Perioperative myocardial ischemia in patients undergoing noncardiac surgery: I. Incidence and severity during the 4 day perioperative period. *J Am Coll Cardiol* 17:843–850, 1991.
5. Mangano D, Wong M, London M, et al. Perioperative myocardial ischemia in patients undergoing noncardiac surgery: II. Incidence and severity during the 1st week after surgery. *J Am Coll Cardiol* 17:851–857, 1991.
6. Oscarsson A, Eintrei C, Anskar S, et al. Troponin T values provide long term prognosis in elderly patients undergoing non-cardiac surgery. *Acta Anaesthesiol Scand* 48:1071–1079, 2004.
7. Eagle K, Berger P, Calkins H, et al. American College of Cardiology/American Heart Association guideline update for perioperative cardiovascular evaluation for noncardiac surgery—executive summary: A report of the American College of Cardiology/American Heart Association Task Force on Practice Guidelines (Committee to update the 1996 guidelines on perioperative cardiovascular evaluation for noncardiac surgery). *Circulation* 39:542–553, 2002.
8. Mangano D, Browner W, Hollenberg M, et al. Long term cardiac prognosis following noncardiac surgery. *JAMA* 268: 233–239, 1992.
9. Kim L, Martinez E, Faraday N, et al. Cardiac troponin I predicts short term mortality in vascular surgery patients. *Circulation* 106:2366–2371, 2002.
10. Polancyk C, Rhode L, Goldman L, et al. Right heart catheterization and cardiac complications in patients undergoing noncardiac surgery. An observational study. *JAMA* 286:309–314, 2001.
11. Sandham J, Hull R, Brandt R, et al. A randomized, controlled trial of the use of pulmonary artery catheters in high risk surgical patients. *N Engl J Med* 348:5–14, 2003.

53 ARRHYTHMIAS

Seth McClennen and Peter J. Zimetbaum

INTRODUCTION

- Postoperative arrhythmias are common, especially after open cardiac surgery. Various patient- and surgery-related factors increase the risk of postoperative arrhythmia (see Chap. 23).

INCIDENCE

- A prospective cohort study of 4181 patients undergoing nonemergent noncardiac surgery found a rate of postoperative supraventricular arrhythmia of 6.1 percent.[1]
- The incidence of postoperative supraventricular arrhythmias after open heart surgery, specifically atrial fibrillation (AF), is especially high. One large meta-analysis estimated the incidence of postoperative AF after coronary artery bypass surgery (CABG) to be 27 percent.[2]
- Postoperative AF after valvular heart surgery is even more common with an incidence between 35 and 50 percent in various studies.[3]

- Postoperative bradyarrhythmias are frequently encountered, most often after valvular heart surgery. In most studies, the incidence varies from 1 percent after CABG to up to 10 percent in patients undergoing aortic valve replacement. Higher rates have been reported after tricuspid valve surgery and multiple-valve surgery.
- A large prospective observational study of more than 10,000 patients undergoing both CABG and valvular heart surgery showed the following odds ratios (OR) and 95 percent confidence intervals (CI) for the risk of receiving a permanent pacemaker during the index hospitalization for each of the following valve replacements[4]:
  Aortic: OR 5.8, CI 3.9 to 8.7
  Mitral: OR 4.9, CI 3.1 to 7.8
  Tricuspid: OR 8.0, CI 5.5 to 11.9
  Double: OR 8.9, CI 5.5 to 14.6
  Triple: OR 7.5, CI 2.9 to 19.3
- Postoperative bradyarrhythmias may also be secondary to vagal reflex in ophthalmologic surgery, spinal anesthesia, and intrascalene block or secondary to endotracheal suctioning in the intubated patient.

TIMING

- The incidence of postoperative AF peaks on postoperative days 2 to 4.[5]
- Postoperative heart block is usually recognized in the immediate postoperative state. It may resolve up to 10 days after the surgery.
- Right-bundle-branch block is the most commonly diagnosed conduction delay after open heart surgery; this is usually recognized in the immediate postoperative state.
- Reentrant supraventricular arrhythmias, such as atrioventricular (AV) nodal reentrant tachycardia, can occur at any time in the postoperative period due to elevated levels of circulating catecholamine.

CAUSES

- ***Mechanical disruption:*** During open cardiac surgery, mechanical disruption of conducting tissue is a major factor in the development of postoperative arrhythmias.
  1. ***Atrial fibrillation:*** Facilitated by high left atrial pressures and mechanical disruption of organized atrial contraction.
  2. ***Complete heart block:*** Often secondary to inadvertent direct surgical injury to the AV node or the His-Purkinje system.
- ***Electrolyte imbalance:*** Can facilitate arrhythmias due to direct effects at the cellular level that change action potential duration (e.g., potassium abnormalities) and hence change refractoriness of tissue.
- ***Hypoxemia/cardiac ischemia:*** Both pulmonary-mediated (e.g., postoperative acute lung injury) and locally mediated (e.g., inadequate local perfusion secondary to arterial vascular disease) impairment in myocardial oxygenation can facilitate arrhythmias in the postoperative state. Reperfusion of ventricular myocardium can also facilitate ventricular tachycardia (VT).
- ***Catecholamine excess:*** In the postoperative state, this can facilitate reentrant arrhythmias such as AV nodal reentrant tachycardia or scar-mediated VT. This is one rationale behind recommendations for aggressive use of perioperative beta blockers to reduce postoperative cardiac risk.

DIAGNOSIS

- For all tachyarrhythmias and bradyarrhythmias, adequate diagnosis and treatment require correct recognition of the rhythm. Therefore for *any* postoperative arrhythmia, clinicians should obtain a hard copy of the rhythm. Telemetry strips are helpful, but 12-lead rhythm strips or an electrocardiogram (ECG) is preferable.
  - Telemetry strips of arrhythmia onset/termination, if possible, can also help in the differential diagnosis.
- Underlying acute medical conditions that may provoke postoperative arrhythmia include pneumonia, pericarditis, pulmonary embolus, various vagal stimuli, and perioperative myocardial infarction.
  - Postoperative AF is very common; in the majority of cases an underlying primary initiating medical condition is not present. However, a routine chest x-ray (to rule out congestive heart failure and occult pneumonia), thyroid function tests, and assessment of left ventricular function (if not available preoperatively) are reasonable. Postoperative AF is usually *not* an ischemic rhythm.
  - Consider drug and alcohol withdrawal in cases of unexplained sinus tachycardia.
  - Postoperative VT is a possible manifestation of acute myocardial ischemia and should initiate a workup including serial cardiac enzymes, ECGs, and possible cardiac catheterization (if myocardial injury is detected or VT is recurrent or incessant).
  - Postoperative bradyarrhythmias should prompt a search for possible vagal contributors, especially in cases where the atrial rate is slow. Common

postoperative vagal stimuli include endotracheal tube suctioning, bronchoscopy, pain, medicines, and spinal anesthetics.

DIFFERENTIAL DIAGNOSIS (SEE TABLES 53-1 AND 53-2)

PHYSICAL FINDINGS

- Perform a cardiac and pulmonary examination to evaluate for possible primary etiologies of arrhythmia.
  1. The jugular venous pressure waveform can be abnormal in any rhythm with AV dissociation (VT, heart block).
  2. Carefully examine the patient with postoperative arrhythmia for signs of congestive heart failure, such as a third heart sound, peripheral edema, or elevated central venous pressure.

LABORATORY TESTING

- Obtain a 12-lead ECG for any newly recognized cardiac arrhythmia if permitted by hemodynamic stability.
- Review telemetry and record the onset and termination of any paroxysmal arrhythmia.
- Obtain an electrolyte panel (including potassium, calcium, and magnesium) for any new atrial or ventricular arrhythmias.
- Measure serum thyroid-stimulating hormone (TSH) for new onset atrial fibrillation or flutter.
- Obtain a chest X-ray to rule out an underlying primary pulmonary abnormality.

TREATMENT

- The treatment of postoperative arrhythmias includes direct therapy (e.g., antiarrhythmic medications) and indirect therapy (e.g., treatment of underlying primary pathology that is triggering arrhythmia).
- Treatments for the arrhythmias discussed below are reviewed in Table 53-3.
- The management of benign postoperative arrhythmias—including atrial ectopy, ventricular ectopy, sinus bradycardia, and AV Wenckebach rhythm—is usually expectant.
- Sinus tachycardia is usually a secondary rhythm: its treatment should focus on the primary stimulus for the tachycardia. Common stimuli include pain, anxiety, occult hypovolemia, infection, hypoxia, hypercarbia, alcohol withdrawal, anemia, and congestive heart failure.
- Atrial fibrillation is the most commonly encountered postoperative arrhythmia. Management consists of the following:
  - ***Rate control:*** This is usually the initial approach. Spontaneous conversion rates up to 30 percent have been reported.[6,7] Commonly employed medications

TABLE 53-1 Differential Diagnosis of Postoperative Arrhythmias: Tachycardia and Ectopy

RHYTHM	TELEMETRY/ECG FINDINGS	CLINICAL PEARLS
Sinus tachycardia	Sinus mechanism on electrocardiogram (ECG)	Gradual increase in rate.
Atrial/ventricular (AV) ectopy	Sporadic rhythm with either interpolated beats or subsequent pauses after ectopic beats	Wide-complex ectopy may represent either ventricular beats or aberrantly conducted supraventricular beats.
Atrial fibrillation (AF)	Irregular ventricular rhythm with undulating fibrillatory baseline	Can be regularized at faster rates or in patients on digoxin.
Atrial flutter	Regular or irregular ventricular response, with underlying regular "sawtooth" ECG pattern	Atrial fibrillation may organize into atrial flutter after administration of antiarrhythmic medications.
Reentrant supraventricular tachycardias (AV–nodal reentrant tachycardia and bypass tract tachycardia)	Acute onset and termination. Regular, fixed P-R interval (P waves may not be readily evident)	Both may occur in the high-catecholamine postoperative state.
Ectopic atrial tachycardia	Acute onset and termination. Regular, fixed P-R interval	Will never terminate with a P wave alone.
Multifocal atrial tachycardia	Multiple (at least three) P-wave morphologies with varying P-R interval	Often degenerates to AF in the postoperative state.
Nonsustained ventricular tachycardia (VT)	Three or more beats of ventricular origin, monomorphic or polymorphic	
Sustained wide-complex tachycardia	Regular or irregular rhythm with QRS duration over 120 ms	Consider and treat as VT until proven otherwise.

TABLE 53-2 Differential Diagnosis of Postoperative Arrhythmias: Bradycardia, Conduction Disturbances, and Heart Block

RHYTHM	TELEMETRY/ECG FINDINGS	CLINICAL PEARLS
Sinus node dysfunction	Regular or irregular bradycardia with sinus mechanism	Slowest rates often noted during sleep and at night.
AV Wenckebach	Fixed atrial rate with varying P-R interval. "Regularly irregular" ventricular rhythm with group beating	Often noted during sleep and at night, usually with slow (<75 bpm) atrial rate.
Junctional rhythm	Bradycardia with narrow-complex ventricular rhythm, no obvious P waves	Regular rhythm. Retrograde P waves or simultaneous antegrade P waves may be "buried" in the QRS complex.
New bundle-branch block (left or right)	Typical left or right bundle pattern on ECG	
High-grade or complete heart block	Regular ventricular rhythm with narrow- or wide-complex escape. Dissociated atrial rhythm usually noted	Lack of complete regularity rules out *complete* heart block. Fast atrial rates with block should suggest infranodal (His-Purkinje) disease.

TABLE 53-3 Treatment and Outcomes of Newly Diagnosed Postoperative Arrhythmias

ARRHYTHMIA	SPECIFIC RECOMMENDATIONS	OUTCOMES
Atrial/ventricular ectopy	Rule out electrolyte abnormalities. No treatment indicated.	May increase risk of subsequent sustained atrial and ventricular arrhythmias. Does not increase risk for myocardial infarction or death.
Sinus tachycardia	Rule out pain, anxiety, occult hypovolemia, infection, hypoxia, hypercarbia, alcohol withdrawal, anemia, congestive heart failure. Rate control is rarely indicated. Treat the underlying condition. If complications of tachycardia are suspected (e.g., congestive heart failure secondary to diastolic dysfunction), administer intravenous diltiazem or metoprolol.	Rates are slower after treatment of primary pathology (e.g., antipyretics for fever, transfusion for anemia, pain control, etc.).
Atrial fibrillation (AF)	Initially control rate with beta-blocking or calcium channel blocking agents. Administer digoxin if relative hypotension prevents administration of the above medications. Anticoagulate with heparin followed by warfarin if AF > 48 h duration if surgical bleeding risk is acceptable. Perform direct-current cardioversion (DCCV) if there is hemodynamic instability, severe symptoms, or contraindications to anticoagulation. Use biphasic defibrillators if available, as they achieve successful cardioversion with less energy. Place defibrillator pads in anteroposterior orientation, as shown in Fig. 53-1. Consider pharmacologic conversion with amiodarone: this is successful in 50 to 90% of cases. Consider ibutilide (conversion rate 30 to 40%), disopyramide, or propafenone in the conversion of post–cardiac surgery AF if amiodarone is contraindicated. Consider ibutilide pretreatment prior to electrical cardioversion. Continue antiarrhythmic medications for 4 to 6 weeks in patients with persisting or recurrent AF. Follow patients on antiarrhythmic medications after discharge to monitor Q-T interval and sinus rate. One simple way to follow is with daily asymptomatic recordings from a continuous-loop event recorder.	AF increases risk of embolic cerebrovascular accidents, hypotension, and pulmonary edema. Spontaneous conversion rates in-hospital are 15 to 30% after open cardiac surgery. All antiarrhythmic drugs are associated with proarrhythmic effects. These are most pronounced in the elderly, those with a history of myocardial infarction, and those with impaired left ventricular function. Spontaneous conversion rates at one month after open cardiac surgery approach 90%.

(continued)

TABLE 53-3 Treatment and Outcomes of Newly Diagnosed Postoperative Arrhythmias *(Continued)*

ARRHYTHMIA	SPECIFIC RECOMMENDATIONS	OUTCOMES
Atrial flutter	Treat initially with rate control, as with atrial fibrillation. Anticoagulate if no conversion to normal sinus rhythm (NSR) in 48 h if surgically acceptable bleeding risk. Attempt atrial overdrive pacing with epicardial leads, if present, to convert to NSR. Concomitant ibutilide or procainamide may enhance efficacy. DCCV in presence of hemodynamic instability, severe symptoms, or contraindications to anticoagulation. Administer 1 mg intravenous ibutilide for pharmacologic cardioversion (up to 78% conversion rate). If atrial flutter is refractory to medical control or persists in the extended postoperative state, consider radiofrequency ablation.	Rate control of atrial flutter is often more difficult than that of atrial fibrillation. Early DCCV may be required. 47 to 78% conversion rates of post–cardiac surgery atrial flutter occur with ibutilide. Atrial overdrive pacing terminates up to 95% of postoperative atrial flutter.
Reentrant supraventricular arrhythmias: atrioventricular nodal reentrant tachycardia, and atrioventricular reentrant tachycardia (AVNRT, AVRT)	Treat these regular narrow-complex tachycardias initially with vagal maneuvers (carotid sinus massage), followed by adenosine, beta blockers, or calcium channel blockers. Perform DCCV if patient is hemodynamically unstable and refractory to adenosine. Initiate chronic standing-dose beta blockade or calcium channel blockade if there is recurrent arrhythmia. Consider electrophysiologic study and ablation if arrhythmia is recurrent or uncontrolled (usually not in the immediate postoperative state).	
Multifocal atrial tachycardia	Search for underlying pulmonary complications. Rate control with beta blockers or calcium channel blocking agents. Consider suppressing arrhythmia with amiodarone. DCCV ineffective.	
Ectopic atrial tachycardia	Search for underlying pulmonary complications or digitalis intoxication. Atrial tachycardias associated with AV block (e.g., 2:1 AV block) suggest digitalis intoxication. Rate control with beta blockers or calcium channel blocking agents. Consider suppressing arrhythmia with amiodarone. DC cardioversion may be attempted, though only case reports have been published. Recurrences in the postoperative state are not uncommon.	Postoperative atrial tachycardias are often transient, related to the acute postoperative metabolic state. Recurrent atrial tachycardias may be amenable to catheter ablation in the extended postoperative state.
Nonsustained ventricular tachycardia (NSVT)	Rule out secondary causes such as electrolyte abnormalities or myocardial ischemia. Administer beta blockers to reduce episodes of NSVT. No specific therapy is indicated for patients with hemodynamically insignificant NSVT. Consider amiodarone, procainamide, or lidocaine for symptomatic or hemodynamically significant NSVT; however, no data exist regarding the outcome of short-term therapy with these agents in the postoperative state.	Consider electrophysiologic study, with ICD placement if positive, if NSVT is recognized more than 4 days after open cardiac surgery in any patient with coronary artery disease and an ejection fraction less than 40%.
Sustained wide-complex tachycardias	Consider all wide-complex tachycardias to be ventricular in origin in absence of convincing evidence to the contrary. Obtain a 12-lead ECG in all hemodynamically tolerated wide-complex tachycardias. If available, record tracings from epicardial wires to aid in diagnosis. Perform DCCV in all hemodynamically unstable wide-complex tachycardias; use biphasic defibrillators if available, as they require less energy for cardioversion and result in less myocardial damage.	90% of wide-complex tachycardias in patients with coronary artery disease are ventricular in origin. Prior to the widespread use of implantable defibrillators, patients post-CABG who experienced unexpected sustained ventricular arrhythmias resulting in hemodynamic compromise had an in-hospital mortality over 40%. Recurrent ventricular tachycardia after postoperative day 4 is usually considered an indication for an electrophysiologic

(continued)

TABLE 53-3 Treatment and Outcomes of Newly Diagnosed Postoperative Arrhythmias *(Continued)*

ARRHYTHMIA	SPECIFIC RECOMMENDATIONS	OUTCOMES
	Obtain initial hemodynamic support for persistent ventricular tachycardia with epinephrine or vasopressin. Administer intravenous amiodarone or lidocaine after cardioversion for arrhythmia suppression.	study (at the least) and probable implantation of an ICD.
Sinus node dysfunction, AV Wenckebach, and junctional rhythms	Do not administer specific therapy if patient is hemodynamically stable. Do not withdraw epicardial pacing abruptly, as this may precipitate sinus bradycardia or sinus node arrest; gradually reduce pacing rate. Identify initiators such as laryngoscopy, endotracheal suctioning, pain, medicines, and spinal anesthetics. Administer intravenous atropine if hemodynamic instability is present.	Usually self-limited once causative stimulus is removed.
New left- or right-bundle-branch block	Rule out occult myocardial ischemia with serial enzymes and ECGs. If sinus tachycardia or AF with rapid ventricular response is present, control rate with AV-nodal agents; often new bundle-branch block is rate-related.	Little or no impact on overall prognosis. New left-bundle-branch block may be a marker of myocardial damage and has been associated with worse outcomes in some studies.
High-grade or complete heart block	Discontinue negative chronotropic (rate slowing) medications. Administer intravenous atropine. Initiate transcutaneous pacing immediately if hypotension is present and atropine is unsuccessful. Do not rely on transcutaneous pacing for any significant time period; place a temporary transvenous pacing wire.	Initial observation with a temporary ventricular pacing wire is appropriate; a permanent pacemaker is indicated if heart block persists for 7 to 14 days postoperatively. Recent retrospective data suggest that patients with heart block persisting for >48 h after valvular surgery are unlikely to recover; early pacemaker implantation may be considered.

are beta-adrenergic blockers, calcium channel blockers, and digoxin. Beta blockers are usually the preferred first-line medicine because of their other cardioprotective effects. The target heart rate should be less than 100 beats per minute.

- ***Anticoagulation:*** This is essential in order to reduce the risk of thromboembolic complications. In the absence of contraindications, anticoagulate if AF is present for more than 48 h and for recurrent postoperative AF. Continue anticoagulation for at least 4 to 6 weeks postoperatively (longer if AF is recurrent or persistent). Begin heparin and warfarin simultaneously and discontinue heparin once the international normalized ratio (INR) is therapeutic for at least 1 day.[7]
- ***Conversion/maintenance of sinus rhythm:*** Acute conversion (synchronized shock via biphasic defibrillator) is indicated for patients with hemodynamic instability, severe symptoms, uncontrollable tachycardia, or if there are contraindications to anticoagulation. Cardioversion pads are placed to ensure a transatrial electrical vector (AP position; see Fig. 53-1). After conversion, amiodarone is most commonly employed as an antiarrhythmic in the postoperative state.

- ***Atrial flutter:*** Management of rate control and anticoagulation is similar to that of AF.
  - Rate control is often more difficult than in AF because of the regular tachycardiac atrial rate.

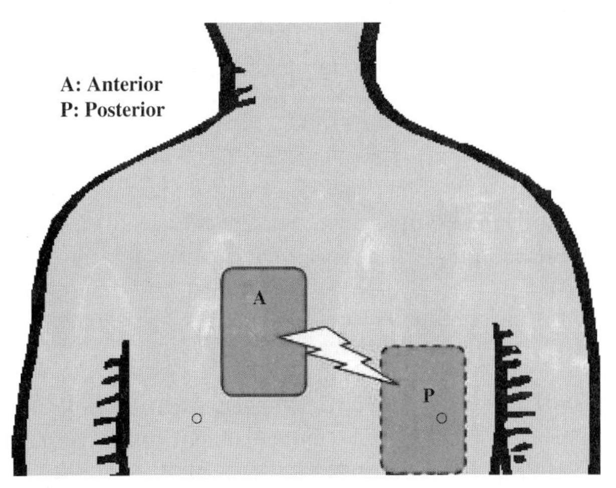

FIG. 53-1 Optimal placement of defibrillator pads for DC cardioversion of atrial fibrillation.

- Rhythm-control options are different than in AF, as atrial overdrive pacing (to convert to sinus rhythm) and ibutilide are both good options for conversion that are not as effective in AF.[7]
- Recurrent atrial flutter should prompt consideration of electrophysiology study and ablation for a definitive cure.

- Reentrant supraventricular arrhythmias: AV nodal reentrant tachycardia (AVNRT) and atrioventricular reentrant tachycardia (AVRT).
  - Initial treatment consists of vagal maneuvers and/or adenosine.
  - These rhythms can be suppressed with beta-adrenergic blocking medications or calcium channel blockers.
  - Recurrent reentrant tachyarrhythmias are an indication for electrophysiology study and ablation.
- Multifocal atrial tachycardia and ectopic atrial tachycardia are usually due to a primary extracardiac cause (similar to sinus tachycardia).
  - Rate control is appropriate during an evaluation for underlying cause.
  - Amiodarone may suppress these arrhythmias and should be used in cases of refractory tachycardia or severe symptoms.
  - Cardioversion is ineffective for multifocal atrial tachycardia.

NONSUSTAINED VT

- This may be secondary to metabolic abnormalities or myocardial ischemia. We do not recommend short-term suppression with antiarrhythmic agents unless the patient is severely symptomatic.
- In patients with coronary artery disease, ejection fraction <40 percent, and nonsustained VT after postoperative day 4 (in the post–cardiac surgery patient) or after noncardiac surgery, an electrophysiologic study is indicated to assess risk for placement of an implantable cardioverter-defibrillator (ICD).[8]

SUSTAINED WIDE-COMPLEX TACHYCARDIAS

- These should be considered ventricular tachycardia until proven otherwise. Obtain a 12-lead ECG for all patients with a hemodynamically tolerated rhythm.
- Cardioversion is usually indicated.

NEW LEFT- OR RIGHT-BUNDLE-BRANCH BLOCK

- This may occur in the immediate postoperative state after cardiac surgery.
- A transition from narrow- to wide-complex conduction any time after surgery is often rate-related but confers an increased risk for the development of heart block, requiring a permanent pacemaker.[9]

HIGH-GRADE HEART BLOCK

- This is not uncommon in the patient who has undergone cardiac surgery, especially among those undergoing concomitant valvular surgery.
- In patients with heart block for over 48 hours postsurgery, strongly consider early implantation of a dual-chamber permanent pacemaker.[10]

REFERENCES

1. Polanczyk CA, Goldman L, Marcantonio ER, et al. Supraventricular arrhythmia in patients having noncardiac surgery: Clinical correlates and effect on length of stay. *Ann Intern Med* 129:279–285, 1998.
2. Andrews TC, Reimold SC, Berlin JA, Antman EM. Prevention of supraventricular arrhythmias after coronary artery bypass surgery. A meta-analysis of randomized controlled trials. *Circulation* 84:III236–III244, 1991.
3. Creswell LL. Postoperative atrial arrhythmias: Risk factors and associated adverse outcomes. *Semin Thorac Cardiovasc Surg* 11:303–307, 1999.
4. Gordon RS, Ivanov J, Cohen G, Ralph-Edwards AL. Permanent cardiac pacing after a cardiac operation: Predicting the use of permanent pacemakers. *Ann Thorac Surg* 66:1698–1704, 1998.
5. Sloan SB, Weitz HH. Postoperative arrhythmias and conduction disorders. *Med Clin North Am* 85;1171–1189, 2001.
6. Maisel WH, Rawn JD, Stevenson WG. Atrial fibrillation after cardiac surgery. *Ann Intern Med* 135:1061–1073, 2001.
7. VanderLugt JT, Mattioni T, Denker S, et al. Efficacy and safety of ibutilide fumarate for the conversion of atrial arrhythmias after cardiac surgery. *Circulation* 100:369–375, 1999.
8. Buxton AE, Lee KL, Fisher JD, et al. A randomized study of the prevention of sudden death in patients with coronary artery disease. Multicenter Unsustained Tachycardia Trial Investigators. *N Engl J Med* 341:1882–1890, 1999.
9. Caspi Y, Safadi T, Ammar R, et al. The significance of bundle branch block in the immediate postoperative electrocardiograms of patients undergoing coronary artery bypass. *J Thorac Cardiovasc Surg* 93: 442–446, 1987.
10. Kim MH, Deeb GM, Eagle KA, et al. Complete atrioventricular block after valvular heart surgery and the timing of pacemaker implantation. *Am J Cardiol* 87:649–651, A10, 2001.

54 PNEUMONIA AND ATELECTASIS

Ahsan M. Arozullah and Gerald W. Smetana*

INTRODUCTION

- Postoperative pulmonary complications (PPCs) are a major source of morbidity and mortality. The contribution to overall perioperative morbidity in most published series is similar to that of cardiac complications. In unselected patients undergoing major noncardiac surgery, the incidence of PPCs averages 7 percent.
- Risk factors for postoperative pulmonary complications include both patient- and procedure-related factors. Strategies to reduce this risk exist throughout the perioperative period. See Chap. 24 for a discussion of these considerations.

DEFINITIONS

- Major postoperative PPCs are those that contribute to morbidity, mortality, and length of stay. The most important of these include pneumonia, atelectasis, respiratory failure (prolonged mechanical ventilation), and exacerbation of underlying chronic obstructive pulmonary disease (COPD). This chapter focuses on pneumonia and atelectasis.
- Minor PPCs are tallied in many studies, but these do not consistently contribute to morbidity or length of stay. Examples of these include fever and cough, hypoxemia, bronchospasm, and airway-management problems in the immediate postoperative period in the postanesthesia care unit.
- Explicit definitions of postoperative pneumonia and atelectasis are necessary in research studies in order to assure that authors across different studies are describing similar patients with similar expected outcomes and morbidity.
- In practice, clinicians need not apply definitions with the same degree of rigor in evaluating individual patients. However, these definitions serve as a useful guide in considering the possibility of a major PPC.

*Dr. Arozullah is supported as a Research Associate in the Advanced Career Development Award Program of the VA Health Services Research and Development Service.

PNEUMONIA

- Physical findings are less specific for pneumonia in the postoperative patient than in other settings and may overlap with those of atelectasis.
- One proposed clinical definition is rales or dullness to percussion on examination plus at least one of the following: new onset of purulent sputum or change in the character of sputum, isolation of organism from blood culture, or isolation of pathogen from transtracheal aspirate, bronchial brushing, or biopsy.[1]
- The Centers for Disease Control and Prevention (CDC) defined nosocomial pneumonia employing a combination of diagnostic criteria. These criteria have been used to define postoperative pneumonia as nosocomial pneumonia that develops following surgery.[2]
- However, the CDC definition did not specify that a pathogenic organism must be isolated. This has led some researchers to criticize the criteria as too broad, leading to the overdiagnosis of pneumonia (Table 54-1).
- Research definitions are often constrained by the difficulty of establishing a confident diagnosis of pneumonia through retrospective review of charts of varying quality. In day-to-day practice, culture confirmation of an organism is not always available, as a productive cough may not be present, sputum cultures may be contaminated by oropharyngeal flora, and bronchoscopy is rarely indicated solely for the purpose of obtaining specimens for culture.
- In practice, in considering the possibility of postoperative pneumonia, clinicians should always obtain a chest radiograph.

TABLE 54-1 Diagnostic Criteria for Postoperative Pneumonia

Criterion 1: Rales or dullness to percussion on chest examination and any one of the following:
a. New onset of purulent sputum or change in sputum character
b. Organism isolated from blood culture
c. Pathogen isolated from transtracheal aspirate, bronchial brushing, or biopsy
OR
Criterion 2: New or progressive infiltrate, consolidation, cavitation, or pleural effusion on chest x-ray and any one of the following:
a. Items a, b, or c listed above in criterion 1.
b. Isolation of virus or detection of virus antigen in respiratory secretions
c. Diagnostic antibody titers
d. Histopathologic evidence of pneumonia

SOURCE: Centers for Disease Control and Prevention.

- The definition of postoperative pneumonia is a new or progressive pulmonary infiltrate on chest radiography in the setting of fever or new pulmonary symptoms or examination findings.
- Ventilator-associated pneumonia is defined as pneumonia that develops during mechanical ventilation after more than 48 h since intubation.
- Separate diagnostic criteria for pneumonia have been proposed for patients receiving mechanical ventilation (Table 54-2).

ATELECTASIS

- Fever, cough, dyspnea, and abnormal findings on chest examination may accompany atelectasis.
- These findings overlap those of pneumonia; therefore it is not possible to diagnose atelectasis based on clinical evaluation alone.
- The diagnosis of postoperative atelectasis requires a chest radiograph that shows segmental or subsegmental volume loss and collapse.

TABLE 54-2 Diagnostic Criteria for Ventilator-Associated Pneumonia

Definite pneumonia

New, progressive, or persistent infiltrate; purulent tracheal secretions; and one of the following:

1. Radiographic evidence of pulmonary abscess and positive needle aspirate
2. Histologic proof on open lung biopsy or at autopsy (abscess formation or consolidation with polymorphonuclear neutrophil accumulation) plus culture of $>10^4$ microorganisms per gram of lung tissue

Probable pneumonia

New, progressive, or persistent infiltrate; purulent tracheal secretions; and one of the following:

1. Quantitative culture of lower respiratory tract secretions obtained by bronchoalveolar lavage or protected specimen brush
2. Positive blood culture of an organism found within 48 h of isolation of the same organism in lower respiratory tract secretions

Definite absence of pneumonia

Patient does not meet the criteria for definite pneumonia with one of the following:

1. Autopsy examination within 3 days of a clinical suspicion of pneumonia showing no histologic signs of lung infection
2. Definite alternative cause with no significant bacterial growth on the reliable respiratory specimen
3. Cytologic identification of a process other than pneumonia (i.e., lung cancer) without significant bacterial growth on the reliable respiratory specimen

Probable absence of pneumonia

Lack of significant growth on a reliable respiratory specimen with either:

1. Resolution without antibiotic therapy of one of the following: fever, radiographic infiltrate, or radiographic infiltrate and a definitive alternative diagnosis
2. Persistent fever and radiographic infiltrate with a definite alternative diagnosis established

INCIDENCE

PNEUMONIA

- Most studies of PPC rates have grouped all PPCs together and have not distinguished between rates of pneumonia and other clinically important PPCs.
- In the development cohort (n = 160,805) of the largest study to date, 1.5 percent of veterans undergoing major noncardiac surgery developed postoperative pneumonia.[1] In this study, the 30-day mortality rate was tenfold higher among patients who developed postoperative pneumonia than among those without postoperative pneumonia.

ATELECTASIS

- Atelectasis may be either segmental or subsegmental. Most subsegmental atelectasis is of no clinical consequence and represents a minor, transient, and clinically inapparent abnormality on the chest radiograph.
- Segmental atelectasis is a major PPC that can contribute to morbidity. Few studies have separated rates of atelectasis from other PPCs. Rates vary substantially across different surgical sites (see Chap. 24).
- Atelectasis rates are much higher if one includes those episodes with no clinical sequelae. Using these criteria, up to 30 percent of patients undergoing upper abdominal surgery and nearly 90 percent of patients undergoing cardiac surgery will develop atelectasis.
- When limited to atelectasis requiring treatment, the incidence is lower. For example, in a study of 1055 patients undergoing nonthoracic surgery who attended a preadmission clinic, 5 (0.5 percent) developed atelectasis requiring bronchoscopic intervention.[3]

TIMING

- Atelectasis that occurs in the first 48 h is often transient and subclinical. Atelectasis that is clinically evident more than 48 h after surgery is likely to contribute to morbidity and require therapy.
- Pneumonia can occur at any time during the postoperative period. However, the likely pathogens causing pneumonia vary depending on the postoperative period.
- Ventilator-associated pneumonia is a distinct clinical entity with a polymicrobial etiology and higher mortality

rates than non-ventilator-associated pneumonia. The incidence is highest during the first week of ventilation and decreases in following weeks. The case fatality rate among patients with this entity ranges from 20 to 50 percent.[4]

- Ventilator-associated pneumonia is divided into early- (<72 h since intubation) and late-onset (≥72 h since intubation) types. *Pseudomonas aeruginosa*, methicillin-resistant *Staphylococcus aureus*, and *Acinetobacter baumannii* are more common pathogens in late-onset ventilator-associated pneumonia than in early-onset ventilator-associated pneumonia.[4]

CAUSES

- With a few exceptions, risk factors for postoperative pneumonia and atelectasis are the same as those for PPCs overall (see Chap. 24).
- Important patient-related risk factors include cigarette use, COPD, poor exercise capacity, and increasing medical comorbidity as measured by the physical status classification of the American Society of Anesthesiologists (ASA). Based on limited evidence, obstructive sleep apnea is probably also a risk factor.
- The most important factor influencing rates of postoperative pneumonia and atelectasis is the surgical site. As a general rule, incisions closer to the diaphragm carry greater risk. Atelectasis rates are highest after cardiac surgery. Repair of thoracic, esophageal, upper abdominal, and abdominal aortic aneurysms are also high-risk surgeries. In addition, the veterans' study referenced above found neck surgery, neurosurgery, and vascular surgery to be risk factors for postoperative pneumonia.[1] The adjusted odds ratios were, respectively, 2.30, 2.14, and 1.29. Whether laparoscopic abdominal surgeries confer lower risks for pneumonia and atelectasis is controversial; however, a decrease in risk is likely.
- General anesthesia is associated with higher PPC rates than epidural or spinal anesthesia.
- Routine use of postoperative nasogastric tubes after abdominal surgery increases the risk of PPCs, including pneumonia and atelectasis. Selective use (based on abdominal distention or nausea) minimizes this risk. The odds ratios for pneumonia and atelectasis are 0.49 and 0.46, respectively.[5]
- Postoperative mechanical ventilation is a risk factor for pneumonia but not for atelectasis. Reintubation is a risk factor for ventilator-associated pneumonia.
- The primary mechanism for the development of PPCs is a decrease in lung volumes after surgery. Therefore subclinical atelectasis may precede and be a risk factor for postoperative pneumonia itself.

DIAGNOSIS

- The diagnosis of postoperative pneumonia is made through a combination of clinical findings, radiologic findings, and laboratory testing, including microbiologic cultures.
- Clinical findings include fever (>101.5°F, 38.6°C), rales or crackles on lung examination, increased leukocyte count (>15,000/μL), and occasionally worsening hypoxemia.
- Radiologic findings on chest x-ray usually include lobar or multilobar interstitial infiltrates with or without pleural effusions.
- Microbiologic tests initially include blood cultures as well as Gram's stain and cultures of sputum. One major challenge to diagnosing pneumonia using routine sputum cultures is that the oropharynx is colonized rapidly by potential pathogens shortly after hospitalization. Although these pathogens may be introduced into the lung through small-volume aspiration of gastric contents, endotracheal intubation, or nasotracheal suctioning, isolates from sputum cultures may represent colonizing rather than infective organisms.
- Arriving at an accurate diagnosis of pneumonia can be challenging, particularly among patients receiving mechanical ventilation.
- Alternative methods for isolating pathogens include endotracheal aspirates, bronchial brushings using protected-brush catheters, bronchoalveolar lavage (BAL), and biopsy. These methods may be particularly useful in patients receiving mechanical ventilation, when clinical factors and chest x-ray findings do not provide a clear diagnosis, and for patients who deteriorate despite empiric antibiotic therapy.[6,7]
- Endotracheal aspirates enhance diagnostic accuracy when combined with quantitative cultures. Lavage of 5 mL of normal saline producing $>10^4$ bacteria per milliliter has been shown to be diagnostic for pneumonia. The production of <100 bacteria per milliliter excluded the diagnosis of pneumonia.[6]
- In addition, consider studies to isolate viral antigen in respiratory secretions, antibody titers, and histopathologic evidence of viral pneumonia, particularly in patients undergoing transplant surgery or those who are immunosuppressed.

DIFFERENTIAL DIAGNOSIS

- Several other conditions may mimic pneumonia in the postoperative setting. Chest radiograph findings of an infiltrate or pleural effusion may represent congestive heart failure, pleural effusions, pulmonary infarct, lung cancer, preexisting granulomas or nodules, and/or lung abscess.

- A particular challenge is to distinguish ventilator-associated pneumonia from acute respiratory distress syndrome (ARDS). ARDS is characterized by severe hypoxemia, diffuse pulmonary infiltrates, diminished lung compliance, and the absence of left heart failure.[8]
- Both direct and indirect lung injury can cause ARDS. Examples of direct lung injury include aspiration pneumonia, near drowning, inhalation injury, and pulmonary contusion. Examples of indirect lung injury include sepsis, multiple transfusions after shock and resuscitation, and pancreatitis. Pulmonary contusion is a common cause of ARDS in trauma patients.
- Since patients with ARDS often meet standard diagnostic criteria for pneumonia, it can be challenging to distinguish between the two. This is particularly true in trauma patients with multiple wounds, whose sputum cultures and chest radiographs may be difficult to interpret.
- Under these circumstances, quantitative culture techniques may be beneficial, as positive culture results often precede changes on chest radiography. Bronchoscopy with BAL and/or protected specimen brush sampling may be necessary to make an accurate diagnosis of pneumonia in these patients.[8]
- In one study, ventilated patients with clinical evidence of pneumonia underwent bronchoscopy with quantitative BAL. If the culture demonstrated 10^5 colony-forming units (CFU) per milliliter or greater, pneumonia was the presumed diagnosis and antibiotics were continued. Conversely, if the culture demonstrated $<10^5$ CFU per milliliter, empiric therapy was stopped. Using this strategy, the overall rate of ventilator-associated pneumonia was only 39 percent.[9]
- This strategy resulted in a false-negative rate of 7 percent; importantly, however, mortality among those initially diagnosed with pneumonia and those diagnosed later were not significantly different, indicating that this strategy may be a reasonable intermediate approach to the diagnosis and treatment of ventilator-associated pneumonia. Quantitative BAL had a sensitivity of 89 percent, specificity of 100 percent, and positive predictive value of 100 percent. Clinical criteria had 100 percent sensitivity, 14 percent specificity, and 43 percent positive predictive value.[9]
- Gram's stain of the sputum has poor correlation with sputum culture results. Gram's stain of the BAL had a sensitivity of only 57 percent and a diagnostic accuracy of 60 percent; this test does not appear to be helpful in guiding initial antibiotic therapy.
- Base empiric antibiotic therapy on the common pathogens found in individual intensive care units (ICUs) and surgical wards. The recommended empiric therapy will likely change over time, as the pathogens responsible for early pneumonias (within 7 days postoperatively) are often different from those responsible for later pneumonias (occurring after 7 days postoperatively).

TREATMENT

PNEUMONIA

- Once postoperative pneumonia is suspected, there are several approaches to treatment. Since confirmatory evidence such as culture results take 2 to 3 days to complete, nearly all primary therapy of postoperative pneumonia is empiric. Antibiotic coverage should be narrowed and targeted once culture and sensitivity results become available.
- The choice of initial empiric therapy matters, as several studies have found higher mortality rates when initial empiric therapy was inappropriate.
- The National Nosocomial Infection Surveillance (NNIS) system reported that the most common pathogens for ventilator-associated pneumonia were *P. aeruginosa* and *S. aureus;* the prevalence of each was 17.4 percent. The NNIS also noted higher resistance patterns in ICUs compared with hospitals at large.[10]
- Several local sources of information about the ICU-specific and hospital-specific sensitivity and resistance patterns are commonly available through microbiology laboratory service and infection control service. Prior studies have found that this information is critical in making sound decisions about initial empiric therapy because there is tremendous variation in predominant organisms and their resistance patterns even among ICUs located within the same hospital.
- Other factors that influence primary antibiotic choice include previous antibiotic use and the timing of the development of pneumonia. Antibiotic-specific considerations include pharmacodynamics, tissue penetration, and toxicity.
- The American Thoracic Society (ATS) has produced a consensus statement regarding the treatment of nosocomial pneumonia, which provides a useful framework for making initial choices of empiric antibiotic treatment.[11]
- Risk factors for classifying pneumonia as severe include ICU admission, respiratory failure, rapid radiographic progression, multilobar infiltrates or cavitations,

severe sepsis with hypotension and/or end-organ dysfunction, acute renal failure, recent abdominal surgery, witnessed aspiration, head trauma, and diabetes mellitus.

- The ATS defines mild-to-moderate nosocomial pneumonia as having no risk factors or early-onset severe pneumonia. The core organisms associated with pneumonia in these patients include enteric gram-negative bacilli (nonpseudomonal) such as *Enterobacter* species, *E. coli*, *Klebsiella*, and *Proteus* species; *Serratia marcescens; Haemophilus influenzae*; methicillin-sensitive *S. aureus; and Streptococcus pneumonia.*
- Core antibiotics for initially treating these patients included second- or third-generation cephalosporins; beta-lactam/beta-lactamase inhibitor combinations; or fluoroquinolones for patients allergic to penicillin.
- Severe nosocomial pneumonia was defined as having risk factors with early- or late-onset pneumonia. The core organisms for these patients include those listed above plus one of the following: *P. aeruginosa*, *Acinetobacter* species, and possibly methicillin-resistant *S. aureus (*MRSA).
- The core antibiotics for treating these patients included an aminoglycoside or antipseudomonal fluoroquinolone (e.g., ciprofloxacin) plus one of the following: antipseudomonal penicillin, beta-lactam/beta-lactamase inhibitor combination, ceftazidime or cefoperazone, or imipenem. Consider adding vancomycin in circumstances where MRSA is prevalent and/or when pneumonia is more severe.

ATELECTASIS

- The treatment of postoperative atelectasis includes maneuvers that enable or encourage lung expansion, with the intention of preventing progression to pneumonia.
- Chest physical therapy—including deep-breathing exercises, moving about the bed, and ambulating once medically stable—can improve lung function postoperatively. Use incentive spirometry coupled with preoperative training, particularly for patients at high risk for developing pneumonia.
- Deep-breathing exercises, incentive spirometry, and intermittent positive pressure breathing (IPPB) appear to be equivalent in treating atelectasis. Use chest physical therapy and incentive spirometry in conscious patients. While each modality is effective, the combination of modalities does not appear to provide additional benefit.[12]
- For unconscious or sedated patients, consider using IPPB or continuous positive airway pressure (CPAP). When hypoxemia is present, provide supplemental oxygen in addition to CPAP.
- Perform bronchoscopy when atelectasis leads to lobar collapse on chest radiography and fails to respond to more conservative measures. Use mechanical ventilation and reintubation in patients with worsening hypercarbia who are at risk for potential respiratory failure.

REFERENCES

1. Arozullah AM, Khuri SF, Henderson WG, et al. Development and validation of a multifactorial risk index for predicting postoperative pneumonia after major noncardiac surgery. *Ann Intern Med* 135:847–857, 2001.
2. Horan TC, Gaynes R. Surveillance of nosocomial infection, in Mayhall CG (ed), *Hospital Epidemiology and Infection Control*. Philadelphia: Lippincott, Williams & Wilkins, 2004: pp 1659–1702.
3. McAlister FA, Bertsch K, Man J, et al. Incidence of and risk factors for pulmonary complications after non-thoracic surgery. *Am J Resp Crit Care Med* 171:514–517, 2005.
4. Hubmayr RD. Statement of the 4th international consensus conference in critical care on ICU-acquired pneumonia. Chicago, May 2002. *Intens Care Med* 28:1521–1536, 2002.
5. Cheatham ML, Chapman WC, Key SP, et al. A meta-analysis of selective versus routine nasogastric decompression after elective laparotomy. *Ann Surg* 221:469–476, 1995.
6. Polk HC, Mizuguchi NN. Multifactorial analyses in the diagnosis of pneumonia arising in the surgical intensive care unit. *Am J Surg* 179(suppl 2A):31S–35S, 2000.
7. Grossman RF, Fein A. Evidence-based assessment of diagnostic tests for ventilator-associated pneumonia. *Chest* 117(4)(suppl):177S–181S, 2000.
8. Croce MA. Diagnosis of acute respiratory distress syndrome and differentiation from ventilator-associated pneumonia. *Am J Surg* 179(suppl 2A):26S–30S, 2000.
9. Croce MA, Fabian TC, Waddle-Smith L, et al. Utility of Gram's stain and efficacy of quantitative culture for posttraumatic pneumonia: A prospective study. *Ann Surg* 227: 743–755, 1998.
10. Fabian TC. Empiric therapy for pneumonia in the surgical intensive care unit. *Am J Surg* 179(suppl 2A):18S–25S, 2000.
11. Hospital-acquired pneumonia in adults: Diagnosis, assessment of severity, initial antimicrobial therapy, and preventive strategies: A consensus statement, American Thoracic Society. *Am J Respir Crit Care Med* 153:1711–1725, 1995.
12. Lawrence VA, Cornell JE, Smetana GW. Strategies to reduce postoperative pulmonary complications after non-cardiothoracic surgery: Background review for an American College of Physicians guideline. *Ann Intern Med* 2006. In press.

55 DEEP VENOUS THROMBOSIS AND PULMONARY EMBOLISM

Daniel J. Brotman and Amir K. Jaffer

INTRODUCTION

INCIDENCE

- Venous thromboembolism (VTE) is a common and morbid complication after surgery. Approximately 2 million cases of deep venous thrombosis (DVT) and 200,000 deaths due to pulmonary embolism (PE) occur every year in the United States. Half of these cases and deaths occur in surgical patients and half in medical patients.[1]
- The prevalence of postoperative VTE varies based on patient-related risk factors for VTE (see Table 46-1), the type of surgery (surgery-specific risk) (see Table 46-2), and finally the type and amount of prophylaxis. These are all discussed in more detail in Chap. 46.
- VTE is often silent. Clinical trials of routine postoperative venography have demonstrated that many postoperative DVTs are clinically inapparent.

TIMING

- Most symptomatic postoperative DVTs occur after hospital discharge.
- Reliance on signs and symptoms of early DVT is not adequate, as the first manifestation of VTE may be a fatal PE. In addition, screening for postoperative DVT is unreliable and expensive.
- Therefore the best strategy to prevent both postoperative VTE and its chronic sequelae, such as postphlebitic syndrome, is to recommend universal VTE prophylaxis for almost all surgical patients. See Chap. 46 for a complete discussion of VTE prophylaxis.

CAUSES

- Key mechanisms by which surgery may precipitate VTE include:
  - Immobility, which, during anesthesia and after surgery, may precipitate stasis of blood in the venous system.
  - Tissue trauma elicits systemic inflammation, activates hemostasis, and causes a hypercoagulable state.
  - Tissue trauma may damage the veins directly (e.g., damage to leg veins during knee replacement or damage to pelvic veins during hysterectomy).
  - The supine position and anesthesia itself may lead to stasis of blood and delayed clearance of clotting factors from the lower extremities.

DIAGNOSIS OF POSTOPERATIVE VTE

- Individual symptoms and signs of DVT (such as swelling or leg pain) and PE (dyspnea, tachypnea, hypoxia, or chest pain) are nonspecific in the general population in that other conditions (such as infection and heart failure) can lead to similar findings. Their predictive value for the diagnosis of VTE may be even lower in postoperative patients for the following reasons:
  - Third spacing of fluids and tissue trauma may lead to leg swelling and pain, particularly in patients who have undergone lower extremity surgery. These findings may mimic DVT.
  - Volume overload, myocardial ischemia, atelectasis, and postoperative pneumonia may cause hypoxia, dyspnea, tachycardia, and chest pain, therefore confounding the diagnosis of PE.

DIFFERENTIAL DIAGNOSIS

- In entertaining the diagnosis of postoperative PE, the differential diagnosis includes the following:
  - ***Volume overload,*** which may cause postoperative hypoxia and dyspnea, especially (but not exclusively) in patients with preexisting heart failure. Because elevated levels of B-type natriuretic peptide (BNP) may result from right ventricular overload in the setting of PE, an elevated BNP does not distinguish between PE and volume overload. Volume overload may also lead to lower extremity edema. When this condition is asymmetrical, it suggests the possibility of DVT.
  - ***Atelectasis*** may cause postoperative hypoxia. The latter can also be seen with PE.
  - ***Myocardial ischemia*** occurring in the postoperative setting may cause dyspnea and chest pain. Hypoxia may result if the ischemia causes systolic or diastolic myocardial dysfunction. Elevated cardiac enzymes may indicate myocardial ischemia, but can also occur due to right ventricular strain in the setting of hemodynamically important pulmonary emboli. This is particularly true for cardiac troponin levels.
  - ***Postoperative pneumonia*** may lead to dyspnea, fever, tachypnea, and chest discomfort, all of which are also seen in patients with PE. Productive purulent sputum and preexisting lung disease (such as chronic

TABLE 55-1 Clinical Model for Predicting Pretest Probability of Deep Venous Thrombosis

FINDING	POINTS*
Active cancer (treatment ongoing, or within previous 6 months, or palliative)	1
Paralysis, paresis, or recent plaster immobilization of the lower extremities	1
Recently bedridden for more than 3 days or major surgery within 4 weeks	1
Localized tenderness along the distribution of the deep venous system	1
Entire leg swollen†	1
Calf swelling by more than 3 cm when compared with the asymptomatic leg (measured 10 cm below the tibial tuberosity)†	1
Pitting edema (greater in the symptomatic leg)	1
Collateral superficial veins (nonvaricose)	1
Alternative diagnosis as likely or greater than that of deep venous thrombosis	−2

*A composite score of 3 or higher indicates a high probability of deep venous thrombosis; 1 or 2 suggests a moderate probability; and 0 or lower indicates a low probability.
†Among patients with symptoms in both legs, the more symptomatic leg is used.
SOURCE: Adapted from Wells et al.,[2] with permission.

TABLE 55-2 Clinical Model for Predicting Pretest Probability of Pulmonary Embolism

FINDING	POINTS*
Clinical signs and symptoms of deep venous thrombosis, including at least leg swelling and pain with palpation of the deep veins	3
An alternative diagnosis is less likely than pulmonary embolus	3
Heart rate >100 beats per minute	1.5
Immobilization or surgery in the previous 4 weeks	1.5
Previous venous thromboembolism	1.5
Hemoptysis	1
Malignancy (on treatment, treated in the last 6 months, or palliative)	1

*A composite score of less than 2 indicates a low probability of PE; 2 to 6 suggests a moderate probability; and greater than 6 indicates a high probability.
SOURCE: Adapted from Wells et al.,[3] with permission.

obstructive pulmonary disease) may indicate an infectious etiology for these symptoms.
  - ***Hypoventilation*** due to narcotic analgesia may also lead to postoperative hypoxia.

CLINICAL FINDINGS

- Postoperative VTE is common following major surgery and may lead to serious morbidity and even death. Therefore clinicians must consider this diagnosis even when signs or symptoms have low specificity and could be due to another diagnosis. This is a "can't miss" diagnosis.
  - The rules of clinical prediction may be helpful in assessing the likelihood of postoperative thrombosis (Tables 55-1 and 55-2).[2,3]
- If clinical assessment suggests the possibility of VTE, one should perform objective diagnostic tests.

LABORATORY AND RADIOGRAPHIC TESTING

- Likelihood ratios for various noninvasive diagnostic tests used in the evaluation of VTE are presented in Table 55-3. Some of these tests might be less accurate in the postoperative setting.
- If PE is suspected, obtain *either* a helical CT or a ventilation/perfusion lung scan. A bilateral duplex ultrasound of the lower extremity may supplement other tests.
  - The likelihood ratio for a positive study by helical CT exceeds 7.1 if multiple, unambiguous, large filling defects are seen. However, confirmatory pulmonary angiography may be indicated in a patient with a low pretest suspicion of PE and only one or two small filling defects on computed tomography (CT).[4,5]
  - Helical CT has the advantage of clarifying other possible diagnoses that could explain the clinical presentation (e.g., pulmonary edema or infiltrate). However, it does require intravenous iodinated contrast, which places patients at risk for renal toxicity.
  - Interpret test results within the context of the pretest clinical suspicion of PE. If the diagnostic test is negative in the setting of a high clinical likelihood of PE, the posttest probability remains moderate and additional testing is necessary.
  - Since the majority of clinically important PEs arise from the large veins in the legs, a duplex ultrasound of the lower extremity is often appropriate in the evaluation of PE. But if this is negative, the diagnosis of PE should still be pursued, as PEs can also arise from the pelvic veins, for which duplex ultrasound is not a good test.
  - If the diagnosis of PE remains in question following noninvasive testing, obtain a pulmonary angiogram. This applies particularly to patients in whom the risk of empiric anticoagulation is higher than average.
- If DVT is suspected, obtain a compression ultrasound of the lower extremity.
  - If clinical suspicion for DVT is high and the ultrasound is negative, obtain a repeat ultrasound about 1 week after the initial study. This is particularly important in

TABLE 55-3 Approximate Likelihood Ratios of Commonly Used Diagnostic Tests for the Evaluation of VTE in the Postoperative Setting

DIAGNOSTIC TEST	LIKELIHOOD RATIO*	COMMENTS
D-dimer	N/A	Not recommended in the postoperative setting.*[6]
Helical chest CT[9]		No reason to except limited accuracy in postoperative setting, but accuracy is user-dependent.[5] Best for ruling in or ruling out large (central) emboli. The likelihood ratio for a positive study may greatly exceed 7.1 if multiple, unambiguous, large filling defects are seen. However, confirmatory pulmonary angiography may be indicated in a patient with a low pretest suspicion of PE and only 1 or 2 small filling defects on CT. May reveal alternate source of dyspnea, hypoxia, or chest pain.
Negative study	0.29	
Positive study	7.1	
Nuclear lung scan[10]		Patients with known pulmonary disease (such as COPD) may be unlikely to have normal or near-normal scans. In the post-operative setting, conditions such as atelectasis or pneumonia may adversely affect test performance.
High probability	23	
Intermediate	0.87	
Low probability	0.26	
Normal/near-normal	0.17	
Duplex ultrasound[11]		Accuracy may be lower for distal DVT, for asymptomatic DVT, and for postoperative surveillance (primarily due to lower sensitivity).
Negative	0.05	
Positive	24	
Magnetic resonance[12] venography		Limited data available to date; promising new technique but not available in most centers. These likelihood ratios require validation in future studies.
Negative	0.05	
Positive	11	
Pulmonary arteriography	N/A	Considered the "gold standard" test for PE, but it is invasive, with an approximately 1% risk of serious adverse events. Interobserver agreement for individual subsegmental PEs may be < 70%.[13]
Venography	N/A	Considered the "gold standard" for DVT, but it is invasive and may precipitate thrombosis and other local vascular complications.

*When likelihood ratios were not specifically reported, they were calculated using standard formulas. Likelihood ratios are interpreted as follows using Bayes theorem:

(Pretest odds of disease) × (likelihood ratio for given finding) = (posttest odds of disease)

COPD = chronic obstructive pulmonary disease; CT = computed tomography; DVT = deep venous thrombosis; N/A = not applicable; PE = pulmonary embolism.

centers where a systematic examination of the calf veins is not part of the ultrasound protocol, since calf-vein thrombi may be missed and may propagate if left untreated.

- We do not recommend D-dimer testing in postoperative patients with suspected DVT or PE, since normal D-dimer results are uncommon in this setting and may not help to exclude the diagnosis of VTE.[6]

INITIAL TREATMENT

- Prompt initiation of anticoagulant therapy is essential in the management of acute VTE except in those patients who are either actively bleeding or in whom the risk of bleeding outweighs the benefits of anticoagulation. For these patients, consider an inferior vena cava (IVC) filter, as discussed below.
- Currently, several groups of drugs are available to treat acute DVT and PE:
  - Unfractionated heparin (UFH).
  - Low-molecular-weight heparins (LMWHs).
  - Factor-Xa inhibitors (pentasaccharides).
  - Parenteral direct thrombin inhibitors (DTIs), which are approved for use in patients with acute VTE in the setting of heparin-induced thrombocytopenia (HIT).
- Table 55-4 outlines the regimens that are currently FDA-approved for VTE treatment.
- LMWHs have several advantages. They can be dosed subcutaneously once or twice daily with more predictable pharmacokinetics and bioavailability. They cause HIT less frequently (about 1 percent) than UFH (about 2 to 3 percent), and in most clinical situations do not require laboratory monitoring.

TABLE 55-4 FDA-Approved Initial Therapy for Venous Thromboembolism

Unfractionated heparin	
Use normogram: 80 U/kg ideal body weight bolus followed by continuous IV drip 18 U/kg/h. Goal: aPTT* = 60–80	
Low-molecular-weight heparin	
Enoxaparin 1 mg/kg SC every 12 h, enoxaparin 1.5 mg SC every 24 h, or tinzaparin 175 IU/kg SC every 24 h	
Factor Xa-inhibitor	
Fondaparinux	5 mg SC daily if weight is <50 kg
	7.5 mg SC daily if weight is 50–100 kg
	10 mg SC daily if weight is >100 kg

*May vary from institution to institution. Maintain activated partial thromboplastin time (aPTT) in therapeutic range, which must correspond to heparin levels of 0.3–0.7 U/mL.

- Studies and meta-analyses that have compared LMWHs with UFHs suggest decreased mortality for patients treated with LMWHs. This is especially true in cancer patients. Based on these studies and the above advantages, it is our preference to use a LMWH over UFH to treat acute VTE, and this practice is supported by the most recent recommendations of the American College of Chest Physicians.[7]
- IVC filters may be permanent or retrievable. The removable IVC filters are attractive options for patients with transient contraindications to anticoagulation therapy. Examples include the postoperative patient or the patient who has just undergone a procedure involving the central nervous system (CNS) who may be at high risk for postoperative bleeding within the first 24 to 96 h after major surgery but in whom the risk of anticoagulation may be acceptable after this period.
- Thrombolysis for acute PE is usually contraindicated in the setting of recent surgery. However, one should consider either surgical embolectomy or thrombolysis with tissue plasminogen activator (t-PA), streptokinase, or urokinase for patients with extreme hemodynamic instability due to PE and are at risk for imminent death.

MAINTENANCE THERAPY

- Debate over the appropriate starting dose of warfarin continues, since more recent evidence suggests that a starting dose of 10 mg daily may achieve a therapeutic international normalized ratio (INR) faster than a 5-mg dose without increasing the risk of bleeding or thromboembolic complications. This can minimize the time on heparin therapy.
- However, previous randomized trials have suggested that patients are more likely to have a therapeutic INR 3 to 5 days after the initiation of warfarin with a 5-mg dose rather than a 10-mg dose, in part owing to a higher risk of supratherapeutic INR values with the higher dose.
- We recommend that, in deciding on the starting dose, clinicians consider patient-specific factors such as age, body size, concomitant medications, and comorbid conditions. Some commonly encountered medications that may necessitate a lower starting dose include amiodarone, trimethoprim/sulfamethoxazole, and metronidazole. Lower starting doses may also be reasonable in patients with recent surgery, liver disease, congestive heart failure, or poor nutritional status and in frail elderly patients.
- Choosing the duration of warfarin therapy requires estimating the risks of recurrent and fatal VTE off warfarin and the competing risks of major and fatal bleeding on therapy. Making this decision requires tailoring the therapy to the individual patient.
- The rate of recurrent VTE at 1 year (after 3 months of therapy) is approximately 3 to 5 percent for patients with reversible risk factors such as surgery or trauma. This risk is low compared to that of patients with unprovoked VTE, whose risk of recurrence may be as high as 10 percent at 1 year after completing 6 months of warfarin therapy, while patients with cancer may have a recurrence rate as high as 20 percent at 1 year after completing 6 months of therapy.
- Therefore, in the absence of cancer, treat patients with postoperative DVT with warfarin for 3 months and those with extensive ileofemoral DVT or PE for 6 months.
- Consider treating patients who have cancer with warfarin indefinitely unless the cancer is cured or the disease is deemed to be in remission. In addition, given the high rates of warfarin-resistant thrombosis and warfarin-associated bleeding in patients with cancer, LMWHs can be used to treat VTE over the long term.[8]
- Finally, we endorse the use of below-knee compression stockings (30 to 40 mmHg at the ankle) in patients with acute DVT, because studies show a 50 percent risk reduction of postthrombotic sequelae at 2 years.

CONCLUSIONS

- VTE is a common and serious complication after surgery.
- Perioperative VTE prophylaxis is an important strategy to prevent this sometimes fatal condition. Consideration of prophylaxis should be part of the routine preoperative evaluation.

- Maintain a high level of suspicion for this disease in the postoperative setting and use the rules of clinical prediction to identify patients who will benefit from diagnostic testing.
- Prompt initiation of anticoagulant therapy is important to prevent recurrent thromboembolic events.
- For patients in whom anticoagulant therapy is contraindicated, consider IVC filters in the setting of VTE.
- The usual duration of warfarin therapy is 3 months for postoperative DVT and 6 months for PE.

REFERENCES

1. Goldhaber SZ, Tapson VF, Committee DFS. A prospective registry of 5,451 patients with ultrasound-confirmed deep vein thrombosis. *Am J Cardiol* 93(2):259–262, 2004.
2. Wells PS, Anderson DR, Bormanis J, et al. Value of assessment of pretest probability of deep-vein thrombosis in clinical management. *Lancet* 350(9094):1795–1798, 1997.
3. Wells PS, Anderson DR, Rodger M, et al. Derivation of a simple clinical model to categorize patients' probability of pulmonary embolism: Increasing the model's utility with the SimpliRED D-dimer. *Thromb Haemost* 83(3):416–420, 2000.
4. Remy-Jardin M, Baghaie F, Bonnel F, et al. Thoracic helical CT: Influence of subsecond scan time and thin collimation on evaluation of peripheral pulmonary arteries. *Eur Radiol* 10(8):1297–1303, 2000.
5. Domingo ML, Marti-Bonmati L, Dosda R, Pallardo Y. Interobserver agreement in the diagnosis of pulmonary embolism with helical CT. *Eur J Radiol* 34(2):136–140, 2000.
6. Brotman DJ, Segal JB, Jani JT, et al. Limitations of D-dimer testing in unselected inpatients with suspected venous thromboembolism. *Am J Med* 114(4):276–282, 2003.
7. Buller HR, Agnelli G, Hull RD, et al. Antithrombotic therapy for venous thromboembolic disease: The Seventh ACCP Conference on Antithrombotic and Thrombolytic Therapy. *Chest* 126(3 suppl):401S–428S, 2004.
8. Lee AY, Levine MN, Baker RI, et al. Low-molecular-weight heparin versus a coumarin for the prevention of recurrent venous thromboembolism in patients with cancer. *N Engl J Med* 349(2):146–153, 2003.
9. Safriel Y, Zinn H. CT pulmonary angiography in the detection of pulmonary emboli: A meta-analysis of sensitivities and specificities. *Clin Imaging* 26(2):101–105, 2000.
10. Value of the ventilation/perfusion scan in acute pulmonary embolism. Results of the prospective investigation of pulmonary embolism diagnosis (PIOPED). The PIOPED Investigators. *JAMA* 263(20):2753–2759, 1990.
11. Kearon C, Ginsberg JS, Hirsh J. The role of venous ultrasonography in the diagnosis of suspected deep venous thrombosis and pulmonary embolism. *Ann Intern Med* 129(12):1044–1049, 1998.
12. Fraser DG, Moody AR, Morgan PS, et al. Diagnosis of lower-limb deep venous thrombosis: A prospective blinded study of magnetic resonance direct thrombus imaging. *Ann Intern Med* 136(2):89–98, 2002.
13. Stein PD, Athanasoulis C, Alavi A, et al. Complications and validity of pulmonary angiography in acute pulmonary embolism. *Circulation* 85(2):462–468, 1992.

56 FLUID AND ELECTROLYTE DISORDERS

Jennifer C. Kerns

INTRODUCTION

- Fluid and electrolyte disorders are common in the postoperative period and can lead to significant morbidity and mortality if not promptly recognized and treated.[1]
- These disorders may be preexisting, but frequently arise during the perioperative and immediate postoperative period.
- Postoperative fluid and electrolyte disorders are particularly common in patients undergoing intestinal surgery (because of the role of the gastrointestinal system in providing the body with water and electrolytes) and in patients with preexisting renal insufficiency or acute renal failure (because of the role of the kidneys in maintaining water and electrolyte balance).
- This chapter reviews the most common postoperative fluid and electrolyte disorders, including causes, diagnosis, and treatment.

HYPOVOLEMIA

Hypovolemia is an important postoperative complication; it can lead to hypotension, electrolyte disturbances, acute renal failure, or even shock.

ETIOLOGY

- Postoperative hypovolemia usually results from decreased sodium/water intake (due to restricted perioperative oral intake and inadequate maintenance intravenous fluids) combined with continued sodium/water losses (perioperative insensible losses, e.g., from respiration, evaporation from an open incision; perioperative blood loss; and normal renal losses).

- Postoperative hypovolemia may also be exacerbated by excessive gastrointestinal losses such as those due to nasogastric suction after intraabdominal procedures or to diuretic therapy (which may, for example, have been used inappropriately to increase declining urine output).
- Rarely, hypovolemic shock may occur as a result of perioperative hemorrhage.

DIAGNOSIS

Hypovolemia is a clinical diagnosis; a careful history and physical will establish it. A basic chemistry panel and urine osmolality may help to confirm the clinical picture. The most common findings of hypovolemia are as follows:

- Symptoms:
  - Increased sensation of thirst
  - Postural dizziness
  - Easy fatigability or muscle cramping
- Signs:
  - Dry oral mucous membranes
  - Poor skin turgor or dry skin in usually moist areas (such as the axilla)
  - Decreased urine output (patients without renal dysfunction should produce urine at a minimal rate of 0.5 mL/kg/h)
  - Orthostatic hypotension or tachycardia
- Laboratory findings:
  - Increased blood urea nitrogen (BUN), with or without an increased creatinine, over the patient's baseline
  - A ratio of BUN to creatinine of >20:1 suggests prerenal azotemia and supports the diagnosis of hypovolemia
  - Increased urinary osmolality (normal kidneys will concentrate the urine to >400 mosmol/kg in a hypovolemic state)

TREATMENT

The mainstay of treatment is intravenous volume repletion.

- Use an isotonic crystalloid solution for most cases [such as normal saline (0.9% NaCl) or lactated Ringer's solution]. Crystalloid solutions will replete intravascular volume deficits and are significantly less expensive than colloid solutions such as albumin or hetastarch.
  - Several systematic meta-analyses support the use of crystalloid solutions, even in patients with congestive heart failure or hypoalbuminemia. For example, in a large meta-analysis of randomized controlled trials that compared colloids with crystalloids in critically ill patients (including trauma patients, patients with burns, and postoperative patients), resuscitation with colloids compared to crystalloids did not reduce the risk of death.[2]
- If hypernatremia coexists, use hypotonic fluids (such as half-normal saline, or 0.45% NaCl) unless hypovolemia is severe (see "Hypernatremia," below).
- Use blood products for patients in whom the hypovolemia is due to acute hemorrhage. Remember that a decreased hematocrit may not occur for 4 h or more, so this is a clinical (not a laboratory) diagnosis early in the course.
- During volume repletion, watch for the development of pulmonary edema in patients with congestive heart failure (CHF) and end-stage renal disease.
  - While it is important to watch for the development of pulmonary edema, a preexisting diagnosis of CHF or renal disease should not preclude the use of intravenous fluids to treat hypovolemia. One study that examined rates of postoperative CHF exacerbations found that intraoperative fluctuations in mean arterial pressure increased the probability, while intraoperative administration of higher net volumes of fluid was actually associated with decreased risk.[3]

HYPERVOLEMIA

Hypervolemia is a common postoperative complication that, when severe, can lead to decreased absorption from the gut (due to bowel edema) and/or hypoxemia (due to pulmonary edema).

ETIOLOGY

- Intraoperative fluid shifts (due to tissue trauma, endotoxemia, proinflammatory cytokines, etc.) may result in intravascular hypovolemia requiring repletion despite interstitial hypervolemia.[4]
- Excessive administration of perioperative intravenous fluids and/or blood products may lead to postoperative hypervolemia, especially in patients with preexisting renal dysfunction, congestive heart failure, cirrhosis, or hypoalbuminemia. However, it can be difficult to determine what is "excessive."
  - The role of intraoperative pulmonary artery (PA) catheters to guide fluid administration has long been debated. Multiple randomized controlled trials have examined the use of PA catheters, including a large trial of almost 4000 high-risk patients.[5] These studies

establish that intraoperative PA catheters do not reduce perioperative mortality and should not be a routine strategy to reduce risk in high-risk patients.

DIAGNOSIS

Hypervolemia is a clinical diagnosis: laboratory testing is generally not helpful. The most common symptoms and signs of hypovolemia are as follows:

- Symptoms:
  - "Swollen" extremities
  - Dyspnea
  - Nausea or abdominal discomfort (due to bowel edema and/or passive hepatic congestion)
- Signs:
  - Peripheral/dependent edema
  - Hypoxemia or dependent rales on pulmonary auscultation
  - Elevated jugular venous pressures
  - Weight gain (daily weights are helpful to monitor volume status)

TREATMENT

- If the patient is eating, restrict dietary sodium to <2 g daily.
- Avoid or minimize sodium-containing intravenous fluids.
- In patients with moderate to severe edema or hypoxemia, consider using a loop diuretic such as furosemide to promote sodium and fluid loss (watch for hypokalemia).
  - The use of intravenous albumin to enhance diuresis in hypoalbuminemic patients is controversial. Although several studies have shown no benefit, these reports did not include patients with severe hypoalbuminemia (e.g., serum albumin <2.0).
- In oliguric or anuric patients, consider hemodialysis with hemofiltration for volume removal.
- Mechanical ventilation may be necessary in severe cases of hypervolemia with associated hypoxemia.

HYPONATREMIA

Postoperative hyponatremia is common. It may be mild and asymptomatic, or it may be severe enough to cause seizures and cerebral edema. This section focuses on acute postoperative hyponatremia, its causes, and its treatment.

ETIOLOGY

- When hyponatremia occurs after surgery, it is usually a result of the administration of hypotonic fluids (like half-normal saline, or 0.45% NaCl) during a period of increased antidiuretic hormone (ADH) secretion due to hypovolemia, pain, and/or stress.[6] The elevation of ADH levels leads to excessive water retention by the kidneys and results in hyponatremia. When the patient is volume-replete but remains hyponatremic due to excessive ADH release, this is called the syndrome of inappropriate ADH (SIADH).
  - Neurosurgical patients as well as patients with certain pulmonary conditions (such as intrathoracic tumors or acute respiratory failure) are at higher risk for developing SIADH than the general surgical population, although all surgical patients are at risk.
- Hyponatremia may also occur as a result of renal salt wasting. This may be due to the use of thiazide diuretics or may occur as a result of cerebral salt wasting (CSW), a syndrome similar to SIADH that occurs in neurosurgical patients but is thought to involve a separate natriuretic hormone in addition to ADH.
- Patients undergoing transurethral prostatectomy frequently develop hyponatremia due to the substantial absorption of sodium-free hypotonic irrigant solutions.[6]

DIAGNOSIS

The diagnosis of hyponatremia requires a careful history and physical examination and measurement of a serum sodium level <135 meq/L. Measure the urinary electrolytes in order to calculate the fractional excretion of sodium (FENa); this may help to determine the etiology, as described below.

- Clinical manifestations are more common with acute severe hyponatremia that develops over hours; they result from dysfunction of the central nervous system (CNS):
  - Headache
  - Confusion
  - Nausea/vomiting
  - Depressed reflexes
  - Seizures/coma
  - Cerebral edema with brainstem herniation
  - Permanent brain damage or death
- Patients who develop hyponatremia because of SIADH or absorption of hypotonic irrigant solutions are usually euvolemic, while patients with hyponatremia due to CSW will be hypovolemic. Thiazide use can lead to a euvolemic or a hypovolemic hyponatremia.

$$\text{FENa (percent)} = \frac{\text{urine Na} \times \text{plasma creatinine}}{\text{plasma Na} \times \text{urine creatinine}} \times 100$$

FIG. 56-1 Formula for the calculation of the fractional excretion of sodium (FENa) in hyponatremic patients.

- If the etiology is not clear from the clinical scenario, measure the urinary electrolytes and calculate FENa (Fig. 56-1).
  - Most causes of acute postoperative hyponatremia (including SIADH, thiazide use, and CSW) will be associated with a urine Na >40 meq/L and a FENa >1 percent.
  - Hyponatremia due to massive absorption of salt-free irrigants (as may be the case in postprostatectomy patients) may reveal a urine Na <25 meq/L and a FENa <1 percent.

TREATMENT[6]

- Restrict oral intake of electrolyte-free fluids (like juice or water). This may be adequate therapy for asymptomatic patients with serum Na concentration >125 meq/L.
- In symptomatic, hypovolemic patients, replace volume and Na simultaneously with intravenous normal saline (0.9% NaCl). Measure serum Na levels approximately every 4 to 6 h. If the duration of hyponatremia is unknown or greater than 1 to 2 days, allow the serum Na to increase at a rate no faster than 0.5 meq/L/h (or 10 to 12 meq/L/day) in order to minimize the risk of osmotic demyelination.
- For symptomatic patients who are euvolemic or hypervolemic, gentle use of hypertonic saline (3% NaCl) may be necessary. This is generally combined with furosemide, which limits the development of hypervolemia and produces a hypotonic urine equivalent to approximately half-normal saline. These mechanisms promote the correction of hyponatremia. Again, ensure that the rate of correction is no faster than 0.5 meq/L/h in order to minimize the risk of osmotic demyelination.
- For severe acute hyponatremia (with ominous CNS effects including seizures/coma), use hypertonic (0.3%) NaCl, and correct the serum sodium at a rate of 1 to 2 meq/L/h. Slow the rate down to 0.5 meq/L/h (as above) as soon as life-threatening manifestations abate.
- Figure 56-2 provides equations to estimate the appropriate rate of infusion of 3% saline.

HYPERNATREMIA

Postoperative hypernatremia is less common than hyponatremia and is almost always due to hypovolemia.

$$\text{Change in serum Na} = \frac{513 - (\text{current serum Na})}{0.5(\text{wt. in kg}) + 1}$$

$$\text{Change in serum Na} = \frac{513 - (\text{current serum Na})}{0.6(\text{wt. in kg}) + 1}$$

FIG. 56-2 Formulas for the calculation of the effect of 1 L of 3% saline on the serum sodium for men and women, respectively.

ETIOLOGY

- Unreplaced water loss. This is usually due to a combination of perioperative restriction of oral intake, insensible water losses, gastrointestinal losses (e.g., due to nasogastric suction), and the use of isotonic maintenance fluids like normal saline.
- Central diabetes insipidus may occur after neurosurgical procedures that disrupt the hypothalamus (e.g., craniopharyngioma resection). The loss of ADH (normally secreted by the hypothalamus) leads to excessive free water loss in the kidney.
- After hypotonic diuresis (e.g., with the use of mannitol to decrease intracranial pressure in neurosurgical patients, or with loop diuretics such as furosemide). The urine tends to be hypotonic, and if the lost free water is not replaced, hypernatremia may occur.
- After infusion or ingestion of a large Na load (e.g., hypertonic saline infusion or irrigation of hepatic hydatid cysts).

DIAGNOSIS

Hypernatremia is a serum sodium level >145 meq/L. Measure the urine osmolality to distinguish diabetes insipidus from other causes of hypernatremia.

- Clinical manifestations frequently result from CNS dysfunction[7]:
  - Extreme thirst
  - Orthostatic hypotension and other signs of hypovolemia
  - Confusion
  - Seizures/coma
  - Intracerebral hemorrhage due to brain shrinkage
- In hypernatremic patients with normal renal function, the urine osmolality will generally be above 700 to 800 mosmol/kg. The one exception is in the case of diabetes insipidus. In these patients, urine osmolality is inappropriately low because they lack the effects of ADH (and thus the ability to concentrate their urine and retain free water).

$$\text{Free-water deficit (L)} = 0.6 \times [\text{wt in kg}] \times [(\text{serum Na}/140) - 1]$$

FIG. 56-3 Formula for the calculation of the free-water deficit in hypernatremic patients.

TREATMENT

The mainstay of therapy is replacement of the free-water deficit.

- If the patient is able to drink (or receive tube feeds), increase the amount of free water that he or she takes in. If the hypernatremia is very mild and asymptomatic, this may be the only therapy needed.
- Calculate the free-water deficit (Fig. 56-3). If the patient is symptomatic, replace this volume of water, and add an additional allowance for continued water losses, intravenously as D_5W or hypotonic saline. Use isotonic saline only when hypovolemia is severe and intravascular volume replacement takes first priority.[7] Check the serum sodium every 4 to 6 h. If the duration of hypernatremia is unknown or longer than 1 day, allow the serum sodium to increase at a rate no faster than 0.5 meq/L/h (or 10 to 12 meq/L/day) in order to minimize the risk of cerebral edema.
- In patients with neurosurgery-induced central diabetes insipidus, correct the ADH deficiency through hormone replacement with desmopressin (a molecule very similar to ADH).

HYPERKALEMIA

As many as 1 to 1.5 percent of inpatients with chronic renal disease will develop life-threatening degrees of hyperkalemia.[1] This postoperative electrolyte disturbance is asymptomatic and therefore will remain undetected unless sought.

ETIOLOGY

Potassium is absorbed by the gut; under normal conditions, it is excreted almost milliequivalent for milliequivalent by the kidneys. Even when potassium intake is significantly increased, normal kidneys will quickly adapt and maintain normokalemia. Most cases of postoperative hyperkalemia arise in patients with significant preexisting renal dysfunction (or acute renal failure), but there is usually a second inciting event that prevents renal adaptation.

- Most cases of hyperkalemia are iatrogenic[8]; physician-prescribed supplemental potassium chloride (KCl) is the most common offender. Medications that are well known to cause hyperkalemia (and should be used with caution in patients with renal dysfunction) include:
  - KCl
  - ACE inhibitors
  - Angiotensin receptor blockers
  - Potassium-sparing diuretics
  - NSAIDs
  - Digoxin
  - Cyclosporine
  - Tacrolimus
  - Trimethoprim
  - Pentamidine
- Significant tissue breakdown (and subsequent release of intracellular potassium into the blood) is another cause of postoperative hyperkalemia, even in patients without renal dysfunction. This may result from burns, trauma, rhabdomyolysis, malignant hyperthermia, and other similar responses to neuromuscular blocking agents.
  - Malignant hyperthermia is an inherited disorder that is precipitated by anesthesia. The depolarizing muscle relaxants such as succinylcholine (which causes simultaneous contractions of skeletal muscles) and inhalational anesthetic agents (which alter the integrity of muscle cell membranes) can trigger this syndrome, in which the skeletal muscles undergo protracted spasm and become hypermetabolic, creating acidemia and hyperkalemia.[9]
  - Hyperkalemia can also occur after succinylcholine use in patients with major tissue trauma, denervating disorders/injuries (like amyotrophic lateral sclerosis, cerebrovascular accident, or major nerve injury), and muscular dystrophy. Burn injuries and/or soft tissue trauma may also predispose to succinylcholine-induced hyperkalemia.[9]
- Postoperative acidemia may also create hyperkalemia. This is due to the shift of intracellular potassium into the extracellular space in exchange for hydrogen ions (see Chap. 57).

DIAGNOSIS

Hyperkalemia is a serum potassium >5.0 meq/L. Hemolysis may falsely elevate the measured potassium levels; if this is suspected, repeat the measurement. Obtain an electrocardiogram (ECG) immediately after establishing a diagnosis of hyperkalemia.

- Patients with hyperkalemia are asymptomatic. It has been said that the first symptom of hyperkalemia is death.
- The most significant effect of high extracellular potassium levels is cardiac. Hyperkalemia affects the

membrane excitability of cardiac muscle cells and can cause progressive dysrhythmias and cardiac arrest.

- The earliest effect on the ECG is usually narrowing and symmetrical peaking (*tenting*) of the T wave. The QT interval is shortened at this stage, due to decreased duration of the action potential (Fig. 56-4).
- Progressive hyperkalemia reduces atrial and ventricular resting membrane potentials, leading to a widened QRS and decreased P-wave amplitude. Prolongation of the PR interval can occur; second- or third-degree AV block may follow. P waves may disappear altogether, leaving the patient in a junctional rhythm.
- Severe hyperkalemia leads to eventual asystole, sometimes preceded by a slow undulatory ventricular rhythm that resembles sine waves.

TREATMENT[1,8]

Hyperkalemia is a medical emergency. As soon as the serum potassium level returns, obtain an ECG and consider placing the patient on continuous cardiac telemetry.

- If ECG changes are present, administer intravenous calcium gluconate. This will rapidly stabilize the myocardium and buy time for potassium-lowering treatments to work.
  - Note that hypercalcemia (or rapid infusion of calcium) may actually precipitate digoxin-related dysrhythmias.
- Methods that will rapidly decrease potassium levels by shifting it into the intracellular space include:
  - Infusion of intravenous insulin (plus intravenous glucose to prevent hypoglycemia)
  - Use of inhaled beta agonists
  - Infusion of intravenous sodium bicarbonate
- Methods to permanently remove excess potassium from the body include:
  - Potassium-binding resins like sodium polystyrene sulfonate (Kayexalate)
    - Note that this is usually combined with sorbitol and is contraindicated, due to risk of bowel necrosis, in patients who have undergone bowel surgery.
  - Loop diuretics
  - Hemodialysis
- Ensure that the patient's diet is potassium-restricted, that intravenous fluids are potassium-free, and that any nonessential medications known to cause hyperkalemia are discontinued (see above).

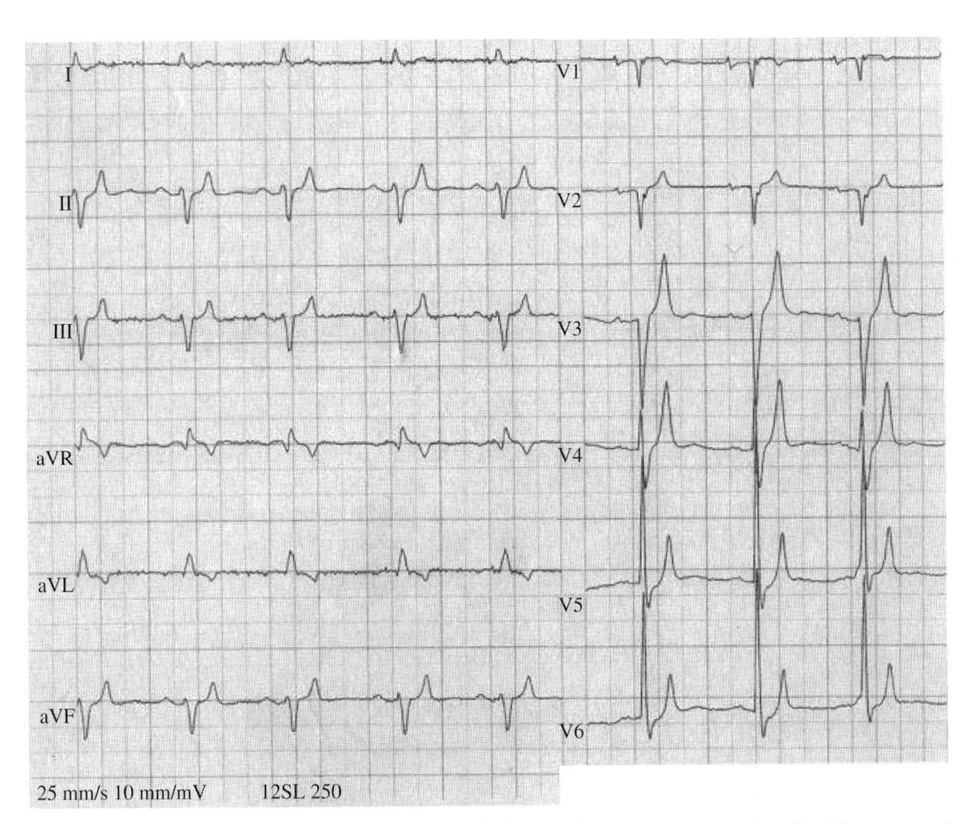

FIG. 56-4 Classic ECG changes associated with hyperkalemia (symmetrical peaked T waves and a shortened QTc interval). (Adapted from Van Mieghem et al.,[11] with permission.)

HYPOKALEMIA

Hypokalemia, like hyperkalemia, is usually asymptomatic, especially when mild. It is one of the most common electrolyte disturbances and occurs in over 20 percent of hospitalized patients.[10]

ETIOLOGY

- Postoperative hypokalemia usually results from the combination of decreased intake (e.g., due to perioperative dietary restriction) and increased losses (e.g., due to diarrhea or medications). Medications that promote renal potassium loss include:
  - Diuretics
  - Intravenous antibiotics including penicillins, gentamicin, amphotericin B
  - Mineralocorticoids (fludrocortisone)
  - High-dose glucocorticoids
- Hypokalemia may also result from increased shift of potassium to the intracellular space, as occurs during the use of inhaled beta agonists or with alkalemia (see Chap. 57).

DIAGNOSIS

Hypokalemia is a serum potassium level <3.6 meq/L. While the cardiac effects of hypokalemia tend to be less worrisome than those associated with hyperkalemia, obtain an ECG if the patient is symptomatic or has underlying heart disease or if the serum potassium level is <3.0.

- Hypokalemia is usually asymptomatic, but when it is significant, it may cause generalized weakness, constipation, muscle cramping, and even rhabdomyolysis or an ascending paralysis.
- Cardiac effects are infrequent but may be significant in patients with cardiac ischemia or digoxin toxicity; in these patients, hypokalemia may potentiate dysrhythmias.
  - ECG changes may include flattened T waves, prominent U waves, and occasionally ST-segment depression or supraventricular tachycardia.

TREATMENT[8,10]

The mainstay of treatment is potassium replacement. The few indications for intravenous replacement include cardiac dysrhythmias, rhabdomyolysis, paralysis, and severe diarrhea. Treat most other patients with oral replacement if possible. The goal serum potassium concentration should be approximately 4.0 meq/L.

- Infuse intravenous potassium chloride (KCl) at a maximum rate of 20 meq/h through a central line (or 10 meq/h through a peripheral line). Monitor the patient's cardiac rhythm during intravenous replacement. To reassess replacement needs, repeat measurement of the serum potassium level after administering a maximum of 60 meq.
- Give oral KCl in divided doses (usually twice daily) and limit the dose to 40 meq at a time owing to the high incidence of dyspepsia.
- Hypomagnesemia can potentiate potassium losses by the kidney and, to ensure success, should be corrected before potassium repletion.
- Minimize the use of medications that cause potassium depletion. If a known offender must be used, consider daily scheduled potassium replacement or the addition of a potassium-sparing diuretic in patients who require regular diuretic therapy.

REFERENCES

1. Yee J, Parasuraman R, Narins RG. Selective review of key perioperative renal-electrolyte disturbances in chronic renal failure patients. *Chest* 115(5 suppl): 149S–157S, 1999.
2. Alderson P, Schierhout G, Roberts I, Bunn F. Colloids versus crystalloids for fluid resuscitation in critically ill patients. *Cochrane Database Syst Rev* 2: CD000567, 2000.
3. Charlson ME, MacKenzie CR, Gold JP, et al. Risk for postoperative congestive heart failure. *Surg Gynecol Obstet* 172(2): 95–104, 1991.
4. Rosenthal MH. Intraoperative fluid management: What and how much? *Chest* 115(5 suppl):106S–112S, 1999.
5. Sandham JD, Hull RD, Brant RF, et al. A randomized, controlled trial of the use of pulmonary-artery catheters in high-risk surgical patients. *N Engl J Med* 346(1):5–14, 2000.
6. Adrogue HJ, Madias NE. Hyponatremia. *N Engl J Med* 342(21):1581–1589, 2000.
7. Adrogue HJ, Madias NE. Hypernatremia. *N Engl J Med* 342(20):1493–1499, 2000.
8. Gennari FJ. Disorders of potassium homeostasis: Hypokalemia and hyperkalemia. *Crit Care Clin* 18(2):273–288, 2002.
9. Halaszynski TM, Juda R, Silverman DG. Optimizing postoperative outcomes with efficient preoperative assessment and management. *Crit Care Med* 32(4 suppl):S76–86, 2004.
10. Gennari FJ. Hypokalemia. *N Engl J Med* 339(7):451–458, 1998.
11. Van Mieghem C, Sabbe M, Knockaert D. The clinical value of the ECG in noncardiac conditions. *Chest* 125(4):1561–1576, 2004.

57 ACID-BASE DISORDERS

Jennifer C. Kerns and Maninder Kohli

INTRODUCTION

THE PROBLEM

- In order to function properly, the body normally maintains the arterial blood pH within a narrow window between 7.35 and 7.45. The respiratory and renal systems provide this regulation.
- Acidemia is an arterial pH less than 7.35, while alkalemia is an arterial pH greater than 7.45. Either of these two physiologic states can lead to a myriad of problems involving the central nervous system (CNS) and cardiovascular system. Severe acidemia or alkalemia can lead to death if untreated.
- Acidosis is a bodily process leading to acidemia, while alkalosis is a particular process leading to alkalemia. There are four basic types of acid-base disorders: respiratory acidosis, respiratory alkalosis, metabolic acidosis, and metabolic alkalosis.
- The four disorders may occur alone (a simple disorder) or in combination (a mixed disorder). This chapter covers the peri- and postoperative causes, diagnosis, and treatment of each of the four simple acid-base disorders.

INCIDENCE

- Although the overall incidence is unclear, acid-base disturbances are extremely common postoperative complications and are nearly universal in mechanically ventilated and critically ill patients.
  - One prospective study found that 87.5 percent of patients had normal acid-base balance before general surgery but that over 50 percent developed a metabolic alkalosis as a postoperative complication.[1]

TIMING

- Acid-base disturbances may be preexisting, may occur during anesthesia and surgery, or may develop for the first time after surgery. This chapter focuses primarily on acid-base disorders that occur during surgery and as postoperative complications.

CAUSES

The causes for each of the four simple disorders are discussed in detail below.

DIAGNOSIS

- Physical findings tend to be nonspecific and generally do not aid in making a diagnosis.
- Laboratory testing is the key to diagnosis. Identification of an acid-base disturbance simply requires the concomitant measurement of an arterial blood gas and a serum chemistry panel (Fig. 57-1). The arterial pH will always indicate the primary (or most dominant) disorder. A pH less than 7.35 indicates an acidosis (whether respiratory or metabolic), while a pH greater than 7.45 indicates an alkalosis (whether respiratory or metabolic).

TREATMENT

Treatment of the acid-base disorders varies depending on the type of disorder and its etiology. The treatment options for each disorder are discussed separately below.

THE FOUR MAJOR ACID-BASE DISORDERS

RESPIRATORY ACIDOSIS

DEFINITION/DIAGNOSIS

A respiratory acidosis is a process that leads to an arterial blood pH less than 7.35 and a concomitant $Paco_2$ greater than 40 to 45 mmHg.

ETIOLOGIES

- ***Decreased release of CO_2 from the respiratory system:*** Impaired ventilatory drive (due to anesthetic agents[2] or excessive oxygen therapy in a patient with chronic compensated hypercarbia), airway or endotracheal tube obstruction, inappropriately low ventilator settings, obstructive lung disease (emphysema or severe asthma), restrictive lung disease, obesity or marked ascites (via restriction of diaphragm), neuromuscular diseases, pulmonary edema.
- ***Increased production of CO_2:*** Malignant hyperthermia, extensive burn injury, laparoscopic surgery[3] with associated insufflation/systemic absorption of CO_2.

CLINICAL CONSEQUENCES/PHYSICAL FINDINGS

- ***CNS effects:*** Anxiety, confusion, dyspnea, narcosis with somnolence progressing to coma, intracranial hypertension with headache and papilledema.
- ***Cardiovascular effects:*** Due to increased sympathetic tone and adrenal catecholamine output, these effects include hypertension, tachycardia, increased cardiac output, and dysrhythmias.
- ***Hyperkalemia:*** Due to the release of intracellular potassium in exchange for extracellular hydrogen ion,

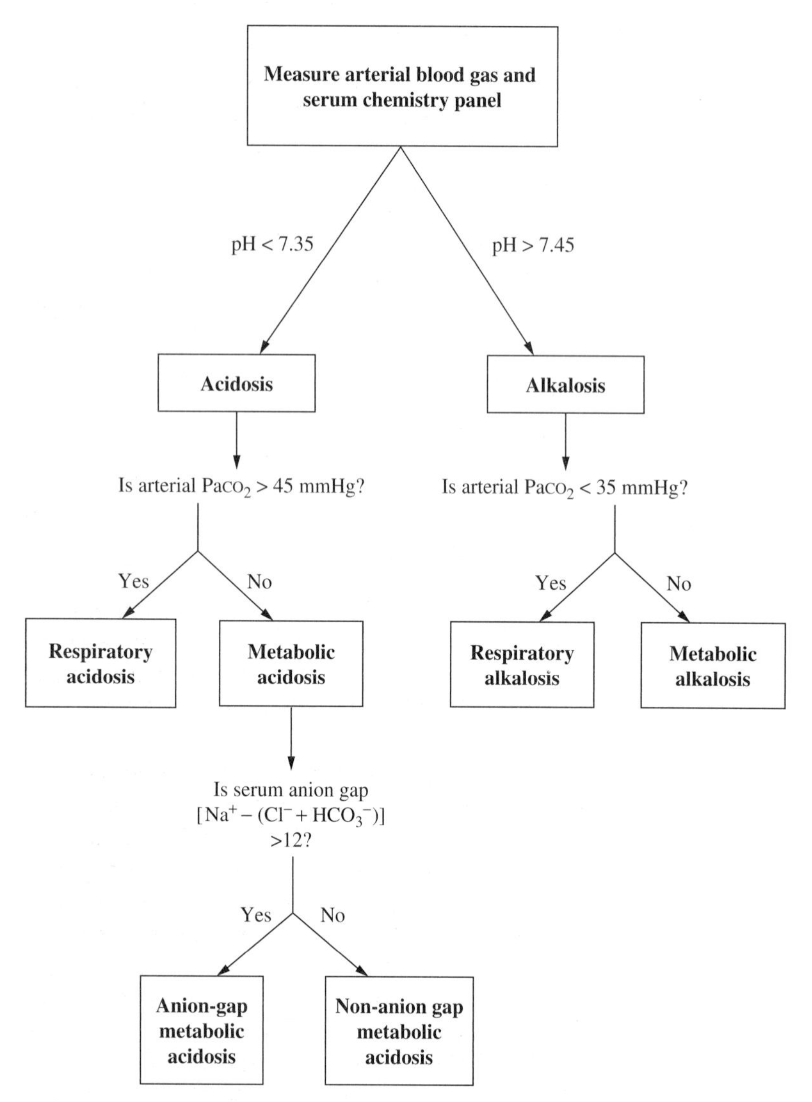

FIG. 57-1 Diagnostic algorithm for simple acid-base disorders.

hyperkalemia can predispose to dysrhythmias and lead to cardiac arrest.

Treatment

Treatment is to return the $Paco_2$ to baseline, usually approximately 40 mmHg:

- ***Increase minute ventilation:*** In an intubated patient, adjust ventilator settings (tidal volume, respiratory rate); in a spontaneously breathing patient, the use of noninvasive mask ventilation [continuous positive airway pressure (CPAP) or biphasic positive airway pressure (BiPAP)] or even intubation for controlled ventilation may be required.
- ***Reverse or minimize the use of drugs that impair ventilatory drive:*** Such drugs include neuromuscular blocking agents[2] and opioids or benzodiazepines used to excess; ventilatory drive may also be impaired by the excessive use of oxygen therapy in patients accustomed to chronic hypercarbia.
- ***Use supplemental oxygen in patients with concomitant hypoxemia:*** Use caution in patients with chronic compensated hypercarbia; the goal in these patients should be to return their $Paco_2$ to their own baseline, which may be significantly higher than 40 mmHg.
- ***Treat coexisting metabolic acid-base disorders.***

RESPIRATORY ALKALOSIS

Definition/Diagnosis

A respiratory alkalosis is a process that leads to an arterial blood pH greater than 7.45 and a concomitant $Paco_2$ less than 35 to 40 mmHg.

Etiologies

- ***Increased release of CO_2 from the respiratory system (hyperventilation):*** Inappropriately high ventilator settings (which may be intentional in patients undergoing craniotomy, in order to induce cerebral vasoconstriction and thereby decrease intracranial pressure); patient-related causes such as pain or anxiety; sepsis; hypoxemia; brain injury; cirrhosis; pregnancy.

- ***Decreased metabolic rate:*** This may be due to anesthetic drugs[2] or hypothermia.

Clinical Consequences/Physical Findings

- ***CNS effects:*** Dizziness, confusion, or coma; neuromuscular irritability leading to tetany or seizures. Intracranial vasoconstriction that results from hypocapnia can lead to regional cerebral ischemia in patients with preexisting impairment of cerebral blood flow.[2]
- ***Cardiovascular effects:*** Increased sensitivity to digitalis; predisposition to ventricular dysrhythmias and subsequent cardiac arrest.
- ***Hypokalemia:*** Due to the shift of potassium into cells in exchange for hydrogen ion, hypokalemia is particularly common during neurosurgery when furosemide or mannitol are used.[2] It can cause ventricular dysrhythmias and cardiac arrest as well as muscle weakness or cramping.
- ***Impairment of oxygen delivery to tissues:*** Alkalemia shifts the hemoglobin-oxygen dissociation curve to the left, compromising the release of oxygen to tissues and thus predisposing to tissue ischemia.

Treatment

Treatment is to return the Pa_{CO_2} to baseline (approximately 40 mmHg).

- ***Treat the underlying etiology:*** In spontaneously breathing patients, hypoxemia may be treated with supplemental oxygen, or treat pain/anxiety with analgesics/anxiolytics.
- ***Decrease minute ventilation*** in mechanically ventilated patients by adjusting ventilator settings (primarily respiratory rate and/or tidal volume).
- ***Treat coexisting metabolic acid-base disorders.***

METABOLIC ALKALOSIS

Definition/Diagnosis

A metabolic alkalosis is a process leading to an arterial blood pH greater than 7.45 and a concomitant serum bicarbonate (HCO_3^-) greater than 24 to 28 mmol/L. Although it is not necessary for diagnosis, measurement of urinary chloride concentration may be helpful in determining treatment approach (see below).

Etiologies[1,2]

In one study, approximately 50 percent of general surgical patients developed postoperative metabolic alkalosis, usually due either to hypovolemia or excessive bicarbonate from transfusion of fresh-frozen plasma.[1,4]

Loss of H^+ and Cl^- Ions

- Gastrointestinal (GI) losses (loss of hydrochloric acid from protracted emesis or nasogastric suction).
- Renal losses (thiazide and loop diuretics; hypersecretion of aldosterone, which may be due to hypovolemia or Cushing's disease).
- Metabolism of excessive lactate or citrate (such as occurs during the intravenous administration of lactated Ringer's solution or massive intraoperative transfusion of blood products containing citrate as a preservative).

Excessive HCO_3^- Intake/Retention

- Renal retention due to hypovolemia [decreased glomerular filtration rate (GFR) leading to inappropriately high reabsorption of bicarbonate[2]]. This is commonly called a "contraction alkalosis."
- Intrinsic renal diseases (e.g., Bartter's syndrome).
- Excessive bicarbonate intake (e.g., after massive transfusion, the lactate and citrate contained in blood products is rapidly metabolized to bicarbonate).

Clinical Consequences/Physical Findings

- ***CNS effects:*** Decreased ventilatory drive (and subsequent hypercarbia with its resultant CNS consequences as outlined above). This may complicate weaning from mechanical ventilation,[2,4] and can lead to frank apnea when combined with opioid analgesia. Neuromuscular irritability (tetany or seizures) may occur.
- ***Hypokalemia:*** Due to intracellular potassium flux, renal losses associated with HCO_3^- reabsorption, or diuretics, hypokalemia leads to a predisposition to cardiac dysrhythmias as well as muscle weakness or cramping.
- ***Hyperlactatemia:*** This is a benign finding (often mistaken for an indication of tissue ischemia) that disappears with correction of the alkalemia.

Treatment

Treatment depends on the underlying cause but usually starts with the administration of intravenous normal saline (unless contraindicated).

- ***Measure urinary chloride if the underlying etiology is unclear.*** Urinary Cl^- is markedly decreased (<10 mmol/L) in the setting of hypovolemia or gastric losses; these patients will generally respond to replacement of volume with intravenous normal saline.
- ***Replace Cl^- with intravenous normal saline*** (0.9% NaCl), or either KCl or $CaCl_2$ in patients in whom volume replacement is contraindicated (e.g., congestive heart failure with pulmonary edema).
- ***Consider using acetazolamide*** to increase renal proximal tubular loss of bicarbonate in patients who are not responsive to Cl^- replacement; be aware that acetazolamide may exacerbate hypokalemia.

- ***Intravenous hydrochloric acid or ammonium chloride*** may be used in rare cases of severe metabolic alkalosis, as when serum bicarbonate exceeds 50 mmol/L (do not use this strategy without the help of a renal or critical care consultant).

METABOLIC ACIDOSIS

DEFINITION/DIAGNOSIS

- A metabolic acidosis is a process leading to an arterial blood pH less than 7.35 and a concomitant serum bicarbonate below 20 to 24 mmol/L.
- The metabolic acidoses are a complex group of disorders with many different causes; they can be divided into two main groups: "anion-gap acidoses" (anion gap >12), and "non–anion gap acidoses" (anion gap ≤12).
- Calculate the anion gap (AG) from the patient's serum basic chemistry panel using the following equation:

$$AG = [Na^+] - [Cl^- + HCO_3^-]$$

- The normal range for the AG is 9 to 12; thus, an AG of 13 or more is elevated and consistent with the "anion-gap metabolic acidoses." In this case, additional laboratory tests (such as serum lactate, ketones, blood urea nitrogen, and so on) may help to determine the underlying cause.

ETIOLOGIES

See Table 57-1 for a comprehensive list of causes:

- ***Anion-gap acidoses:*** The most common causes in the postoperative patient include renal failure and lactic acidosis (usually due to tissue ischemia, as from hypoxemia, cardiopulmonary bypass, or hypotension/shock).

TABLE 57-1 Common Causes of Metabolic Acidoses

INCREASED ANION GAP ACIDOSIS	NON–ANION GAP ACIDOSIS
Lactic acidosis (e.g., from shock or tissue ischemia)	Prolonged diarrhea
Uremia (renal failure)	Primary adrenal insufficiency (hypoaldosteronemia)
Ketoacidosis (from diabetes, alcohol, or starvation)	Bilious losses (percutaneous drainage or nasogastric tube suction)
Paraldehyde, methanol, or ethylene glycol ingestion	Excessive administration of normal saline (intravenous NaCl)
Rhabdomyolysis	Potassium-sparing diuretics (like spironolactone)
Alcohol intoxication	Renal tubular dysfunction (RTA)
Aspirin toxicity	Enterostomy or ureteroenterostomy
Carbon monoxide or cyanide poisoning	Acetazolamide therapy

- ***Non–anion gap acidoses:*** The most common cause in the postoperative patient is excessive administration of intravenous saline.[5]
  - Although the clinical relevance of such a saline-induced non–anion gap acidosis is debatable, several studies of patients undergoing surgery have suggested that those who developed a hyperchloremic (non–anion gap) metabolic acidosis after the administration of a 0.9% saline solution had significantly greater blood loss than patients given buffered fluids such as lactated Ringer's solution.[6,7]

CLINICAL CONSEQUENCES/PHYSICAL FINDINGS

- ***CNS effects:*** Somnolence, confusion, coma; increased ventilatory drive/tachypnea.
- ***Cardiovascular effects:*** Impaired cardiac contractility (especially when pH <7.2); hypotension; myocardial irritation with a resultant predisposition to dysrhythmias.
- ***Hyperkalemia:*** Due to the release of intracellular potassium in exchange for extracellular hydrogen ion, hyperkalemia can predispose to dysrhythmias and lead to cardiac arrest.
- ***Impaired muscle strength and endurance:*** Weakness of the diaphragm and respiratory muscles may contribute to respiratory compromise and/or failure (and worsened acidemia).
- ***Impaired uptake of oxygen by hemoglobin*** (compromised oxygen-carrying capacity, which may exacerbate tissue ischemia and lactic acidosis).
- ***Possible propensity toward intraoperative/postoperative blood loss.***[6,7]
- Frequently the effects of the underlying etiology are worse than the acidosis itself (e.g., lactic acidosis resulting from tissue ischemia).

TREATMENT

- Correct the underlying cause.
- Temporizing therapies may include the following:
  - ***Mechanical ventilation to facilitate respiratory compensation*** (increase minute ventilation by increasing respiratory rate and/or tidal volume).
  - ***Replacement of serum bicarbonate*** with oral potassium citrate or sodium citrate (which is metabolized to bicarbonate, and is frequently used in patients with acidosis due to renal etiologies).
    - In severe cases (e.g., arterial pH <7.15), consider intravenous sodium bicarbonate; however, the benefit of this is controversial.[8] Theoretically, improving the pH may mitigate some of the harmful effects of acidemia; however, little evidence supports this. Studies examining the use of intravenous $NaHCO_3$ in surgical patients are lacking, but a systematic review of the use of $NaHCO_3$ in hypoxemic lactic

acidosis during cardiopulmonary resuscitation[9] and several studies in diabetic ketoacidosis[8,10] have all failed to show a benefit in clinical outcomes.

REFERENCES

1. Okusawa S, Aikawa N, Abe O. Postoperative metabolic alkalosis following general surgery: Its incidence and possible etiology. *Jpn J Surg* 19(3):312–318, 1989.
2. Miller RD, ed. *Anesthesia,* 5th ed Philadelphia: Churchill Livingstone 2000:1404–1413.
3. O'Malley C. Physiologic changes during laparoscopy. *Anesthesiol Clin North Am* 19(1):1–19, 2001.
4. Webster NR, Kulkarni V. Metabolic alkalosis in the critically ill. *Crit Rev Clin Lab Sci* 36(5):497–510, 1999.
5. Waters JH, Miller LR, Clack S, Kim JV. Cause of metabolic acidosis in prolonged surgery. *Crit Care Med* 27(10): 2142–2146, 1999.
6. Waters JH, Gottlieb A, Schoenwald P, et al. Normal saline versus lactated Ringer's solution for intraoperative fluid management in patients undergoing abdominal aortic aneurysm repair: An outcome study. *Anesth Analg* 93(4):817–822, 2001.
7. Martin G, El-Moalem H, Bennett-Guerrero E, et al. Comparison of intraoperative blood loss in patients undergoing major surgery using Hextend, Hespan, and lactated Ringer's solution (abstr). *Anesthesiology* 91:A166, 1999.
8. Peixoto A. Critical issues in nephrology. *Clin Chest Med* 24(4):561–581, 2003.
9. Levy MM. An evidence-based evaluation of the use of sodium bicarbonate during cardiopulmonary resuscitation. *Crit Care Clin* 14(3):457–483, 1998.
10. Viallon A, Zeni F, Lafond P, et al. Does bicarbonate therapy improve the management of severe diabetic ketoacidosis? *Crit Care Med* 27(12):2690–2693, 1999.

58 RENAL FAILURE

Maninder Kohli and Jennifer C. Kerns

INTRODUCTION

- Acute renal failure (ARF) is an important postoperative complication that contributes to perioperative morbidity and mortality. More than 25 percent of all episodes of hospital-acquired renal insufficiency occur in surgical patients.[1]
- The mortality of postoperative ARF ranges from 25 to 90 percent despite important technological advances in renal replacement therapy and intensive care support.[2]

INCIDENCE

- Postoperative renal failure is common. For example, the incidence was 0.6 percent in a large VA database of patients undergoing noncardiac surgery.[3]
- ARF occurs more frequently in patients undergoing cardiac surgery, with an overall incidence of about 8 percent.[4]

TIMING

- Postoperative ARF usually develops within a few days after surgery.
- Patients with sustained hypotension, volume depletion, or bladder/ureteral injury may rapidly develop a decline in the glomerular filtration rate (GFR) after the precipitating event.
- In contrast, nephrotoxin-mediated ARF typically develops after a delay of several days.

RISK FACTORS

- Preoperative renal disease is one of the strongest predictors of postoperative renal failure. Important predisposing factors for renal disease include diabetes, hypertension, and immunologic renal disease.
- Other significant medical comorbidities that increase risk are advanced age and congestive heart failure.
- Surgical procedures that increase risk are cardiac, aortic, and vascular procedures, as well as surgery for obstructive jaundice (see Chap. 34).

CAUSES

- Table 58-1 lists the principal causes and differential diagnosis of acute postoperative renal failure.

TABLE 58-1 Differential Diagnosis of Postoperative Renal Failure

Prerenal causes
Intraoperative hypotension
Volume depletion
Sepsis
Congestive heart failure
Renal causes
Post–ischemic acute tubular necrosis
Drug-induced nephritis
Radiocontrast dye
Hemoglobinuria
Myoglobinuria
Postrenal causes:
Tubular obstruction
Bladder dysfunction
Pelvic/ureteral obstruction

- ***Sustained hypotension*** from various causes is one of the most common etiologies of postoperative ARF. Severe perioperative fluid and blood loss, prolonged anesthetic time and aortic cross-clamp time, positive-pressure ventilation, and cardiopulmonary bypass are among the predisposing factors for postoperative hypotension and ARF. Disruption of afferent arteriolar autoregulation with nonsteroidal anti-inflammatory drugs (NSAIDs) and efferent constriction with angiotensin-converting enzyme (ACE) inhibitors and angiotensin receptor blockers (ARBs) can further reduce renal mean arterial pressure.[5]
- Inflammatory mediators in patients with *gram-negative sepsis* can reduce systemic vascular resistance and cause renal vasoconstriction, with a resulting decline in renal function.[5]
- ***Prolonged postsurgical ischemia*** and sepsis can lead to postoperative acute tubular necrosis (ATN).
- ***Cholesterol embolization*** from cardiopulmonary bypass and aortic surgery can cause renal dysfunction.
- Injury to the deep renal medulla from *nephrotoxins* (such as aminoglycosides and iodinated contrast media) can lead to significant tubular damage several days after the exposure. Acute drug-induced interstitial nephritis is an occasional cause of intrinsic postoperative ARF.
- ***Postoperative bladder dysfunction*** can occur in patients with benign prostatic hyperplasia and neurogenic bladder. Ureteral injury, papillary necrosis, and retroperitoneal hematoma are important considerations in postrenal causes of postoperative ARF.[6]

DIAGNOSIS

- The diagnosis of postoperative renal insufficiency is frequently delayed. Decreased urinary output may be the first sign of ARF, although many patients have nonoliguric renal insufficiency. Moreover, symptoms manifest only after the occurrence of significant renal dysfunction.
- Symptoms and signs of ARF include reduced oral intake, vomiting, flank pain, mental status changes, hypertension, and volume overload.
- Measurements of serum chemistry, urinary osmolality, and electrolytes and examination of the urinary sediment are mandatory in the evaluation of postoperative renal failure.
- Calculate the creatinine clearance using the Cockroft-Gault equation (Appendix A). This provides a reasonable estimate of the GFR.
- Determine the fractional excretion of sodium in order to distinguish between ATN and renal hypoperfusion (Table 58-2 and Appendix A).

TABLE 58-2 Differentiating Prerenal and Renal Azotemia

	PRERENAL	RENAL
Urinary osmolality (mOsm/kg)	>50	<350
Urinary/plasma osmolality	>1.3	<1.1
Urinary sodium (meq/L)	<20	>40
Urinary/plasma creatinine	>40	<20
Fractional excretion of sodium (FENa)	<1%	>1%

- Hyaline casts (concentrated Tamm-Horsfall mucoproteins) are nonspecific and may indicate hypoperfusion. Often, the presence of brown granular casts suggests ATN. White blood cells can indicate urinary tract infection, and eosinophiluria suggests interstitial nephritis or cholesterol embolization.
- Variations in serum sodium levels can lead to mental status changes.
- Impaired renal concentrating ability, salt wasting, hypotonic fluids, and the postoperative syndrome of inappropriate antidiuretic hormone (SIADH) can lead to hyponatremia.
- Hypernatremia can develop from the inability to replace free water losses during the polyuria phase of recovery of renal function.
- Perform a renal ultrasound if there is a strong suspicion of urinary tract obstruction. Older men with benign prostatic hyperplasia and patients who have undergone urologic or gynecologic procedures are at a higher risk for developing postrenal causes of postoperative ARF.

TREATMENT

- The mainstays of therapy for patients with postoperative ARF are supportive and include the following:
  - Hydration
  - Correction of acid-base disturbances
  - Monitoring serum electrolytes: sodium, potassium, phosphate, and calcium
- Maintain cardiac output and raise mean arterial pressure (MAP) to at least 90 mmHg to optimize renal perfusion in patients with prerenal azotemia. Hydrate patients who are hypotensive, are clinically volume-depleted, and have a fractional excretion of sodium <1.
- In oliguric or anuric patients who are euvolemic, be cautious with aggressive hydration so as to avoid volume overload.
- The use of diuretics is controversial. One should probably use diuretics after volume status has been corrected, and then only in moderate doses for a short time.[7]
- A controlled trial found that the use of low-dose dopamine provided no protection from renal dysfunction.[8] We do not recommend this strategy.

- Discontinue nephrotoxins and avoid radiologic procedures involving iodinated contrast media. Consider alternatives for aminoglycosides, NSAIDs, ACE inhibitors, ARBs, and potassium-sparing diuretics.
- Hydration can also minimize pigment-induced ARF. The strategy of urinary alkalinization with bicarbonate and forced diuresis with mannitol is controversial in such patients. In a recent study of trauma patients with rhabdomyolysis, the use of bicarbonate and mannitol did not reduce the incidence of renal failure, need for dialysis, or mortality.[9]
- The role of atrial natriuretic peptide (ANP) in the management of patients with ATN is uncertain. A large study randomly assigned critically ill patients with ATN to an infusion of synthetic ANP (anaritide) or placebo. No improvement occurred in dialysis-free survival (43 versus 47 percent, respectively).[10]
- Theoretically, initiation of dialysis can delay the return of renal function due to several detrimental effects, such as reduced urinary output, induction of hypotension, and complement activation from a blood-dialysis membrane interaction. We recommend renal replacement therapy for patients with severe perturbations complicating postoperative renal failure, including volume overload, pulmonary edema, severe acidosis, uremia (blood urea nitrogen >140), and refractory hyperkalemia.
- It is unknown whether the timing or adequacy of dialysis influences survival in patients with postoperative ARF. The indications for urgent dialysis and maintenance of dialysis in the postoperative patient with renal failure are the same as for patients in other settings.
- Base the selection of dialysis (hemodialysis versus continuous), the frequency and intensity of dialysis (daily versus intermittent), and the degree of ultrafiltration on available modalities and the hemodynamic stability of the patient.[5]
- The mortality of patients requiring postoperative dialysis is disturbingly high. In a study of patients undergoing cardiac surgery, 8 percent developed postoperative ARF.[4] Mortality among the patients who required dialysis was 28 percent, compared with a mortality of 1.8 percent in patients with postoperative ARF who did not require dialysis. However, of the patients who survive dialysis, over 80 percent eventually recover sufficient renal function to discontinue dialysis.[5]

SUMMARY

- Postoperative renal failure is a major morbid event associated with significant mortality. Preexisting chronic kidney disease is the most important risk factor.
- Be alert to the risk of developing this complication, since signs and symptoms may not be apparent.
- Implement appropriate diagnostic and treatment strategies as soon as the diagnosis is apparent. The most important strategies are avoidance of nephrotoxins and restoration of adequate perfusion pressure. When indicated, promptly initiate renal replacement therapy.

APPENDIX A

COCKROFT-GAULT EQUATION

Creatinine clearance (mL/min) for women

$$= \frac{[140 - \text{age (years)}] \times \text{weight (kg)}}{\text{serum creatinine } (\mu\text{mol/L})}$$

Multiply result by 1.22 for male patients.

FRACTIONAL EXCRETION OF SODIUM

$$\frac{\text{Urinary Na} \times \text{serum creatinine}}{\text{Serum Na} \times \text{urinary creatinine}} \times 100 = \text{FENa}$$

ESTIMATED WATER DEFICIT

$$[\text{Weight (kg)} \times 0.6] \times [1 - (140/\text{serum Na})]$$

REFERENCES

1. Liano F, Pascual J. Epidemiology of acute renal failure: A prospective, multicenter community-based study. *Kidney Int* 50(3):811–818, 1996.
2. Carmichael P, Carmichael AR. Acute renal failure in the surgical setting. *A NZ J Surg* 73(3):144–153, 2003.
3. Chertow GM, Henderson W, Khuri S, et al. Acute renal failure after non-cardiac surgery: Results from the national VA surgical risk study. *J Am Soc Nephrol* 8:123A, 1997.
4. Conlon PJ, Stafford-Smith M, White WD, et al. Acute renal failure following cardiac surgery. *Nephrol Dial Transplant* 14:1158, 1999.
5. Edwards BF. Postoperative renal insufficiency. *Med Clin North Am* 85:1241–1254, 2001.
6. Joseph AJ, Cohn SL. Perioperative care of the patient with renal failure. *Med Clin North Am* 87:193–210, 2003.
7. Lamiere N, Vanholder R, Van Biesen W. Loop diuretics for patients with acute renal failure: Helpful or harmful. *JAMA* 288:2599, 2002.
8. Bellomo R, Chapman M, Finfer S, et al. Low-dose dopamine in patients with early renal dysfunction: A placebo-controlled randomized trial. *Lancet* 356:2139, 2000.
9. Brown CV, Rhee P, Chan L, et al. Preventing renal failure in patients with rhabdomyolysis: Do bicarbonate and mannitol make a difference? *J Trauma* 56(6):1191–1196, 2004.
10. Allgren RL, Marbury TC, Rahman SN, et al. Anaritide in acute tubular necrosis. *N Engl J Med* 336:828, 1997.

59 ANEMIA AND BLEEDING

Kurt Pfeifer and Jeffrey L. Carson

INTRODUCTION

Anemia occurs frequently after surgery. Prompt evaluation is necessary to determine potential causes and provide appropriate treatment.

- Blood loss from the surgical procedure is the most common cause of postoperative anemia. However, anemia may result from a variety of other postoperative care-related and patient-specific factors.

INCIDENCE

- Anemia is a very common problem, both in the preoperative and postoperative settings. Exact estimates of incidence are difficult to determine due to heterogeneity of patients and procedures.
- Even with meticulous intraoperative hemostasis, all surgical patients sustain some degree of blood loss (Table 59-1). Estimates of intraoperative hemorrhage can be misleading; a number of studies have demonstrated up to a threefold difference between estimated and calculated/measured surgical blood loss.[2]
- Postoperative hemorrhage occurs in approximately 2 percent of patients undergoing laparoscopic procedures.[3] The incidence in major open surgeries ranges from <1 percent to virtually 100 percent (i.e., coronary artery bypass grafting).

TABLE 59-1 Typical Intraoperative Blood Loss for Various Surgeries

TYPE OF SURGERY	ESTIMATED, CALCULATED, OR MEASURED	BLOOD LOSS (mL)
Coronary artery bypass grafting	Measured	500
Craniofacial resections	Measured	1000
Gastric bypass		
Laparoscopic	Estimated	50
Open	Estimated	250
Hip arthroplasty	Calculated	2100
Hip fracture repair	Estimated	750
Knee arthroplasty	Calculated	2000
Laryngectomy	Measured	250
Lumbar spinal fusion	Estimated	500–1000*
Radical cystectomy	Estimated	500 in men, 1400 in women[1]
Radical neck dissection	Measured	500
Radical prostatectomy		
Laparoscopic	Estimated	400
Open	Estimated	750
Transurethral resection of prostate	Measured	500

*Amount of blood loss is directly proportional to the number of levels fused.

TIMING

- Anemia and bleeding can occur at any point during postoperative recovery. The proximity of these findings to the time of surgery may indicate likely causes.
- Anemia in the immediate postoperative period is most commonly due to surgical blood loss plus hemodilution from perioperative intravenous fluids. Bleeding during this period is most commonly caused by inadequate intraoperative hemostasis, but medication-induced inhibition of hemostasis (prophylaxis for deep venous thrombosis or the use of platelet inhibitors) and preexisting coagulopathies may contribute to blood loss.[4]
- New-onset anemia in the days to weeks following surgery may be due to surgical site bleeding, hemorrhage from another site (i.e., gastrointestinal bleeding), inadequate erythropoiesis, or, rarely, hemolysis. Bleeding and anemia during this period are often caused by postoperative medications that affect coagulation or platelet function.

CAUSES

ANEMIA

- Anemia in any clinical setting can be divided into four categories of causes: loss, increased destruction, or reduced production of red blood cells (RBCs) and iatrogenic (phlebotomy for blood tests).
- In the postoperative period, the most common cause of newly diagnosed anemia is surgery-related hemorrhage. However, one must maintain a high index of suspicion for other causes. Table 59-2 lists common causes of perioperative anemia, divided into the categories described above.

BLEEDING

- Perioperative bleeding may result from inadequate surgical site hemostasis but is frequently caused or potentiated by concomitant bleeding disorders. These disorders can be iatrogenic or may predate surgery; they can be further divided into abnormalities of primary (platelet-mediated) and secondary (coagulation cascade-mediated) hemostasis.
- Common causes of iatrogenic postoperative hemorrhage are medication-related disorders of hemostasis. These may be due to interference with primary hemostasis [i.e., inhibition of platelet function by nonsteroidal

TABLE 59-2 Selected Causes of Anemia

CAUSE OF ANEMIA	CLINICAL FEATURES/PATHOPHYSIOLOGY
Blood loss	
Surgical blood loss	Most common cause. Related to surgical blood loss or injury that led to surgery.
Bleeding from other sites	GI bleeding most common.
Increased destruction (hemolytic anemia)	Uncommon cause. High LDH and low haptoglobin sensitivity of 90%; normal LDH and haptoglobin 92% specificity.
Enzyme deficiency	Hemolysis from G6PD precipitated by infection, drugs (i.e., sulfa), or diabetic ketoacidosis.
Hemoglobinopathy	Sickle cell, thalassemia.
Membrane defect (spherocytosis)	Spherocytes seen on peripheral smear.
Hypersplenism	Results from sequestration of RBCs.
Infections	Systemic infections.
Microangiopathic	DIC and TTP. Peripheral smear shows fragmented cells.
Autoimmune hemolytic anemia warm or cold antibodies	Systemic lupus erythematosus associated with warm antibodies. Most common drugs penicillins and methyldopa.
Posttransfusion	
Decreased production	
Nutritional (iron, B_{12}, folate)	Iron deficiency is the most common cause of anemia and is associated with hypochromic microcytic cells. B_{12} and folate deficiency result in macrocytic cells.
Bone marrow disease	Aplastic anemia, pure RBC aplasia, myelodysplasia, or infiltration with tumor.
Suppression of bone marrow	Results from drugs, cancer chemotherapy, or irradiation.
Low hormone levels stimulating RBC production	EPO (chronic renal failure), hypothyroidism, and hypogonadism.
Iatrogenic	Repeated phlebotomy for blood tests.

DIC = disseminated intravascular coagulation; EPO = erythropoietin; G6PD = glucose-6-phosphate dehydrogenase deficiency; LDH = lactic dehydrogenase; RBC = red blood cell; TTP = thrombotic thrombocytopenic purpura.

anti-inflammatory drugs (NSAIDs) and heparin-induced thrombocytopenia] or secondary hemostasis (i.e., due to vitamin K antagonists and thrombin inhibitors).

- Inherited coagulopathies may be previously unknown during preoperative evaluation; these include von Willebrand's disease (vWD), the hemophilias, and factor XIII deficiency.[5] Severe liver disease, chronic renal failure, and certain cancers may cause acquired coagulopathies.
- Certain specific surgical settings lead to acquired and often complex abnormalities of hemostasis. These include cardiopulmonary bypass, massive transfusion, prostate surgery, and disseminated intravascular coagulation (DIC).[4]
- Although hemorrhage at the surgical site should be a primary consideration in any patient with postoperative blood loss, gastrointestinal, gynecologic, occult hemorrhage (i.e., retroperitoneal) remains a significant possibility and must be evaluated when evidence fails to identify surgical site bleeding.

DIAGNOSIS

DIFFERENTIAL DIAGNOSIS

ANEMIA

- Acute decreases in hemoglobin levels most commonly result from the loss of RBCs due to the surgical procedure or the injury that led to surgery.
- Slowly falling hemoglobin levels immediately after surgery are still most often due to ongoing bleeding from the surgical wound or as a result of fluid equilibration. Hemolysis is an uncommon cause.
- Failure to recover weeks after surgery is consistent with impaired ability to produce RBCs.
- Causes of inadequate erythropoiesis are often known before surgery but may also remain occult until the stress of surgery unmasks them. Table 59-2 summarizes those clinical scenarios where one should suspect these uncommon causes of anemia.

BLEEDING

- The differential diagnosis of bleeding can be challenging, as more than one factor may contribute to hemorrhage, and the possible causes of a bleeding disorder are much broader than those of anemia.
- The differential diagnosis of postoperative bleeding includes four general categories: (1) surgery-related, (2) medication-related, (3) inherited coagulopathies, and (4) systemic disorders and other causes (Table 59-3).

PHYSICAL FINDINGS

- Physical examination plays a relatively minor role in the evaluation of postoperative anemia and bleeding. However, vital signs remain a critical part of the evaluation, as hemodynamic instability indicates a high potential for complications and dictates the speed and setting of the remainder of the evaluation.
- Investigation of the surgical site and other areas for signs of bleeding is obviously an important means of quickly ascertaining a cause for anemia. Typical findings of anemia, such as pallor (particularly of the mucous membranes), provide little direction regarding the cause of anemia.

TABLE 59-3 Differential Diagnosis of Postoperative Bleeding

CAUSE OF POSTOPERATIVE BLEEDING	CLINICAL FEATURES/PATHOPHYSIOLOGY
Surgery-related	
Inadequate local hemostasis	Bleeding restricted to operative site (i.e., soaking bandages, large output from drains).
Postprostatectomy hemorrhage	Excessive hematuria due to local hyperfibrinolysis from presence of urokinase at surgical site.
Excessive fibrinolysis in abdominal aortic aneurysm repair and liver transplantation	Systemic hyperfibrinolysis caused by mesenteric ischemia.
Cardiopulmonary bypass syndrome	Systemic reduction of coagulation and fibrinolytic factors and inhibition of platelet function.
Medication-related	
Heparin/low-molecular-weight heparin	Inhibition of factor Xa.
HIT	Immune-mediated destruction of platelets.
Vitamin K antagonists	Inhibited synthesis of vitamin K–dependent coagulation factors.
Thrombolytic agents (i.e., tissue plasminogen activator)	Generation of excess plasmin, which degrades fibrin, fibrinogen, and factors V and VIII.
NSAIDs/beta-lactam antibiotics	Induction of platelet dysfunction.
Inherited coagulopathies[*]	
von Willebrand's disease	Dysfunctional or inadequate levels of von Willebrand factor causing abnormal platelet aggregation.
Hemophilia	Inadequate levels of factor VIII (hemophilia A) or IX (hemophilia B).
Factor XIII deficiency	Inadequate levels of factor XIII, causing fibrin clot.
Systemic disorders	
DIC	Consumption of coagulation factors by indiscriminate activation of coagulation pathways.
Liver disease	Inadequate synthesis of coagulation factors and plasmin inhibitors.
Uremia	Induction of platelet dysfunction.
Other causes	
Massive transfusion	Severe bleeding necessitating rapid replacement of platelet-depleted blood products, leading to thrombocytopenia.
Posttransfusion purpura syndrome	Exposure to blood products causing an immune response to the platelet antigen HPA-1a, which leads to platelet destruction.
Vitamin K deficiency	Inadequate synthesis of vitamin K–dependent coagulation factors.

DIC = disseminated intravascular coagulation; HIT = heparin-induced thrombocytopenia; NSAIDs = nonsteroidal anti-inflammatory drugs.
[*]Only a handful of examples are listed here.

- In patients with postoperative bleeding, the physical examination may provide more benefit in determining a cause of the hemorrhage. Palatal or skin petechiae may indicate an abnormality with platelet number or function, while purpuric lesions and oozing at surgical and vascular access sites point to disruption of secondary hemostasis. Rectal and genital examination can help to identify nonsurgical sources of hemorrhage.

LABORATORY TESTING

Anemia

- Serial hemoglobin and hematocrit will provide insight into the rate of bleeding and the cause. In patients with surgical blood loss, the blood count should stabilize within 1 or 2 days of surgery.
- If the hemoglobin level continues to fall in the absence of bleeding, examine the following: complete blood

count (CBC), reticulocyte count, peripheral smear (looking for characteristic changes of hemolysis), lactate dehydrogenase (LDH), and haptoglobin (looking for the possibility of hemolysis). An abnormal LDH and haptoglobin has 90 percent sensitivity and 92 percent specificity for hemolysis.
- If a defect in erythropoiesis is suspected based on inadequate recovery in the blood count, evaluation can proceed as outlined in Chap. 30.

BLEEDING

- Evaluation of postoperative bleeding should begin with a platelet count, prothrombin time (PT), and partial thromboplastin time (PTT).
- Abnormalities in any of these values trigger a more thorough evaluation, as described in Chap. 31.
- Special considerations for bleeding occurring in postoperative patients are disseminated intravascular coagulation (DIC), heparin-induced thrombocytopenia (HIT), and primary fibrinolysis. Laboratory evaluation for each of these conditions requires more specialized testing.
- ***DIC:*** No laboratory test can reliably rule in or rule out DIC. Rather, the diagnosis is based on the combination of history, physical examination, and laboratory data. At a minimum, the diagnosis of DIC requires laboratory evidence of both thrombin generation and the consumption of platelet and coagulation factors.
  - The diagnosis of DIC is supported by elevation of PT and PTT and decreases in fibrinogen level, platelet count, thrombin time, and antithrombin level. Each of these is relatively nonspecific and insensitive.
  - Diagnose thrombin generation by the presence of D-dimers, fibrinopeptide A, prothrombin fragment 1.2, thrombin-antithrombin complex, and protamine paracoagulation assay for fibrin monomer. All but the last of these can be elevated in the postsurgical setting, thereby making these tests relatively unhelpful for the diagnosis of DIC. Protamine paracoagulation assay for fibrin monomer is not affected by the postoperative state, but it is not readily available or reliable unless performed by specialized laboratories.
- ***HIT:*** Consider this diagnosis in any patient who develops a 30 percent or greater decline in platelet count or has an unexpected thromboembolic event within 4 to 14 days (earlier if previously exposed to heparin products) of receiving unfractionated or low-molecular-weight heparin (LMWH).[6]
  - Other diagnostic tests include an assay for platelet-associated immunoglobin (IgG), platelet serotonin release assay, and platelet factor IV enzyme-linked immunosorbent assay (ELISA). Both the platelet-associated IgG and platelet serotonin release assays have a high specificity (close to 100 percent) but have substantially less sensitivity (50 to 81 percent and 85 to 94 percent, respectively). Platelet factor IV ELISA is commercially available and has a sensitivity of >90 percent and specificity of 92 percent.
- ***Excessive fibrinolysis:*** For patients with chronic liver disease who are undergoing procedures that can induce excessive fibrinolysis, confirm this problem by finding increased levels of tissue plasminogen activator and reduced euglobulin lysis time and alpha$_2$-antiplasmin levels.

TREATMENT

ANEMIA

- Supplement nutritional deficiencies.
- Blood transfusion remains the mainstay of treatment for anemia that is critical.
- No consensus exists regarding the indications for blood transfusion in the surgical setting. Data from intensive care unit (ICU) patients indicate that transfusion at a hemoglobin concentration of 7 g/dL is as safe as or perhaps safer than a threshold of 10 g/dL.[7]
- Patients with cardiovascular disease may be less tolerant of anemia and require a higher transfusion trigger, but the data are conflicting.
- See Chap. 30 for a thorough discussion of RBC transfusion.
- The role of erythropoietin is limited in the typical patient with normal bone marrow function, since adequate stores of nutrients (iron, B_{12}) are usually present or can be replaced, and blood transfusion is effective in situations requiring prompt treatment.
- For Jehovah's Witnesses and other patients who refuse transfusion, consider the use of erythropoietin to correct hemoglobin concentrations rapidly. The dose of epoetin alfa is 300 U/kg/day for 15 days. Administer iron orally, when possible, or intravenously if oral medications are not permitted or critically low hemoglobin levels are present. In these circumstances, administer sodium ferric gluconate complex intravenously, 125 mg daily for eight doses.
- ***Hemolysis:*** Avoid and eliminate triggers (i.e., penicillins).

BLEEDING

- Collaborate with surgical colleagues and consider the role of immediate surgical reexploration pending the results of medical evaluation for other causes of bleeding. In some cases, angiography or computed tomography (CT) angiography to identify arterial bleeds at the surgical site may be helpful to guide therapy.
- If the source of bleeding is not related to the surgical site and a systemic cause of bleeding is apparent, focus

TABLE 59-4 Summary of Treatments for Different Causes of Postoperative Hemorrhage

CAUSE OF BLEEDING	TREATMENT
Thrombocytopenia	Stop potential causative medications and agents causing platelet dysfunction. Transfuse platelets to maintain counts >50,000.
HIT	Stop heparin-based agents. *No platelet transfusion.* Stop warfarin therapy and give vitamin K orally. Start alternative anticoagulant.
Massive transfusion	Transfuse platelets to maintain counts >100,000 if bleeding and >50,000 if none.
Posttransfusion purpura syndrome	IVIg.
Platelet dysfunction	Stop potential causative medications.
Uremia-induced	Maintain hematocrit ≥30. Cryoprecipitate or desmopressin. Platelet transfusion as last resort.
Cardiopulmonary bypass-induced	None; self-limited.
Coagulopathy	For life-threatening hemorrhage of any cause, consider recombinant factor VIIa.
Inherited coagulopathies	See Chap. 31.
Heparin therapy	Protamine.
LMWH therapy	Protamine if last dose within 8 h.
Fondaparinux therapy	*No antidote.*
Vitamin K–antagonist therapy	Vitamin K IV and FFP. Prothrombin complex concentrate or recombinant VIIa if life-threatening.
DIC	Transfuse platelets to maintain counts >20–50,000 Transfuse cryoprecipitate to maintain fibrinogen level >100 mg/dL. Transfuse FFP to maintain INR <1.5.
Liver disease	Vitamin K PO or IV. Transfuse FFP to maintain INR <1.5.
Excessive fibrinolysis	
Thrombolytic therapy	Transfuse platelets and cryoprecipitate. EACA, tranexamic acid, or aprotinin IV.
Postprostatectomy	EACA IV or PO.
Cardiopulmonary bypass	Prophylactic EACA, tranexamic acid, or aprotinin IV.

DIC = disseminated intravascular coagulation; EACA = epsilon-aminocaproic acid; FFP = fresh-frozen plasma; INR = international normalized ratio; IVIg = intravenous immunoglobulin; HIT = heparin-induced thrombocytopenia; LMWH = low-molecular-weight heparin.

treatment on the specific source of bleeding. Involve subspecialists (i.e., gastroenterology, gynecology) in considering invasive evaluation and treatment for non-surgical sources of bleeding.

- When abnormalities of coagulation are identified, treatment should be directed at the specific hemostatic defect. See Table 59-4 for a summary of treatments of postoperative bleeding.

THROMBOCYTOPENIA

- Immediately discontinue any possible causative agents, including heparin, LMWH, and H_2 antagonists. Also stop any medications that inhibit platelet function (i.e., NSAIDs, clopidogrel).
- In general, maintain a platelet count of 50,000 or greater for any postoperative patient with bleeding (including those with DIC).[8] Except in patients with HIT and thrombotic thrombocytopenic purpura (TTP), administer platelet transfusions to achieve this. In these conditions, platelet transfusion is contraindicated, and other treatments must be initiated with the assistance of hematology consultants.
- ***Massive transfusion:*** For patients who have undergone massive transfusion (two or more blood volumes), administer prophylactic platelet transfusions to maintain a platelet count of 50,000. If bleeding is present, use a higher transfusion threshold of 100,000.
- ***Posttransfusion purpura syndrome (PTP):*** The treatment of choice for PTP is intravenous immunoglobulin (IVIg) administered over 2 to 5 days. Response to this therapy is often rapid and is effective in 85 percent of patients.[8] Platelet transfusions may be utilized as a stopgap measure when the patient is experiencing life-threatening hemorrhage, but the benefit is likely to be small even with large doses.
- ***HIT:*** After discontinuing all heparin-based medications, start the patient on a direct thrombin inhibitor (lepirudin, bivalirudin, or argatroban), fondaparinux, or a heparinoid to prevent thrombosis.[6] Perform ultrasonography of the lower limbs to detect subclinical deep venous thrombosis. Patients receiving vitamin K antagonists (warfarin) should receive vitamin K to reduce the risk of thrombosis potentiation by these agents. Do not resume warfarin therapy until platelet counts are greater than 100,000, and then provide at least 5 days overlap with alternative anticoagulation.

PLATELET DYSFUNCTION

- Discontinue medications that inhibit platelet function (i.e., NSAIDs, clopidogrel).
- Screen for and treat conditions such as uremia and liver disease, which can cause platelet dysfunction.
- Consider either cryoprecipitate or desmopressin for patients with uremia.
- Desmopressin and prophylactic platelet transfusions have not demonstrated a significant benefit in the treatment of transient platelet dysfunction following cardiopulmonary bypass.
- Consider platelet transfusions only when the above therapies have failed and bleeding persists.

COAGULOPATHY

- Treatment of inherited coagulopathies is similar in the preoperative and postoperative settings and is covered in Chap. 31.
- ***Heparin, LMWH, and fondaparinux:*** In the setting of significant postoperative bleeding, stop all anticoagulants immediately. The effects of unfractionated heparin will disappear within 2 h of discontinuation; but if severe bleeding is present, administer protamine sulfate to immediately reverse anticoagulation. Protamine reverses the effects of LMWH incompletely, and anticoagulant activity persists for up to 12 to 18 h following the last dose of LMWH. If bleeding is severe, administer protamine within 8 h of the last dose.[9] Beyond that time frame, carefully weigh the benefits of protamine therapy against the risks. Fondaparinux has a half-life of approximately 16 h and cannot be reversed with protamine sulfate. A recent report suggested value for the use of recombinant factor VIIa to reverse bleeding in a patient on LMWH therapy.
- ***Vitamin K antagonists:*** Patients with postoperative hemorrhage while being treated with a vitamin K antagonist require interventions beyond medication cessation to resolve bleeding. All such patients should receive intravenous vitamin K and fresh-frozen plasma (FFP) with the goal of achieving and maintaining an international normalized ratio (INR) <1.5 as quickly as possible. If the patient's hemorrhage is life-threatening, consider prothrombin complex concentrate or recombinant factor VIIa.
- ***DIC:*** The mainstay of therapy remains treatment of the underlying cause and aggressive basic supportive measures. However, the administration of blood products is warranted to prevent sequelae. Give platelet transfusions to maintain a platelet count >20,000, or > 50,000 in the presence of significant bleeding. Transfuse cryoprecipitate to maintain a fibrinogen concentration >100 mg/dL. Administer FFP for patients who have significant hemorrhage and elevation of PT/PTT. In this setting, transfuse FFP to achieve a target INR of <1.5 or resolution of hemorrhage. Heparin and LMWH may have a role in a small subset of patients with thrombosis-predominant DIC (i.e., chronic DIC, acute promyelocytic leukemia). Antithrombin and activated protein C concentrates may also have a role in therapy, but supportive evidence is limited.
- ***Liver disease:*** For patients with severe liver disease and evidence of synthetic dysfunction, give vitamin K orally to maximize the liver's limited production of coagulation factor. In the setting of postoperative hemorrhage, FFP may temporarily reverse a patient's coagulopathy. If there is evidence of excessive fibrinolysis, consider the use of antifibrinolytics, as described below.

EXCESSIVE FIBRINOLYSIS

- ***Thrombolytic therapy:*** Patients can develop acute thrombotic complications following surgery and may require thrombolytic therapy (tissue plasminogen activator). In addition to generating fibrinolysis, thrombolytic therapy also causes thrombocytopenia. If bleeding ensues, immediately stop thrombolytic therapy (if possible) and give cryoprecipitate, platelet transfusion, and antifibrinolytics [i.e., epsilon-aminocaproic acid (EACA), tranexamic acid, and aprotinin].
- ***Postprostatectomy hemorrhage:*** Several studies have demonstrated the efficacy of EACA in reducing postprostatectomy hemorrhage. EACA can be administered either orally or intravenously; base the duration of therapy on the duration of urinary bleeding.
- ***Cardiopulmonary bypass:*** Multiple studies have demonstrated significant reduction in postoperative hemorrhage with the use of EACA, tranexamic acid, and aprotinin. These agents are rapidly becoming part of standard cardiopulmonary bypass protocols. In these protocols, one starts antifibrinolytics by continuous infusion prior to skin incision and continues their use for the duration of the procedure. Although feared, no significant increase in thrombotic complications has been identified.

REFERENCES

1. Lee KL, Freiha F, Presti JC, et al. Gender differences in radical cystectomy: Complications and blood loss. *Urology* 63(6): 1095–1099, 2004.
2. Rosencher N, Kerkkamp HE, Macheras G, et al. OSTHEO Investigation. Orthopedic Surgery Transfusion Hemoglobin European Overview (OSTHEO) study: Blood management in elective knee and hip arthroplasty in Europe. *Transfusion* 43(4):459–469, 2003.
3. Schafer M, Lauper M, Krahenbuhl L. A nation's experience of bleeding complications during laparoscopy. *Am J Surg* 180(1): 73–77, 2000.
4. McKenna R. Abnormal coagulation in the postoperative period contributing to excessive bleeding. *Med Clin North Am* 85(5):1277–1310, 2001.
5. Francis CW, Kaplan KL. Hematologic problems in the surgical patient: Bleeding and thrombosis, in Hoffman R, Benz EJ, Shattil SJ, et al (eds). *Hematology: Basic Principles and Practice,* 3d ed. Philadelphia: Churchill Livingstone, 2000: 2385–2386.
6. Comunale ME, Van Cott EM. Heparin-induced thrombocytopenia. *Int Anesthesiol Clin* 42(3):27–43, 2004.
7. Hebert PC, Wells G, Blajchman MA, et al. A multicenter, randomized, controlled clinical trial of transfusion requirements in critical care. Transfusion Requirements in Critical Care

Investigators, Canadian Critical Care Trials Group. *N Engl J Med* 1999:340:409–417.
8. British Committee for Standards in Haematology, Blood Transfusion Task Force. Guidelines for the use of platelet transfusions. *Br J Haematol* 122(1):10–23, 2003.
9. Weitz JI, Hirsh J, Samama MM. New anticoagulant drugs: The seventh ACCP conference on antithrombotic and thrombolytic therapy. *Chest* 126(3):265S–286S, 2004.

60 JAUNDICE

Kaleem M. Rizvon and Calvin L. Chou

INTRODUCTION

- Approximately 25 to 75 percent of patients develop liver functions test abnormalities postoperatively. These abnormalities are most commonly isolated, minor elevations. However, significant jaundice with total bilirubin elevations of more than 2.5 mg/dL may occur.

INCIDENCE

- The incidence of postoperative hepatic dysfunction varies with patient- and procedure-related risk factors.

Patient-Specific Risks

- ***History of liver disease:*** A significant portion of patients with cirrhosis develop jaundice after surgery. Perioperative risk varies with the level of hepatic dysfunction as determined by the Child-Pugh score.
- ***Cardiac dysfunction*** increases the risk of ischemic hepatic injury in patients who have postoperative hypotensive episodes. In one prospective study, ischemic hepatitis occurred more often in patients with low cardiac output and increased central venous pressure.[1] In another report, the majority of the patients who developed ischemic hepatitis had evidence of cardiac disease, which often led to passive congestion of the liver.[2]
- ***Use of total parenteral nutrition (TPN)*** in the perioperative period can cause jaundice, either due to cholestasis or the accumulation of fat in the liver. Prolonged administration may cause steatohepatitis, micronodular cirrhosis, pigment gallstones, and acalculous cholecystitis.
- ***Other patient-specific risks*** include renal failure, advanced age, obesity, chronic obstructive pulmonary disease, and preoperative infections.

Surgery-Specific Risks

- ***Cardiac surgery:*** Cardiac surgery confers a high risk of postoperative jaundice; the incidence is 20 to 25 percent.[3] Postoperative jaundice is more common among patients who undergo multivalve surgery as opposed to those who have coronary bypass surgery.
- ***Upper abdominal surgery:*** The incidence of hepatic dysfunction is less than 1 percent after elective abdominal surgery. Cholecystectomy increases the risk of extrahepatic biliary obstruction and bile duct injury. Iatrogenic bile duct injury is more common after laparoscopic cholecystectomy than after open procedures.[4] Retained bile duct stones are present in 1 to 5 percent of patients after cholecystectomy.
- Other procedure-related risk factors include hypotensive episodes, blood product transfusion, certain anesthetic agents, and medications.

TIMING

- The time course of postoperative jaundice varies widely. Examples of etiologies during different time frames include:
  - Soon after surgery (due to ischemic hepatitis)
  - Weeks after surgery (secondary to drugs)
  - Months after surgery (secondary to complications of surgery such as stricture formation)

CAUSES

- Table 60-1 summarizes common causes of postoperative jaundice.

TABLE 60-1 Causes of Postoperative Jaundice

Bilirubin overproduction
Multiple packed-red-cell transfusions
Hematoma resorption
Gilbert's syndrome
Hemolysis
Congenital: glucose-6-phosphate deficiency, sickle cell anemia
Acquired: mechanical heart valves, mismatched blood transfusions, drug-induced hemolysis
Hepatocellular injury
Ischemic hepatitis
Anesthetic agents
Drugs
Viral hepatitis
Sepsis
Cholestasis
Extrahepatic cholestasis: cholecystitis, choledocholithiasis, biliary duct stricture
Intrahepatic cholestasis: sepsis, benign postoperative jaundice
Miscellaneous causes
Total parenteral nutrition

OVERPRODUCTION OF BILIRUBIN

- The liver conjugates approximately 250 mg of bilirubin each day and has considerable capacity to excrete two or three times this load before hyperbilirubinemia manifests.
- In some common postoperative states, bilirubin production far exceeds this capacity, and jaundice results. Some common causes of bilirubin overproduction are:
  - ***Blood transfusions:***About 10 percent of a unit of packed red cells hemolyzes within hours of transfusion. Multiple packed-red-cell transfusions can thus result in elevated levels of bilirubin.
  - ***Hematoma resorption:*** Extravasation of blood during surgery can increase the bilirubin load to levels much higher than those normally produced daily.

HEMOLYSIS

- ***Congenital:*** Those with glucose-6-phosphate (G6PD) deficiency who receive sulfa drugs and those with hemoglobinopathies such as sickle cell anemia are examples of patients with congenital diseases that increase the risk of postoperative jaundice. Unconjugated bilirubin rises after surgery in patients with Gilbert's syndrome due to hepatic UDP-glucuronyl transferase deficiency.
- ***Acquired:*** Mismatched blood transfusions, medications such as penicillin, and traumatic hemolysis secondary to a prosthetic valve or disseminated intravascular coagulation may all cause postoperative jaundice.

HEPATOCELLULAR INJURY

- ***Ischemic hepatitis:*** Also known as shock liver, this can occur quickly after surgery. It is commonly due to episodes of hypotension during surgery, though it is much more common in hypotensive patients with cardiac dysfunction.
- ***Anesthetic agents:*** Haloalkanes used as inhalational anesthetic agents can cause varying degrees of hepatotoxicity.
  - Halothane and methoxyflurane cause liver injury more often than other agents, such as isoflurane and desflurane.
  - Halothane undergoes about 100 times more biotransformation than isoflurane. A metabolite of halothane, trifluoroacetyl chloride, binds to the endoplasmic reticulum of the hepatocyte, promoting immune-mediated liver injury.[5]
  - Halothane can cause mild hepatic injury, an increase in aminotransferases, and cholestasis within 3 days of exposure. With multiple exposures, a more severe form of hepatic injury occurs, with more than a tenfold elevation of aminotransferases, coagulopathy, and jaundice.
  - Risk factors for halothane hepatitis include obesity, age over 60 years, female gender, multiple exposures, and short intervals between exposures.
- ***Drugs:*** Many drugs may potentially cause hepatic injury. Although jaundice and hepatic dysfunction usually occur a few weeks after surgery, an early rapid decline in liver function can occur with acetaminophen toxicity, especially in patients who chronically abuse alcohol. In addition to halothane, other agents that can cause a hepatitis-like picture include isoniazid, phenytoin, methyldopa, and dantrolene.
- Viral hepatitis can occur weeks after surgery, either from reactivation of preexisting infection or, rarely, a new infection from the transfusion of packed red blood cells or other blood products.
- Sepsis can cause jaundice due to both hepatocellular injury and cholestasis.

CHOLESTASIS

- Extrahepatic causes include injury to the biliary tree, resulting in stricture formation and obstruction, as well as both calculous and acalculous cholecystitis.
- Intrahepatic causes include sepsis, drugs, and benign postoperative jaundice.
- As first described by Schmid,[6] benign postoperative jaundice occurs due to the combined effects of anesthesia, hypotension, and blood loss without a specific cause for jaundice. It is characterized by significant elevations of bilirubin (in some cases as high as 40 mg/dL), mostly of the conjugated type; elevated alkaline phosphatase; normal or minor elevations of transaminases; and a benign clinical course. Coagulopathy may occur occasionally but is reversible with vitamin K therapy.

MISCELLANEOUS CAUSES

- TPN can cause steatosis of the liver and biliary diseases such as calculous and acalculous cholecystitis.
- Nutritional deficiencies, hormonal imbalances, excessive caloric intake, and bacterial overgrowth in the small intestines can all cause hepatic dysfunction in patients on TPN.[7]

DIAGNOSIS

DIFFERENTIAL DIAGNOSIS

- Postoperative jaundice can be due to any of the causes mentioned above.
- Take into account the timing; medication history, including anesthetic agents; type of surgery; perioperative hypotension; infections; and blood transfusions.

- Obtain appropriate laboratory and radiologic testing with consultation for advanced procedures such as endoscopic retrograde cholangiopancreatography (ERCP) and surgery. Figure 60-1 depicts an algorithmic approach to diagnosis.

PHYSICAL FINDINGS

- Examine carefully for stigmata of chronic liver disease, such as ascites, splenomegaly, palmar erythema, gynecomastia, spider angiomata, and encephalopathy.

LABORATORY TESTING

- A complete blood count may show anemia secondary to hemolysis or blood loss after surgery, thrombocytopenia due to hypersplenism in cirrhosis, and leukocytosis due to perioperative infections.
- A peripheral smear will also show schistocytes in some patients with immune-related hemolytic processes.
- Liver-related tests are important in differentiating the causes of jaundice.
- In patients with hemolysis, the bilirubin is mostly of the indirect type, with an increased reticulocyte count, increased levels of lactate dehydrogenase, and decreased or absent levels of haptoglobin.
- Increased transaminases due to hepatocyte injury are characteristic of ischemic hepatic injury. Transaminases rise quickly, along with a less dramatic increase in serum bilirubin. The levels decrease rapidly after reaching a plateau. Other potential causes of transaminase elevations in this setting include anesthetic toxicity, drug toxicity (such as that due to acetaminophen), and infectious etiologies (such as viral hepatitis).
- Elevated alkaline phosphatase usually indicates biliary stasis. Conjugated hyperbilirubinemia often coexists in this setting.
- Coagulopathy is associated with a number of conditions after surgery and requires vitamin K supplementation and administration of fresh-frozen plasma.
- Elevated amylase and lipase levels will help to confirm a suspected diagnosis of pancreatitis.
- In considering this diagnosis, obtain serologies for viral hepatitis.
- In considering the diagnosis of autoimmune hepatitis, measure autoimmune markers such as antinuclear antibody, anti–smooth muscle antibody, antimitochondrial antibody, and anti-liver-kidney microsomal enzyme antibodies.

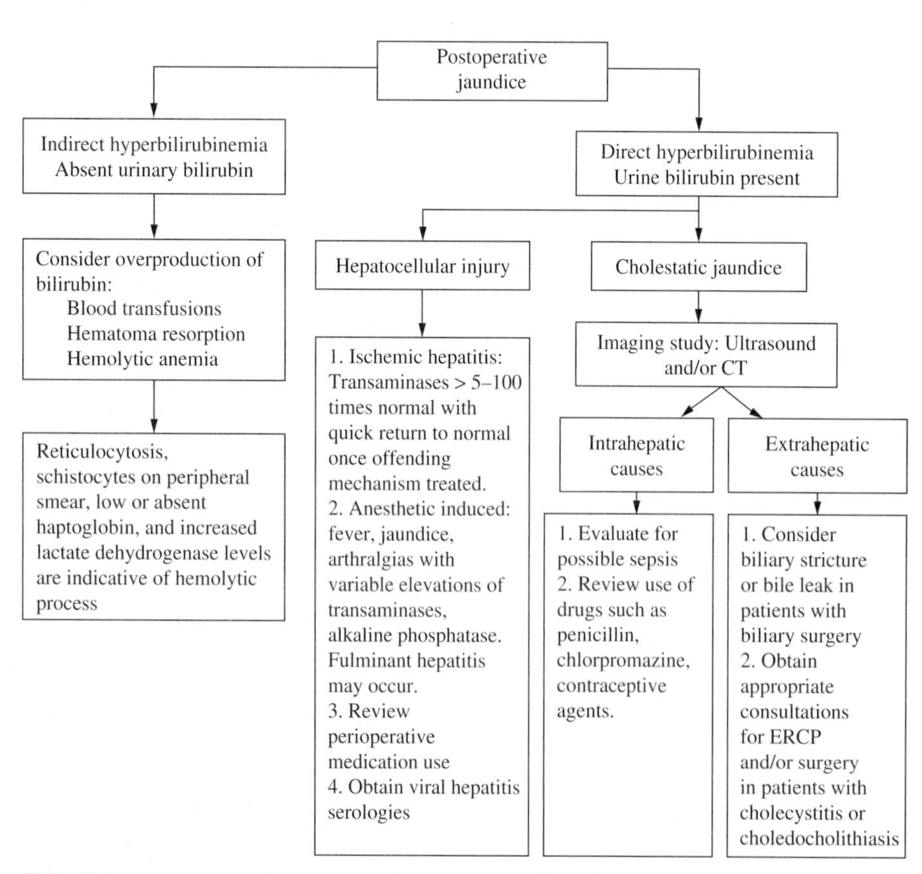

FIG. 60-1 Approach to the patient with postoperative jaundice.

IMAGING STUDIES

- Imaging studies are helpful in the evaluation of patients with cholestatic liver test abnormalities.
- Abdominal ultrasonography and computed tomography of the abdomen will readily identify choledocholithiasis as well as common bile duct or intrahepatic ductal dilatation and assist in further management.
- Perform magnetic resonance cholangiopancreatography (MRCP) or endoscopic retrograde cholangiopancreatography (ERCP) in patients with suspected extrahepatic obstruction. Select ERCP for patients who require sphincterotomy for alleviation of biliary obstruction.
- In select patients, consider a liver biopsy to further characterize the pathologic process. As this procedure carries some morbidity, obtain a liver biopsy only for patients in whom the causative factors remain unclear and for whom the results may change management. Centrilobular necrosis is characteristic of ischemic hepatitis due to increased susceptibility of hepatocytes in this region to hypoxia. The biopsy findings in patients with halothane-induced liver injury include panlobular necrosis and stromal collapse, as seen in patients with fulminant viral hepatitis.

TREATMENT

- General treatment goals include careful observation of patients with postoperative jaundice for further deterioration. Once a possible etiology is established, avoid further insult to the liver and biliary tree.

OVERPRODUCTION OF BILIRUBIN

- ***Hemolysis:*** Avoid stressors that can prolong the underlying process (for example, sulfa drugs in patients with G6PD deficiency, or dehydration and hypoxemia in patients with sickle cell disease).
- ***Gilbert's syndrome:*** With other liver function tests in normal range, elevated bilirubin tends to be asymptomatic. Treatment of underlying infection and hydration with avoidance of starvation will improve bilirubin levels.

HEPATIC INJURY

- ***Ischemic hepatitis:*** Although little can be done to treat ischemic hepatitis once it has begun, avoid hepatotoxic medications and hypoxia in order to minimize the risk of additional hepatic injury.

ACETAMINOPHEN TOXICITY

- Early administration of *N*-acetyl cysteine is important.
  - Start with a loading dose of 140 mg/kg PO.
  - 70 mg/kg PO every 4 h until 17 doses have been administered. For patients who are unable to tolerate the medication orally, an intravenous preparation is available.
- Careful monitoring for further deterioration with development of encephalopathy is essential.
- The King's College criteria[8] for liver transplantation in patients with acetaminophen toxicity are:
  - pH ≤7.3 irrespective of the stage of encephalopathy
  - Prothrombin time of >100 s
  - Serum creatinine of >3.4 mg/dL in patients with grade III or IV encephalopathy

CHOLESTASIS

- ***Sepsis:*** Treatment of the underlying infection will lead to the gradual resolution of jaundice.
- ***Benign postoperative cholestasis:*** The course is benign, but the elevation of bilirubin can be quite high, with normal aminotransferases. Coagulopathy may be present; it is usually mild and reversible with vitamin K supplementation.

BILIARY OBSTRUCTION

- Perform ERCP with sphincterotomy if biliary obstruction is due to choledocholithiasis after cholecystectomy.
- In patients who have developed biliary strictures, place biliary stents in order to relieve jaundice.
- For patients who require surgery for relief of obstruction, three factors predict postoperative mortality[9]:
  - Hematocrit <30 percent
  - Serum bilirubin >11 mg/dL
  - Malignant cause of obstruction
- The absence of all three factors confers a perioperative mortality of 5 percent.
- When all three factors are present, perioperative mortality approaches 60 percent.

- ***Cholecystitis:*** Perform open or laparoscopic cholecystectomy. In patients who are critically ill and have acalculous cholecystitis, consider cholecystostomy as a lower-risk treatment strategy.[10]

REFERENCES

1. Henrion J, Descamps O, Luwaert R, et al. Hypoxic hepatitis in patients with cardiac failure: Incidence in a coronary care unit and measurement of hepatic blood flow. *J Hepatol* 21: 696–701, 1994.
2. Seeto RK, Fenn B, Rockey DC. Ischemic hepatitis: Clinical presentation and pathogenesis. *Am J Med* 109(2):109–113, 2000.

3. Chu CM, Chang CH, Liaw YF, et al. Jaundice after open heart surgery: A prospective study. *Thorax* 39(1):52–56, 1984.
4. Davidoff AM, Pappas TN, Murray EA, et al. Mechanisms of major biliary injury during laparoscopic cholecystectomy. *Ann Surg* 215(3):196–202, 1992.
5. Brown BR Jr, Gandolfi AJ. Adverse effects of volatile anaesthetics. *Br J Anaesth* 59(1):14–23, 1987.
6. Schmid M, Hefti ML, Gattiker R, et al. Benign postoperative intrahepatic cholestasis. *N Engl J Med* 18;272:545–550, 1965.
7. Chung C, Buchman AL. Postoperative jaundice and total parenteral nutrition associated hepatic dysfunction. *Clin Liver Dis* 6(4):1067–1084, 2002.
8. Harrison PM, O'Grady JG, Keays RT, et al. Serial prothrombin time as prognostic indicator in paracetamol induced fulminant hepatic failure. *BMJ* 27;301(6758):964–966, 1990.
9. Dixon JM, Armstrong CP, Duffy SW, et al. Factors affecting morbidity and mortality after surgery for obstructive jaundice: A review of 373 patients. *Gut* 24:845–852, 1983.
10. Molina EG, Reddy KR. Postoperative jaundice. *Clin Liver Dis* 3(3):477–488, 1999.

61 STROKE AND SEIZURES

James B. Lewis, Jr., and Frank Lefevre

STROKE

INTRODUCTION

- Stroke is a broad term encompassing several pathophysiologic processes (Table 61-1). Stroke is the sudden onset of a neurologic deficit caused by a vascular deficit that persists for more than 24 h.
- The frequency of different types of stroke in the perioperative period approximates the frequency of stroke in general (see Table 61-1), with perhaps a greater proportion of embolic strokes occurring perioperatively.[1]
- The clinical presentation of stroke in the perioperative period may be less straightforward than at other times. Postoperative immobility and/or medication effects may obscure and modify the typical symptoms. In addition, patients may be less able to communicate new symptoms due to postoperative pain, other postoperative symptoms, and medication effects.

INCIDENCE AND RISK FACTORS

- The overall risk of postoperative stroke following general surgery is low at 0.2 to 0.7 percent.[2] However, a number of risk factors at the patient and procedural levels confer an increased risk for perioperative stroke.
    - Patients with a prior history of stroke or transient ischemic attack (TIA) are at higher risk for perioperative stroke. This risk was approximately 3 percent in one large series of patients with a history of cerebrovascular disease undergoing general surgery.[2]
    - The risk of recurrent perioperative stroke is also related to the timing of the prior stroke. Although exact numbers are lacking, most experts consider the risk of recurrent stroke highest in the 2 weeks following an initial event and increased for up to several months (see Chap. 37).
    - Another important risk factor for perioperative stroke is atrial fibrillation, which is present in up to one-third of patients with perioperative stroke. Advanced age, hypertension, diabetes, and smoking are also risk

TABLE 61-1 Stroke in the Perioperative Period

TYPE OF STROKE	FREQUENCY	PERIOPERATIVE RISK FACTORS	CLINICAL CONSIDERATIONS
Ischemic stroke	80%		
Thrombotic	60%	Hypercoagulability of surgery Hypoperfusion Poor blood pressure control	Avoid blood pressure reduction unless extreme degrees of elevation Avoidance of dehydration, hypovolemia
Embolic	20%	Atrial fibrillation Other cardiac arrhythmias Myocardial infarction Hypercoagulability of surgery Long bone fracture	Perioperative anticoagulant management for patients with preexisting atrial fibrillation Appropriate monitoring for cardiac arrhythmias and events
Hemorrhagic stroke	20%		
Intracranial hemorrhage	15%	Poor blood pressure control Anticoagulants, antiplatelet agents Septic emboli Iatrogenic; e.g., arterial injury	Careful blood pressure control Judicious use of anticoagulants, antiplatelet medications
Subarachnoid hemorrhage	5%	Poor blood pressure control Iatrogenic; e.g., arterial injury	Careful blood pressure control

factors. Hypertension is present in one-half or more of patients presenting with perioperative stroke. For patients over 65 years of age, the incidence of postoperative stroke is 1 to 2.5 percent.[3]
   - Significant carotid stenosis probably increases the risk of postoperative stroke due to the inability to adequately increase blood flow in the face of increased demands. However, interventions to reduce stroke risk in this circumstance, such as prophylactic carotid endarterectomy, have not been shown to improve outcomes. Therefore it is unlikely that preoperative testing for carotid stenosis is indicated for most patients[3] (see Chap. 37).
- The types of surgeries associated with the highest rates of perioperative stroke are cardiac, carotid, and aortoiliac procedures. For these types of surgery, the overall rate of perioperative stroke is 1 to 5 percent.[3]
   - Carotid endarterectomy and certain neurosurgical procedures have high rates of perioperative stroke due to specifics of the surgical procedure.[4] These clinical situations are unique in that the procedure itself confers the additional risk of stroke. Also, the stroke risk varies with some of the procedural aspects, such as the precise location of neurosurgery. For example, removal of a tumor that is contiguous with a major blood vessel may involve a high risk of stroke, whereas a similar tumor not involving blood vessels may have a much lower risk. In these types of circumstances, surgical planning and risk assessment is ideally handled in conjunction with a neurologist, the surgeon, and/or other appropriate subspecialists.
   - Many studies have estimated the rate of neurologic events following coronary artery bypass grafting (CABG). The overall rate of stroke following CABG is 2 to 5 percent; approximately 2 percent of patients undergoing CABG develop major, permanent disability due to perioperative stroke. However, the overall rate of neurologic symptoms is much higher. Approximately 20 percent of patients have a measurable neurologic disability following CABG, and up to 40 percent of patients may show changes on neuropsychiatric testing.[3] The physiologic mechanisms and long-term sequelae of these neurologic phenomena, sometimes referred to as post-pump syndrome, are poorly understood and are an area of active investigation.

TIMING

- Strokes can occur at any time in the perioperative period, but they do so most commonly within several days of the procedure. In one study of 61 postoperative ischemic strokes at the Mayo Clinic over a 10-year period, the median procedure-to-stroke interval was 2 days. Ten of the strokes (16 percent) occurred intraoperatively, and the range was 0 to 16 days after surgery.[5]

DIAGNOSIS

- The approach to the diagnosis of postoperative stroke is similar to that in the nonoperative setting, with some important distinctions. The presenting signs and symptoms are the same, most commonly a new focal motor deficit, cognitive deficit, or speech difficulties.
- However, a variety of physiologic derangements, physical limitations, and medication effects in the postoperative period may obscure the typical clinical presentation. The patient may be less aware of new neurologic symptoms or may be less likely to consider them important. Conversely, these same postoperative factors may cause symptoms that mimic a stroke, as when psychoactive medications cause weakness and confusion.
- Therefore the clinical signs and symptoms of stroke are *less* sensitive and *less* specific in the postoperative period.
- Nevertheless, the recognition and diagnosis of perioperative stroke should be given high priority. Surgical teams caring for the patient may be unfamiliar with the clinical manifestations of postoperative stroke, and the generalist consultant can augment the surveillance role.
- Obtain appropriate neuroimaging studies to promptly evaluate any new neurologic deficits that suggest the possibility of postoperative stroke. Magnetic resonance imaging (MRI) is usually the preferred neuroimaging test, since it has the highest sensitivity for acute strokes. Computed tomography (CT) may be more available and is adequate to rule out acute hemorrhagic stroke. However, CT will not detect most acute ischemic strokes, and a repeat CT will be necessary in 48 to 72 h if suspicion for ischemic stroke remains despite initially negative CT findings.

TREATMENT

The medical consultant should institute strategies to reduce the risk of stroke in the preoperative period and continuing postoperatively and beyond. These interventions will parallel those intended to reduce the risk of postoperative vascular complications in general, including myocardial infarction (MI). See Chap. 37 for a discussion of preventive strategies.

- In the postoperative period, direct efforts at surveillance for neurologic symptoms, optimal control of blood pressure, and prompt recognition of any new neurologic signs.

- Prompt recognition of stroke is important because of the increasing number of acute interventions that may improve outcomes (such as the use of thrombolytics and/or neuroprotective agents).[4] The management of acute stroke is increasingly complex. Comanagement with a specially trained stroke team, whenever available, is optimal. Management in an acute stroke unit leads to better outcomes compared to care on a general care ward.
  - Determine the optimal acute treatment of stroke in conjunction with an individual with expertise in acute stroke treatment. Some of the treatment decisions, especially the use of thrombolytic agents, are complicated by the bleeding risk in the postoperative period. On the other hand, do not automatically dismiss a potentially beneficial intervention without a thorough consideration of the risks and benefits of the particular situation.
  - In the subacute period (several days to several weeks), attention shifts from the management of acute problems to the rehabilitation challenges that encompass both postoperative and poststroke needs.
  - Also in this period, prevention of and attention to medical complications of stroke are particularly important. Some of these include lung-expansion techniques to prevent pneumonia, early ambulation, and prophylaxis for deep venous thrombosis. Prompt recognition and treatment of medical complications during this period is an important role for the generalist consultant.

SEIZURES

INTRODUCTION

- Epilepsy is defined as *recurrent* seizures due to either a genetic or central nervous system (CNS) abnormality. This is distinguished from a seizure due to an underlying correctable physiologic disorder. The overall incidence of epilepsy in the general population is about 1 percent. Although the complete classification of seizures is extensive, the key part of it is the division of seizures into focal (partial) and generalized.[6]
- Focal seizures originate in one hemisphere and are subdivided into simple partial, with preservation of consciousness, and complex partial, with loss of consciousness. Complex partial seizures may have associated automatisms. The occurrence of an aura preceding the seizure favors the diagnosis of a partial seizure.
- Generalized tonic-clonic seizures may begin as a partial seizure with subsequent secondary generalization or may originate simultaneously in both cortices, i.e., primary generalized seizures. Generalized (tonic-clonic) seizures without a focal origin are much more characteristic of seizures due to metabolic causes. Incontinence and a postictal phase with confusion, exhaustion, and generalized weakness are characteristic of the tonic-clonic seizure.
- Status epilepticus is defined as a seizure persisting for more than 30 min. repetitive seizures occurring without resolution of the postictal phase. Any seizure lasting more than 5 min should receive emergent treatment.

INCIDENCE

- The medical literature provides no data regarding the incidence of seizures in the perioperative period. However, metabolic derangements occurring during the perioperative period, surgery on the brain itself, and any brain injury related to surgery predispose to seizures.
- Specific surgeries carry an increased risk of seizures: e.g., cerebral aneurysm clipping, 21 percent (includes onset, preoperative, postoperative, and late-onset seizures); craniotomy, 20 percent or more; liver transplantation, 6 percent; stereotactic brain surgery, 2 to 3 percent; coronary artery bypass surgery, 6 percent; and bone marrow transplantation, 7 percent. Stroke itself carries about a 9 percent risk of seizure, with about half of these events occurring within 24 h of the stroke.

TIMING

- The timing of the seizure during the perioperative period is of importance. Seizures that occur immediately postoperatively are more often due to metabolic derangements. Seizures that occur 2 weeks or more after surgery often herald the onset of a true seizure disorder. This is particularly true for patients who underwent intracranial neurosurgery.

CAUSES

- For both patients with epilepsy and those with seizures but without epilepsy, many metabolic factors can precipitate seizures. These include hypoglycemia, hyperthyroidism, hyponatremia, hypomagnesemia, uremia, end-stage liver disease, medications (high-dose penicillins, meperidine, others), hypocalcemia, drug and alcohol withdrawal, drug toxicity, sepsis, CNS infection, and malignant hyperthermia.
- Intraoperative seizures have occurred rarely with inhalational anesthetic agents such as sevoflurane and enflurane. However, do not attribute postoperative

seizures beyond the recovery room to general anesthesia. Seizures may rarely occur after the administration of local anesthetics such as lidocaine.

- Perioperative structural CNS injury and/or cerebral anoxia can create a substrate for a seizure and occasionally subsequent epilepsy. Examples include surgical injury to cortical brain tissue, brain hemorrhage, stroke, prolonged hypotension with cerebral anoxia, and hyperperfusion injury with carotid endarterectomy.

DIAGNOSIS

- For the patient with the new onset of seizures perioperatively, determination of the cause is the key to management. Obtain a careful history including an assessment of risk factors and a description of the seizure episode. TIAs, migraines with auras, basilar migraines, and syncope with a jerking movement or two (myoclonus) can mimic a seizure. Risk factors for a seizure include known epilepsy, drug and alcohol abuse, and chronic liver or renal disease. Talking with family members may help to discover a history of alcohol or other substance abuse.
- Perform a neurologic examination to identify evidence of any neurologic deficits. Postictal paresis (Todd's paralysis) may occur in a patient with a seizure. The paresis lasts for only a few minutes and points to a partial seizure with generalization rather than a primary generalized seizure.

LABORATORY TESTING

- Laboratory testing should include electrolytes, antiepileptic drug levels as appropriate, liver and renal function tests, serum glucose, and a toxicology screen.
- For a patient with known epilepsy, a subtherapeutic antiepileptic drug level and absence of metabolic abnormalities may end the diagnostic evaluation. However, perform neuroimaging, especially in the patient without known epilepsy, if no obvious etiology is apparent.
- Individualize the workup of the patient who seizes due to an apparent metabolic abnormality. Neuroimaging and electroencephalography occasionally uncover a CNS abnormality in these patients. The metabolic abnormality has unmasked the seizure focus.
- If immediately available, MRI is the test of choice for the evaluation of new-onset seizures, since it is more sensitive in detecting most structural abnormalities. Obtain an electroencephalogram (EEG) if new-onset epilepsy is suspected. Perform a lumbar puncture only if there is suspicion of meningitis.
- Status epilepticus is a medical emergency that requires prompt diagnosis and treatment. Although all of the preceding evaluation is necessary in this condition, it is critical to initiate treatment immediately. Prolonged seizures can lead to metabolic derangements such as acidosis and rhabdomyolysis as well as neuronal cell injury. Mortality rates still remain above 20 percent; long-term mortality is even higher.
- Although status epilepticus is usually clinically apparent, in some situations, as in "comatose" patients, the internist must maintain a high index of suspicion for this diagnosis. In one study, 8 percent of comatose patients without overt seizure activity proved to have status epilepticus on EEG monitoring.[7] An EEG revealing continuous seizure activity establishes the diagnosis of status epilepticus.

TREATMENT

- Treatment depends upon the etiology. If a patient has a known seizure disorder, measure the blood level of his or her antiepileptic medication and increase the dosage if the level is subtherapeutic. Side effects of antiepileptic drugs are more important in limiting dosing than are blood levels.
- If the patient has a new structural lesion (invasive neurosurgical procedure, new stroke, or other brain lesion), then initiate intravenous loading with phenytoin or another antiepileptic agent.
- If the cause appears to be metabolic or drug-induced, no chronic treatment is necessary other than correction of the metabolic disturbance. This is particularly true in the case of alcohol withdrawal with no structural or EEG abnormality.
- Clinical or EEG evidence of a focal seizure with or without generalization usually requires chronic antiepileptic medication.
- Surgical site injury from a seizure can be a concern for all patients with tonic-clonic seizures. Promptly administer an intravenous benzodiazepine for all patients who are actively seizing postoperatively so as to minimize the risk of surgical site injury.
- Table 61-2 lists the first- and second-generation antiepileptic medications. Although second-generation antiepileptic agents are touted as having fewer side effects and drug interactions,[8] they are not more effective, nor do they improve quality of life as compared with first-line agents. Good initial choices for primary generalized or partial seizures are phenytoin, carbamazepine, valproate, and topiramate.
- Physicians often choose phenytoin because it offers convenient intravenous and oral loading. Administer an intravenous load with 15 to 20 mg/kg at a rate less

TABLE 61-2 Antiseizure Medications

ANTIEPILEPTIC GENERIC NAME	BRAND NAME	SEIZURE TYPE*	INITIAL OR LOADING DOSE	MAINTENANCE OR MAXIMAL DOSE	DOSING INTERVAL	THERAPEUTIC RANGE	TOXICITIES, COMMENTS
Carbamazepine	Tegretol Carbatrol Epitol	Partial General	2–3 mg/kg	10–25 mg/kg/d	bid–qid	4–12 μg/mL	Hyponatremia, drug interactions, aplastic anemia
Ethosuximide	Zarontin	Absence	500 mg/d	1.5 gm	qd–bid	40–100 μg/mL	Nausea, drowsiness
Phenobarbital		Partial General	90–180 mg	90–180 mg	qd–bid	10–40 μg/mL	Sedation, rash
Phenytoin	Dilantin	Partial General	20 mg/kg IV at <50 mg/m 400 mg PO	5 mg/kg/d	qd–tid	10–20 μg/mL	Hypersensitivity, nystagmus, drug interactions
Primidone	Mysoline	Partial General	100–125 mg hs	250 mg tid–qid	tid–qid	4–12 μg/mL	Sedation, rash
Valproate	Depakene Depakote Depacon	Partial General Absence	15 mg/kg/d	60 mg/kg/d	bid–qid	50–150 μg/mL	Weight gain, hepatotoxicity, nausea
Felbamate	Felbatol	Partial; not first-line	400 mg tid	3600 mg/d	bid–qid	NA	Aplastic anemia, liver failure
Gabapentin	Neurontin	Partial	300 mg/d	3600 mg/d	tid	NA	Drowsiness, dizziness
Lamotrigine	Lamictal	Partial General Absence	50 mg/d	250 mg bid	bid	NA	Rash, valproate interaction, somnolence, diplopia
Levetiracetam	Keppra	Partial General	500 mg bid	3000 mg/d	bid	NA	Dizziness, sedation, headache
Oxcarbazepine	Trileptal	Partial General	300 mg bid	2400 mg/d	bid–tid	NA	Somnolence, few drug interactions, hyponatremia
Tiagabine	Gabitril	Partial	4 mg/d	32–56 mg/d	bid–qid	NA	Dizziness, tremor, abdominal pain
Topiramate	Topamax	Partial General	50 mg/d	200 mg bid	bid	NA	Weight loss, memory impairment, acidosis
Zonisamide	Zonegran	Partial General Absence	100–200 mg/d	600 mg/d	qd–bid	NA	Somnolence, sulfa derivative, renal stones

*Partial seizures refer to simple and complex partial seizures with or without secondary generalization. General seizures refer to primary generalized tonic-clonic seizures.

than 50 mg/min. Alternatively, one can use an oral load of 15 to 20 mg/kg by giving 300 to 400 mg every 2 to 4 h.

- Remember that hypersensitivity to phenytoin places patients at increased risk for similar reactions to phenobarbital and carbamazepine. Valproate and topiramate are good choices in this setting.
- If status epilepticus is present, basic principles of resuscitation apply. Obtain intravenous access, secure the patient's airway, and provide for adequate ventilation. Table 61-3 details the stepwise management.[9] Fosphenytoin has advantages over phenytoin since it may be given at 150 mg/min and causes less hypotension and arrhythmias. Management of status epilepticus ideally requires the assistance of a neurologist and often an anesthesiologist.
- Prevention of seizures in the patient with known epilepsy is important. Perioperative goals are to maintain therapeutic blood levels of antiepileptic drugs and to avoid any known precipitants of seizures, such as the metabolic factors noted in the introduction above. See Table 61-2 for a list of optimal therapeutic levels of antiepileptic drugs. See Chap. 12 for the use of prophylactic antiepileptic agents in patients undergoing intracranial surgery.
- Adjust phenytoin levels for serum albumin and renal failure that impairs protein binding. If the patient already has a measurable phenytoin level, the dose in milligrams per kilogram required to attain a therapeutic level is the desired concentration minus the measured concentration (both in μg/mL).
- Continue all seizure medications throughout the perioperative period. If the patient is unable to tolerate orally or nasogastrically delivered medications, substitute one of the following intravenous antiepileptic drugs: phenytoin, phenobarbital, fosphenytoin, or valproate.

TABLE 61-3 Management of Status Epilepticus

Step 1
Assess airway, breathing, and circulation.
Administer oxygen; monitor cardiac rhythm, oxygen saturation, and vital signs.
Establish intravenous line with normal saline.
Perform bedside glucose test.
Draw blood for AED levels, complete blood count, electrolytes, calcium and magnesium, glucose, and toxicology screen.
Give thiamine 100 mg and, if indicated, 50% dextrose, 50 mL IV.
Obtain history and perform physical examination.
Step 2
Give lorazepam 0.1 mg/kg IV up to 2 mg/min (4 mg/dose maximum) or diazepam 0.25 mg/kg IV up to 5 mg/min (10 mg/dose maximum).
Repeat in 10 min if seizures persist.
Give fosphenytoin 20 phenytoin equivalents (PE)/kg loading dose up to 150 PE/min.
If seizures persist, give additional fosphenytoin 5–10 PE/kg to a total dose of 30 PE mg/kg or serum concentration of 30 μg/mL.
Step 3
Intubate, place arterial line, and draw arterial blood gas and phenytoin level.
Consider phenobarbital 20 mg/kg IV at 100 mg/min.
Step 4
Consider pharmacologic coma with pentobarbital 5–8 mg/kg loading dose followed by continuous infusion of 2–4 mg/kg/h titrated to burst suppression for 6–48 h.
Alternatively, give midazolam 0.2 mg/kg loading dose followed by continuous infusion beginning at 1 μg/kg/min increasing by 1 μg/kg/min every 15–30 min up to 10 μg/kg/min.

Modified from Goetz,[9] with permission.

REFERENCES

1. Warlow C, Sudlow C, Dennis M, et al. Stroke. *Lancet* 362: 1211–1224, 2003.
2. Lefevre F, Woolger JM. Surgery in the patient with neurologic disease. *Med Clin North Am* 87:257–271, 2003.
3. Kelley RE. Stroke in the postoperative period. *Med Clin North Am* 85:1263–1276, 2001.
4. Blacker DJ. In-hospital stroke. *Lancet Neurol* 2:741–746, 2003.
5. Limburg M, Wijdicks E, Eelco F, Hongzhe L. Ischemic stroke after surgical procedures: Clinical features, neuroimaging, and risk factors. *Neurology* 50:895–901, 1998.
6. Chang BS, Lowenstein DH. Epilepsy. *N Engl J Med* 349: 1257–1266, 2003.
7. Towne AR, Waterhouse EJ, Boggs JG, et al. Prevalence of nonconvulsive status epilepticus in comatose patients. *Neurology* 54:340–345, 2000.
8. French JA, Kanner AM, Bautista J, et al. Efficacy and tolerability of the new antiepileptic drugs. Report of the Therapeutics and Technology Assessment Subcommittee and Quality Standards Subcommittee of the American Academy of Neurology and the American Epilepsy Society. *Neurology* 62:1252–1273, 2004.
9. Goetz CG. *Textbook of Clinical Neurology,* 2d ed. Philadelphia: Saunders, 2003.

62 DELIRIUM

Margaret Beliveau-Ficalora and Jeffrey R. Allen

INTRODUCTION

- Delirium is a common complication in the perioperative setting, especially among elderly patients. Confounding factors may result in overlooking or delaying the diagnosis of postoperative delirium.

- In certain high-risk populations, especially patients with hip fracture, delirium may exist preoperatively. Preoperative delirium portends a worse prognosis for functional recovery after surgery.
- Postoperative delirium increases the risk of a number of adverse outcomes. For many patients, the development of postoperative delirium leads to longer lengths of hospital stay and an increased likelihood of posthospital institutionalization.
- Patients with hip fractures who develop postoperative delirium are less likely to recover their prefracture walking ability and are more likely to become dependent in activities of daily living (ADLs).[1]
- Multiple studies have demonstrated that patients who develop postoperative delirium have a higher 1-year mortality than those without delirium.

INCIDENCE

- In patients over 65 years of age, the incidence of postoperative delirium ranges from 10 to 60 percent. The type of surgery is a major determinant of the overall incidence of postoperative delirium. The more stressful the surgical procedure, the higher the risk of delirium.

TIMING

- Delirium develops most often on the second to fifth postoperative days. It may be difficult to identify delirium on the first postoperative day due to the residual effects of anesthesia.

CAUSES

- Many predisposing factors increase the risk of postoperative delirium. These include preoperative, intraoperative, and postoperative factors.

PREOPERATIVE FACTORS

- ***Advanced age:*** Vision and hearing loss are common among patients above 70 years of age. Difficulty seeing and hearing may increase the risk of illusions or hallucinations.
- ***Preexisting dementia and cognitive dysfunction:*** Many studies have confirmed that patients with preexisting dementia are at high risk for the development of postoperative delirium.
    - These patients are often frail and require careful monitoring for potential precipitants of delirium in the perioperative setting. This may be the most important preoperative risk factor.
- ***Preexisting psychiatric disorders:*** Patients who have discontinued their psychoactive medications in the perioperative period are at increased risk for postoperative delirium.
    - Alterations in serotonergic and noradrenergic neurotransmitters may predispose patients with anxiety or depression to postoperative delirium.
    - For example, up to 80 percent of depressed patients in one study developed postoperative delirium.[2]
- ***Preoperative polypharmacy:*** Many drugs have been implicated in the development of postoperative delirium. These include narcotic analgesics, especially meperidine; antidepressants; cardiac drugs such as beta-blockers and digoxin; corticosteroids; H_2-receptor blockers; baclofen; and other psychotropics drugs, such as lithium, benzodiazepines, and the phenothiazines. Toxic levels of any of these drugs will increase the risk of delirium.
- ***Untreated hypothyroidism***.[3]
- ***Drug and alcohol dependence:*** Withdrawal from alcohol or drugs increases the risk of postoperative delirium. In particular, benzodiazepines and opioid analgesics can be associated with withdrawal symptoms. Screen elderly patients for substance abuse or iatrogenic drug use before surgery.
- ***Prolonged surgical procedure*** (over 4 to 6 h).
- ***Cancer patients receiving chemotherapy.***[4]
- ***Seizure disorders:*** Patients with seizure disorders who are off anticonvulsant drugs perioperatively are at increased risk for delirium. Be alert for the possibility of nonconvulsive seizures presenting as delirium.
- ***Chronic pain syndromes:*** Risk may be due to analgesic withdrawal.

PROCEDURES INCREASING THE RISK OF POSTOPERATIVE DELIRIUM[5]

- Cardiac surgery (especially for patients who have been placed on a heart bypass machine)
- Ophthalmic surgery (16 percent of patients who receive a postoperative eye patch develop delirium)
- Hip replacement surgery and hip fractures (40 to 60 percent of patients develop postoperative delirium)
- Transplant surgery (due to immunosuppressant medications including cyclosporine, tacrolimus, and corticosteroids)
- Hysterectomy and abortion (delirium likely due to sense of loss)
- Transurethral prostatectomy (TURP) (due to hypoosmolarity and glycine toxicity)

INTRAOPERATIVE FACTORS

- ***Type of surgery:*** Certain types of surgery confer an intrinsically higher risk of delirium.
  - Cardiac surgery increases the risk for cerebral ischemia. This will put the elderly patient at risk because of decreased brain reserve and decreased tolerance of hypoxia.
  - Orthopedic procedures, especially femoral neck fractures.
  - Cataract surgery may predispose to delirium because of sensory deprivation.
  - Major vascular procedures, especially those with long aortic cross-clamp times.
- ***Anesthesia:***
  - Anticholinergic drugs are commonly used in anesthesia. Elderly patients are particularly susceptible to these drugs, and one should use them with extreme caution.
  - In elderly patients, whenever possible, use drugs with shorter half-lives that cause fewer residual effects. The residual effects of some intraoperative anesthetic and analgesic agents (e.g., barbiturates, opioid analgesics, local anesthetics) can last up to 72 h. These agents may induce a postoperative delirium.
  - Most studies have found little or no difference in the incidence of postoperative delirium based on the type of anesthesia (i.e., general, regional, or spinal).

POSTOPERATIVE FACTORS

- ***Hypoxia:*** Surgery and anesthesia can lead to a profound ventilation/perfusion mismatch, especially in the first 48 to 72 h. Surgery in close proximity to the diaphragm (thoracic, upper abdominal) is particularly likely to create this mismatch. Elderly patients may be particularly intolerant of hypoxia because of their limited neurologic and pulmonary reserve.
- ***Pain:*** Inadequate analgesia may precipitate delirium in elderly patients with marginal cognitive function. Narcotic analgesics may also contribute to the development of delirium.
- ***Anemia:*** A hematocrit below 30 confers an increased risk of postoperative delirium.[6]

DIAGNOSIS

DIFFERENTIAL DIAGNOSIS

- Delirium is an acute confusional state. See Table 62-1 for the differential diagnosis of delirium. Hallmarks of the diagnosis include the following:
  - Acute onset (hours to days)
  - Fluctuating course during the day
  - Symptoms worse at night
  - Fluctuating levels of consciousness and attention
  - Perceptual disturbances (hallucinations or illusions)
  - Altered sleep-wake cycle
  - Increased or decreased psychomotor activity
- Clinicians may easily recognize the hyperactive variant of delirium by the presence of hypervigilance and agitation.

TABLE 62-1 Differential Diagnosis of Postoperative Delirium

Central nervous system
Stroke
Transient ischemic attack
Seizure
CNS infection
Organ-system dysfunction
Congestive heart failure
Renal failure
Liver disease
Respiratory failure
Myocardial infarction
Nutritional deficiency
B_{12} deficiency
Folate deficiency
Malnutrition
Thiamine deficiency
Fluid and electrolytes
Dehydration
Fluid overload
Hyponatremia
Hypercalcemia
Fever and infection
Wound infection
Pneumonia
Urinary tract infection
Central nervous system infection
Clostridium difficile colitis
Urinary tract
Urinary retention
Urinary tract infection
Sensory and sleep deprivation
Vision and hearing deficits
Frequent room changes
Poor or excessive lighting
Noise
Frequent awakenings
Endocrine
Hyperglycemia
Hypoglycemia
Hyperthyroidism
Adrenal insufficiency
Drugs
Alcohol or benzodiazepine withdrawal
Anticholinergic agents
Narcotics
Excessive or inadequate analgesia

- The clinical presentation of the hypoactive variant may be more subtle. These patients may simply appear depressed or tired and the delirium may go unrecognized.
- It is essential to distinguish delirium from dementia, depression, and underlying psychotic illness.
  - A key point is knowledge of the patient's baseline mental status. Preoperative assessment should include a brief evaluation of the patient's cognitive function.
  - Many short, easily administered tests can help establish the presence of preexisting dementia.
  - The Folstein Mini-Mental Status Exam and the Confusion Assessment Method (CAM) are both useful tools that focus on the patient's cognitive abilities. The Folstein may be more applicable to establishing a baseline of dementia in patients the clinician is concerned about. The CAM may be particularly relevant for patients who appear confused after surgery. This assessment method focuses on key features of the diagnosis of delirium: acuity of onset with fluctuating course, inability to attend to the environment, disorganized thinking, and changes in the level of consciousness.[7]
  - Question patients and family members about confusion and other cognitive difficulties.
- After establishing a diagnosis of postoperative delirium, undertake a search for the underlying cause.
- The mnemonic CONFFUSED can help sort through the most common underlying causes.
- ***C = Central nervous system (CNS):*** Consider stroke, transient ischemic attack, seizures, and infectious etiologies (meningitis, encephalitis). Perform a careful screening neurologic evaluation in all patients with postoperative delirium. Evidence from the history and physical examination should trigger consideration of neuroimaging. For example, new neurologic deficits or a history of head trauma should prompt consideration of computed tomography or magnetic resonance imaging of the head.
- ***O = Organ-system dysfunction:*** Consider heart failure, renal failure, liver disease, respiratory failure, and myocardial infarction. Delirium may be the first and only sign of these conditions.
- ***N = Nutritional deficiency:*** Vitamin B_{12} deficiency, folate deficiency, malnutrition, and thiamine deficiency (Wernicke-Korsakoff psychosis) can all contribute to postoperative delirium.
- ***F = Fluids and electrolytes:*** Consider the possibilities of dehydration, fluid overload, hyponatremia, and hypercalcemia.
- ***F = Fever and infection:*** The most common infectious causes of postoperative delirium are wound infection, pneumonia, urinary tract infection, and CNS infections.
- ***U = Urinary tract:*** Urinary retention and urinary tract infection can both cause delirium.
- ***S = Sensory deprivation and sleep disturbance:*** Elderly patients are particularly susceptible to environmental changes. They are also more likely to suffer from baseline problems of hearing and vision. Frequent room changes, poor or excessive lighting, and high levels of ambient noise all put the elderly patient at risk. Missing glasses or hearing aids may make the environment difficult to interpret. Frequent awakenings for medications, vital sign checks, and dressing changes will all contribute to sleep deprivation.
- ***E = Endocrine:*** Delirium may result from hyper- or hypoglycemia or thyroid disease, especially hyperthyroidism.
- ***D = Drugs:*** Withdrawal from alcohol or benzodiazepines may precipitate delirium. Anticholinergic agents and narcotics can also cause delirium. Excessive or inadequate analgesia can be a contributing factor.

HISTORY AND PHYSICAL EXAMINATION

- A careful history and physical examination remain the cornerstones of assessment.
- However, it may be difficult to obtain a detailed history from a confused patient.
  - Question patients and families at length about pain. This includes not only pain at the surgical site but also chest pain and headache.
  - Also seek other symptoms such as dyspnea.
  - Undertake a careful and thorough review of all perioperative medications, including the use of alcohol.
- Physical examination finding are generally nonspecific.
  - Evidence of heart failure or respiratory failure may be obvious.
  - Focal neurologic deficits suggest underlying CNS involvement.
  - Fever or hypotension may indicate underlying sepsis or infection.
  - Carefully inspect wounds and assess for skin breakdown as part of the physical examination of the patient with postoperative delirium.
  - Hypertension and tachycardia may suggest the possibility of a withdrawal syndrome.

LABORATORY TESTING

- Baseline laboratory testing should include a complete blood count (CBC), electrolytes, renal function, blood sugar, calcium, and urinalysis.
  - Obtain additional testing only as indicated by the history and physical examination. Consider thyroid function, vitamin B_{12}, and folate in the appropriate settings.

  - Obtain an electrocardiogram (ECG) and cardiac enzymes in patients with a history of coronary artery disease, especially if signs or symptoms suggest myocardial ischemia.
  - Obtain blood and urine cultures and chest x-ray if infection is suspected.
  - Drug levels can help rule out toxicities.
- ***Neuroimaging*** should not be part of the baseline workup. Reserve neuroimaging for patients in whom delirium is persistent and for which no underlying cause is apparent. Consider early neuroimaging for patients with a history of trauma (especially head trauma). Patients with new focal neurologic deficits should also undergo neuroimaging.
- ***Lumbar puncture*** is rarely necessary in the perioperative setting. Perform a lumbar puncture in patients with fever and confusion if no other cause for confusion is apparent after initial evaluation. Neurosurgical patients with postoperative delirium may also require lumbar puncture if fever and/or elevated white blood cell count is present.
- ***An electroencephalogram (EEG)*** is not necessary as part of the initial evaluation of delirium. Obtain an EEG only when no other etiology is apparent and if subclinical seizures are suspected. Some metabolic or infectious etiologies may have characteristic EEG patterns (hepatic encephalopathy, uremia, herpes simplex encephalitis), but most often these processes can be recognized without the EEG.

TREATMENT

- Target the management of postoperative delirium to the underlying etiology whenever possible.
- Table 62-2 provides a summary of treatment strategies for postoperative delirium.
- Maintain patients in a quiet environment with emphasis on continuing a normal sleep/wake cycle, and provide reassurance. In the intensive care unit (ICU) setting, this is often difficult, and frequent reorientation is necessary.
- Pain control is critical.
  - Although it is extremely important to treat postoperative pain adequately, remember that narcotic analgesics can cause or exacerbate delirium.
  - Nonnarcotic analgesic medications [nonsteroidal anti-inflammatory drugs (NSAIDs), tramadol, and acetaminophen] as well as local anesthetic therapy (lidocaine patch, self-infusing anesthetics at the surgical site) can be very useful in these situations.
- Search for reversible causes, as described earlier in this chapter.
- Discontinue medications with CNS toxicity.
  - Narcotic analgesics are the most common cause of postoperative delirium in elderly patients.
  - Assess the ongoing need for the following medications which may cause mental status changes: corticosteroids, meperidine, anticholinergics, and cimetidine.[5]
- One-on-one supervision can provide reassurance and reorientation and maintain an extra component of patient safety. This helps to avoid the use of restraints, which can increase agitation.
- Use neuroleptics to control agitation and anxiety[8]:
  Haloperidol 0.5 to 2.0 mg PO, IV, or IM every 8 to 12 h
  Risperidone 0.25 to 1 mg PO every 12 h
- Treat alcohol withdrawal with benzodiazepines (e.g., lorazepam 0.5 to 2.0 mg every 4 to 6 h, depending on the severity of symptoms). Thiamine (100 mg IV) can prevent Wernicke's encephalopathy.[5]
- In patients with delirium caused by medication overdose, consider the following antidotes if hemodynamic instability exists or patient safety is compromised:
  Benzodiazepines: Flumazenil 0.2 mg IV every minute (1 mg maximum)
  Opioids: Naloxone (use extremely small doses such as 0.04 mg IV every 5 to 15 min)
  Anticholinergic medications: Physostigmine 1 mg IV
- Patients who develop postoperative neurologic impairments require a thorough medical evaluation to accurately determine the etiology and develop an effective treatment plan.
- Anticipate postoperative delirium based on risk factors in order to minimize the morbidity associated with this condition.

TABLE 62-2 Treatment of Postoperative Delirium

TREATMENT STRATEGY	RECOMMENDATION
Reassurance/quiet setting	1:1 supervision as needed for safety
Adequate pain control	Consider nonnarcotic analgesics
Eliminate or decrease medications with CNS toxicity	Examples include opioid analgesics, corticosteroids, cimetidine, meperidine,[9] anticholinergic medications
Neuroleptics to control agitation/anxiety	Haloperidol 0.5–2.0 mg q 8–12 h Risperidone 0.25–1.0 mg PO q 12 h
Treat alcohol withdrawal	Lorazepam 0.5–2.0 mg PO q 4–6 h (adjust as needed) Thiamine 100 mg IV

REFERENCES

1. Marcantonio ER, Flacker JM, Michaels M, Resnick NM. Delirium is independently associated with poor functional recovery after hip fracture. *J Am Geriatr Soc* 48(6):618–624, 2000.

2. Gustafson Y, Brannstrom B, Berggren D, et al. A geriatric-anesthesiologic program to reduce acute confusional states in elderly patients treated for femoral neck fractures. *J Am Geriatr Soc* 39:655–662, 1991.
3. Ladenson PW, Levin AA, Ridgeway EC, et al. Complications of surgery in hypothyroid patients. *Am J Med* 77(2):261–266, 1984.
4. Silberfarb PM. Chemotherapy and cognitive defects in cancer patients. *Annu Rev Med* 34:35–36, 1983.
5. Merli GJ, Weitz HW. *Medical Management of the Surgical Patient*, 2d ed. Philadelphia: Saunders, 1998:55–58.
6. Marcantonio ER, Goldman L, Orav EJ, et al. The association of intraoperative factors with the development of postoperative delirium. *Am J Med* 105:380–384.
7. Inouye SK, Van Dyck CH, Alessi CA, et al. Clarifying confusion: The Confusion Assessment Method. *Ann Intern Med* 113: 941–948, 1990.
8. Jackson KC, Lipman AG. Drug therapy for delirium in terminally ill patients. *The Cochrane Library,* issue 2. Chichester, UK: Wiley, 2004.
9. Adunsky A, Levy R, Heim M, et al. Meperidine analgesia and delirium in aged hip fracture patients. *Arch Gerontol Geriatr* 35(3):253–259, 2002.

63 PAIN MANAGEMENT

William Wertheim and
Paul H. Willoughby

INTRODUCTION

- Perioperative pain is a principal concern of patients and a central management issue for physicians who provide perioperative care.
- Poorly controlled pain leads to patient dissatisfaction and contributes to increased morbidity and mortality. Depression, anxiety, and fear are among the emotional tolls. Patients with undertreated pain may limit their mobility and have excess adrenergic tone, leading to an increase in pneumonia, myocardial infarction, and hypercoagulability.[1]
- Proper management, including appropriate pharmacologic management and regional analgesic techniques, can improve function and shorten length of hospital stay.
- Most hospitals have an acute pain service of some sort. Acute pain services can be instrumental in managing perioperative pain and eliminating or reducing a major source of patient concern.
- Resources may range from a nurse whose responsibility is to address institutional pain management requirements to a complete acute pain service (APS) that includes physicians, nurse practitioners, nurses, psychologists, and pharmacists. Although anesthesiologists often fill the physician role, physicians from a variety of areas may participate in an APS. Some of this change relates to mandates from accreditation agencies (such as the Joint Commission on Accreditation of Health Organizations) and hospitals governing the evaluation, assessment, and management of pain. In some states, pain evaluation and management is regulated by law.[2]

INCIDENCE

- Pain in the postoperative period is nearly universal. Most patients experience moderate or mild pain that is readily manageable with the means outlined below. However, postoperative pain remains undertreated; one recent British study reported that up to one-fifth of patients had suboptimal pain control.[3]

TIMING

- The APS directs most of its attention to the postoperative period. Preexisting medical conditions and any history of chronic pain syndromes should be considered in evaluating patients with postoperative pain. The treating clinician should begin addressing analgesia as soon as the patient is awake; keeping in mind that the effects of spinal or epidural anesthesia may be longer in duration than those of general anesthesia.

CAUSES

- Minor surgical procedures tend to cause less postoperative pain and may respond to less intense therapy or nonpharmacologic therapy, such as cryotherapy or ice.
- More invasive surgeries may require narcotics and invasive analgesic techniques.[4,5]
- Barriers to pain relief include both people and processes that interfere with appropriate pain therapy. Patients may not wish to ask a busy nurse for medication or may be concerned about addiction or side effects.
- Nurses may find that administering medications "as needed" (PRN) is time-consuming; they may also withhold medication because of concerns about addiction. Physicians may be reluctant to order narcotics for fear of addiction or from concern about compliance with conflicting regulations.
- Orders that require patients to ask for medication and systems that delay medication dosing are also barriers.[1]
- The most challenging patients are those with preexisting pain, narcotic tolerance, and poor coping skills. The clinician should carefully elicit a history that includes details of prior drug use, prior pain syndromes, and social and emotional support.

- Consider the location, quality, and quantity of pain; alleviating and exacerbating factors; daily variation; functional impairment; level of disability; and previous treatment. Elicit a history of prior surgeries and responses to pain therapies. Distinguish true medication allergy from unpleasant side effects (for example, narcotic-induced nausea may be prevented with antiemetics). Poor experience with regional techniques is the main predictor of patients' refusal to have regional techniques in future surgeries.
- Patients with chronic pain syndromes often develop exacerbation of their pain due to positioning and psychological stress related to the surgical procedure. For example, individuals with chronic low back pain are susceptible to pain after lying on an operating room table or bed for prolonged periods. Patients with complex regional pain syndromes may develop spread of pain to new surgical areas. This necessitates the use of regional analgesic techniques either with epidural analgesia or peripheral nerve blockade.
- Obtain a history of previous illicit or therapeutic narcotic use. Document previous narcotic dose requirements in order to estimate postoperative narcotic requirements. Patients who are tolerant of narcotics will often require invasive means of pain control for even mild to moderately painful procedures.[1]
- Depressed patients are likely to report higher pain scores for any given surgery. Continue antidepressant medications in the perioperative period and consider psychiatric consultation for complex cases.

DIAGNOSIS

- If patients are able to verbalize, the diagnosis of postoperative pain is straightforward. For accurate titration of medications and appropriate management of the subjective symptom of pain, use a standardized numeric scale. For patients who cannot read or write, pictorial demonstrations are also effective.[4] A sudden or unexpected increase in pain should raise the question of infection or other postsurgical complications; patients with chronic pain from other causes may also have worsening symptoms due to immobility, positioning, or physiologic stress.

TREATMENT

INFLUENCE OF MEDICAL COMORBIDITIES (TABLE 63-1)

- Medical comorbidities affect the selection of analgesia. Avoid acetaminophen in patients with liver dysfunction; also avoid nonsteroidal anti-inflammatory drugs (NSAIDs) and cyclooxygenase-2 (COX-2) inhibitors in patients with renal dysfunction. Use NSAIDs cautiously if at all in patients with a history of peptic ulcer disease.
- Patients with chronic respiratory disease, particularly those with ventilatory defects, may require modification of medication choice to avoid excessive sedation and blunting of the respiratory drive. Patients who lack the cognitive ability to understand patient-controlled analgesia (PCA) or who are physically unable to press a button are not eligible for PCA. Severe neurologic dysfunction, infection at the block site, and coagulopathies are relative contraindications to regional anesthesia.[1,4]

TABLE 63-1 Complications of Pain Management Strategies

TREATMENT	COMPLICATIONS
Local cryotherapy, heat	Local discomfort
Acetaminophen	Hepatic toxicity
Nonsteroidal anti-inflammatory drugs	Gastrointestinal hemorrhage Bleeding tendency
Oral or parenteral opiates	Respiratory depression Nausea, vomiting Constipation Pruritus
Regional or epidural anesthetics	Respiratory depression Nausea, vomiting Constipation Pruritus Bradycardia Hypotension Urinary retention Infection Sensory or motor block

IMPACT OF PREOPERATIVE MEDICATIONS

- ***NSAIDs:*** NSAIDs are not a contraindication for regional techniques but should be discontinued before surgery if possible. Aspirin impairs platelet function for 7 to 10 days after administration; it is safe to continue naproxen and ibuprofen up to 48 to 72 h before surgery.
- ***Thrombolytic therapy:*** Regional anesthesia is contraindicated within 10 days of use of thrombolytic therapy.
- ***Warfarin:*** Anticoagulation modifies the approach to pain management. If regional anesthesia is contemplated, consider the impact of anticoagulation medications on pain treatment strategies. For patients on warfarin, assess the risks of transiently discontinuing therapy. If holding anticoagulation during the perioperative period is contraindicated, then discontinue warfarin and administer unfractionated heparin (see below). Do not give subcutaneous unfractionated heparin for 1 h

after placement or removal of an epidural or spinal catheter. Delay removal of any catheters until 2 to 4 hours after discontinuing heparin.

- ***Low-molecular-weight heparin (LMWH):*** Because of their effectiveness in providing anticoagulation, length of effect, and difficulty in reversing anticoagulation, LMWHs are exceptionally difficult to use when a regional analgesic procedure is planned. If a regional technique is particularly bloody, delay initiation of therapy for 24 h. Otherwise, begin therapy 8 to 24 h after surgery, depending on the medication and dosing schedule. Delay regional anesthesia or catheter removal for 12 to 24 h after the last dose of LMWH.
- ***Antiplatelet medications:*** The risk of complications from antiplatelet medications (thienopyridine derivatives such as ticlopidine and clopidogrel) and platelet GP IIb/IIIa antagonists (abciximab, eptifibatide, tirofiban) is relatively unknown.
- ***Direct thrombin inhibitors:*** No specific recommendations are available for newer medications such as direct thrombin inhibitors and fondaparinux. The FDA has required black-box warnings similar to those of LMWH as a precautionary measure, without any evidence. Regional anesthesia is relatively contraindicated for patients who are receiving a combination of anticoagulation medications due to higher rates of hematoma.

APPROACH TO PAIN MANAGEMENT

- PCA devices have replaced intermittent dosing of narcotics for moderately painful surgery.
- Epidural analgesia is very effective for thoracic, abdominal, and lower extremity surgery.
- Peripheral nerve blocks with local anesthetic infusions are effective for surgery on the extremities.
- Surgeons may place catheters in the wound in order to administer continuous infusions of local anesthetic.
- Many institutions have developed surgery-specific algorithms. Knowledge of each institution's pathways can aid the practitioner in preparing the patient before the procedure.
- The World Health Organization published a stepladder of pain therapy for cancer management in the 1970s. One can also apply the principle of increasing the number and strength of medications and treatment to implement the management of acute pain. However, in acute pain management, there is little time for gradually increasing treatments. The physician should anticipate the level of therapy needed for each patient and planned surgery.[5]
- Begin with the most benign pain-control strategies and build in intensity as needed. Consider the use of lower doses of multiple therapies so as to minimize the side effects of each therapy.
- One option for acute postsurgical pain is cryotherapy. This is a device through which cold water flows continuously. Ice packs can also be useful, but frostbite injury can occur.
- Heat is effective for chronic pain and muscular pain that is not associated with surgical insult. Shoulder pain is frequent after thoracotomy and can be treated with heat. Exacerbation of muscular pain due to positioning during surgery is also amenable to this form of therapy.

SPECIFIC ANALGESICS

- ***Acetaminophen and NSAIDs*** are effective medications in preventing postoperative pain. Acetaminophen is devoid of platelet effects and therefore preferred. All of these agents decrease narcotic requirements and can improve patient satisfaction. For moderate-severe pain, order around-the-clock dosing during the patient's waking hours so as to minimize gaps in pain control.
- ***Opiates:*** The next level of therapy involves the use of opiates and opioids. The route of administration depends on the severity of the pain and the patient's ability to take oral medications.
  - The preferred route of administration is oral; intravenous is the next choice. If these routes are not available, intramuscular or rectal administration can be employed.
  - For severe pain, intravenous administration is more efficacious and reliable. The oral route is most appropriate when pain is mild, the patient has been made comfortable with short-acting intravenous medications, or the patient's narcotic requirements have been determined with intravenous therapy. Of note, transdermal fentanyl has a black-box warning against its use in the treatment of acute pain. Although it is useful for chronic pain, fentanyl's long latency of effect and dissipation when removed precludes its use in the postoperative setting.[6]
  - All narcotics need to be titrated to effect. There is a sixfold variation in opiate requirements among narcotic-naive patients.
- ***Morphine*** is the most frequently used intravenous narcotic. It is inexpensive and widely available.
  - Its half-life is 2 to 3 h and it reaches its peak effect within 20 to 40 min. Administer a loading dose of 0.1 mg/kg in divided doses, as many patients will experience relief at less than full loading doses. Typically this is given in divided doses to avoid hypotension. Usually in adults, give 2 to 5 mg IV Q 10 min until comfortable up to 0.1 mg/kg.
  - Hypotension may occur in patients who receive large doses, are hemodynamically unstable, are volume-depleted, or are elderly. A localized area of redness

along the injection site is not an allergic reaction but represents histamine release. Flushing the catheter with saline will minimize this reaction.
  - Morphine is metabolized in the liver into morphine-6-glucuronate and morphine-9-glucuronate, which are excreted into the kidneys. At high doses, these metabolites can cause respiratory depression. One should therefore avoid high doses of morphine in patients with renal failure.
- ***Hydromorphone*** is a synthetic opiate in the morphine class with roughly the same half-life as morphine but without the histamine release or active metabolites. This makes it useful for patients with renal failure. Parenteral hydromorphone is seven times as potent as morphine.
- ***Meperidine*** has fallen into disfavor and is best reserved for the treatment of shivering. Its metabolite normeperidine causes central nervous system (CNS) hyperexcitability, which can lead to seizures. Normeperidine has a half-life of 15 to 20 h and is not dialyzable. Treatment for less than 3 days to a total of 10 mg/kg/day is acceptable. Higher doses can lead to seizures. It is difficult to give in high doses intravenously due to the cardiac effects of this agent. Disadvantages include pain with intramuscular use, inconsistent absorption, and risk with repeated dosing. For these reasons, other narcotics are preferred in the treatment of postoperative pain.
- ***Fentanyl*** and other shorter-acting narcotics have a limited role for intravenous use outside the operating arena. They are useful for short procedures or pain of brief duration. Due to their low therapeutic ratios, they are generally reserved for physician administration or for the intensive care unit. Appropriate starting doses of fentanyl are 25 to 50 μg. When given rapidly and in high doses, muscular rigidity, particularly in the chest wall, may occur.

PATIENT-CONTROLLED ANALGESIA

- Patient-controlled analgesia (PCA) has replaced intermittent doses of narcotics for the treatment of postoperative pain in most institutions. It safely allows patients to titrate the narcotic to their own individual requirements. Although it is more expensive to administer PCA than to use intermittent doses, patients are generally more satisfied with PCA. It decreases barriers to pain relief and minimizes nursing work.[7–9]
- PCA may consist of intermittent or "demand" doses of medication or demand doses plus a continuous infusion. The demand dose should be large enough to provide pain relief from one or two pushes of the demand button. It also must be small enough to avoid overdose or unwanted side effects. The lockout interval prevents repetitive dosing in too short a period of time. Short lockout intervals of about 10 min with small demand doses are more effective than long lockout periods of 30 min with larger demand doses.
- A continuous infusion can be useful in some patients. When a narcotic-naive patient has an extremely painful surgery, a small continuous infusion can decrease the number of demands. For moderately painful surgery, a background infusion only increases the total amount of narcotic used without decreasing the number of demands.
- In selected patients, use a 1- or 4-h dosing limit to control the total amount of narcotic given in that period of time. This strategy limits the amount of narcotic in patients with addiction histories. It also provides notice that the patient must be reevaluated by a physician or APS, as he or she may have unexpectedly higher narcotic requirements. Pain is a symptom, and sometimes patients who reach their limit actually have pain that requires medical attention and evaluation.
- Almost every narcotic and analgesic can be administered via a PCA device. Even mixtures with antiemetics have been created.
- Because acute postoperative pain improves over time, direct conversion from PCA is unnecessary. Equivalent dosing tables are available, but one may also consider decreasing the amount of narcotic over time. If patients have high narcotic requirements, one may use long-acting agents while also ordering shorter-acting agents for breakthrough pain.
- In the hospital, use long-acting agents and around-the-clock scheduling even for patients with low requirements, so as to ensure timely pain relief. Use shorter-acting medications for breakthrough pain. Newer agents, including oxycodone CR and morphine CR, require only one dose to achieve a steady state. Other preparations of morphine and methadone require multiple doses before a steady state is achieved. Transdermal fentanyl requires more than 24 h to achieve a steady state.

REGIONAL ANALGESIC TECHNIQUES

- Several options exist for either neuraxial (spinal, epidural) or regional analgesia that offer a number of benefits to the patient. Such techniques may allow the use of lower doses of systemic analgesia and hence less medication side effects. Such a reduction, particularly with reduced opiate administration, reduces postoperative gastrointestinal and pulmonary complications and may also reduce cardiac complications.[6,10,11]
- Either inject a single dose of an agent into the epidural space or place a catheter. Both opiate infusions (such as

fentanyl, sufentanil, morphine, or hydromorphone) and local anesthetic agents such as bupivacaine, ropivacaine, and levobupivacaine are effective. Achieve optimal pain reduction with a combination of epidural local anesthetics and opiate analgesics. Some experience exists with clonidine or epinephrine as adjuvants. Epidural analgesia may also be delivered via a patient-controlled device. Side effects include hypotension, motor block, nausea, vomiting, and pruritus.

- In selected patients, peripheral regional analgesia is effective. One can administer either a single-dose injection or a continuous infusion by catheter. The locus of the block may involve a nerve plexus; infiltration of a surgical wound; paravertebral, intercostal, or interpleural administration for thoracic analgesia; or intraarticular administration. Opiates, local anesthetic agents, and NSAIDs are all effective.

REFERENCES

1. Carr DB, Jacox AK, Chapman RC, et al. *Clinical Practice Guideline: Acute Pain Management: Operative or Medical Procedures and Trauma*. Rockville, MD: Agency for Health Care Policy and Research, U.S. Department of Health and Human Services, 1992.
2. American Society of Anesthesiologists. Practice guidelines for acute pain management in the perioperative setting: A report by the American Society of Anesthesiologists Task Force on Pain Management, Acute Pain Section. *Anesthesiology* 82:1071, 1995.
3. Dolin SJ, Cashman JN, Bland JM. Effectiveness of acute postoperative pain management: I. Evidence from published data. *Br J Anaesth* 89:409–423, 2002.
4. Ready LB, Odin R, Chadwick HS, et al. Development of an anesthesiology-based post-operative pain management service. *Anesthesiology* 68:100–106, 1988.
5. Kehlet H, Wilmore DW. Multimodal strategies to improve surgical outcome. *Am J Surg* 183:630, 2002.
6. Jin F, Chung F. Multimodal analgesia for postoperative pain control. *J Clin Anesth* 13:524, 2001.
7. Macintyre PE. Safety and efficacy of patient-controlled analgesia. *Br J Anaesth* 87:36, 2001.
8. Walder B, Schafer M, Henzi I, et al. Efficacy and safety of patient-controlled opioid analgesia for acute postoperative pain: A quantitative systematic review. *Acta Anaesthesiol Scand* 45:795, 2001.
9. Crews JC. Multimodal pain management strategies for office-based and ambulatory procedures. *JAMA* 288:629, 2002.
10. Rigg JR, Jamrozik K, Myles PS, et al. Epidural anaesthesia and analgesia and outcome of major surgery: A randomised trial. *Lancet* 359:1276, 2002.
11. Rodgers A, Walker N, Schug S, et al. Reduction of postoperative mortality and morbidity with epidural or spinal anaesthesia: Results from overview of randomised trials. *BMJ* 321:1493, 2000.

INDEX

Note: Page numbers followed by *f* or *t* indicate figures or tables, respectively.

B

Q

R